Classic Cases
in Medical Ethics

Accounts of Cases That Have Shaped Medical Ethics,
with Philosophical, Legal, and Historical Backgrounds

Classic Cases in Medical Ethics

Accounts of Cases That Have Shaped Medical Ethics, with Philosophical, Legal, and Historical Backgrounds

SECOND EDITION

Gregory E. Pence

Professor of Philosophy
School of Medicine
University of Alabama at Birmingham

McGraw-Hill, Inc.

New York   St. Louis   San Francisco   Auckland   Bogotá   Caracas   Lisbon
London   Madrid   Mexico City   Milan   Montreal   New Delhi   San Juan
Singapore   Sydney   Tokyo   Toronto

This book was set in Palatino by The Clarinda Company.
The editors were Cynthia Ward, Judith R. Cornwell, and Susan Gamer;
the production supervisor was Elizabeth J. Strange.
The cover was designed by Karen K. Quigley.
R. R. Donnelley & Sons Company was printer and binder.

CLASSIC CASES IN MEDICAL ETHICS
Accounts of Cases That Have Shaped Medical Ethics,
with Philosophical, Legal, and Historical Backgrounds

This book is printed on recycled, acid-free paper
containing 10% postconsumer waste.

1 2 3 4 5 6 7 8 9 0   DOC   DOC   9 0 9 8 7 6 5 4

ISBN 0-07-038094-5

Library of Congress Cataloging-in-Publication Data

Pence, Gregory E.
    Classic cases in medical ethics: accounts of cases that have
shaped medical ethics, with philosophical, legal, and historical
backgrounds   Gregory Pence. —2nd ed.
        p.   cm.
    Includes bibliographical references and index.
    ISBN 0-07-038094-5
    1. Medical ethics—Case studies.   I. Title.
R724.P36   1995
174'.2—dc20

94-41691

About the Author

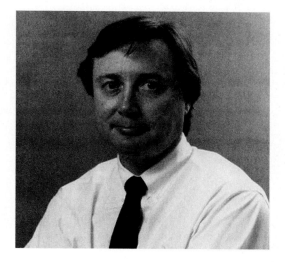

GREGORY E. PENCE is Professor in the Department of Philosophy and School of Medicine at the University of Alabama at Birmingham. For over a decade, he served on the Institutional Review Board on human experimentation. He is a past Chair of the Board for Birmingham AIDS Outreach. He has published in *Bioethics, Journal of the American Medical Association, American Philosophical Quarterly, Canadian Journal of Philosophy*, the *New York Times, Newsweek*, and the *Wall Street Journal*. He has twice won teaching awards, and he has given many talks on bioethics in places that include China and Israel.

Contents

PART FOUR
Classic Cases about Individual Rights and the Public Good

CHAPTER 14   Involuntary Psychiatric Commitment: Joyce Brown

CHAPTER 15   Preventing Teenage Pregnancy: Bertha

Contents

Preface

Although the heart of *Classic Cases in Medical Ethics* is still the detailed, famous cases themselves, the discussion sections have now been greatly expanded; thus this second edition can function not only as a casebook but also as a textbook.

There are other significant changes as well. Several new cases have been added: Nancy Cruzan, Larry McAfee, Jack Kevorkian, the "God committee" in Seattle, Baby Theresa, Kimberly Bergalis, and reform of the American medical system. Three of these—the Cruzan case, Dr. Kevorkian, and medical care in the United States—are covered in brand-new chapters. A great deal of additional important material appears in the "Background" and "Update" sections: for example, Chapter 6 summarizes decisions by the Supreme Court about abortion since *Roe v. Wade*; Chapter 16 discusses hereditary breast cancer; Chapter 17 examines various controversies about AIDS.

Almost every chapter of the first edition has been extensively rewritten, for one reason or another: arguments have been improved; new developments have taken place and have now been given better summations; more accurate facts and medical details have become available; errors spotted by alert readers have been corrected. The most extensive changes appear in the chapters on death and dying, teenage pregnancy, presymptomatic testing for genetic disease, and AIDS.

•

I have been teaching some version of this material for nearly 20 years, and during that time I have taught more than 3,000 undergraduates and 3,000 medical students. As a teacher, I have come to appreciate the *mastery approach,* which endeavors to give students a sense of achievement—mastery—in a field. Bioethics, or medical ethics, is an exciting subject for students, but it can also be confusing; many students find that the question "What did you learn?" is not always easy to answer. This book is written so that a student who has read it can answer, "A lot! Let me tell you about the issues raised by the case of . . ."

By some accounts, bioethics reached its thirtieth birthday in 1992. This means that it is already history for some students—students who were not born when it began. Bioethics instructors must now teach students who were not born when the "God committee" became famous in 1962, or even a decade later when the story of the Tuskegee study broke; most students know nothing about the Karen Quinlan case, which took place in 1975.

Students' ignorance is often not their own fault. As we all know, it is easier to assume knowledge than to impart it. In bioethics, at least, this book hopes to remedy that problem.

Acknowledgments

Physicians who helped on this book include Ronald Cranford, Arnold Diethelm, Norman Fost, Roy Gandy, Keith Georgeson, Seymour Glick, Patricia Goode, Tom Huddle, Donald Kahn, Joanne Lynn, Luis R. Marcos, Max Michael, Paul Palmisano, James Pittman, Sarah Polt, Michael Saag, Norman Shumway, and Arthur Zitrin. The surgeon Roy Gandy has given generously of his time to help me with the chapters on surgery.

Philosophers who helped on this new edition include Albert Jonsen, Harold Kincaid, Loretta Kopelman, James Rachels, Robert Redmon, William Ruddick, and Peter Singer. Peter Singer graciously read most of the manuscript in its penultimate stage and made many helpful suggestions.

I have received much help from the National Reference Center for Bioethics Literature, especially from Pat Milmoe McCarrick, Anita Nolan, and Sue Meinke; the people there have always gone out of their way to help me.

Others who helped include Richard Bleiler; Russ Fine; Nat Hentoff; the American Fertility Society; and my wife, Patricia Rippetoe.

I benefited from the comments and suggestions of the publisher's reviewers: J. Lee Cooke, Bloomsburg University; Paul Durbin, Jefferson Medical College; Patricia Flynn, Saint Mary's College of California; Drew Leder, Loyola College in Maryland; Douglas C. Long, University of North Carolina at Chapel Hill; and Ronald F. White, College of Mount Saint Joseph.

At McGraw-Hill, Cynthia Ward has nurtured this book. Judith Cornwell has painstakingly read every page; her careful attention to the arguments and style greatly improved this second edition. Susan Gamer, a senior editing supervisor at McGraw-Hill, showed a genius for organization and detail that transformed the final version of the book into something of which we can both be very proud. I am grateful to all for their help on the second edition.

Gregory E. Pence

Classic Cases
in Medical Ethics

Accounts of Cases That Have Shaped Medical Ethics,
with Philosophical, Legal, and Historical Backgrounds

PART ONE

Classic Cases about Death and Dying

CHAPTER 1

Comas

Karen Quinlan and Nancy Cruzan

Two of the most famous cases of medical ethics in the United States were those of Karen Quinlan and Nancy Cruzan. The Quinlan case began in 1975, and despite its fame, some of the real issues it represented remained misunderstood for a long time. The Cruzan case, 15 years later, resulted in an important decision by the Supreme Court in 1990. This chapter describes each case, the ethical issues, and how those issues evolved in the years between the two cases.

BACKGROUND: MORAL DISAGREEMENT AND MORAL REASONING

As we shall see, the Quinlan and Cruzan cases directly involved *moral disagreement:* that is, conflicting standards of morality and conflicting judgments about particular issues. In the case of Karen Quinlan, for example, the nuns who were administrators at the hospital believed that morality is founded on unchanging standards given by God, whereas Karen's parents and their parish priest believed that moral rules must change in order to be compassionate. In the case of Nancy Cruzan, the attorney general of Missouri believed far more than Nancy's parents did that the state should protect vulnerable incompetent patients. Indirectly, these cases also involved general philosophical questions about morality: Where does morality come from? Is there such a thing as moral "truth"? If different standards exist by which to judge an issue, how are we able to live together?

When reasonable people need to discuss moral conflicts and general questions about morality, philosophical reflection can sometimes help. For instance, we can ask (as Socrates asks in the dialogue *Euthyphro*) whether morality depends on a god or gods, or whether it can exist independently. If we believe that morality depends on a deity, we must then go on to ask—to specify—how we know that any particular moral rule is that deity's will. If we turn to a source such as the Bible, we need to ask which of various interpretations we will choose, and how we will justify that choice. To engage in such *moral reasoning,* it is useful to consider several concepts.

Moral Pluralism

One common "solution" to moral conflict is simply to accept that a certain irreducible amount of moral diversity exists in everyday life. This idea is sometimes called *moral pluralism* or simply *pluralism*.

Moral pluralism has a great deal to recommend it. First, when we consider that, for example, the world has several major religions, each with billions of adherents, not all of us will be confident enough to assert that only our own religion is true or that followers of other religions are condemned. Religion, of course, is only one example of such disagreement; there are a multitude of others, including the issues discussed in this book: death and dying; conception and birth; experimentation; the individual versus the public good. Second, even if we did feel confident that our own beliefs or judgments about such issues were best, it is an undeniable *fact* that people disagree greatly over them. Therefore, publicly adopting an attitude of complete certainty about our own ideas can make us seem moralistic, arrogant, prejudiced, and closed-minded. Moral pluralism, on the other hand, gives us a chance to demonstrate, rather than simply announce, the value of our ideas; also, it gives us a chance to recognize what is valuable in other people's ideas. We may have a thing or two to learn (and this book may help us do that).

Moral Truth

Pluralism raises the question whether there is or is not such a thing as "truth" in ethics. It is worth noting that this question goes back at least as far as the fifth century before the Christian, or Common, era (B.C.E.), when Socrates debated it with the Sophists; and it has also been a primary focus of ethical theory throughout the second half of the twentieth century. In part, this question has to do with the limitations of reasoning in ethics. Although "moral truth" is a rather difficult concept and is not the subject of this book, saying something about it at this point will be helpful.

Moral philosophers differ greatly about whether there is any truth at all in ethics. *Moral skeptics* believe that no objective ethical truth is possible. Against this is the position that a moral idea or statement can be true; ethical theories which hold that moral statements can be true (or false) in some objective way include *cognitivism, realism,* and *naturalism.* In theories like these, however, moral truth is not necessarily characterized by universal agreement. To put this second position another way, the premise, "If a statement is morally true, everyone will agree about it" does *not* necessarily hold. (This idea is not really startling: consider that in science there are also truths which are known only to a small, highly educated elite.) The ancient Greeks, for instance, developed a naturalistic ethical theory called *perfectionism,* which assumed that people will not always agree about moral truths because some people are wiser or more sensitive than others.

Worldviews and Moral Issues

A *worldview* is a comprehensive concept of life: worldviews include overall philosophies of life such as religions, political theories like Marxism or feminism, psychological theories like Freudianism or behaviorism, and specific ethical theories like utilitarianism. It is sometimes thought that a worldview will provide answers or solutions to all moral issues, but this is not necessarily true.

To begin with, some people believe that no one "worldview" such as an ethical theory could be good enough to capture the complicated reality of contemporary moral life—though as a practical matter, we may be able to find small bits of truth even without discovering a true worldview or developing a completely satisfactory ethical theory. If we refused to act without the moral certainty of a worldview, we would be paralyzed. In actuality, throughout our lives we do formulate moral judgments as best we can when we make decisions and face crises: when we marry, give birth, raise children, and bury our dead. We may not be certain about what we should do, but most of us get by.

Also, keep in mind that most of us do not arrive at adulthood with a "pure" worldview. Most of us have actually inherited bits and pieces of different worldviews from different cultures, views which may have been reshaped or discarded by larger, pluralistic societies. Though there are some "total communities" (such as the Amish, Orthodox Jews, Jehovah's Witnesses, conservative Catholics, and the Primitive Baptist Church), even those of us who are raised in them may question our worldviews when confronted with very different moral ideas—as we typically are when we enter a college or university.

Nor is it necessarily a bad thing that we don't have one all-encompassing worldview, because most such worldviews are simplistic and rigid. In bioethics, good judgments require knowledge of complex concepts, general facts, and specifics of each case, and the ability and willingness to balance different values. To impose a single, absolute worldview on an issue in bioethics would violate the rights of those involved and would therefore lead to many undesirable outcomes.

Similarly, it is not necessarily a bad thing that we can't figure out one monistic answer to a question such as "What makes an act right?": people and people's lives may be more complex than monistic answers to such questions would allow. Absorbing different aspects of several worldviews gives us more flexibility to adapt to changing situations in the modern world. Accepting parts of many ethical theories gives us different insights into moral issues without binding us to one rigid view.

Intuition and Moral Reflection

Suppose that we think in terms of moral pluralism, understand that moral "truth" (if it exists at all) may not presuppose universal agreement, and recognize that for most people a "worldview" may not solve moral issues. How, then, is reasoning possible in ordinary morality?

The answer, as suggested above, is pragmatic, or practical. Not all of us have to agree on everything in order to agree on one particular thing. We can take specific cases one at a time; within each case, we can take specific arguments one at a time; and within each argument, we can sometimes even take specific premises one at a time.

In ethics, basic, core beliefs are called *intuitions.* We all carry intuitions around inside us, and these come from many sources, including our own feelings. Ethical reasoning must always start somewhere, and intuitions are often our basis for accepting or rejecting premises in moral arguments; sometimes our intuitions themselves can serve as premises in such arguments. Some of our intuitions "go together"—in which case they are said to be *consistent*—but some contradict each other. We always need to see what our intuitions imply, how they may contradict other intuitions, how they compare with known facts, and how they compare with the views of people we respect.

In essence, "seeing" these aspects of our intuitions is *moral reflection*. Moral reflection is what allows us to accept or reject each premise of an argument; it is what allows us to find a good answer in a specific case. We should not be surprised if the premises we accept or reject, and the decisions we make in specific cases, vary as we gain more knowledge and experience in life; and we should not be surprised if some of our decisions change as a result of the process of moral reflection itself.

Moral reflection is a slow process, and it will not please those zealots who are impatient for moral progress and who want to uplift humanity rapidly by achieving moral consensus. But given the limitations on our powers of reasoning in ethics, we may have no other choice than to adopt this slow process. Even if we accept moral pluralism, even if we cannot discover moral "truth," and even if we cannot develop a single worldview or a perfect ethical theory, we still need rules by which to live. We still need to live with people who have different ideas, without thinking of those people as evil or terrible—and without resorting to force to solve our disagreements.

Delimiting Moral Issues

Mill's principle of harm   The nineteenth-century political philosopher John Stuart Mill wrote *On Liberty* in 1859. This classic work contains an admirable distinction between private life and public morality—a distinction based on the concept of "harm."

Mill believed that a civilized society must promote certain ideals and discourage certain vices. He also believed that a society can do this while granting individuals a sphere of private belief and action immune from interference by government. Mill saw that the power of the nation-state can be dangerous when used against the individual, and he held that governments and their agents—such as the police—should be forbidden to meddle in private life. Equally, he held, the majority should be prevented from becoming tyrannical: it should be forbidden to impose its social or religious beliefs on a dissenting minority.

Where is the line to be drawn between private life and public morality? Mill's rough rule of thumb is called his *harm principle*. According to this principle, private life encompasses those actions of an adult (or adults together) that are purely personal and that do not put other people at risk of harm.

In private life, as defined by this principle of harm, there should be no interference by government—even for a person's own good. For example, consider a certain form of sexual activity between two consenting adults: even if other people consider this activity "immoral," for Mill it will not be a "moral question" if no one else is affected.

Personal life, morality, public policy, and legality   Building on Mill's work, this book will make a distinction among four areas: (1) personal life, (2) morality, (3) public policy, (4) legality.

Issues of *personal life* (the first area) are purely private and affect no one else.

When someone else is affected, issues move from the personal area to the second area, the realm of *morality*.

When society attempts to promote certain values while at the same time tolerating individuals' personal disagreement with those values, issues move into the third area, *public policy*. Actions in the area of public policy—like those in the area of morality—do affect other people's interests. However, "negative" actions in this area are not necessarily considered "immoral"; similarly, if some "positive" action is encouraged by public policy, omitting to perform that action would not be considered "immoral." For example, consider alcohol. Though society tends to discourage drinking (as by taxation) and regulate it (alcohol cannot be sold to minors), people may in general drink without being seen as "immoral." For another example, consider adoption. Society would like adults to adopt needy children (and may offer tax incentives to encourage adoption), but no one thinks it "immoral" for a childless couple not to adopt a baby.

When society decides to promote certain actions and discourage certain other actions without tolerating individual disagreement, issues move into the fourth area, *legality*. In this area, some actions (such as paying taxes) are compulsory and others (theft, murder) are forbidden. Omitting a legally compulsory action or committing a legally forbidden action is punishable by the force of the state. In general, the more harmful an action is considered, the more likely it is to fall into the area of legality.

The effect of these distinctions is to limit the range of morality from two ends: first, by carving out a zone of private, personal life; and second, by allowing society to encourage and discourage behaviors without explicit moral judgment. In summary, then:

- *Personal life:* Concerns actions that are purely private and affect no other person (or persons).
- *Morality:* Concerns interpersonal actions—situations where one person's actions affect other people.
- *Public policy:* On the one hand, concerns actions which affect other people negatively, but which society tolerates, though it attempts to discourage such actions (as by education). On the other hand, concerns actions which affect other people positively and which society attempts to encourage (as through incentives).
- *Legality and illegality:* Concerns positive actions which are, by law, compulsory; and negative actions which are, by law, forbidden. Penalties (such as fines and incarceration) are imposed for omitting compulsory actions or performing forbidden actions.

Here are some further examples: smoking is a personal issue; smoking in your child's room is a moral issue; taxing tobacco products heavily is a public-policy issue; prohibiting the sale of cigarettes to minors is a legal issue. To repeat:

according to these distinctions, *not every issue is moral.* An issue such as masturbation, or littering in one's own car, or individual and family religious beliefs is not a moral issue at all.

•

It should be understood that although these distinctions will be used in this text, they would not be recognized—as Mill's more general distinction might not be recognized—in some evaluative frameworks or "worldviews." For example, a fanatical teetotaler might see no reason to tolerate drinking by anyone, even in private; and Roman Catholicism forbids the use of contraceptive devices by married couples (a stand reaffirmed by the pope in 1993). There are various reasons for such disagreement. In some worldviews, everything in life may be seen as a moral issue: that is, the "personal" area is always the "moral" area. Other frameworks may make a distinction between "personal" and "moral" issues but may come to different conclusions about what actually falls into each area; for example, such a framework might consider not only harm to others but also "self-harm" as a matter of morality. Another framework might assume that there is simply no such thing as "self-harm" distinct from harm to others, that when we harm ourselves we also in some sense harm others.

As we shall see, the Quinlan case may have arisen in part because the hospital and the Catholic hierarchy on the one hand and Karen Quinlan's family on the other did not agree on a distinction between personal and moral issues. It is worth pointing out, in this regard, that other religiously affiliated hospitals may reject distinctions assumed by a patient or a patient's family and mandate their own values within their own walls. Patients and families need to be aware of this, since they may not agree with the policies of a hospital to which they have been referred.

THE QUINLAN CASE

The Medical Situation: Karen Quinlan's Coma

In April of 1975, Karen Quinlan had just turned 21. She was a perky, independent young woman, and she had recently left her adoptive parents' home in New Jersey—against their wishes—and moved in with two male roommates a few miles away. Karen's friends saw her as a wild, free spirit; they thought she lived recklessly and said she took illegal drugs. (A friend alleged that Karen had taken heroin, cocaine, and methadone—though Karen's parents denied this.[1]) Once, Karen lost control of her car going around a curve, went over a cliff, slid down a ravine, and walked away unhurt; she told her parents that it was no big deal.

On April 15, a few nights after moving out of the family home, Karen celebrated a friend's birthday at a local bar. After a few gin and tonics, she suddenly seemed faint and was taken home. Her friends put her to bed, where she immediately slept. When they checked on her 15 minutes later, she wasn't breathing. (Her friends never said why they had felt a need to check her condition.) While one of her roommates called an ambulance, the other started mouth-to-mouth resuscitation. Though Karen did not respond to this, a policeman did later get her breathing, and her color returned—but she did not regain consciousness.

When Karen was admitted, after midnight, to the intensive care unit (ICU) at Newton Memorial Hospital in New Jersey, a bottle of Valium was found in her purse; some pills were missing from it, suggesting that Karen had consumed both Valium and alcohol that evening. Karen had also been dieting, perhaps fasting, for several days (at admission, she weighed only 115 pounds).

Valium (diazepam) is a benzodiazapine (so are Librium, Ativan, and Xanax). Benzodiazapines are a class of antianxiety drugs that act on specific nerve receptors in the brain. Barbiturates (or "downers"), by contrast, act more globally to depress the central nervous system. Both benzodiazapines and barbiturates are *synergistic* in that the effect of each intensifies in combination with alcohol. Also, alcohol *potentiates* barbiturates and antianxiety drugs: that is, the combined effect of alcohol and one of these drugs is greater than the sum of the two effects independently. (For example, let us say that one drink is equivalent in effect to 5 milligrams—mg—of Valium. However, a driver is far more dangerous after consuming one drink plus 5 mg of Valium than after consuming simply two drinks.) The effects of drugs are further accelerated when there is no food in the intestine; and Karen, as noted above, may have been fasting.

The later court transcript has contradictory evidence about what drugs were in Karen's bloodstream. Robert Morse, the attending physician, testified that "She had some barbiturates, which was normal, 0.6 milligrams; toxic is 2 milligrams, and the fatal dose about 5 milligrams percent" [sic].[2] Julius Korein, the consulting neurologist hired by the Quinlans, testified that Karen's medical chart said the drug screen on April 15 "was positive for quinine, negative for morphine, barbiturates, and other substances. A subsequent test for Valium and Librium was positive."[3] (Librium was not mentioned by anyone else.) The court prosecutor, George Daggett, said that Karen had taken tranquilizers with alcohol shortly before becoming unconscious.[4] The Quinlans denied that the drug screen showed barbiturates. They said, "The early urine and blood samples, taken on the day Karen was brought to the hospital, revealed only a 'normal therapeutic' level of aspirin and the tranquilizer Valium in her system."[5]

It is most likely that Karen had taken barbiturates, benzodiazapines, or both, in combination with alcohol. Then their cumulative effects, on an empty stomach, suppressed her breathing and caused *anoxia*—loss of oxygen to an area, in this case the brain—which in turn caused irreversible brain damage. (This was how the actor River Phoenix died in 1993.)

Nine days after Karen's admission to Newton Memorial, her medical status was unchanged and she was transferred to St. Clare's, a larger Catholic hospital in Denville, New Jersey, which (unlike Newton) had neurologists on its staff.

A respirator (also called a *ventilator*) kept Karen breathing during her first days of hospitalization; it also prevented aspiration of vomit into the lungs, which could cause pneumonia. When the respirator forced air into her lungs, Karen would sometimes choke and sit bolt upright with her arms flung out and her eyes open and wild; at these times, she appeared to her parents to be in intense pain. Eventually, Karen's breathing approximated normal, but her lungs did not fully expand to "sigh volume." At less than "sigh volume," some sacs of the lungs will become infected, and so Karen needed a larger, more powerful respirator, the MA-1, which would periodically expand her lungs fully to the "sigh."

Unfortunately, the MA-1 required a tracheotomy (a hole in the trachea or throat area), to which Karen's mother, Julia Quinlan, reluctantly agreed.

Karen Quinlan, of course, was in a coma. The word *coma*, however, is extremely vague and means different things to different people. In this case, although the patient was comatose, her eyes sometimes opened and sometimes she would suddenly seem to laugh or cry. But her eyes were *disconjugate*, i.e., they moved in different, random directions at the same time; and though the eyes still "worked," she was thought to be *decorticate*: her brain could not receive input from her eyes. Despite popular belief to the contrary, under New Jersey law Karen was not brain-dead in 1975. She had "slow-wave"—*not* isoelectric, or "flat"—electroencephalograms (EEGs). Technically, she was in what later came to be called a *persistent vegetative state* (PVS). PVS is a generic term covering a type of deep unconsciousness that is almost always irreversible if it persists for a few months. Over the next 5 months, Karen's posture would begin to show the kind of neurological damage seen in stroke victims; her muscles would become rigid and contracted, and her weight would drop drastically.

At one time, a patient in such a condition would eventually starve to death; but crude intravenous and nasogastric feeding tubes had begun to be used in the late 1960s. Initially, Karen was nourished by an intravenous feeding tube; but as her condition persisted, this became impractical because the rigidity of her muscles made it difficult to insert and reinsert the tube into her veins. By September of 1975 (5 months after her admission), she was on a nasogastric feeding tube. Julia Quinlan disliked this feeding tube:

> They were feeding her a high caloric diet—which seemed completely unreasonable, especially since her body didn't always accept the food. Often she would vomit. . . . And she was more agitated than she'd ever been. I wouldn't have thought it possible that Karen's head could writhe so much. It was as though her body was in a vise, and her head was caught in a whirlpool.[6]

In fact, it was the combination of this invasive feeding tube and the respirator that, for many people, would come to symbolize an oppressive "medical technology," unnaturally prolonging dying.

Karen's sister, Mary Lou, knew that Karen was unconscious but wasn't prepared for what she saw when she visited the hospital:

> Whenever I thought of a person in a coma, I thought they would just lie there very quietly, almost as though they were sleeping. Karen's head was moving around, as if she was trying to pull away from that tube in her throat, and she made little noises, like moans. I don't know if she was in pain, but it seemed as though she was. And I thought—if Karen could ever see herself like this, it would be the worst thing in the world for her.[7]

A lawyer testified that in September of 1975 Karen looked as follows:

> Her eyes are open and move in a circular manner as she breathes; her eyes blink approximately three or four times per minute; her forehead evidences very noticeable perspiration; her mouth is open while the respirator expands to ingest

oxygen, and while her mouth is open, her tongue appears to be moving in a rather random manner; her mouth closes as the oxygen is ingested into her body through the tracheotomy and she appears to be slightly convulsing or gasping as the oxygen enters her windpipe; her hands are visible in an emaciated form, facing in a praying position away from her body. Her present weight would seem to be in the vicinity of 70-80 pounds.[8]

Given her condition, there was little chance that Karen would ever regain consciousness; but St. Clare's was giving her a "1 in a million" chance of recovery—a chance that some people say hospitals must offer. The question what was to be done with her arose, and she was moved out of the ICU and placed in a corner of the emergency room (ER), where the staff could respond if she vomited. Since her heart was strong, she no longer needed the ICU's cardiac monitor, and the ER was a logical, if somewhat cold, solution—though it upset her father, Joseph Quinlan, who wanted her back in the ICU.

It took Karen's family many months to agree among themselves that Karen would never regain consciousness. Finally, however, they accepted that Karen was beyond hope: that her mind was gone, that her life was over, that she was dead. They also agreed that she would never have wanted her body to continue in this condition. According to the Quinlans, Karen had twice said that if anything terrible happened to her, she did not want to be kept alive as a vegetable on machines. Their parish priest also helped them, assuring them that according to Pope Pius XII, "extraordinary means" (like the MA-1 respirator) are not morally required of Catholics.

And so the Quinlans decided to remove the respirator and let Karen's body die. They had no idea that their months-long struggle to reach this decision would be the easy part.

The Legal Battle

The legal environment   The legal environment at the time of the Quinlan case needs to be explained, especially the effect of a case in Massachusetts, that of Kenneth Edelin (this case is discussed in detail in Chapter 6).

Abortion had been legalized in 1973, when the Supreme Court decided in *Roe v. Wade* that states could pass laws banning abortion only *after* viability of the fetus. The Court did not state that a fetus is a "person" at viability, but its decision did stipulate where states could draw the line between legal and illegal abortions.

At that time, Kenneth Edelin was a senior resident in obstetrics at Boston City Hospital, where he performed a very late second-trimester abortion by hysterotomy at the request of a pregnant teenage girl. In 1975, in a sensationalistic trial, Edelin was convicted of manslaughter: the jury understood *Roe v. Wade* to mean that a viable fetus is a person, believed that Edelin had not done everything possible to save a viable fetus, and thus found that he had acted illegally. Edelin was sentenced to 1 year of probation and was at risk of losing his license if his appeal was denied.

Edelin had been convicted just a few weeks before Karen Quinlan's admission to St. Clare's; as the Quinlan case developed during 1975, his appeal was pending, and things looked bad for him. All this influenced the Quinlan case, since the lawyers involved must have seen the parallels. In Edelin's case, a patient wanted him to kill a "being" who might legally be considered a "person." In the Quinlan case, parents were asking their daughter's physicians to promote her death, when she was legally still a "person." Possibly, the lawyers for Karen's doctors saw Edelin's conviction as having established a precedent.

Moreover, in 1975 the American Medical Association (AMA) equated with-drawing a respirator in order to allow death to occur ("letting die") with "euthanasia" ("mercy killing")—and equated euthanasia with murder. It is also important to stress that in early 1976, there had as yet been no legal decisions clarifying the rights of patients or their families in cases about death and dying.

The doctors in Karen Quinlan's case, Robert Morse and his colleague Arshad Javed, were (like Kenneth Edelin) just beginning their medical careers. Morse had completed his residency in neurology only 10 months earlier; Javed had graduated from a medical school in Pakistan and had completed an American fellowship in pulmonary medicine 2 years before being assigned to Karen's case. Obviously, neither of them had any long experience with unconscious brain-injured patients. It is not hard to understand why, in the context of Edelin's con-viction, Morse and Javed became nervous about possibly crossing the line between legality and illegality. Morse also feared a possible malpractice suit, if the Quinlans later changed their minds about their request to have Karen's respi-rator disconnected. One definition of malpractice in the United States is "depar-ture from normal standards of medical practice in a community"; and in 1975— when almost all physicians felt it their duty to continue care until the last moment—actively assisting in the death of a comatose patient would certainly have been such a departure.[9]

The Quinlan case in the courts   Before describing how the Quinlan case fared in the courts, it will be helpful to give an overview of possible stages of a court case. In a state case, the first stage takes place in a court of limited jurisdiction: a probate, district, or municipal court. After judgment is delivered there, an appeal can be directed to a circuit court. Next, there are state appellate courts (e.g., in Alabama the Court of Civil Appeals and the Court of Criminal Appeals). At the state level, the court of last resort is usually called the *state supreme court* (though in New York it is the Court of Appeals). Federal cases are heard in a separate court system. Intermediate steps in this system include district courts of appeals (such a court often has three judges). Nationally, the court of last resort is the Supreme Court of the United States. State or federal cases can be tried either as violations of civil law (such as malpractice cases) or as violations of criminal law (such as assault and battery cases). Homicide and manslaughter are defined by each state's criminal code, and such definitions differ from state to state. Brain-death clauses and "letting die" clauses in state statutes describe *exceptions* to homicide.

To get Karen's respirator disconnected, Joseph Quinlan sought counsel at a Legal Aid office (Karen, since she was no longer a minor and was indigent, was eligible for Legal Aid). The lawyer was Paul Armstrong, and to the Quinlans, Armstrong was a young, idealistic attorney ready to take on City Hall. Their case was first heard by Judge Robert Muir of a New Jersey probate court, and there were no intermediate appeals because the New Jersey Supreme Court agreed to hear the case immediately. (State supreme courts sometimes hear a case immediately when the case may set a precedent.)

The simplest and easiest legal route for the Quinlans would have been to obtain guardianship of Karen and then have her moved to another hospital, where the respirator could have been disconnected. Armstrong may have botched the case by not pursing this quiet strategy; instead, he raised the dramatic issue of letting Karen die:

> In the hands of a conscientious but regrettably inexperienced 30-year-old lawyer, Paul Armstrong, the Quinlan family got very dubious legal advice. For the question of *guardianship* could have been pursued prior to and separate from the question of *treatment refusal.*[10]

By announcing to Judge Muir that Joseph Quinlan wanted to disconnect Karen's respirator, Armstrong tied Muir's hands. A guardian must protect the interests of his or her ward; in this case, the ward was a vulnerable patient, and the question whether that patient was still a "person" had by no means been settled. Given Armstrong's announcement, Muir could not have appointed Joseph Quinlan Karen's guardian without begging the question whether Karen was a person and thus prejudging the case. (*Begging the question* is assuming the truth of what should be proven.) Consequently, Muir appointed another lawyer, Daniel Coburn, as Karen's guardian *ad litem* ("for this suit or action"); Coburn thus became the advocate for an incompetent patient.

Armstrong, then, needed to find an argument for letting Karen die. He originally argued, incorrectly, that Karen was legally brain-dead. Muir scolded him and made it clear that since Karen's brain stem was still functioning, she did not meet New Jersey's "total brain" standard of death—although neurologists testified that her condition was "irreversible" and that her chances of returning to normal were "minuscule." (Standards of brain death are discussed below.) Nor was Armstrong able to argue successfully on the basis of a "right to die." The Constitution of the United States does not mention a "right to die"; and at that time, no Supreme Court decision had said anything about such a right even for competent patients, much less for incompetent patients like Karen Quinlan.

Armstrong's ultimately successful argument for allowing the Quinlans to have Karen's respirator disconnected was based on the Constitution's implied *right to privacy.* The phrase *right to privacy* is perhaps misleading, since it seems to imply only private behavior; in fact, it refers to the right of a person to decide purely personal issues without interference from government. A constitutional right to privacy was first recognized by the Supreme Court in 1965 in *Griswold v. Connecticut,* when it found unconstitutional state laws banning physicians from giving contraceptives to married couples.

The opening statement by Karen's guardian, Daniel Coburn, in Judge Muir's court included the following commentary:

> I have one simple role in this case . . . and that is, to do every single thing that I can do as a skilled professional to keep Karen Quinlan alive. . . .

We talk about facts. Karen Quinlan is not brain dead. She's nowhere near being "brain dead," if that's the accepted standard. . . .

There's another facet. . . . There are thousands of Karen Quinlans out there. I've received thousands of phone calls from all over the world about people . . . where there was no hope, and they recovered. They have been brain damaged, and they are educable, although they may have some retardation. But they are still alive. These people don't want Karen Quinlan dead. I don't want Karen Quinlan dead. . . .

As to the theory that she's not really leaving this earth—that she's just getting to the next world a little bit sooner—in all frankness to the court, and I'm not trying to be flippant, my attitude is that if the Quinlans want an express, I'm going to take the local. . . .

As far as the legal basis for this, I've heard "death with dignity," "self-determination," "religious freedom"—and I consider that to be a complete shell game that's being played here. This is euthanasia. Nobody seems to want to use the word. I'm going to use the word, whether it's euthanasia or a variation of it. . . .

One human being, by conduct, or lack of conduct, is going to cause the death of another human being.[11]

Ralph Porzio, the flamboyant attorney for Karen's doctor Robert Morse, implored Judge Muir "not to impose an execution—a death sentence" on Karen. He asked, "Once you admit that a person is alive, legally and medically, and once you make a determination that a life must come to an end, then where do you draw the line?"[12] Porzio held that Karen should not be killed on the basis of someone else's assessment of her quality of life: "Fresh in our minds are the Nazi atrocities. Fresh in our minds are the human experimentations. Fresh in our minds are [sic] the Nuremberg Code." Porzio cited the sanctity of life as "the cornerstone of Western culture . . . and our Western religions," and asserted that turning off Karen's respirator would be "like turning on the gas chamber." He said that he didn't "care where the idea [of mercy killing] comes from, whether it comes from Rome or from Mecca or from Salt Lake City, the end result is still the same." He also compared Morse's refusal to disconnect the respirator to the civil disobedience of Socrates and Thomas More. He reminded the Court that "we are not gods." In closing, he held nothing back:

> So let us then, as in this hour of trial as we begin, so conduct ourselves that when the eyes grow dim and when our own lives shall fade, and when men and women in some distant day shall gather to warm their hands over the fires of memory, they may look back—they may look back and say of us: They searched for truth, they nurtured justice, they knew compassion; but above all, above all, they walked with honor and wore the garments of understanding.

Morse himself testified that there was no medical precedent allowing him to disconnect Karen's respirator. The neurologist Julius Korein, testifying for the Quinlans, said that he had seen about 50 patients in PVS and that all of them were better off than Karen; he described Karen as having no mental age at all and as being like "an anencephalic monster."[13] Fred Plum, the consulting neurologist for the other side, confirmed Korein's diagnosis; Plum described Karen as "lying in bed, emaciated, curled up in what is known as flexion contracture. Every joint was bent in a flexion position and making one tight sort of fetal position. It's too grotesque, really, to describe in human terms like fetal."[14] (Plum's graphic testimony did not seem to penetrate public awareness, and no photographs of Karen in the hospital were available. During the wait for the verdict, the Quinlans were offered $10,000 by a national tabloid "as a starting point" for a picture. They refused—wanting their daughter to be remembered as she had lived rather than in her comatose condition—and the hospital's hired security force kept photographers out. Thus most people did not understand the nature of her deterioration, and some artists even portrayed her as a normal girl resting peacefully.)

In November 1975—almost 7 months after Karen's original admission—Judge Muir decided that Coburn should continue as Karen's guardian and that the respirator should not be disconnected. Muir said that Karen's own wishes were unknown because they had never been written down, and that her parents' testimony about her wishes could not be taken as final if it entailed her death. He also ruled that no constitutional "right to die" existed.

Several weeks later, the New Jersey State Supreme Court heard the case. In the higher court, testimony about the role of physicians in deciding matters of life and death became prominent. For one thing, the justices expressed surprise at the importance placed by physicians on the distinction between disconnecting a respirator and not starting it. At the time, the official position of AMA was that it was permissible not to put a patient on a respirator; but once a patient was on a respirator, it was not permissible to take that patient off if the intention was to allow death to occur. The justices found this line of reasoning "rather flimsy."

Additionally, the lawyers for the physicians argued that once a physician accepted a patient, an absolute duty to pursue the patient's welfare became "attached" to the physician, such that the physician could never, ever pursue death. However, Julius Korein (the neurologist who had testified for the Quinlans in the lower court) now testified again, revealing "company secrets" among physicians. Korein described how physicians used "judicious neglect" in letting terminal patients die; he said that this was an "unwritten standard" in medicine. With his testimony in this case, Korein made public a standard that had previously been discussed only within medicine.

The justices also pressed the hospital's lawyers about the physician-patient relationship. Why couldn't Morse and Javed allow Karen to be transferred to another hospital, where other physicians could disconnect her? The lawyers for the hospital hemmed and hawed and tried to come up with an answer. Finally, they said that St. Clare's thought that to do so would be immoral.

In January 1976, after 2 months of deliberation, the New Jersey Supreme Court ruled unanimously in favor of the Quinlans. It held that the implied right to privacy under the Constitution was broad enough to allow the family of a dying incompetent patient to decide to let that patient die by disconnecting life support. Because the Supreme Court of the United States had never made a comparable decision, New Jersey was thus the first to apply the right to privacy in a case of "letting die." The New Jersey court also allowed Joseph Quinlan to become Karen's guardian, suggested (though it did not require) an advisory role for ethics committees in future cases, and gave legal immunity to Morse and Javed for disconnecting Karen's life support.

The aftermath   At both the lower-court and the higher-court level, the Quinlan case generated immense publicity; and it involved many different county, state, and hospital officials and private lawyers. AMA and many physicians hated not only the publicity but the presence of lawyers; most physicians felt that tragic cases like Karen's should be kept out of the courts. (Somewhat inconsistently, however, physicians also wanted immunity from prosecution before they would break new ground in cases involving dying patients.)

In April 1976, 4 months after the higher-court decision, Karen Quinlan was still alive. By then, decubitus ulcers had eaten through her flesh, and her hip bones were exposed. Why Karen was still alive at this point is one of the least understood and most interesting aspects of this case.

According to the Quinlans, Morse resisted implementing the decision of the New Jersey Supreme Court, because "this is something I will have to live with for the rest of my life."[15] A nun who worked in an administrative position was more blunt: "You have to understand our position, Mrs. Quinlan. In this hospital we don't kill people."[16] To this, Julia Quinlan replied, "Why didn't you tell me 10 months ago? I would have taken Karen out of this hospital immediately." The administrators at St. Clare's were not by any means alone in their position. Catholic hospitals saw the *Quinlan* decision as another step down a slippery slope that had started 3 years earlier with the American legalization of abortion in 1973. During the trial, the Vatican theologian Gino Concetti had criticized the Quinlans: "A right to death does not exist. Love for life, even a life reduced to ruin, drives one to protect life with every possible care."[17] A pulmonary specialist at Catholic University in Rome said that removal of the respirator "would be an extremely dangerous move by her doctors, and represents an indirect form of euthanasia."[18]

Instead of simply disconnecting Karen's respirator, therefore, Morse and Javed decided to try to "wean" her from it. The tired, confused Quinlans and their inexperienced lawyer seem not to have understood what this meant, and the real implications would become painfully clear over the next 10 years. (A more experienced lawyer would have obtained a writ of *habeus corpus*—literally, "you should have the body"—which is designed to protect Americans from false imprisonment. A writ of habeus corpus can be issued by a local judge, and it works very quickly; if they had gotten such a writ, the Quinlans could have transferred Karen to a hospital where she would have been allowed to die.) Eventually, Javed had Karen off the respirator for 4 hours; then, after intensive work over many weeks, for 12 hours. By late May of 1976, Karen was off the respirator altogether. This weaning created some confusion in the general public: some people took it to mean that Karen had gotten better; others took it to mean that Karen's physicians had "pulled the plug" and that a miracle must have occurred because she hadn't died—but both impressions were false.

Now, St. Clare's hospital wanted to transfer Karen immediately to any other facility, and a desperate search for a nursing home ensued. The New Jersey Medicaid office forced one nursing home to accept Karen on June 9, 1976—at this point, Karen had been unconscious for 14 months. Joseph Fennelly, who felt that some doctor had an obligation to help the family, was the only physician in New Jersey who would accept Karen as a patient. Fennelly argued that the medical profession had helped create this problem, adding that physicians were often cowards in such cases, "too afraid of their medical skins" to act humanely.[19]

It was not until June 13, 1986, after more than 10 years in the nursing home, that Karen Quinlan's body was declared dead. For several months before that, Karen had had pneumonia; at the end, the Quinlans declined antibiotics to reverse it. Julia Quinlan maintained a vigil at her daughter's bedside and was there at the last moment of Karen's biological life.

Paul Armstrong became famous and later tried other "right to die" cases before the New Jersey Supreme Court. Robert Morse died when his small plane crashed in 1987.

THE CRUZAN CASE

Nancy Cruzan's case led to a landmark decision by the United States Supreme Court in June 1990.[20] Before this decision, 20 states had recognized the right of competent patients to refuse medical life support, and all these states (with the exception of New York and Missouri) had recognized the right of surrogates to make decisions for incompetent patients.[21] The *Cruzan* decision, however, was the first decision by the United States Supreme Court to explicitly recognize the rights of dying patients.

The Patient: Nancy Cruzan's Coma

Nancy Cruzan, then age 24, lost control of her car around midnight on a lonely, icy country road in Missouri on January 11, 1983.[22] She was thrown 35 feet from the car and landed face-down in a water-filled ditch. Paramedics arriving on the scene found that her heart had stopped. They injected a stimulant into the heart and then shocked it into restarting; but because her brain had been anoxic for perhaps 15 minutes, Nancy Cruzan was in PVS.[23]

For 7 years, Nancy remained in this state. Over time, her body became rigid and her hands curled tightly, so that her fingernails were like claws. Her care cost the state of Missouri $112,000 a year. Karen Quinlan had been kept alive by both a respirator and a feeding tube; but Nancy Cruzan was sustained by only a feeding tube, which was needed because she could not swallow.

The Case

Nancy Cruzan's feeding tube became the point at issue in the Cruzan case. Legally or morally, is a PVS patient "owed" food and water? Karen Quinlan's parents evidently thought so; they never withdrew the nutrition that kept Karen's body alive. Nancy's parents, Joe and Joyce Cruzan, thought otherwise: they sought permission in court to disconnect their daughter's feeding tube.

The Supreme Court's first decision on death and dying   In discussing the Cruzan case, it is necessary to understand three standards of legal evidence. The minimum standard is *preponderance of evidence;* a more rigorous standard is *clear* *and convincing evidence;* the most rigorous standard—the standard used for serious felonies—is *beyond a reasonable doubt.*

The Cruzans won their case in probate court; but upon direct review, the Missouri Supreme Court reversed the decision, and this reversal had to do with the standard of clear and convincing evidence. The Missouri Supreme Court held that the state had an interest in preserving life—regardless of "quality of life"—and that before medical support could be withdrawn from an incompetent patient, there must be *clear and convincing evidence* of the patient's wishes. The Missouri Supreme Court said that citing vague and unreliable recollections by Nancy's parents and friends about what she would have wanted was not enough to meet the demanding standard of clear and convincing evidence.

It was in reviewing this Missouri decision that the United States Supreme Court began to recognize a right of a *competent* patient to decline medical treatment, even if such refusal will lead directly to the patient's death. Thus *Cruzan* was the first time the Supreme Court decided that the Constitution gives Americans a "liberty interest" to be free of unwanted medical support. The reporter covering the Supreme Court for *The New York Times* wrote:

> The framers of the Constitution, who prohibited the Government from depriving a person of "life" or "liberty" without due process of law, had little reason to envision a day when the very act of sustaining a life might itself be a deprivation of liberty.[24]

And yet, she went on to say, modern medical technology had done precisely that. The Supreme Court also found that withdrawing a feeding tube was not different from withdrawing any other kind of life-sustaining medical support. Hence some state laws permitting forgoing or withdrawing respirators but not artificial nutrition were unconstitutional.

With regard to *incompetent* patients, the Supreme Court held in *Cruzan* that a state could, but need not, pass a statute requiring the "clear and convincing" standard of evidence about what a formerly competent patient would have wanted done if he or she went into a permanent coma. Because Missouri had such a standard, its law was constitutional. However, since the Cruzan family had not met that standard, Nancy Cruzan's feeding tube could *not* be removed.

How did the Supreme Court see its first decision on death and dying? Justice Sandra Day O'Connor wrote in her concurring opinion, "Today we decide only that one state's practice does not violate the Constitution. The more challenging task of crafting appropriate procedures for safeguarding incompetents' liberty interests is entrusted to the 'laboratory' of the states."[25] She thus suggested that state legislatures and state courts should seek a balance between the rights of families to make such decisions for incompetent relatives and the obligation of a state to protect the interests of incompetents.

The *Cruzan* decision said nothing about another category where a state might make a law about withdrawing medical treatment: the death of "never competent" patients, such as people with profound mental retardation. Because of past abuses, it is reasonable to expect that only state laws with the most rigorous standards of proof about such cases will pass the Supreme Court's review. The

Supreme Court might even require for such cases the same standard used in criminal law—"beyond a reasonable doubt."[26]

To summarize the three standards of evidence:

1. Preponderance of evidence (most permissive)
2. Clear and convincing evidence (permitted by *Cruzan*)
3. Beyond a reasonable doubt (least permissive;
   perhaps necessary with incompetents)

Reactions to *Cruzan*   Reactions to the Supreme Court's decision in *Cruzan* ran along two lines: legal commentators were on the whole positive whereas medical commentators were negative.

Most legal scholars supported the new conservative position of the Rehnquist Court on its role with regard to the Constitution. The proper function of the Supreme Court, according to the law professor Charles Baron, was not as a "super legislature" over the states or even "to promulgate uniform rules of state law. The U.S. Supreme Court should only have the power to strike down state laws that conflict with federal law, and the U.S. Constitution."[27] That is, not every bad or undesirable state law is necessarily unconstitutional.

Another law professor, John Robertson, went so far as to say that Nancy Cruzan could not be harmed and hence had no interests in the case. Robertson argued that the real claim in *Cruzan* had nothing to do with Nancy Cruzan's right to die or right to privacy (her "liberty interests"); the case was about the Cruzan *family's* right to be free of the emotional burden of maintaining her body in a state institution.[28]

Both Baron and Robertson agreed that the previous legal standard of *substituted judgment* (the standard applied by the New Jersey Supreme Court in *Quinlan*) was a mockery in such cases,

> . . . [leading] us to pretend that we are merely complying (however reluctantly) with the wishes of the patient. The result in most states is mere lip service to substituted judgment. Almost any evidence is deemed sufficient to establish a preference for death over PVS. Or families are empowered to express patient preferences for death—with few questions asked.[29]

A different kind of reaction came from physicians who worked with families of vegetative and hospice patients. Although they understood the points about constitutional law, these physicians intensely disliked the decision and emphasized the misery that families had to endure because of laws like those in New York and Missouri. A neurologist and ethicist, Ronald Cranford, said:

> We should realize what the law is in Missouri . . . that once medical treatment is started (at least for artificial nutrition and hydration), it can't be stopped. [And to allow such a state to use the "clear and convincing standard" is] "unworkable, unfair, and cruel to so many families who will experience the utter helplessness of the Cruzans. It will place an enormous burden on society, which will spend hundreds of millions of dollars each year for a condition that no one in their right mind would ever want to be in."[30]

The hospice physician Joanne Lynn and the bioethicist Jacqueline Glover emphasized that the Missouri and New York laws—now permissible, according to the Supreme Court—essentially meant that "the suffering of the patient and family, the costs, the kind of life that can be gained, are all to count for nothing. If life can be prolonged, then it will have to be."[31]

The aftermath   Five months after the Supreme Court's decision in *Cruzan*, on December 14, 1990, Nancy Cruzan's feeding tube was removed legally, and she died. Nancy had been divorced just before her accident, and she had some friends who knew her only by her married name, Nancy Davis. When her case first became widely known, these people had not realized that she was the woman the headlines and news stories were referring to.[32] Later, as nationwide publicity grew, they learned who Nancy Cruzan was and came forward. The appeals process was already under way by that time, and the judges were discussing larger issues; but after the major decision, the case was reheard in a lower court because Nancy's friends were offering new testimony. In that hearing, the lower court decided that the state's "clear and convincing" standard for evidence had now been met.[33]

ETHICAL ISSUES

Communication and Control

The Quinlan and Cruzan cases involved not only moral conflicts but also conflicts about control and management of medical treatment.

In the Quinlan case, one such issue had to do with Karen's transfer from a small community hospital—Newton Memorial—to St. Clare's. When the Quinlans were initially approached about transferring Karen, they didn't understand what the consequences of the transfer might be. At a local hospital, patients and families are often dealing with physicians they know, trust, and may have chosen themselves. Once patients are transferred to a large, impersonal, "tertiary care" hospital, by contrast, they will be dealing with medical personnel who are strangers, who are assigned to their cases by the luck of the draw, and whose sense of professionalism may conflict with the family's decisions or wishes.

Another issue—which often arises when a patient is transferred—has to do with hospital policies, since different hospitals and many specialties have their own internal rules. Ideally, of course, hospitals would post their policies, including those about care of the dying, and inform patients and their families in advance about such policies. In reality, however, patients and families are rarely informed about hospital policies before an admission or transfer takes place. For example, when the Quinlans were asked to give their "informed consent" and sign papers allowing Karen to have the tracheotomy required for the MA-1 respirator, they were not aware of St. Clare's policy: once a patient was on such a respirator, the respirator could not be removed. How could a hospital obtain "informed consent" from a family facing a crucial decision without giving the family such information? Similarly, the Cruzans may not have realized that state-run hospital facilities in Missouri would not remove a feeding tube from a PVS patient.

Another issue involved Medicaid, the medical coverage designed for poor people. Karen Quinlan and Nancy Cruzan, as incompetent adults, could be declared bankrupt and thus were eligible for Medicaid; and both the Quinlans and the Cruzans accepted state Medicaid payment for their daughters' care. In accepting Medicaid benefits, however, they may not have realized that now state health officials and bureaucrats could make life-and-death decisions for Karen and Nancy.

Still another issue concerns whose concept of "death" will control a case when a patient is incompetent and the question of withdrawing support arises. Karen Quinlan was not *legally* dead, and her family disagreed with the hospital about which *evaluative* standard of death to apply: evaluatively, the Quinlans believed that Karen was already dead, whereas the hospital wanted to be more cautious.

There may be other evaluative conflicts. In the Cruzan case, Missouri applied a stringent standard in trying to determine Nancy Cruzan's own wishes with regard to withdrawing her feeding tube and rejected the evidence the Cruzans offered. The Cruzans and the state also disagreed in their assessment of risks and benefits involved in Nancy's treatment.

Standards of Brain Death

People have always feared that they might be declared dead prematurely and buried alive. In the eighteenth century, there were gruesome stories about exhumations that found frantic scratches on the inside lids of coffins. In the nine-teenth century, some legislatures required a delay before burial; and in 1882 an undertaker named Kirchbaum attached periscopes to coffins so that a person who woke up after being buried might signal for help.[34]

For thousands of years, the definition of death included cessation—almost simultaneously—of breathing and heartbeat. When breathing stopped, cardiac anoxia (lack of oxygen) would begin; this would be followed by cessation of the heart and then by ischemia (lack of blood flow to an area). Ischemia of the brain destroys brain tissue very rapidly. This is the traditional *whole-body standard* (or criterion) of death.

The whole-body standard became inappropriate when ventilators were developed that allowed artificial respiration of brain-damaged patients; using heart-lung machines, crude bodily functions could be maintained without most brain functions. In 1967, the surgeon Christiaan Barnard transplanted Denise Darvall's heart into a dying patient named Louis Washkansky (this case is dis-cussed in Chapter 10), and the question arose whether the donor had really been dead before her heart was removed, since she had been sustained on a heart-lung machine until then. A new standard of death was needed to determine when organs could be removed from a still "living" body.

Brain death—an alternative to whole-body death—was first described in the medical literature in 1959.[35] There is more than one standard of brain death.

In 1968, shortly after Barnard's transplant operation (this timing was not a coincidence), an ad hoc committee at Harvard Medical School developed the *Harvard criteria* of brain death.[36] The Harvard criteria operationally defined brain death as behavior that indicated unawareness of external stimuli, lack of bodily movements, no spontaneous breathing, lack of reflexes, and two isoelectric (nearly flat) electroencephalogram (EEG) readings 24 hours apart. These criteria required a loss of virtually all brain activity (including the brain stem, and hence breathing). The Harvard criteria were exceedingly cautious: no one declared dead by these criteria has ever regained consciousness. (As the saying goes, "If you're Harvard dead, you're *really* dead.") The extreme conservatism of the Harvard standard is well known, and regretted, by people waiting for organ transplants from donors who must be declared brain-dead: relatively few potential donors—dying patients with healthy organs—have met the Harvard standard during the last 25 years. (Patients who have been comatose for a long time may be more likely to meet that standard, but they do not have healthy, transplantable organs at death.)

Another standard of brain death is the "higher person" criterion, or—as we shall call it in this book—the *cognitive criterion*. This criterion identifies a philosophical core of properties of "persons" and assumes that without such a core, a human body is no longer a person; the core properties commonly include reason, memory, and self-awareness. For example, neurological disorders like Huntington's disease destroy brain cells at a high rate, so that not much of the "higher person" is left. The cognitive criterion has the greatest potential to generate organs for transplantation. So far, however, this criterion has been considered both controversial and vague and has not been legally adopted by any state—although countless families in fact act on it when they agree to reduce treatment to speed a patient's death.[37]

A third standard of brain death, the *irreversibility standard*, falls between the Harvard and cognitive criteria. According to this standard, death occurs simply when unconsciousness is irreversible. Operationally, this judgment would be made by a neurologist and another physician. The irreversibility standard would allow PVS patients to be declared dead after several years (perhaps, in some cases, after several months). At the time of the first heart transplant in 1968—7 years before the Karen Quinlan case—this standard was thought to be too broad. One problem with the irreversibility standard is that at least seven patients have recovered after being in PVS for over 1 year. It is true that these seven patients were exceptional: in a study by the Multi-Society Task Force on PVS, they were the only ones of 434 adults with traumatic head injuries to regain consciousness and make a good recovery after so long a time in PVS.[38] It is also true that no patient has recovered after 30 months in PVS (both Karen Quinlan and Nancy Cruzan were in PVS longer than that). The study by the task force concluded that "recovery of consciousness from a posttraumatic persistent vegetative state is unlikely after 12 months in adults and children," implying that medical maintenance of PVS patients after 1 year is futile because unconsciousness is then permanent. Nevertheless, the exceptions represent a warning against quick judgments that a patient's condition is "irreversible"; and even if they suggest that the chance of recovery is only something on the order of 7 in 434 (less than 1 in 60), some people would want to be given this chance. To date, no state has accepted the irreversibility standard.

The *Uniform Brain Death Act* (UBDA) attempted to provide a consistent definition of brain death which all states could use—so that, for instance, a patient could not be "dead" in New Jersey, be taken across the George Washington Bridge, and be declared "resurrected and alive" in New York.[39] According to the UBDA standard, death occurs when there is irreversible loss of *all* brain function. Not all states have accepted the UBDA criterion, however. As noted earlier in this chapter, a state's statutes concerning brain death are exceptions to its laws concerning homicide. Because definitions of homicide and penalties for homicide vary from state to state (these are not matters of federal law), it follows that laws dealing with brain death—and related laws about suicide and withdrawing care from dying patients—also vary from state to state. One reason why not all states have accepted UBDA is that the act may not have gone far enough. If it had been in effect in New Jersey during the Quinlan case or in Missouri during the Cruzan case, it would not have changed the outcome. Both Karen Quinlan and Nancy Cruzan had a functioning brain stem, and so neither of them would have met the UBDA standard of brain death.

To sum up standards of brain death:

- *Harvard criteria.* Operational definition based on loss of nearly all brain functioning, with two nearly flat EEGs. Conservative; least conducive to transplantable organs.
- *Cognitive criterion.* Definition based on loss of "core properties"—mental capacities without which a body is no longer to be considered a "person." Most liberal; most conducive to organs for transplant.
- *Irreversibility standard.* Defines death as occurring when unconsciousness is irreversible (operationally, when PVS has lasted over 1 year). Less conservative than the Harvard criteria but not so liberal as the cognitive criterion; moderately conducive to obtaining organs for transplant.
- *Uniform Brain Death Act (UBDA).* Defines death as occurring when there is irreversible loss of all brain function. Conservative; not conducive to transplantable organs.

In the two decades since the Karen Quinlan case, people have become more educated about death and dying, and the concept of brain death has contributed to a radical change in our ideas concerning the end of life. One remarkable fact which became widely known during the Quinlan case—and was again revealed when videotapes of patients like Nancy Cruzan were televised—is that a person whose heart is beating and whose eyes are open and moving may, by certain standards, nevertheless be dead. In former times, people believed that death was marked by some uniform, metaphysical event which had physical manifestations and was perhaps the counterpart of an event at the beginning of life, when a sperm and egg became an embryo or when a fetus became a person; some people would have described these metaphysical events as the entrance and departure of a soul. The occurrence of such metaphysical events cannot be proven, however; and even if they do occur, they have no physical manifestations. Today, people have come to believe that the definition of death is not a matter of discovery but rather, to a significant extent, a kind of decision that families and their physicians can make.

Mercy

In a case like Karen Quinlan's or Nancy Cruzan's, *mercy* may become a factor. A person arguing from mercy might appeal to something like the "golden rule": "If I ended up in a condition like Karen's or Nancy's, I would want to die, and I hope that those around me would be merciful enough to let me die. If I could somehow possibly be 'conscious' in such a state, I wouldn't want to go on. I wouldn't want to be imprisoned in such a body for months or years. That would be worse than being buried alive, because if I were buried alive I would die after only a few days. Mercy requires us to make dying humane, not an endless torture."

The Quinlans and the Cruzans did argue that allowing Karen and Nancy to die would be the merciful thing to do. The issue of mercy is relevant in these and similar cases because we can't know for certain that such patients do not *feel*—we cannot be certain that they do not experience sensations such as pain and discomfort; we may not even be certain that they do not experience distress, fear, frustration, loss, or other tormenting emotions.

For example, Karen Quinlan's limbs were at first tied down, but her head moved violently, as if she were trying to dislodge the nasogastric feeding and ventilator tubes. Also, some of Karen's family—and their lawyer—said that Karen looked as if she were in pain. Julia Quinlan said, "[It] seems as if she's in pain by her facial expressions"; and, "They say she doesn't feel pain, but I wondered if they really knew."[40] The question whether these phenomena were intentional behavior or merely reflexes is a philosophical as well as a medical issue. *Intentional behavior* would indicate an organism seeking some goal, such as freedom from pain, and might even indicate awareness.

As the seventeenth-century philosopher René Descartes noted, consciousness in others is always an *inference* from outward behavior; it cannot be directly observed. Unconsciousness, or lack of consciousness, is also an inference. If we claim—as some people do—that flies aren't conscious, this is an inference from flies' behavior; and as far as flies are concerned, we can make such inferences easily. In the case of a human being, however, a lot is at stake if we are wrong.

Consider, for example, that a condition called the *locked-in syndrome* has only recently been recognized. Patients in this state are so extensively paralyzed that they can control nothing except blinking their eyes, but these patients are just as conscious as any normal person. This syndrome may have led to some live burials in the past. Could anything be more terrible to imagine than that? Perhaps; suppose that Karen Quinlan's mind was alive for 10 years inside her apparently comatose body.

Neurologists feel confident that patients in Karen Quinlan's condition are not conscious. In a similar case, that of Paul Brophy in 1986, the American Academy of Neurology wrote:

No conscious experience of pain and suffering is possible without the integrated functioning of the brain stem and cerebral cortex. Pain and suffering are attributes of consciousness, and PVS patients like Brophy do not experience them. Noxious stimuli may activate peripherally located nerves, but only a brain with the capacity for consciousness can transfer that neural activity into an experience.[41]

According to the Multi-Society Task Force on PVS, scanning devices show that brain activity of PVS patients is far below that of patients with locked-in syndrome, and extensive neurological examinations of PVS patients during autopsies have revealed deep lesions incompatible with awareness.[42]

Although these neurological findings may be reassuring, however, they do not resolve the issue of mercy. Eventually, the cases of Karen Quinlan and Nancy Cruzan came to symbolize mercy as an issue for both patients and families. These cases seemed to represent an inversion of values in medicine: instead of doing what families wanted, medicine did what bureaucracies required; instead of a dignified death, breathing machines and feeding tubes maintained existence; instead of a quick death, there was the slow withering over a decade of an emaciated body. For many people, these two deaths were merciless.

PVS Patients: Costs of Care

A comprehensive study in 1994 estimated that in the United States between 10,000 and 25,000 adults and between 4,000 and 10,000 children were in PVS.[43] Costs per patient per year ranged between $24,000 and $120,000.[44] The longest case of PVS so far has been that of Rita Greene, who became comatose in 1952, at age 24, after open-heart surgery and died in D.C. General Hospital in the District of Columbia in 1991.[45]

PVS patients usually require round-the-clock monitoring by private nurses. Karen Quinlan and Nancy Cruzan, for example, required 24-hour nursing (in case an airway became clogged, leading to suffocation), expectorants and anticonvulsive drugs, changes of urinary catheters and tubes removing fecal waste, flexing of their muscles to prevent contractions, washing the body, brushing the teeth, treating dental cavities to prevent lethal mouth infections, and treating other infections with antibiotics.

When a hospital is left with a PVS patient after having done all it can, these facts create moral dilemmas for the hospital and the family. What is to be done with the patient? Few nursing homes will admit PVS patients, since the care these patients require is far beyond what most such homes can provide; and in any case there is virtually no medical insurance that would cover long-term care of a PVS patient in a nursing home. Hardly any family can afford this care, which might easily cost $100,000 a year, and no one will reimburse the hospital for it. In the event, many PVS patients simply remain in limbo in American hospitals, since legally and ethically they cannot be dumped into the streets to die.

It is hard to feel sorry for St. Clare's, which forced the Quinlans to keep Karen's body alive and then did not want to pay for the course of action its own policies had demanded—just as, in the Cruzan case, it is hard to feel sorry for the state of Missouri, which argued for keeping her body alive and would have had to pay for her care if that argument had prevailed. Still, what to do about caring for PVS patients is a broader issue than whether or not an institution like St. Clare's deserves our sympathy.

In this regard, it is relevant to note that Karen Quinlan's social worker did try to transfer her to a state psychiatric hospital, so that St. Clare's would not have to bear the cost of her care; but the state institutions lacked respiratory therapists and respirators and therefore would not accept her. Not having such resources is usually a matter of state public policy; that is, it is part of the state's decision making on issues of medical distributive justice. Usually, when a state does not provide certain treatments, this reflects a judgment that the chances of recovery are too small to justify the cost. It is both a vice and a virtue of the American medical system that no particular individuals can be identified who make such judgments—which in effect are judgments to deny those treatments to certain patients.

Another issue of costs of PVS has to do with the system of reimbursing hospitals on the basis of "diagnostically related groups" (DRGs). Under this system, which began in 1983, a hospital receives a fixed sum for each patient's care; if care continues after that sum is exhausted, the hospital will lose money. Given this system, will cost pressures discourage physicians from doing everything possible for PVS patients? Might physicians tend to tell the family that a patient's condition is "terminal" or "hopeless" when in fact the patient may have some small chance of recovering and leading a normal life?

Kinds of Medical Support

In the years between the Quinlan case and the Cruzan case, physicians and philosophers debated whether certain levels of medical support had moral significance. Could a dying patient be harmed by not receiving extraordinary support? Could such a patient be harmed by not receiving *ordinary* support? Is a patient "morally owed" food and water as "humane care" in all circumstances? If acting to hasten death (for instance, by giving an overdose of morphine to a cancer patient in pain) is immoral, is it also immoral to hasten death by inaction (by not starting chemotherapy, for example)? In the terminology then current, would "passive euthanasia" (inaction) be equivalent to "active euthanasia" (action)? Would "forgoing" medical support be equivalent to "withdrawing" support that has already been initiated?

The flames of these controversies rose high at times and in some quarters are still burning today. The following discussion outlines three of the major issues.

Extraordinary versus ordinary care   In 1957, a group of anesthesiologists asked Pope Pius XII what they owed to dying patients. The pope said that they need not take "heroic" steps to keep such patients alive: patients were owed merely ordinary, but not extraordinary, care.

One problem with distinguishing between ordinary and extraordinary care is that the word *care* is equivocal: in medical contexts, it can refer to either compassion or technology, though undoubtedly the pope meant technology. As a result, "ordinary" compassion is sometimes seen as requiring "extraordinary" technology. That equation, however, should not be made without thought, for it is based on an assumption that a completely compassionate act cannot include, or take the form of, stopping extraordinary medical support. In other words, patients should expect and receive compassion, but categories of technology should not define it.

A second problem is that "ordinary" and "extraordinary" care are end points of a continuum that shifts with medical progress. In 1967, when Christiaan Barnard first transplanted a human heart, his heart-lung bypass machine was considered "extraordinary." That machine was the forerunner of the large, bulky ventilator which kept Karen Quinlan breathing. Today, miniaturized ventilators have been developed—some small enough to be used with premature babies—and have become common. Because many seriously ill patients now are ventilated at some point, yesterday's "extraordinary" has become today's "ordinary."

Artificial nutrition and hydration During the 1960s, artificial feeding of comatose patients was considered a temporary treatment. Patients unable to swallow were nourished by means of flexible plastic tubing which conveyed artificial, carefully balanced liquid nutrients to the gastrointestinal (GI) tract. Eventually, however, this treatment became an accepted way of indefinitely sustaining the bodies of dying and chronically ill patients.

In the 1980s, some people believed that whatever might be said about "extraordinary" and "ordinary" care in the future, providing food and water at least would always be considered ordinary and humane. Such basic care was felt to be owed to PVS patients despite their problematic moral status; as we have seen, the Quinlans wanted Karen's ventilator disconnected but would have thought it wrong to remove her feeding and hydration tube. The Cruzan case marked a significant change: since Nancy Cruzan was not on a respirator, the issue was simply removing her feeding tube.

There are, of course, arguments for and against withdrawing nutrition and hydration. Some states allow removal of respirators but not withdrawal of artificial nutrition and hydration; and conservative critics see removal of feeding and hydration tubes as the immediate cause of death and hence as "mercy killing." One philosopher argued in 1983 that providing food and water to PVS patients is the ordinary care "that all human beings owe each other"; another argued at about the same time that such feeding involves "the most fundamental of all human relationships," and that "to tamper with, or adulterate, so enduring and central a moral emotion" is "a most dangerous business."[46]

On the other side are those who see artificial feeding either as prolonging the inevitable—dying—or as sustaining the body of a patient who is in fact already dead. People who argue in this way give little weight to the symbolic value of feeding and think that equating withdrawal of nutrition with "murder" is conceptually confused. According to this view, the moral question here is simple: Is artificial feeding and hydration a *benefit* or a *burden* to a patient, to the patient's family, and to the hospital staff?

In considering this moral conflict, some points of fact become relevant. To begin with, it should be noted that, despite "commonsense" ideas to the contrary, neither dehydration nor starvation may be distressing to semiconscious, dying patients. Actually, bedside observations by physicians in geriatric medicine and hospices indicate that patients near death who are not on nutritional support seem more comfortable than similar patients who are on such support. One important national commission noted in 1983 that loss of appetite is "almost the norm in the latter stages of terminal illness" and concluded, "Only rarely should a dying patient be fed by tube or intravenously."[47]

Also, it is necessary to understand the reality of "feeding" a chronically comatose or vegetative patient. This feeding is not like spooning chicken soup into the mouth of a patient who is simply weak or semiconscious. Some vegetative patients have no gag or swallowing reflexes, and so they cannot be fed by mouth. Therefore, an artificial liquid diet must be mechanically introduced into the body. This is done in three basic ways: (1) by a temporary nasogastric tube run up the nostrils and down into the gastrointestinal tract; (2) by a permanent intravenous feeding line, surgically attached to one of the major veins of the chest; (3) by a surgically implanted gastrostomy tube. With many kinds of feeding tubes, patients must be tied down to avoid dislodging the line. All feeding tubes carry the risk of infection; with many, such a large volume of fluid is needed to supply the nutrients that other problems are caused. The "chicken soup" image can distort people's impression of a PVS case. Karen Quinlan's sister, for example, thought that her comatose sister would look like Sleeping Beauty and was shocked by the emaciated figure she saw. By the time of Nancy Cruzan's case in 1990, improvements in artificial feeding would create an opposite effect: PVS patients now had rotund "Porky Pig" faces because of retention of fluids.

Furthermore, artificial feeding usually requires intense medical support. Many physicians involved in caring for PVS patients during the late 1970s decided that artificial nutrition was by no means natural feeding, and that the artificial procedures were not simple "care" but highly sophisticated medical treatment. By the 1990s, most physicians had come to feel that artificial IV feeding lines for PVS patients were comparable to ventilators: both were advanced medical technology.

Not everyone has agreed with the emerging idea that artificial nutrition and hydration are just another form of medical treatment, which can, ethically, be forgone or withdrawn for PVS patients. Several physicians and members of the clergy in conservative religions oppose such withdrawal.[48] However, most state courts now allow withdrawal of artificial nutrition and hydration.

Withdrawing treatment and forgoing treatment   During the last two decades, a central debate has concerned the degree to which a physician may be involved in hastening the death of a dying patient. One cause of this debate was a declaration by AMA in 1973 (two years before *Quinlan*):

> The intentional termination of the life of one human being by another—mercy killing—is contrary to that for which the medical profession stands and is contrary to the policy of the American Medical Association.
>   . . . The cessation of the employment of extraordinary means to prolong the life of the body when there is irrefutable evidence that biological death is imminent is the decision of the patient and/or immediate family.[49]

In this statement, the word *extraordinary* is ambiguous, and AMA policy did not clarify it. Are all patients on ventilators receiving "extraordinary" care? Is a physician who withdraws a dying patient's ventilator with the intent of "termination of life," and without the consent of the family, guilty of "mercy killing"? What if the physician withdraws a feeding tube?

Concern about the possibility of being considered guilty of "mercy killing" led some physicians to *forgo* the use of ventilators and artificial feeding. Since withdrawal of such care might be seen as "intentional termination" of life ("mercy killing"), it was far easier to forgo medical support than to withdraw it. This reasoning created an odd situation, in which physicians would *forgo* the same treatment that they would or could not *withdraw*.

To others, it seemed that patients could be harmed both by AMA's policy and by the interpretation that an extraordinary treatment (like a ventilator) could be forgone but not withdrawn. They believed that because the outcome is never certain, a patient is morally owed extraordinary treatment—both a ventilator and artificial feeding, for example—in order to see if recovery is possible. Also, some people argued that, regardless of whether a ventilator or a catheter was "ordinary" or "extraordinary" medical support, nobody really thought that a physician who withdrew such a device would thus "kill" a terminally ill patient. In such a situation, we would say—if, for instance, the patient had cancer—that he or she had been killed by the *cancer,* not by the physician.

Kinds of Cases

When we engage in moral reasoning about people who are dying, it is helpful to distinguish among different kinds of cases. Consider how a society might ideally make decisions about death and dying. First, the courts would deliberate about *competent adult* patients with terminal diseases, defining these patients' right to refuse treatment. Second, the courts might rule on whether competent adults have a right to refuse medical treatment when they are *not* terminally ill (patients such as Elizabeth Bouvia and Larry McAfee, discussed in Chapter 2, would be in this category). Third, the courts might move to a very different kind of case, in which a surrogate or proxy is making decisions for a patient who once was but is no longer competent—an *incompetent but formerly competent* patient. A fourth kind of situation would include decision making by a surrogate for infant and child patients: in general, the category of *presently incompetent but later to be competent* patients. Finally, the courts would rule on whether or not special standards are needed for *never competent* patients (such as severely retarded babies and adults). Some of these cases raise difficult ethical questions with regard to evaluating "quality of life," since what a competent person may see as an "inferior" quality of life may be perceived differently by an incompetent patient.

In the Quinlan case, the decision of the New Jersey Supreme Court ran two different kinds of cases together, and this evident confusion worried some critics who already saw the case as depreciating the absolute value of life.[50] As we have seen, the New Jersey court based its decision partly on the right to privacy as established by the United States Supreme Court in *Griswold v. Connecticut* in 1965—a right that, in a medical context, would presumably apply only to *compe-*

tent patients. But the ruling that Karen's respirator could be disconnected was also based on the standard of *substituted judgment,* according to which relatives or friends can substitute their judgment for that of an *incompetent* patient.

Consequently, at least two problems were seen with this decision. One was that it was unclear how a family's right to exercise substituted judgment could have been derived from *Griswold.* Critics felt that the New Jersey court had jumped too quickly from married people's right to control their own reproduction (the situation in *Griswold)* to parents' right to let an adult, comatose child die—since there had then been no intervening decisions about whether competent adults (terminally ill or not) had a right to hasten their own death by refusing medical treatment.

Another problem had to do with the standard of substituted judgment itself, which is notoriously loose and subjective.[51] This standard (later used by several other state supreme courts) presumes that decisions made by a patient's family or friends will reflect what the patient himself or herself would have wanted done. In the Quinlan case, however, it was unclear whether Karen Quinlan had ever expressed a wish not to have her life prolonged if she became comatose, or even a wish that her parents should act for her in such a situation.

The Slippery Slope

The Quinlan case thus gave rise to intense concern about the *slippery slope*—a metaphor which has become one of the most powerful ideas in ethics and politics. In this image, some issue or situation (perhaps even society as a whole) is envisioned as perched at the edge of a steep slope, and moral principles are seen as chocks or ledges which prevent it from sliding down. If we remove too many chocks (or sometimes just one chock), a downward slide will begin. The slide may be imperceptible at first, but then it will gain momentum, and as more chocks are removed (or fall under this momentum) the slide will become unstoppable. Inevitably, the slide will end at the bottom of the slope, which is seen as a "pit," a "jungle," moral chaos, or ruin. The slippery slope may refer either to a *prediction about empirical consequences* if some moral change occurs, or to a *linkage in reasoning* if certain premises are accepted.

In cases like Karen Quinlan's, people who think in terms of this metaphor fear that once society allows one kind of death to occur in one kind of situation, it will then allow a second kind of death to occur in a second situation, and then a third kind in a third situation, and so on, plunging down the slippery slope and soon arriving at the bottom, where masses of vulnerable patients will be killed against their wishes. These critics argue that if, say, "quality of life" becomes an acceptable reason for letting a competent patient die, it will next be applied to—imposed on—incompetent patients. Once leukemic adults are allowed to die, leukemic teenagers and children will also be allowed to die; first we allow abortion of a fetus because of Down syndrome, and then we let a newborn with Down syndrome die.

The slippery slope is discussed more in Chapter 3; for now, we should note that it is often used to support a status quo. It can put the onus of proof on those who desire change, to demonstrate in advance that no harm will ensue.

UPDATE

Advance Directives

One of the most controversial ethical and legal aspects of the Quinlan case was whether or not to withdraw medical support when the patient's wishes were not explicitly known. It was the fact that Karen Quinlan's wishes were unproven which led some critics to condemn her family's decision to withdraw her respirator; legal critics also said that, since her wishes were uncertain, the decision in the Quinlan case had abandoned *parens patria,* the ancient duty of courts to protect incompetents (this principle had been accepted in English law for centuries).

It was because of the Quinlan case that written *advance directives* began to become popular, as a way for people to make their wishes known beforehand for the guidance of physicians at some later time. By 1992, 43 states had statutes recognizing some version of advance directives.[52] The decision in the Cruzan case emphasized that such a document would be crucial in meeting the "clear and convincing" standard required by New York and Missouri.

Advance directives can take several forms. A *living will* (sometimes videotaped) informs physicians about conditions under which a person would or would not want medical support continued. A *values inventory* specifies what a person values in life and may be useful to a patient's family and physicians if they must make decisions for that person. A *durable power of attorney* assigns to someone else the right to make financial and life-and-death medical decisions if the person becomes incompetent. In those states which allow it to be applied to medical decisions, durable power of attorney is the most powerful device for protecting the rights of dying people; however, not all states have statutes creating powers of attorney for proxy medical decisions. One possible addition to an advance directive would be which standard of brain death (see above) a person wants to have applied when he or she is declared dead. Some people who have this intention in mind may believe that simply signing a general advance directive will take care of it, but actually specifying a standard within the directive is much more powerful.[53]

In December 1991, all American hospitals were required by the Health Care Financing Administration to ask incoming patients if they had, or wanted to sign, an advance directive. It was hoped that this requirement would increase the use of advance directives, and that it would force hospitals both to specify their policies about honoring such directives and to tell patients about those policies.

Today, although considerable progress had been made, there are still some problems with advance directives. Advance directives often do not cover *nonterminal* though permanent comas; directives often fail to specify whether food and water are included under "unwanted medical treatment"; and (with the exception of durable powers of attorney) some directives do not arrange for a proxy for decision making if a patient becomes incompetent. Also, because such directives are requested only on admission to a hospital, most young people have not signed them. At present, a typical young adult like Nancy Cruzan who is admitted to a hospital with a head injury and becomes a PVS patient has not signed an advance directive.

Ethics of Withdrawing Support

In 1975, Karen Quinlan's physicians—Morse and Javed—were upholding the official position of AMA: that withdrawing medical support from a patient was the same as "active euthanasia." In 1986, AMA changed its policy to reflect a new understanding of chronically comatose patients supported by ventilators and artificial nutrition. Now it is "ethically" possible for a physician, after consulting with the family, to withdraw a ventilator and feeding tubes from an "irreversibly" comatose patient. This new AMA policy did not say that being irreversibly comatose was equivalent to being brain-dead; thus criteria for ethical removal of medical support (according to AMA) may or may not be the same as a state's legal standard of brain death, and a physician could, under AMA policy, remove support from a patient who was not legally dead under a state's laws.

In the Cruzan case, unlike the Quinlan case, the issue was solely removal of a feeding tube. As noted earlier, the Supreme Court stated in *Cruzan* (1990) that it saw no difference between withdrawing artificial nutrition and withdrawing other kinds of medical support. Clearly, American courts and medicine have come a remarkably long way in a very short time in rethinking the ethics of withdrawing support from chronically comatose patients.

Medical Futility

In December 1991, Helga Wanglie, age 87, had been in PVS for 8 months, sustained by a ventilator and a feeding tube, at Hennepin County Hospital in Minneapolis, Minnesota.[54] At this point, a group of physicians at the hospital decided to oppose the wishes of the patient's husband, Oliver Wanglie, who had refused to give his permission for her respirator and feeding tube to be discontinued. The Wanglie case was unusual for two reasons. First, since Helga Wanglie's medical insurance covered her hospitalization almost entirely, the hospital would actually *lose* money by withdrawing artificial life support. Second—and more important—the case involved an ethical and philosophical dispute about whether a medical team could be forced by a family member to continue care it regarded as "futile."[55] When Helga Wanglie died, the legal case ended, and the Hennepin County physicians did not continue to seek a precedent in the courts; however, about half a dozen other cases of medical futility were heard by courts and hospital ethics committees.[56]

During the early 1990s, the concept of *medical futility* was being widely discussed. The issue is evaluative, or semievaluative, but at times this aspect was obscured by the desire of clinical physicians for an objective standard for ending care.[57] It is noteworthy that the bioethicists who brought the Wanglie case were mainly *physician* bioethicists: when bioethics first developed, few physicians entered the field, but this had changed over the previous two decades.

Bioethicists were divided about cases of medical futility. Some of them supported the physicians who sought to withdraw care, arguing that society could not go on indefinitely bearing the enormous costs of such treatment of hopeless patients. Others, however, were distressed that any bioethicists could abandon their original role of championing families and seeking to have physicians and administrators follow families' wishes regarding the care of dying patients.

It should be noted that pressure from families for presumably "futile" care is by no means typical. Most American patients and their families now decline treatment when their physicians advise them that there is no realistic chance of recovery. A study in 1994 that followed over 4,000 patients whose condition was diagnosed as life-threatening or terminal found that only 14 percent of them were resuscitated after being near death. This figure was far less than most physicians predicted and far less than it would have been a decade earlier, when most of those patients would have been resuscitated.[58]

In the same year as this study—1994—the deaths of former president Richard Nixon (of a stroke) and Jacqueline Kennedy Onassis (of cancer) were emblematic of the trend toward declining care in terminal situations. Richard Nixon had left instructions that he was not to be connected to a respirator or resuscitated; and Jacqueline Onassis, when she was told that no further medical treatment would help her, simply went home to die.

An Autopsy on Karen Quinlan

PVS patients may eventually help us learn more about the anatomical basis of human consciousness. Neurologists now believe that consciousness has two dimensions or components: wakefulness (or arousal) and awareness. On this analysis, PVS patients can be described as wakeful but not aware.

In 1994, results of an autopsy on Karen Quinlan's brain were revealed; it showed extensive damage to the thalamus. Before this, wakefulness had been thought to be activated by a series of inputs relayed from the brain stem and thalamus to the cortex. The pattern of damage in Karen's brain, however, suggested that the thalamus has less of a role in arousal than had been thought and more of a role in awareness.[59]

FURTHER READING

Margaret Battin, *The Least Worst Death: Essays in Bioethics at the End of Life,* Oxford University Press, New York, 1993.

Joanne Lynn, ed., *By No Extraordinary Means: The Choice to Forgo Life-Sustaining Food and Water,* expanded ed., 1989, Indiana University Press, Bloomington, 1989.

Pat Milmoe McCarrick, "Scope Note 7: Withholding or Withdrawing Nutrition or Hydration," National Reference Center for Bioethics Literature at the Kennedy Institute of Ethics, Georgetown University, Washington, D.C., updated, November 1986.

CHAPTER 2

Requests to Die

Elizabeth Bouvia and Larry McAfee

This chapter discusses the cases of Elizabeth Bouvia and Larry McAfee, two people with nonterminal physical disabilities who decided that they no longer
wanted to live.

BACKGROUND: PERSPECTIVES ON SUICIDE

Greece and Rome

The ancient Greeks—or at least their aristocrats—strove not simply to live, but to
achieve a life that would exemplify nobility, honor, excellence, and beauty. The
Greeks believed that "the unexamined life is not worth living," and that "the
really important thing is not to live but to live well." This was also their attitude
toward death, and they thought that philosophy would give them the wisdom to
approach death in the same way as life (the word *philosophy* means "love of wisdom"). Plato records Socrates as saying, "True philosophers make dying their
profession, and . . . to them of all men, death is least alarming. . . . So if you see
one distressed at the prospect of dying, it will be proof that he is a lover not of
wisdom but of the body."[1]

Socrates' own death is one of the most famous in history: sentenced to die for
his beliefs, Socrates could have fled his beloved Athens but instead chose to
drink the poison hemlock. At his death scene, he talked about the nature of death
with his friend Cebes. In this discussion, Cebes says that it is easy not to fear
death if one is convinced of life after death, but he himself believes that the soul
"may be dispersed and destroyed on the very day that the man himself dies
[and] may be dissipated like breath or smoke, and vanish away, so that nothing is
left of it anywhere. . . . No one but a fool is entitled to face death with confidence, unless he can prove that the soul is absolutely immortal and indestruc-
tible." Socrates replies that the soul may indeed be immortal, but if it is not, then
death is like a sleep from which one never awakes. If death is sleep, there is nothing to fear in death, because no one will exist who can feel pain or miss life.

(Many people would reply to Socrates that not having a conscious self is exactly what they fear about death.)

Hemlock is a poison that acts (like nicotine) by decreasing circulation at the extremities, creating the sensation of distal numbness, and eventually stopping the heart. During Socrates' and Cebes' abstract discussion, the hemlock has been taking effect on Socrates, working up from his toes to his legs. As the discussion ends, the state poisoner finds that Socrates' thighs are numb and says that Socrates will die in minutes, when the poison reaches the heart. As his friends begin to cry, Socrates says, "Calm yourselves and try to be brave!" He dies moments later. Plato—his admiring follower, and the author of this account—writes, "Such . . . was the end of our comrade, who was, we may fairly say, of all those whom we knew in our time, the bravest and also the wisest and most upright man."

Centuries later, in ancient Rome, the emperor Marcus Aurelius and the "slave philosopher" Epictetus celebrated suicide as more courageous than an undignified life of pain. The Roman Stoics defended the *argument for the open door:* "If the room is smoky, if only moderately, I will stay; if there is too much smoke, I will go. Remember this, keep a firm hand on it, the door is always open."[2] (The argument for the open door would be revived in the twentieth century by the existentialist philosopher Jean-Paul Sartre, who emphasized that choice—even the choice of staying alive each day—is inescapable.[3]) Seneca wrote about old age: "If it begins to shake my mind, if it destroys my faculties one by one, if it leaves me not life but breath, I will depart the putrid or the tottering edifice."[4]

Jesus and Augustine

According to the New Testament, Jesus prohibited killing and advocated pacifism; but the primary focus of his message—contrary to widespread belief—was not to impart a morality to live by but rather to establish a new spiritual relationship with God. His dominant message, as presented in the gospels, is: repent of sin, ask forgiveness of God, be "born again," and be ready for the dawning kingdom of God, which will come very soon. In Matthew, he says to his disciples, "There be some standing here, which shall not die, till they see the Son of Man coming in his kingdom."[5] As Alasdair MacIntyre writes in his *Short History of Ethics:*

> The paradox of Christian ethics is precisely that it has always tried to devise a code for society as a whole from pronouncements which were addressed to individuals or small communities to separate themselves off from the rest of society. This is true both of the ethics of Jesus and of the ethics of St. Paul. Both Jesus and St. Paul preached an ethics devised for a short interim period before God finally inaugurated the Messianic kingdom and history was brought to its conclusion. We cannot, therefore, expect to find in what they say a basis for life in a continuing society.
>
>   . . . St. Paul's dislike of marriage as other than expedient ("It is better to marry than burn") is not so inhumane as unhistorically minded secularists have made it out to be, if it is understood in terms of the pointlessness of satisfying desires and creating relationships which will hinder one from obtaining the

rewards of eternal glory in the very near future. . . . [But] the crucial fact is that the Messianic kingdom did not come, and that therefore the Christian church ever since has been preaching an ethics which could not find application in a world where history had not come to an end.[6]

With regard to morality, then, certain key ideas of the organized religion now called Christianity were actually formed not by Jesus but by later thinkers. Some of these ideas were developed in the fourth century of the Christian or Common era (C.E.), especially by Augustine, who condemned suicide as "detestable and damnable wickedness."

The Bible contains no explicit prohibition of suicide (in fact, it seems to condone the suicides of Saul and Judas), and Augustine based his condemnation on the sixth commandment (Exodus 20:13), best known today as translated in the King James version: "Thou shalt not kill." However, a more accurate translation of either the Hebrew or the Greek words would be: "Thou shalt not commit wrongful killing"—and in this translation the commandment offers much less guidance, because there is a question which killings are "wrongful" and which are not. (Only a few pages after the ten commandments, at Exodus 23:23, God commands Moses to lead the Israelites in attacking neighboring tribes such as the Hittites and does not distinguish between killing enemy soldiers and killing civilians.)

Augustine distinguishes between *private killing* and killing that is carried out at the orders of a divine or divinely constituted authority. Private killing, or killing undertaken "on one's own authority," is never right;[7] but according to Augustine, not all killing is private. God may command a killing, and when this is the case, full obedience is required. Such a command may take two forms: it may come directly from God (as when God commands Abraham to sacrifice Isaac) or it may be required by a just law. With either form, the individual who does the killing does not do it on his or her own authority but is simply an "instrument," a sword in God's hand, and thus is not morally accountable.

This reasoning underlies the permissibility of capital punishment and killing in war: both are performed by people who are acting in accordance with law. The worldly Ambrose had already said that Christians could kill in war, and Augustine went even further by condoning war against heretics. Frederick Russell in *The Just War in the Middle Ages* says that through Augustine, "the New Testament doctrines of love and purity were accommodated to the savagery of the Old Testament and pacifism was defeated."[8]

Augustine apparently did not condone killing in self-defense, although present-day Catholic moral theology does allow it for persons who are not capable of attaining the "higher way" of self-sacrifice.[9]

One problem with Augustine's view is that he gives no explanation of how he knows that certain forms of killing are ordered by God and other forms are forbidden. How do we know that he is not begging the question when he assumes that the sixth commandment forbids suicide? In Protestant Christianity (which of course developed much later than Augustine), this problem becomes even more serious, since the interpretation of God's will is a more individual process.

It may seem natural to ask whether it really matters that Jesus did not talk about suicide, or that Augustine's argument presents difficulties. Does all that have anything to do with modern Christianity? Isn't it enough to know the general intent of Jesus's teachings and the present Christian view about suicide? The answer is, perhaps not.

To begin with, Jesus's original views are open to different interpretations. Also, whatever his original views were, they must differ significantly from modern Christian doctrines, which are complex and vary widely. Furthermore, in its nearly 2,000 years, Christianity itself has become fragmented into different churches, denominations, and sects; and its doctrines have been profoundly interpreted and reinterpreted. Although many Christian theologians and church leaders have made confident assertions, they have often disagreed with each other, and there seems to be no way for us to know which of them—if any—may have discovered the truth.

With regard to applied ethics, such problems increase. Quakers, Mennonites, and the Amish, for example, have always rejected Augustine's position and followed the original pacifism of the early church. How do they know that Augustine was mistaken? Today, some devout Christians support capital punishment but reject suicide. How do they know that suicide is sinful but killing a criminal is not?

Some people, of course, simply believe that "God's will" is whatever they have been taught; and some also believe that questioning "God's will" is blasphemy, an insult to God. This approach is dangerous, however—especially in medical ethics. As Paul Badham writes:

> As Church Historian, I am very conscious of how Christians of previous ages have vehemently denounced medical practices which today no Christian would dream of questioning. For centuries Christians forbade giving of medicine, the practice of surgery, the study of anatomy, or the dissection of corpses for medical research. Later the practice first of inoculation and then of vaccination faced fierce theological condemnation, as did the initial use of quinine against malaria. The introduction of anesthesia, and above all the use of chloroform in childbirth, were seen as directly challenging the divine edict that "in pain you shall bring forth children" (Genesis 3:16), and hence were violently denounced from pulpits throughout Britain and the U.S.A.[10]

It can be added that bioethics today faces problems which could never have been imagined by the people who wrote the Bible: patenting genes, defining brain death, withdrawing advanced medical technology, financing medical care, experimenting on animals. Moreover, if everything has a purpose, then presumably our ability to think critically exists for a purpose. If we believe in God, it is not blasphemy to believe that we were given minds so that we would be able to reflect on these questions and on possible answers. The philosophical approach to bioethics assumes that for those who seek God's will, reasoning and knowledge of history are compatible with their quest.

Western Philosophers

Aquinas   The thirteenth-century philosopher and theologian Thomas Aquinas held that suicide is sinful for several reasons; in fact, he considered it the most dangerous of sins because it left no time for repentance. Aquinas felt that suicide is wrong because life is a gift from God and only God can take life back (ever since, Thomists have argued vigorously for this view). He also argued that suicide hurts the community by depriving it of talented people, and that it is sinful because it deprives children of their parents. Finally, Aquinas said, suicide is unnatural, going against the instinct of self-preservation.

Montaigne, Spinoza, and Donne   Three thinkers who evidently condoned suicide were the French essayist Michel de Montaigne in the sixteenth century, and the Dutch philosopher Baruch Spinoza and the English poet John Donne in the seventeenth. Montaigne concluded his essay "To Philosophize Is to Learn How to Die" by saying, "If we have learned how to live properly and calmly, we will know how to die in the same manner."[11] Spinoza—who was Jewish—wrote, "A free man, that is to say, a man who lives according to the dictates of reason alone, is not led by the fear of death."[12] Donne wrote, "When the [terminal] disease would not reduce us, [God] sent a second and worse affliction, ignorant and torturing physicians."[13]

Hume   In the eighteenth century, the Scottish philosopher David Hume argued that suicide "is no transgression of our duty to God" and made the somewhat humbling observation, "The life of a man is of no greater importance to the universe than that of an oyster."[14] In his famous "Essay on Suicide," he disagreed with Augustine and Aquinas, who had both held that suicide violates the will of God. Especially for dying patients, Hume believed, voluntary death is not a sin: "A house which falls by its own weight, is not brought to ruin by [God's] providence."[15] Hume believed that if God had made the world through the laws of causality—the laws of physics, medicine, etc.—then disease merely expressed the natural working of such laws.

Hume also attacked the idea that suicide is blasphemous. Immanuel Kant (whose views are discussed below) said that we have a "station" in life which is assigned by God and which we must not give up; but Hume replied, "It is a kind of blasphemy to imagine that any created being can [by taking his own life] disturb the order of the world. Any suicide is insignificant to the workings of the universe and it is blasphemy to think otherwise." To Hume, it was self-indulgent to think that the world's smooth functioning required one's own continued existence.

Against Aquinas's argument that suicide harms the community, Hume argued:

> A man who retires from life does no harm to society; he only ceases to do good; which, if it is an injury, is of the lowest kind. All our obligations to do good to society seem to imply something reciprocal. I receive benefits of society, and therefore ought to promote its interests; but when I withdraw myself altogether from society, can I be bound any longer? But [even] allowing that our obligations to do good were perpetual, they have certainly some bounds; I am not obliged to do a small good to society at the expense of a great harm to myself: when then should I prolong a miserable existence, because of some frivolous advantage which the public may perhaps receive from me?

This is also a possible reply to the argument (discussed below) that suicide is wrong because it is—to use Mill's distinction—"other-regarding" and thus may harm people we know.

Kant   The German philosopher Immanuel Kant—Hume's contemporary— strongly opposed suicide. He based this conclusion on several arguments.

First, for Kant an act is right if it represents or is based on a "maxim" (rule) which can be "universalized," that is, a rule we would want everyone to act on. Kant argued that suicide cannot be universalized, because its motive is self-interest (for instance, escaping pain); for Kant, self-interest can never justify an action. Since we cannot universalize the maxim that people may commit suicide, suicide is immoral.

Second, Kant argued that suicide is immoral because people should always be treated as "ends in themselves," never as "mere means." His reasoning here is that treating oneself as an "end" entails recognizing one's own free will as an absolute (rather than a relative) value, but destroying oneself by committing suicide means destroying that freedom of will. "Man's freedom cannot subsist except on a condition which is immutable. This condition is that man not use his freedom against himself to his own destruction."[16]

Third, Kant argued that a person "who does not respect his life even in principle cannot be restrained from the most dreadful vices." In other words, if I do not respect my own life, I cannot really respect anything at all; for example, in order to respect the general principle that life is sacred, I must respect the sacredness of my own life.

Finally, as noted above, Kant held that we have a moral duty to live because our lives are not really our own possession: "Human beings are sentinels on earth and may not leave their posts until relieved by another beneficent hand. God is our owner; we are His property."

Mill   John Stuart Mill presented his principle of harm in *On Liberty* (1859), in one of the most famous passages in western political philosophy:

> [There is] one very simple principle, [that is] entitled to govern absolutely the dealings of society with the individual in the way of compulsion and control, whether the means used is physical force in the form of legal penalties, or the moral coercion of public opinion. That principle is, that the sole end for which mankind are warranted, individually or collectively, in interfering with the liberty of action of any of their number, is self-protection. That the only purpose for which power can be rightfully exercised over any member of a civilized community, against his will, is to prevent harm to others. His own good, either physical or moral, is not a sufficient warrant. . . . The only part of the conduct of any one, for which he is amenable to society, is that which concerns others. In the part which merely concerns himself, his independence is, of right, absolute. Over himself, over his own body and mind, the individual is sovereign.[17]

According to Mill's principle, with regard to our own lives and bodies, we can do whatever we want, so long as others are not harmed. Mill distinguished between *self-regarding* and *other-regarding* acts and argued that only other-regarding acts are subject to moral criticism.

Interestingly, Mill's analysis can be used both for and against suicide. On one hand, it can be can argued that taking one's own life is clearly "self-regarding"; in fact, suicide is often described as the ultimate "private" issue. On the other hand, it can also be argued that one should not commit suicide because suicide is an "other-regarding" act.

It does seem that most acts of suicide are other-regarding in some way: when someone commits suicide, parents, children, friends, colleagues, physicians, students, and others may be affected. In fact, since motives for suicide include spite and malevolence, a suicide may be *deliberately* other-regarding—it may be intended to hurt other people by making them feel guilty, sorry, or incompetent. On the basis of Mill's principle of harm, a suicide motivated by the desire to hurt someone else would obviously not be excusable. However, it is not entirely clear how a suicide that *inadvertently* harmed others would be judged. Very few of our actions are completely self-regarding (this is a general problem with Mill's principle), and it is arguable that anyone who contemplates suicide should be aware of that. As John Donne wrote, "No man is an island, entire of itself; every man is a piece of the continent, a part of the main."

The Modern Era

In the modern era—the late nineteenth century and the twentieth century—suicide has come to be seen, in many respects, as a medical, psychological, or social problem rather than a moral issue. Some nineteenth-century physicians had imputed suicide to heredity, imbalances in body chemistry, or even the shape of the head; around the turn of the century, Émile Durkheim analyzed it in terms of sociology rather than pathology. (Durkheim also broadened the definition of *suicide* to include indirect means.) Today, it is common to consider suicide as associated with emotional disorders such as clinical depression, with developmental problems, and with "social pathology"—that is, group or community problems.

However, there remain contexts in which suicide is discussed, and debated, as a matter of morality; and perhaps the most important of these contexts is illness and debilitation. A century ago, only the poor and people without families went to a hospital to die; today, more than 80 percent of Americans die in hospitals. Before the Harrison Act of 1914, Americans could legally purchase heroin and other opiates to lessen the pain of terminal illnesses such as cancer; today, this is not possible. Before World War II, most people died of sudden-onset, acute diseases such as pneumonia and cholera. Today, most people live longer and die more slowly from emphysema, diabetes, cardiomyopathy, cancer, and coronary artery disease. Because of changes like these, choosing to end one's life has become a prominent issue.

When the American feminist Charlotte Perkins Gillman killed herself in 1935, she left a note saying that she preferred "chloroform to cancer." In an essay published posthumously, she wrote: "The record of a previously noble life is precisely what makes it sheer insult to allow death in pitiful degradation. We may not wish to 'die with our boots on,' but we may well prefer to 'die with our brains on.' "[18]

THE BOUVIA CASE

The Patient: A Woman with Cerebral Palsy

In September 1983, Elizabeth Bouvia was driven by her father from Oregon to Riverside General Hospital in California, where she was diagnosed as suicidal and admitted to the psychiatric ward as a voluntary patient. She stated that she wanted "just to be left alone and not bothered by friends or family or anyone else and to ultimately starve to death." "Death is letting go of all burdens," she said. "It is being able to be free of my physical disability and mental struggle to live."[19] She claimed that she had already attempted suicide at least once.

Elizabeth Bouvia was 25 years old and was almost totally paralyzed from cerebral palsy. She had never had the use of her legs, though she had some control over her right hand (enough to operate a battery-powered wheelchair and to smoke cigarettes) and enough control of her facial muscles to chew, swallow, and speak.

Her life had never been easy. After her parents divorced when she was 5 years old, she lived with her mother only until age 10, when her mother placed her in a children's home. The following account comes from two physicians:

> For their 18th birthday, some children receive cars and gifts. When [Elizabeth Bouvia] turned 18, her father, a postal inspector, told her that he would no longer be able to care for her because of her disabilities. The chief of psychiatry at Riverside says that what she did next showed great drive and promise. She gathered her requisite amount of state aid and lived on her own in an apartment with a live-in nurse. Although she earlier had dropped out of high school, she completed her general equivalency degree and went on to graduate from San Diego State University with a bachelor's degree in 1981. She even entered a master's program at the university's School of Social Work, but left in 1982 over a disagreement about her field work placement.
>
>   . . . For eight months, she worked as a volunteer in the San Diego placement program, but she has never been employed for salary or wages.
>
>   . . . During the last year, Ms. Bouvia faced a series of devastating events. In August, 1982, she married an ex-convict, Richard Bouvia, with whom she had been corresponding by mail. Together they conceived a child, but a few months later she suffered a miscarriage.
>
>   . . . Her husband's part-time job did not provide enough income for the two to live decently, so they called her father to ask for help. He declined to aid them, Richard Bouvia said. They next went to Richard Bouvia's sister in Iowa to ask for help. That did not work out for long, and soon they ended up back in Oregon, where Richard Bouvia still could not find work. At that point, he abandoned her, stating—according to pleadings in the case—that he "could not accept her disabilities, a miscarriage, and rejection by her parents."

. . . A few days later, Elizabeth Bouvia got a ride to Riverside General and wheeled herself into the emergency room, complaining that she wanted to commit suicide.[20]

In addition to her problems with her husband and father, she had severe degenerative arthritis, which caused great pain even though she was paralyzed. As a resident of California (she had lived in Riverside as well as in Oregon), she was eligible for Medi-Cal, a substantial supplement to Medicaid for the indigent.

Elizabeth Bouvia's first attending physician, for the 4 months from September to late December, was Donald Fisher, chief of psychiatry at Riverside Hospital. Since Fisher was unwilling to let her starve herself to death as she intended, she contacted the American Civil Liberties Union (ACLU) and also telephoned a reporter. Richard Scott of Beverly Hills, who was both a physician and a lawyer, took her on as a *pro bono* (charity) case.

The Legal Battle: Refusing Sustenance

In the first hearing—before a California probate judge, John Hews—Fisher testified that he believed his patient would eventually change her mind, that he would not let her starve, and that he would force-feed her if necessary: "The court cannot order me to be a murderer nor to conspire with my staff and employees to murder Elizabeth."[21] Elizabeth Bouvia asked Judge Hews to enjoin the hospital from feeding her.

At this point, the Bouvia case "escalated into a public debate":

Disabled individuals held vigils at the hospital to convince her to change her mind. Bouvia's estranged husband hitchhiked to Riverside from Iowa, retained lawyers, and asked to be named her legal guardian. He charged the ACLU with using his wife as a "guinea pig." She filed for divorce. Columnist Jack Anderson's offer to raise funds for Bouvia's treatment was rebuffed. Richard Nixon sent a letter to Bouvia to "keep fighting." A meeting with President Reagan was discussed. Two neurosurgeons offered free surgery to help her gain the use of her arms. A convicted felon volunteered to shoot her.[22]

In December 1983, the day after the closing arguments had been completed, Judge Hews decided to allow the force-feeding. Hews acknowledged that the patient was "rational," "sincere," and "fully competent"; his decision was based on the probable effects *on others* of allowing her to starve: the "profound effect on the medical staff, nurses, and administration of the hospital," as well as the "devastating effect on other . . . physically handicapped persons."[23] Hews indicated that his decision was influenced by Advocates for the Developmentally Disabled, which had held candlelight vigils outside Riverside Hospital, fearing that if Elizabeth Bouvia died, other disabled people would choose to do the same. This attitude was also expressed by a lawyer at the Law Institute for the Disabled, who asserted that Elizabeth Bouvia symbolized a "social problem" of disabled people (they are told by society that they cannot be productive) and said, "She needs to learn to live with dignity."[24] Elizabeth Bouvia's lawyer described Hews as having accepted "the Chicken Little defense that the sky would fall if Ms. Bouvia wasn't force-fed."[25]

Habeeb Bacchus, associate chief of medicine at Riverside Hospital, became Elizabeth Bouvia's second physician (indigent patients and those in university hospitals have different physicians each month, as the "attending" physician changes). Bacchus was also worried that letting her die would depress other disabled people: "Being allowed to die when there's no need for her to die—this is a dangerous precedent. Patients might wonder, 'Am I next slated to be allowed to die?'"[26] Judge Hews allowed the force-feeding to continue under Bacchus, holding that since the patient was not terminally ill and could live for decades, "there is no other reasonable option."

The columnist Arthur Hoppe felt otherwise:

> I had the feeling that the judge, the doctor, and the hospital had found Elizabeth Bouvia guilty—guilty of not playing the game. It was as though the Easter Seal Child had looked into the camera and said being crippled was a lousy deal and certainly nothing to smile about.[27]

The law professor George Annas also disagreed bitterly with Hews:

> The judge's decision begs the question: Is there a reasonable option? In the adversary proceeding played out in California, no one seemed to search for reasonable options. The county, in fact, consistently took the most extreme position. It continually threatened to eject Ms. Bouvia from the hospital by force, and leave her out on the front sidewalk, hoping someone would pick her up and take her away. Almost from the beginning, the county and hospital made it clear that they did not care whether she lived or died but, because of their own fear of potential legal liability, would not let her die at Riverside Hospital.[28]

Elizabeth Bouvia appealed; while she did, physicians in California argued about her case. Laurens White, who later became president of the California Medical Association, said, "The most troublesome thing about this [case is that] Mrs. Bouvia's First Amendment rights may hit somebody else's medical ethics right between the eyes. . . . Refusal to take water and food is not suicide. Providing care while a patient is doing this is a tough thing, but I think she should have the right to do it. Forcing her to eat is battery."[29] With regard to Fisher's original force-feeding, White said, "He's full of it. . . . He's just completely off the wall about this." Bacchus dug in, however: "It is very simple. Physicians, if they err, should err on the side of saving life. When it comes to criminal charges, wrongful death is more of a crime than battery, so there you have it."[30]

Meanwhile, the force-feeding had of course been going on. At first, plastic tubing was inserted in the patient's mouth, but she bit through it. Thereafter, four attendants would hold her down while tubing was inserted through her nose into her stomach and a liquid diet was pumped in. Annas commented on this gruesome scene:

> I do not believe competent adults should ever be force-fed; but efforts at persuading the individual to change his or her mind, and offering oral nutrition

should continue. If a court determines, however, that invasive force-feeding is required, . . . then to [prevent] hospitals from becoming the most hideous torture chambers, some reasonable limit must be placed on this "treatment."[31]

Elizabeth Bouvia lost her first appeal to have the lower-court decision reversed, and she left Riverside Hospital on April 7, 1984. What happened at that point has been interpreted differently by different commentators.

Two physicians writing in the *Archives of Internal Medicine* gave the following description:

> The standoff continued until April 7, when Ms. Bouvia unexpectedly checked herself out of the hospital. The hospital bill for the 217 days, excluding physicians' fees, was more than $56,000, paid by Riverside County and by the State of California. Ms. Bouvia went to the Hospital del Mar at Playease de Tijuana, Mexico, known for amygdalin (Laetrile) treatments for cancer. She believed the staff would help her die. Her new physicians, however, became convinced that she wanted to live. Two weeks later, Ms. Bouvia left the hospital, hired nurses, and moved to a motel. Three days later, with friends, a reporter, and an intern from Hospital del Mar at her side, she gave up her plan to starve herself to death and took solid food. Ms. Bouvia said that she wanted treatment, including surgery to reduce muscle spasms. As of August 1985, Ms. Bouvia's location and plans were not known. Her case was complicated further by the revelation that the newspaper reporter who covered the case most closely had a contract with Ms. Bouvia for a book, television, and movie rights to her story.[32]

This account emphasizes Elizabeth Bouvia's "unexpected" departure from the hospital, the size of her hospital bill, the fact that the bill was paid for at public expense, the agreement of her Mexican physicians with her American physicians in refusing to honor her wish to die, her seemingly arbitrary decision to give up her plan of starving herself, and her contract with a reporter for book and film rights to her story. (Actually, after a decade, there has been no movie or book.)

In contrast, here is George Annas's account of the same events:

> Two years ago this column dealt with Elizabeth Bouvia's unequal and doomed struggle. . . . After losing both in the hospital and in the courtroom, Ms. Bouvia fled to Mexico on April 7, 1984, to seek her death. She was soon persuaded that Mexican physicians and nurses would be no more sympathetic to her plan than those at Riverside, and so returned to California. Because of the brutal force feeding she had endured at Riverside, she was afraid to return there. Since no other facility would admit her unless she agreed to eat, she resigned herself to eating and entered a "private care" location. There she remained, without incident, for more than a year.[33]

It is interesting to note that differences can also be found in accounts of the earlier events in the Bouvia case. For instance, this is how the inception of the case was described by Derek Humphrey of the Hemlock Society:

> Her troubles multiplied. The graduate school where she had been studying refused to readmit her, and her brother was drowned in a boating accident. Not

long after, Elizabeth had a miscarriage, and she learned her mother was dying of cancer.

. . . Determined once again to be in charge of her fate, she asked her father to take her to the county hospital in Riverside, near Los Angeles (an area where she had friends), for an examination. She checked herself into the psychiatric ward and told physicians she wanted to die by starvation. Elizabeth specifically asked that, until she died, she be looked after normally and given painkillers when her arthritis was troublesome.[34]

The disability advocate Paul Longmore, who argues that the Bouvia case reflects rank prejudice against the disabled, describes the early phases as follows:

The very agencies supposedly designed to enable severely physically handicapped adults like her to achieve independence . . . become yet another massive hurdle they must surmount, an enemy they must repeatedly battle but can never finally defeat.

. . . [When she tried to go on internship,] the SDSU [San Diego State University] School of Social Work refused to back her up. They wanted to place her at a center where she would only work with disabled people. She refused. Reportedly, one of her employers told her she was unemployable, and that, if they had known just how disabled she was, they would never have admitted her to the program. . . .

The attorneys brought in three psychiatric professionals to provide an independent evaluation. None of them had any experience or expertise in dealing with persons with disabilities. In fact, Elizabeth Bouvia had never been examined by any psychiatric or medical professional qualified to understand her life experience. . . . Her examiners prejudicially concluded that because of her *physical* condition she would never be able to achieve her life goals, that her [physical] disability was the reason she wanted to die, and that her decision for death was reasonable. . . . [Judge Hews] too declared that Ms. Bouvia's physical disability was the sole reason she wished to die.[35]

These accounts all appeared in scholarly journals, which would presumably imply objectivity. However, the two physicians seem to be portraying Elizabeth Bouvia as irresponsible; Annas and Humphrey seem to portray her as a helpless heroine fighting a cold bureaucracy; and Longmore apparently sees her as a victim of a prejudiced system and of misguided, do-gooder lawyers. Note also that the physicians refer to her as "Bouvia," Humphrey calls her "Elizabeth," and Longmore uses "Elizabeth Bouvia" or "Ms. Bouvia." The physicians say that "she got a ride" to Riverside, as if she had hitchhiked to some arbitrary location; Humphrey, by contrast, says that her father took her to a place "where she had friends." Longmore emphasizes her desire to be independent; Humphrey emphasizes her physical pain and social trauma. Longmore suggests that society is prejudiced against disabled people and thus that Elizabeth Bouvia's disability is not so much her problem as society's problem. Humphrey writes from a point of view "inside" Elizabeth Bouvia; the physicians write from the viewpoint of hospital staff members who must accept patients presenting "management problems."

On September 22, 1985, Elizabeth Bouvia entered Los Angeles County–USC Medical Center (the hospital with the largest number of beds in the United

States), where a morphine pump was installed to control the pain caused by her worsening arthritis. At this public hospital, her declaration that she would eat and live was evidently accepted; she was not force-fed; and she was not required to socialize with other patients.

After 2 months, however, she was transferred to nearby High Desert Hospital, another public hospital. Although apparently she also ate voluntarily at High Desert, her physicians there decided that she wasn't eating enough and began force-feeding her. Their rationale was that "since she is occupying our space, she must accede to the same care which we afford every other patient admitted here, care designed to improve and not detract from chances of recovery and rehabili tation."[36] Several critics thought it odd to say that a patient who "occupies" hospital "space" must do what the hospital dictates. (That would make an interesting slogan for a hospital's advertising.)

The question whether or not the patient was eating "enough" is of some importance, because she soon petitioned the courts again to have the forced feeding stopped. At this time, she weighed only 70 pounds. A consultant on nutrition had noted on her chart that a weight of 75 or 85 pounds "might be desirable," and her physicians wanted to achieve an ideal weight of 104 to 114 pounds. Keep in mind that because of her paralysis, her muscle mass was slight, and so her ideal body weight would be much lower than normal for a person of her height (5 feet).

At the new hearing, a new judge—Judge Warren Deering— interpreted her weight as evidence of starvation and as "not motivated by a bona fide right to privacy but by a desire to terminate her life."[37] Deering held that the right to privacy (defined as the "right to be left alone") did not apply to suicide by starvation, and that any treatment necessary to preserve life could be forced on her. "Saving her life is paramount," he said.

Elizabeth Bouvia appealed again, and the California Court of Appeal found in her favor. The justices said that she could refuse life-sustaining medical treatment: "A desire to terminate one's life is probably the ultimate exercise of one's right to privacy."[38] Moreover, they found "no substantive evidence to support the [lower] court's decision." Judge Deering (like Judge Hews) had taken into account the fact that this patient could live for decades more, but the appeals court completely dismissed this factor: "This trial court mistakenly attached undue importance to the amount of time possibly available to [Elizabeth Bouvia], and failed to give equal weight and consideration for the quality of that life; an equal, if not more significant, consideration." The appeals court concluded:

> This matter [Deering's decision against Bouvia] constitutes a perfect paradigm of the axiom: "Justice delayed is justice denied." Her mental and emotional feelings are equally entitled to respect. She has been subjected to the forced intrusion of an artificial mechanism into her body against her will. She has a right to refuse the increased dehumanizing aspect of her condition. . . . The right to refuse medical treatment is basic and fundamental. It is recognized as part of the right of privacy protected by both the state and federal constitutions. Its exercise requires no one's approval. It is not merely one vote subject to being overridden by medical opinion.
>
>   . . . [A precedent has been established that when] a doctor performs treatment in the absence of informed consent, there is an actionable battery. The obvi-

ous corollary to this principle is that a competent adult patient has the legal right to refuse medical treatment. [Moreover,] if the right of the patient to self-determination as to his own medical treatment is to have any meaning at all, it must be paramount to the interests of the patient's hospital and doctors. . . . The right of a competent adult patient to refuse medical treatment is a constitutionally guaranteed right which must not be abridged.

. . . In Elizabeth Bouvia's view, the quality of her life has been diminished to the point of hopelessness, uselessness, unenjoyability, and frustration. She, as the patient, lying helplessly in bed, unable to care for herself, may consider her existence meaningless. She is not to be faulted for so concluding. . . . As in all matters, lines must be drawn at some point, somewhere, but that decision must ultimately belong to the one whose life is the issue.

Note especially the statement that *the right of a competent adult patient to refuse medical treatment is a constitutionally guaranteed right which must not be abridged.* With regard to force-feeding, the wording of the decision was very strong:

We do not believe it is the policy of this State that all and every life must be preserved against the will of the sufferer. It is incongruous, if not monstrous, for medical practitioners to assert their right to preserve a life that someone else must live, or more accurately, endure, for "15 or 20 years." We cannot conceive it to be the policy of this State to inflict such an ordeal upon anyone.

Moreover, the appeals court added that "no criminal or civil liability attaches to honoring a competent, informed patient's refusal for medical service."

If nothing else, Elizabeth Bouvia—frail, small, alone, and barely able to move—had won a remarkable victory for other patients. She had wrested from the appeals court the first clear statement (it preceded the *Cruzan* decision by 5 years) that competent, adult patients have a constitutional right to refuse medical treatment in order to die.

The Aftermath

After her victory in court, Elizabeth Bouvia did not kill herself. Some caring people had come forward and offered to help her die. These new friends seem to have showed her that life could be worth living, and gradually she came to change her mind.

THE McAFEE CASE

The Patient: A Quadriplegic Man

Larry McAfee was 29 years old when he became almost completely paralyzed (a C-2 quadriplegic) in a motorcycle accident on May 5, 1985. He had been an adult student at Georgia State University in Atlanta, studying mechanical engineering, and an avid outdoorsman; on weekends, he had often motorcycled with other students in the mountains northwest of Atlanta. His accident occurred while he was riding on a dirt road at less than 10 miles per hour: he hit a curve, fell over his motorcycle, snapped his head, and crushed his two top vertebrae on the bottom of his helmet.

He was left with the use of only his eyes, mouth, and head. He could not clear his throat and sometimes had a sensation of choking. He could not breathe on his own (the muscles that control breathing were also paralyzed) and therefore needed a ventilator. He had no control over his bladder or bowels. He could feel no physical pleasure from any sexual activity, although he still experienced sexual desire. He had never married; according to statistics, single people who suffer spinal-cord injuries like his seldom marry (and those who are married at the time of their injury are almost always divorced later).[39]

The Case: Quality of Care and the Right to Die

In the mass media, the case of Larry McAfee was usually presented as a right-to-die issue involving his own perception of his "quality of life." It should be noted, however, that this perception included his assessment of the quality of his medical care and that the case also involved the rationing of medical care—or, more precisely, what happens when care is *not* rationed.

McAfee had a $1 million health insurance policy, but he remained for over 1 year at the expensive Shepherd Spinal Center in Atlanta, where the average stay for C-1 to C-4 patients was 19 weeks; and later, at his apartment in Atlanta, he insisted on nurses who were 3 times more expensive than home health aides. After 16 months at home, he had used up his insurance benefits.[40] Some members of his family offered to take care of him, but he said that he did not want to be a financial or physical burden to them.

At this point, he was eligible for Medicaid, the fund in each state that pays for medical care for the indigent. According to Aaron Johnson, commissioner of Georgia's Medicaid office, McAfee wanted Georgia to pay for care for him in his apartment and refused to go to a state-controlled nursing home where his care would have been much less expensive.[41] In other words, he wanted to be cared for at pubic expense but according to his own wishes.

Apparently, Larry McAfee was then "dumped" in the Aristocrat Berea nursing home outside Cleveland, Ohio—a facility that provided care for respirator-dependent C-1 patients—with the state of Georgia paying. Officials at Aristocrat Berea said that they had acted in good faith, accepting him on a temporary, short-term basis because they had understood that no bed was available for him in Georgia. After 2 years, when it became clear to them that this had been a "dump," they hustled him onto a plane bound for Georgia, whisked him to the emergency room (ER) at Grady Memorial Hospital in Atlanta (by federal law, patients cannot be denied admission to an ER), and went back to Ohio.

According to the administrator of Aristocrat Berea, Larry McAfee wouldn't make appointments for vocational rehabilitation and was very unhappy over conditions that no other patients complained about: "Larry was very demanding, wanted things precisely the way he wanted them. . . . I had nurses toward the end who just couldn't work with him anymore because they were just extremely,

extremely frustrated."[42] He also noted that McAfee's family and friends were all in Georgia.

McAfee, however, claimed that he had been housed with demented, senile, and brain-damaged patients who, because of tight funds, were being "warehoused"—with only 1 or 2 staff members assigned to supervise as many as 30 to 40 patients. The easiest way to "warehouse" such patients is to keep them heavily sedated. McAfee said that he experienced intense loneliness and received inadequate personal care. "You're just a sack of potatoes," he said.[43]

After he was returned to Atlanta in January 1989, Larry McAfee spent several miserable months in the intensive care unit (ICU) of Grady Memorial Hospital. Though he hated Grady Memorial, no other facility in Georgia would take him. During the summer of 1989, however, officials at Grady Memorial found that the patient—who was then 33 years old—would be accepted by Briarcliff Nursing Home in a suburb of Birmingham, Alabama, and he was voluntarily transferred to Birmingham. (Briarcliff was one of the few nursing homes in the country that accepted ventilator-dependent patients.)

Russ Fine, a disability advocate and director of the Injury Control Research Center at the University of Alabama at Birmingham (UAB), became aware of the case when Larry McAfee called a weekly radio talk show hosted by Fine and his wife, Dee. According to Fine, Larry McAfee's treatment on Medicaid in Ohio, Georgia, and Alabama represents "everything that's wrong about the system that serves [severely] disabled people."[44] When he first met Larry McAfee, Fine was appalled to find him lying in bed staring at the ceiling. The patient had no voice-activated telephone and no television. All he could do was stare "at whatever happened to be in front of his face. From a quality of life standpoint, it was a devastating commentary on a society with a very advanced health-care system."[45] A reporter once arrived to find that McAfee's urinary catheter was not connected to a container and urine was spilling over the floor. Fine says, "These facilities were not equipped to take care of a patient such as Larry, with labor-intensive health-care requirements."[46]

That summer—6 years after a federal appellate court had found in favor of Elizabeth Bouvia—Larry McAfee decided to file suit in court for the right to die. He did not want his ventilator disconnected, since it had once been dislodged accidentally and he had experienced a terrifying sensation of suffocation (in fact, he also had a sense of suffocating at some other times). Instead, he designed a switch, to be connected to his IV line, that would enable him to give himself lethal drugs by blowing in certain ways.

On September 7, 1989, after a heart-wrenching 45-minute hearing in Fulton County Superior Court, Judge Edward Johnson found in Larry McAfee's favor. Johnson ruled that McAfee's physicians could prescribe the drugs that McAfee would then himself switch on to kill himself; McAfee could also have his ventilator disconnected, if he wished. Notably, Johnson wrote that McAfee had "a right to be free from pain at the time the ventilator is disconnected."[47] During the hearing, all the parties had assumed that a decision for McAfee would result in his death within a few days; however, the state of Georgia appealed. On direct appeal, the Georgia Supreme Court affirmed Johnson's decision.

The Aftermath

Larry McAfee did not use his switch device to kill himself. Russ Fine, through his intervention and discussions with McAfee, had convinced McAfee that life could be worth living. However, although McAfee may have decided to live, his problems of care and support were not over. (Financial aspects of these problems are discussed further later in this chapter, in the section on allocation of resources.)

During the summer of 1989, while his assisted-suicide suit was pending in court, Larry McAfee had qualified for additional benefits under a special disability extension of Medicare, but these payments were to end in April 1990. Anticipating that, Fine persuaded officials of Birmingham's United Cerebral Palsy (UCP) to allow him to live temporarily in a nine-person group home run by UCP for the severely disabled; this home had a supported-employment program. Larry McAFee's stay in the UCP home began in April 1990 but was interrupted during May and June, when he was in a private hospital recuperating from surgery to remove a kidney stone. By July 1990, he had returned to the UCP home; but UCP officials had not received the funding they had hoped for and therefore announced that he would have to leave their facility soon. Officials at Grady Memorial Hospital in Atlanta, where he had run up a bill of $175,000, had no intention of taking him back. Under intense pressure from the media, officials in Georgia arranged for him to be transferred—in early July of 1990—to the Medical College of Georgia at Augusta, where he was promised most of what he wanted. The Medical College created an independent-living facility for Larry McAfee and five other disabled patients.

ETHICAL ISSUES

The Concept of Assisted Suicide

Definitions One question raised by the cases of Elizabeth Bouvia and Larry McAfee is what to call the intended action: suicide, rational suicide, assisted suicide, euthanasia, voluntary death, self-deliverance, or something else. To help sort out this semantic welter, two points can be made.

First, *euthanasia* usually means the killing of one person by another (or others) for allegedly merciful reasons. The two cases in this chapter cannot be said to involve euthanasia, then, since in each case the death would be initiated by the person herself or himself. Opponents of suicide sometimes lump it together with euthanasia, but that is a semantic sleight-of-hand designed to win an argument when more rational means have failed.

Second, it is inaccurate to say that a *terminally ill* patient who forgoes medical treatment thereby "commits suicide." It is true that the definition of *suicide* is now often broadened to include indirect ways of bringing about one's own death.[48] Nevertheless, it is still important to maintain the distinction between: (1) cases where an underlying disease is incrementally leading to death, and by choosing not to do everything possible, the patient accepts death at an earlier date; and (2) cases where a competent adult without a terminal illness causes his or her own death. Case 2 is appropriately called *suicide*. (Note also that in case 2 the reason or reasons for suicide will almost invariably be considered irrational by some other person, some other people, or most other people.) One reason to maintain the distinction between forgoing treatment in terminal illness and committing suicide is that if a death is classified as a suicide, many life insurance companies refuse to pay benefits. Another reason is that in many states it is illegal to assist in a suicide. In three important cases—*Saikewicz, Conroy,* and *Colyer*—state supreme courts have decided that withdrawal of treatment in terminal illness is not suicide.[49]

Actually, the issue in the Bouvia and McAfee cases is probably best described as *assisted suicide.* Neither Elizabeth Bouvia nor Larry McAfee had a terminal disease (each could have lived another 20 or 30 years): hence the term *suicide.* They could not easily kill themselves, and so they needed help from others, especially medical staff members: hence the term *assisted.*

Arguments for and against assisted suicide   Defining assisted suicide does not necessarily make it any less controversial. In both of the cases in this chapter, the physicians resisted any role for themselves in assisting suicide, and many people supported them.

Opponents of assisted suicide have stressed that neither Elizabeth Bouvia nor Larry McAfee had a terminal illness (thus neither of them would meet one crucial condition of Hume's argument, a "house falling under its own weight") and that both of them were young. This meant that they might place some hope in medical progress, if they changed their minds and decided to live. It was also argued that neither of them really needed to die in a medical institution—that the duty of physicians and hospitals to comfort the sick and dying does not extend to disabled people who are neither sick nor dying, and that such disabled people cannot claim a "right" to have physicians and nurses help them kill themselves. These critics also point to the role of medicine as a bulwark against death, not a catalyst for dying.

In these two cases, also, opponents of assisted suicide argued that Elizabeth Bouvia and Larry McAfee may not really have wanted to die. Since they did not simply commit suicide quietly but instead made dramatic demands on public institutions, it was suggested, they may have been "acting out" and pleading for attention. In such a situation, medicine cannot just accede to the expressed wish of the patient, because it may not represent the patient's real wishes. It would not seem sensible, much less compassionate, to assist in the suicide of every distraught or depressed patient who comes to an ER and announces a desire to die.

There are also religious arguments against assisted suicide, of course. The Roman Catholic church, for example, opposes "rational suicide"; in 1990, the Catholic theologian Kevin O'Rourke argued that it is based on an illusion—the idea that human beings are totally in control of their lives and destinies.[50] O'Rourke believes that God has a plan for each person, and that this plan never includes suicide.

Advocates for *communitarian ethics* also oppose assisted suicide: they argue that severely disabled people should not simply be allowed to die; rather, society must provide humane institutions where these people can be loved. With regard to the community, opponents of assisted suicide can also argue that how society treats disabled people—whether its attitude is prejudiced or unbiased, what resources it is willing to expend, how it intends to cover the costs, and so on—is not an issue that medicine can solve or should be expected to solve.

On the other side, supporters of assisted suicide in cases like those of Elizabeth Bouvia and Larry McAfee argue that providing such assistance may, appropriately, be the final part of a continuum of good medical care. Normally, leaving a patient untreated—*patient abandonment*—is considered unethical and may even be a crime; and cutting short the "continuum" of care may be seen as a form of abandonment. The fact that a patient does not have a terminal disease is irrelevant, according to this argument. The real issue is whether or not the patient has an acceptable quality of life, and that is an evaluative judgment which can be made only by patients themselves. If physicians or others in effect make this evaluation by refusing to assist in suicide, that may be the worst kind of medical paternalism.

A note on unassisted suicide   It is sometimes asked why patients such as Elizabeth Bouvia and Larry McAfee don't simply go off somewhere and kill themselves. One answer is that it's not easy to commit suicide when you want to die painlessly and aesthetically, and when you need to be sure that you accomplish what you intend. When you are already sick or disabled, suicide becomes even more difficult.

For example, consider the attempted suicide of Robert McFarlane, a national security advisor during the administration of Ronald Reagan, at the time of the Iran-Contra hearings. McFarlane took somewhere between thirty and forty 5- to 10-milligram (mg) tablets of Valium, but he didn't die, and some people inferred that therefore he didn't really want to kill himself. An equally plausible explanation is that he didn't really know how to kill himself; most people don't. In 1985, a physician, Robert Rosier, didn't even know how much morphine to give his terminally ill wife to bring about her death—and if a physician doesn't know, what hope is there for the rest of us?[51]

It is common to infer ambivalent motives whenever a suicide is botched, but that may be mistaken. Emergency room physicians can confirm that most people don't know how to kill themselves. ER medicine is full of stories of bizarre survivals (often related with gallows humor).[52] The hand holding the gun wobbles a fraction of an inch and leaves the would-be suicide a "drooling zombie." "Jumpers" survive the fall from the Golden Gate Bridge because the drugs they have taken to give themselves courage also relax their muscles and thus soften the impact. One jumper—a woman—hits a parked car and not only does not die but does not even lose consciousness. The skirt of an elderly woman jumper catches on a balcony halfway down a skyscraper; she tries to fight off the fireman who reaches her on a ladder; he gets a medal and she gets a straitjacket.

Although suicide attempts by teenagers increased 300 percent between 1967 and 1982, only 1 in 50 attempts succeeded.[53] Elderly people are apparently more knowledgeable, though even they succeed only 1 in 3 times; Miami Beach, a popular retirement city, leads the United States in successful suicides. Women attempt suicide more than men but are less often successful; this may be because men tend to use violent means such as guns whereas women tend to use drugs.

Available methods for committing suicide present a grim picture. To begin with, Valium and other benzodiazapines—which figure prominently in many attempted suicides—rarely cause death when used alone because they are usually taken in insufficient quantities. Instead, the would-be suicide awakes with half his or her IQ.

People who try some other popular methods are just as likely to end up in the ER as dead. Carbon monoxide (CO) poisoning may not work because the car can stall or run out of gas; or the CO may not be concentrated enough to produce death, so that the person ends up in a coma. Slitting the wrists in a warm tub is not easy: the cuts are painful and must be made very deep and in the right place. Nor is this method certain: in the time between unconsciousness and death, the arm may move out of the water and the blood may coagulate. One ER physician observes, "Most slashers just get a trophy: a claw hand."

Some people are discovered in the act of committing suicide, especially those who choose a method that takes several hours. They may then wake up in an ER with a nasogastric tube down the throat, into which syrup of ipecac is pumped to induce vomiting; this is followed by injections of saline solution; next comes gastric lavage—alternate flooding and suctioning out of the stomach—and then granulated charcoal is pumped in to absorb the remaining toxins. These procedures are painful, messy, and unpleasant for patients who return to consciousness while they are in progress.

People may be reluctant to use certain methods if they want to spare the feelings of others, or if they want to be found in a reasonably dignified state after death. For instance, a drug overdose not only decreases respiration but also relaxes bowel and bladder control. Even messier is jumping off a building or shooting oneself in the head. Hanging is not foolproof: it is difficult to do correctly because the neck may not break and the victim, kicking in agony as he or she partially asphyxiates, may not die. If it succeeds, it also relaxes bowel and bladder control; and a man who dies by hanging himself will be found with an erect penis.

Rationality and Competence

One ethical issue in these cases was made famous by a play called *Whose Life Is It, Anyway?* which was later made into a movie (Elizabeth Bouvia had evidently seen the film version). Its hero, Ken Harrison, like Larry McAfee, is a quadriplegic who wants to die. Harrison offers rational arguments for suicide, but a psychiatrist reasons that those arguments are undercut by Harrison's "obvious intelligence." In other words, because Harrison is intelligent and sane enough to formulate a convincing case for suicide, he is too intelligent and sane to really want to die. Or, to put it another way, only if he were irrational would Harrison really decide to die; he could convince the psychiatrist of his rationality only by deciding to live.

In Elizabeth Bouvia's case the psychiatrist Nancy Mullen testified along similar lines: Mullen held that since the patient was seeking suicide, she must be incompetent to make medical decisions about her life and prospects; Mullen said that she herself could conceive of no situation where a person could make a "competent" decision to take his or her own life.[54] Carol Gill, a clinical assistant professor of occupational therapy (who herself used a wheelchair), argued similarly: she criticized ACLU for accepting the decision of "a handful of medical experts" that Elizabeth Bouvia was competent when she decided to starve herself.[55] It should be noted that Gill had not examined Elizabeth Bouvia before concluding that the patient was incompetent.

Mullen, Gill, and the psychiatrist in *Whose Life Is It, Anyway?* were all making the logical error called *begging the question*. A question is "begged" when the answer is assumed to be true rather than proved. In these cases, the "question" or point is whether a decision to die rather than lead an unsatisfactory life is "irrational": that is, whether such a decision indicates mental illness, misinformation, faulty reasoning, or the like. Simply assuming that a decision to die is *necessarily* or *always* irrational—and hence incompetent—begs that question.

This is not to say, of course, that a decision to die is necessarily or always rational. Elizabeth Bouvia, for example, might in fact have been suffering from clinical depression, and psychological tests might have shown this. But Mullen and Gill did not base their arguments on this kind of consideration. They were not Elizabeth's Bouvia's therapists and were not among the professionals who were treating her. Mullen and Gill reacted to the content of the decision itself rather than to any psychological factors which they knew of firsthand and which might have influenced that decision. Actually, three psychiatric professionals who tested Elizabeth Bouvia did find her competent.[56]

With regard to the legal aspects of competence, in the United States a patient must be considered mentally competent until proven otherwise in a legal hearing, and no patient can be held in a hospital against his or her will without having been proven legally incompetent. (Chapter 14 discusses criteria for involuntary psychiatric commitment.) Typically, in a large urban hospital a lower-court judge will spend 1 day every 1 or 2 weeks ruling in competency hearings. In such hearings, two attending psychiatrists or residents usually testify for commitment; indigent patients have court-appointed lawyers.

In practice, hospitals sometimes break the law regarding competence. One well-known case was that of Donald ("Dax") Cowart in Texas in 1973. Cowart, a young bachelor, was burned over 67 percent of his body in a propane-gas explosion. As a former pilot, Dax understood burns and requested a gun to shoot himself when emergency medical technicians arrived at the scene of the explosion. His request was denied, and for 232 days he underwent excruciatingly painful treatments, against his will, in Parkland Memorial Hospital in Dallas. Although he was never declared incompetent, his physicians ignored his refusal to be treated; instead, they honored the wishes of his very religious mother and forced treatment on him. He was left blind, horribly disfigured, and with only partial use of his fingers.[57]

Autonomy

As we have seen, John Stuart Mill (in *On Liberty*) applied his principle of harm to define or delimit private or "self-regarding" actions. Mill held that so far as such actions are concerned, the individual should be *autonomous*; that the source of values is individual experiences and choices (in other words, values are not imposed by the state); and that the state should have no power to force an individual to act for the public good or in even in his or her own best interest. In essence, Mill saw individual rights as conditions limiting what government may do to citizens.

During the early development of bioethics, this concept of individual autonomy became very important in the "patient rights" movement. According to the principle of autonomy, as applied to the right to die, a person who has not been proved incompetent has the right to make decisions about when to end his or her own life. Clearly, applying the principle of autonomy might lead to bad results in some specific cases; its general application, however, may lead to the "greatest good for the greatest number" of patients who want to die. If the principle is not extended to such patients, they can be "forced to live" inside a hospital; and it can be argued that there is little difference between this result and involuntary commitment of competent people to psychiatric wards—a practice for which psychiatrists in the former Soviet Union were widely condemned by their counterparts in the free world.

Applying the principle of autonomy in Elizabeth Bouvia's case, for instance, would suggest that the key question was not whether she was demonstrably "competent" or "incompetent." Instead, the question would be simply whether there was any room for doubt about her incompetence; if there was room for doubt, she would have a right to autonomy and thus she herself rather than anyone else could control the decision to die.

Not everyone, however, would agree that the principle of autonomy resolves a case like Elizabeth Bouvia's. For one thing, some observers considered her unstable—even if there was room for doubt that she was actually "incompetent"—and felt that assisted suicide in her case would therefore set a dangerous precedent. These critics saw something odd in her case: she seemed to want to kill herself only inside a hospital and did not take the opportunity to die outside, in private; and this seemed to indicate that after all there might be some psychiatric problem.

Another criticism related to the concept of autonomy is whether or not it can be genuinely applicable to severely disabled people in American society. We turn next to this issue.

Social Prejudice and Physical Disabilities

The disability advocate Paul Longmore, whose commentary on Elizabeth Bouvia's case was quoted earlier and who is himself a ventilator-dependent quadriplegic, opposes voluntary death among the severely disabled. Longmore believes that the Bouvia case shows how a prejudiced system destroys the independence of disabled people, leaving them in a position where their so-called "autonomous" decisions to die are actually bogus.

By creating intolerable conditions for disabled people, Longmore holds, American society paints them into a corner. Such patients have only one decision left that can be consistent with their former autonomous selves: they can decide to die. Every other decision is made for them by others who keep them passive and dependent. In Longmore's words:

Given the lumping together of people with disabilities with those who are terminally ill, the blurring of voluntary assisted suicide and forced "mercy" killing,
and the oppressive conditions of social devaluation and isolation, blocked opportunities, economic deprivation, and enforced social powerlessness, talk of their
"rational" or "voluntary" suicide is simply Orwellian newspeak. The advocates
of assisted suicide assume a nonexistent autonomy. They offer an illusory self-
determination.[58]

Longmore argues that in a different kind of society or in a different kind of hospital system—where disabled people were given independence and their autonomy was maximized—disabled people would be less likely to choose to die, and
younger disabled people particularly would not make such a choice.

Some critics of autonomy see Elizabeth Bouvia's case as a failure on the part
of society: a lack of caring, a situation in which a patient "slipped through the
cracks" of an impersonal system. These critics see Elizabeth Bouvia as a tragic
figure not primarily because of her physical situation but rather because of her
social situation: even as a hospitalized patient, she remained alone, and it was
her aloneness that underlay her fierce assertion of her right to tear herself away
from life.

On this analysis, to see Elizabeth Bouvia as simply a "right to die" case is to
miss the heart of a much bigger issue. What made Elizabeth Bouvia want to die
was the cumulative effect of centuries of prejudice against people who are physically disabled—prejudice that is virulently expressed in modern American society, which idealizes youth, beauty, sex, athleticism, fitness, and wealth. These are
not the only values that make life worthwhile, but our culture lacks any strong
expression of many other values, such as caring for others, erudition, creativity,
and community.

Longmore argues in this way, and he also attacks several films that seem to
covertly encourage severely disabled people to kill themselves as a highly rational response to their low quality of life. He cites *Annie Hall, Elephant Man,* and
especially *Whose Life Is It, Anyway?* and claims that *Whose Life Is It, Anyway?*
depressed Elizabeth Bouvia.

Specifically, Longmore maintains that Elizabeth Bouvia's problems resulted
in part because she did not receive the maximum payments she was entitled to;
he says that her county is notorious for its stinginess in benefits to disabled people. Furthermore, he says, the hospital where she was supposed to do her internship refused to comply with laws designed to ensure disability rights. He also
believes that Elizabeth Bouvia was strongly discouraged from seeking work or
marrying because benefits are reduced when a disabled person takes a job or
marries. California's In-Home Supportive Services program allowed Elizabeth
Bouvia to manage her own life at home while she was single; when she married,
however, she became ineligible for the program: her husband was now expected
to care for her. Given these circumstances, Longmore thinks it is no wonder that
Bouvia was later divorced or that she became discouraged about completing her
training—for even in the unlikely event that she was able to overcome discrimination and find a job, she would then lose the benefits that allowed her to live on
her own at home. Longmore concludes:

This is a woman who aimed at something more significant than mere self-sufficiency. She struggled to attain self-determination, but she was repeatedly thwarted in her efforts by discriminatory actions on the part of the government, her teachers, her employers, her parents, and her society. Contrary to the highly prejudiced view of the appeals court, what makes life with a major physical disability ignominious, embarrassing, humiliating, and dehumanizing is not the need for extensive physical assistance, but the dehumanizing social contempt toward those who require such aid.

The case of Larry McAfee also raises the issue of social prejudice, although in his case that issue may have been somewhat clouded by his own personality. Was he a demanding, spoiled patient as some people described him, or was he a heroic figure who would rather die than live in the institutional squalor of publicly funded nursing homes?

Russ Fine, the disability advocate who intervened in the McAfee case, clearly feels that Larry McAfee's desire to die was mainly a result of severely inadequate physical and psychological care. Public officials were trying to control costs by requiring patients like Larry McAfee to live in the most cost-effective facilities, but McAfee said that if he couldn't get his own apartment he would rather die. According to Fine, McAfee "was very vocal about inferior nursing care, which was the rule, not the exception, in these marginal health-care facilities that had accepted these contracts."[59] Once, Fine had brought McAfee a Thanksgiving dinner and the two were watching a televised football game while waiting for McAfee's family to arrive. Fine was drowsing in an armchair when he suddenly realized that McAfee had stopped breathing. By the time the family arrived, nurses and aides were swarming over McAfee, trying to get him breathing. When he finally revived, Fine saw tears streaming out of his eyes. "He didn't really want to die," Fine concluded. "He was just terrified."[60]

It should be noted that Larry McAfee, like Elizabeth Bouvia, wanted to work, but this would have made him ineligible for most publicly funded assistance in housing or medical care.

Cases such as Bouvia's and McAfee's suggest that society often does give severely disabled people only three limited, grim choices: to become a burden on their families or friends, to live miserably in a large public institution, or to kill themselves. However, these three are not by any means the only possible options, and it can certainly be argued that society should explore and offer more and better choices.

For instance, small independent-living facilities known as *group homes* can be established; in such a facility (which is probably one of the best formats), a few home health aides can help disabled residents lead productive lives. Both Elizabeth Bouvia and Larry McAfee evidently would have accepted such an arrangement all along, and it would appear a great deal cheaper than the care they did receive.

Not many group homes exist, however, and one of the main reasons is a reaction called NIMBY—"not in my back yard"—that is, neighborhood resistance to such homes. In the case of group homes for the disabled, such resistance seems to be based significantly on prejudice. Neighborhoods sometimes argue that group homes will create dangerous situations and lower property values, but this does not seem very convincing with regard to homes for people like Elizabeth Bouvia and Larry McAfee. Prejudice should surely not be allowed to prevent communities from giving their severely disabled members better choices than imprisonment in hospitals or death.

Allocating Scarce Medical Resources and the Rule of Rescue

The McAfee case involved the issue of funding, and therefore allocation, of medical resources. In this regard, the case illustrated several quirks in our medical system.

As we have seen, Larry McAfee's own private insurance benefits ran out quite soon; thereafter, his care was financed in various ways, principally by Medicaid. It should be noted that levels of Medicaid support are determined by the states and that the level in any state can be too low to cover expenses of nursing-home care. In fact, only a very small number of nursing homes in the United States will admit ventilator-dependent patients like Larry McAfee, and virtually none will take ventilator-dependent Medicaid patients, since reimbursement for these Medicaid patients is so limited. It should also be noted that, according to federal regulations, Medicaid cannot be used for group homes or independent apartments; moreover, with regard to support for communal living for the disabled, Georgia is seen by many disability advocates as one of the least generous states. Medicaid regulations disallowing group and independent living arrangements have drawn considerable opposition: critics such as Paul Longmore have charged that Medicaid works to warehouse disabled people rather than to let them live independently and possibly work.

Social security was another, though modest, source of funding for Larry McAfee's care. Social security (which comprises more than one program) includes federally financed medical care for Americans over 65 (Medicare), and a welfare program for poor retirees and disabled young people—Supplemental Security Income (SSI). In 1992, SSI payments averaged $362 a month and were paid to 5.4 million elderly, disabled, or blind Americans.[61] Larry McAfee's SSI benefits increased his total reimbursement.

Still another source of payments, for a time, was a special extension of the Medicare disability program. This, however, had been repealed by Congress in November 1989 (in order to save money) and expired on April 10, 1990. Before their expiration, these benefits had been used for agency nurses (costing $3,000 a week) while Larry McAfee was in the Briarcliff Nursing Home.

United Cerebral Palsy (UCP) also provided some funding. As has been described above, UCP in Birmingham was persuaded by the disability advocate Russ Fine to admit Larry McAfee to a UCP group home there on a temporary basis. When he entered this group home, UCP initially paid for his agency nurses, but this was in the expectation that federal funding would soon be provided instead.

In Larry McAfee's case, disability advocates argued that he could live more cheaply as well as far more satisfactorily and with far better care in an independent-living facility; and he himself argued that Medicaid should at least help defray the cost of an independent-living facility by contributing the same amount that the Georgia Medicaid program would pay him for a nursing home. Accordingly, officials at UCP and some rehabilitation centers orchestrated an intense national campaign to make an exception for Larry McAfee. Such an exception would take the form of a presidential waiver for McAfee: that is, his care would be federally funded rather than paid for by the state Medicaid program. When Larry McAfee entered the nine-person UCP home on April 11, 1990, it was hoped that the president—then George Bush—would issue such a waiver for him; it was also hoped that the waiver would apply to care he would subsequently receive in Georgia if he returned there.

In mid-May, with the matter of the waiver still unsettled, Larry McAfee entered a hospital in Birmingham for removal of a large kidney stone. Since Medicaid pays for hospital care of acute conditions, this postponed for a while the problem of long-term funding, and he remained in the hospital for a month (an unusually long stay, clearly based on financial rather than medical considerations).

From June 15 to about July 10, Larry McAfee was back in the UCP home; but it had become clear to UCP officials in Birmingham that there would be no presidential waiver, and they had announced to the newspapers that he would have to leave their facility soon. Meanwhile, Russell Fine tried to get the president or the Georgia legislature to accept some kind of group arrangement for him.

About July 10, the Georgia legislature relented, and Larry McAfee was transferred to the Medical College of Georgia; the independent-living facility that was created there for him and the five other patients was an exception to Georgia's disability law and to its state Medicaid plan.

There are obviously a number of issues involved in this financial saga, but let us focus on only one, a phenomenon that bioethicists call the *rule of rescue*. The campaign to obtain a presidential waiver for Larry McAfee provoked considerable criticism and was seen as demonstrating that decisions about who should be helped are too often arbitrary. Two citizens, for instance, were disturbed when McAfee said that he would not return to a nursing home to "vegetate" and wanted Georgia to pay for his private apartment.[62] They complained:

> But why should McAfee be the only one singled out and given special attention, not to be in a nursing home, or that Medicaid should "open up" for? . . . McAfee "understands" that life is preferable, but it must be life with some dignity; in this case, *his* way or no way. McAfee says that if someone else won't pay for him to live *where and how* he chooses, he'd rather be dead. What about all the other people in the same situation?[63]

Critics like these hold that American society will "rescue" only someone like McAfee who manages to get into the national spotlight; it ignores all the others whose needs are just as great. (In McAfee's case, there were some 75,000 to 85,000 others.)

Larry McAfee and Elizabeth Bouvia both illustrate the rule of rescue. When one person's plight is made prominent by the news media, society tends to feel compelled to rescue that person, even if the rescue entails spending enormous amounts of scarce medical resources. In contrast, obscure people quietly go "unrescued" and live in abysmal conditions until they die. The rule of rescue in effect turns some crucial decisions over to the media: the editors of local newspapers and television news departments become gatekeepers, determining who will and will not be rescued. This is hardly the most rational way to distribute scarce medical resources. (The rule of rescue is discussed further in Chapter 12.)

UPDATE

In 1990, as noted in Chapter 1, the United States Supreme Court decided in *Cruzan* that no state may pass a law limiting the right of competent patients to decline medical treatment, even if declining treatment would hasten death. *Cruzan* built on previous appellate court decisions, including *Bouvia* and *McAfee*, and was a resounding victory for advocates of the right of competent adults to control their own death and dying.

In 1991, the Americans with Disabilities Act (ADA) went into effect. This legislation represents one of the most sweeping changes in the history of American law. Although at present it is still widely unenforced, its long-term effects will eventually integrate many Americans with disabilities—including those with cerebral palsy and spinal-cord injuries—into normal life.

A decade after Elizabeth Bouvia's victory in court, her body was described as "gnarled and useless."[64] She was living in California as a Medicaid patient, in a private hospital room with 24-hour care; the cost was $300 a day. A continuous dose of morphine was controlling her pain, and her weight was up to 100 pounds. Her life, she has said, is "a lot of needles and bags," and she spends most of her time watching television. On her own description, she would seem to be resigned to her fate: "I wouldn't say I'm happy, but I'm physically comfortable, more comfortable than before. There is nothing really to do. I just kind of lay here."

Ironically, Richard Scott, the physician and lawyer who represented Elizabeth Bouvia, committed suicide in August 1992. His wife said that he had battled depression for most of his life. When he died, Elizabeth Bouvia said, "Jesus, I wish he could have come in and taken me with him."

In 1993, Larry McAfee's story became the subject of *The Switch*, a CBS television movie. Gary Cole of the television series *Midnight Caller* starred as Larry McAfee; Russ Fine was portrayed only as a talk show host, not as an expert on rehabilitation. The producers had paid Russ and Dee Fine for rights to their story, but the Fines contributed the money to Larry McAfee.[65] In January of 1993, according to Russ Fine, Larry McAfee was "real happy" about the movie and its national premiere. However, to keep the disability payments that funded his home, McAfee himself could not accept any of the profits. A few months later, authorities in Georgia "forgot" to include McAfee's independent-living center in the state budget for such centers. At that time McAfee's center in Augusta housed five other patients and cost $116,000 per year; the overall budget from which it had been omitted was $8.9 million. Once again the Fines contacted the media, pointing out that the cost per person in the independent-living center was only $52 a day, and the Georgia legislature "found" funds to continue the center for another year.

Tragically, in November 1993, Larry McAfee suffered two devastating strokes. The probable cause was a nursing error: a kink in his urinary catheter that caused urine to back up. Because of his paralysis, he could not feel what was happening; and the backup caused toxicity and high blood pressure.[66] McAfee survived but was left with only a little short-term memory. He had been planning to leave the independent-living facility for his own apartment but instead had to leave it for a long-term nursing home in Augusta. This nursing home was just the kind of place and fate that Larry McAfee had wanted to avoid when he won the right to use his "switch" and before he lost the ability to choose to use it.

Dax Cowart, the burn patient who had been treated against his will in Texas, became a millionaire from an out-of-court settlement with the gas company, graduated from law school in 1986, married a nurse he had known in high school, and became interested in two hobbies: ham radio and raising golden retrievers. He also became a frequent speaker for the Society for the Right to Die, arguing that even though he was glad to be alive today with his present blessings, his physicians had been morally wrong to treat him against his wishes. As he once said to this author, "If I should be so unlucky as to be burned that way again, and if I knew what was waiting at the end, I wouldn't go through that pain to get there."[67]

It is, indeed, interesting to note that in the three most famous cases of nonterminal adults who wanted to die in medical facilities, all three patients changed their minds when they had a genuine opportunity to do so.

FURTHER READING

David Hume, "On Suicide" (1755), in Eugene Miller, ed., *Collected Essays of David Hume,* Liberty Classics, Indianapolis, Ind., 1986.

Pat Milmoe McCarrick, "Scope Note 18: Active Euthanasia and Assisted Suicide," *Kennedy Institute of Ethics Journal,* vol. 2, no. 1, March 1992.

James Rachels, *The End of Life,* Oxford University Press, Oxford, 1986.

CHAPTER 3

Physician-Assisted Dying

Jack Kevorkian

This chapter discusses whether physicians should help terminally ill patients die. It focuses on the physician Jack Kevorkian, who has assisted in the death of several patients with terminal illnesses or nonterminal medical conditions that caused great suffering.

The term *physician-assisted dying* is somewhat vague. In this chapter, we will use it very broadly to refer to almost any act by a physician that helps a patient die. Such acts include giving information, writing prescriptions for lethal drugs, administering drugs in lethal dosages, and simply being present in order to act if anything unexpected happens while a patient kills himself or herself.[1] This is in a sense closely related to assisted suicide (discussed in Chapter 2); the main difference is that—as the terms are used in this text—*assisted suicide* involves patients whose condition is nonterminal whereas *physician-assisted dying* typically involves patients whose condition is terminal. (As was noted in Chapter 2, the term *suicide* is not really appropriate when a dying person accepts or brings about an earlier death.)

BACKGROUND: EUTHANASIA

Ancient Greece and the Hippocratic Oath

The Hippocratic oath, which forbids killing by physicians, began in ancient Greece at the time of Socrates. It is often considered the origin of medical ethics, but that common impression was disputed in 1931 by Ludwig Edelstein, a historian of medicine who described Hippocrates as a disciple of Pythagoras.[2] Although Pythagoras is usually thought of as a mathematician—the originator of the Pythagorean theorem—he was also a mystic who worshipped numbers as divine and believed that all life was sacred. As his follower, then, Hippocrates would not have been representative of most Greek physicians. Moreover, the Hippocratic *corpus*, or body of writings, is not even the work of one man named Hippocrates but was developed by a number of his own followers. The practitioners of the Hippocratic school "possessed no legally recognized professional qualifications" and were in competition with gymnastic instructors, drug-sellers, herbalists, midwives, exorcists, and "purifiers."[3]

There have also been misconceptions about the content of the original Hippocratic oath. Today, few medical schools use the original version, and in schools where it is used at all, many parts of it (especially a pagan curse that appears at the end) are changed; also, the version of the oath given at a graduation ceremony does not necessarily reflect the values taught at that school. Let us see what the original oath actually makes physicians promise. Here is the complete text of Edelstein's translation:

> I swear by Apollo Physician and Asclepius and Hygeia and Panaceia and all the gods and goddesses, making them my witnesses, that I will fulfill according to my ability and judgment this oath and this covenant:
>
> To hold him who has taught me this art as equal to my parents and to live my life in partnership with him, and if he is in need of money, to give him a share of mine, and to regard his offspring as equal to my brothers in male lineage, and to teach his art—if they desire to learn it—without fee and covenant; to give a share of precepts and oral instruction and all the other learning to my sons and to the sons of him who has instructed me and the pupils who have signed the covenant and have taken this oath according to the medical law, but to no one else.
>
> I will apply dietetic measures for the benefit of the sick according to my ability and judgment; I will keep them from harm and injustice.
>
> I will neither give a deadly drug to anybody if asked for it, nor will I make a suggestion to this effect. Similarly I will not give to a woman an abortive remedy. In purity and holiness I will guard my life and my art. I will not use the knife, not even on sufferers of stone, but will withdraw in favor of such men as are engaged in this work.
>
> Whatever houses I visit, I will come for the benefit of the sick, remaining free of all intentional injustice, of all mischief and in particular of sexual relations with both female and male persons, be they free or slaves.
>
> What I may see or hear in the course of the treatment or even outside of the treatment in regard to the life of men, which on no account one must spread abroad, I will keep to myself holding such things shameful to be spoken about.
>
> If I fulfill this oath and do not violate it, may it be granted to me to enjoy life and art, being honored with fame among all men for all time to come; if I transgress it and swear falsely, may the opposite of all this be my lot.

This version does include swearing never to help dying patients who request death—and never to perform abortions—but that should be understood in context. Such vows were included because the Hippocratic school wanted to solidify its membership against competing healers; thus the oath also includes swearing not to perform surgery and (medical school instructors take notice!) not to charge students for teaching them the art of medicine.

The prohibition against euthanasia by the Hippocratic school therefore set its members apart from most other physicians in ancient Greece, who were not opposed to letting patients die or even to mercy killing; indeed, many Greek physicians excelled in helping patients die painlessly. There seem to have been two bases for this prevailing attitude that patients could be allowed to die or helped to die. The first reason was philosophical: the Greeks thought that life had certain natural limitations, beyond which it was folly to try to extend living. (The concept of a *meson* or natural limit infused Greek culture, particularly architecture and theater. To attempt to go beyond *meson* was *hubris*—arrogance—and invited the gods to strike one down.) The second reason was practical: physicians at that time simply did not know very much; also, they worried about being shown up by competitors. Consequently, they would often let terminal patients die in peace rather than attempt to heal them.

Still, the Hippocratic oath symbolizes an ancient tradition of self-sacrifice and respect for human life. It also symbolizes commitment to the patient's welfare over the physician's convenience. Today, when too many physicians (even one is perhaps "too many") seem driven by money, have affairs with their patients, and divulge their patients' confidences, it seems wise to retain this symbolic commitment.

The Nazis: Involuntary "Euthanasia"

"Euthanasia" in Nazi Germany is often invoked in debates about physician-assisted dying. German physicians during the Nazi era killed 90,000 patients in the name of "euthanasia" because of presumed mental or physical "inferiority" such as retardation. A related program, the so-called "final solution" to the problem of "cleansing" Germany of "racially inferior" non-Aryan stock, was kept more secret at the time: this was the program under which the Nazis killed approximately 6 million Jews, 600,000 Poles, thousands of Gypsies, and thousands of homosexuals.

Leo Alexander, a New York psychiatrist who was an observer at the Nuremberg trials, argued in 1949 that the Nazis' "euthanasia" of people with disabilities and the later Nazi genocide—the mass murder of Jews and others—can both be traced to the same beginning: acceptance by German physicians of the idea that some people, because their quality of life is poor, are better off dead than alive. This line of reasoning is an example of the *slippery slope,* introduced in Chapter 1. According to Alexander, from the moment when a mentally vegetative person was first killed, Germany and German medicine followed a downward plunge that ended in the death camps:

> The beginnings at first were a subtle shifting in emphasis in the basic attitude of the physicians. It started with the acceptance of the attitude, basic in the euthanasia movement, that there is such a thing as life not worthy to be lived. This attitude in its early stages concerned itself merely with the severely and chronically sick. Gradually, the sphere of those to be included in this category was enlarged to encompass the socially unproductive, the ideologically unwanted, the racially unwanted and finally all non-Germans. But it is important to realize that the infinitely small wedged-in lever from which this entire trend of mind received its impetus was the attitude toward the nonrehabilitable sick.[4]

In 1986, another New York psychiatrist, Robert Jay Lifton, argued similarly, although the "first step" is different in Lifton's analysis:

The Nazis justified direct medical killing by use of the . . . concept of "life unworthy of life," *lebensunwertes Leben*. While this concept predated the Nazis, it was carried to its ultimate racial and "therapeutic" extreme by them.

. . . Of the five identifiable steps by which the Nazis carried out the destruction of "life unworthy of life," coercive sterilization was the first. There followed the killing of "impaired" children in hospitals, and then the killing of "impaired" adults—mostly collected from mental hospitals—in centers especially equipped with carbon monoxide. The same killing centers were then used for the murders of "impaired" inmates of concentration camps. The final step was mass killing, mostly of Jews, in the extermination camps themselves.[5]

Alexander and Lifton are often cited by people who are opposed to physician-assisted dying, and also by some people who are opposed to "letting die" or assisted suicide. These people argue that if any patient is allowed to die or helped to die—even an irreversibly comatose patient (like Karen Quinlan in Chapter 1) or a suffering patient who asks for death (like Elizabeth Bouvia in Chapter 2)—then society will slide down a slippery slope and end by killing all kinds of patients. Many of these commentators emphasize that in Nazi Germany, it was physicians, especially professors in elite medical schools, who took the first step.

Not everyone accepts this argument, however. Some of those who disagree with Alexander, for example, hold that German medicine had been blatantly racist since early in the twentieth century; and that the eventual mass murders did not result from a subtle, initially imperceptible shift in attitudes but rather were a manifestation of widespread overt racism in the general population as well. Moreover, whatever steps led to the Nazi "euthanasia" program, it can be argued that the Nazi program had nothing in common with concepts like physician-assisted dying. In Nazi Germany, the term *euthanasia* camouflaged atrocities (eventually, it hardly even pretended to camouflage these atrocities). Nazi "euthanasia" was murder: its victims all died involuntarily; no terminal patients were ever helped to die voluntarily.

Voluntary Euthanasia in the Netherlands

The Netherlands has been the first country to decriminalize physician-assisted suicide in the postwar era. Interestingly, this country was occupied by the Nazis during World War II, and Dutch physicians actively resisted the Nazi murder programs at that time.

The decriminalization of voluntary euthanasia began in 1971 when the mother of the physician Geertruida Postma suffered a cerebral hemorrhage. The hemorrhage left the elderly woman partially paralyzed, deaf, and with gross speech deficits; to prevent falls, she had to be kept tied to a chair in her nursing home. According to Postma, her mother repeatedly begged for death. Finally, Postma said, "When I watched my mother, a human wreck, hanging in that chair, I couldn't stand it anymore."[6] Postma first injected morphine to induce unconsciousness, then killed her mother by injecting curare, and then informed the authorities. She was found guilty of murder but was given only a suspended sentence.

Two years later, in 1973, the Royal Dutch Medical Association developed the following guidelines, which were accepted by Dutch prosecutors and which have been used by Dutch physicians for the past two decades:

1. Only physicians may practice voluntary euthanasia.
2. Requests must be made by competent patients.
3. Decisions by patients must be unambivalent, repeated, and well-documented.
4. The practicing physician must consult another physician.
5. The patient must not be pressured into his or her decision.
6. The patient must be in unbearable pain or suffering, without probability of change.
7. No other measures may be available that would improve the condition and would also be acceptable to the patient.

Notice that these guidelines do not explicitly allow a physician to kill a vegetative patient, such as Karen Quinlan; nor do they allow a physician to kill a patient who is severely retarded, even at the family's request. Note also that the patient's condition does *not* have to be terminal. It should be pointed out that, technically, both assisted suicide and mercy killing by physicians are still illegal.[7] Over the last two decades, the Netherlands has moved closer and closer to legalization without actually arriving at it.

For several reasons, the Dutch guidelines may not be readily generalizable to the United States. First, certain unique features of Dutch law should be taken into consideration. Legal cases in the Netherlands are decided not by juries but by professional judges appointed for life. Five attorneys general, and 200 public prosecutors under them, can decline to prosecute on their own authority. The legal system is thus not vulnerable to pressure from fringe groups or to emotional appeals to jurors. Second—and very important—everyone in the Netherlands has free medical care, paid for by heavy taxes; thus no physician, patient, or family ever needs to think of ending life to ease the financial burden of care. Third, the typical Dutch patient has a physician who makes house calls, who has had a relationship with him or her for years, and who may be the one that will actually carry out his or her request for assisted death. Finally, malpractice cases against physicians are rare, and large awards to plaintiffs who win such cases are even rarer; as a result, Dutch physicians do not practice "defensive medicine."

More than two-thirds of the Dutch people endorse these guidelines,[8] and the country as a whole seems remarkably satisfied. If this has been an "ethics lab" for an experiment in physician-assisted dying, then no slide down a slippery slope has occurred—at least not as the Dutch themselves see their society—and the continuation of these practices in the Netherlands is not in doubt.

After two decades, Dutch physicians have assisted in the deaths of between 2,000 and 3,000 thousand patients per year (the population of the Netherlands is 15 million).[9] Physician-assisted death has been accepted as an occasional duty by most Dutch physicians, who see it as the last part of a continuum of lifelong care of each patient according to his or her own wishes.[10] Only 4 percent of Dutch physicians have categorically refused to assist patients in dying.[11] Of the patients who have asked for physician-assisted death, most were in the final weeks of life when they made the request.[12] Almost 85 percent had cancer; the rest were in the last stages of AIDS, multiple sclerosis, or other terminal degenerative diseases involving paralysis. Most have been in their sixties rather than in their seventies or eighties.[13]

There has naturally been some vocal opposition, especially from people who consider the new practices a "descent into barbarity."[14] There have also been more specific concerns. In 1991, the Remmelink Commission reported that more than 1,000 deaths a year had been hastened by physicians without the explicit written consent of the patient. According to the researchers, these "can best be characterized as concerning patients who were near death and clearly suffering grievously";[15] but opponents emphasized that in such cases the original guidelines had already been exceeded. In the early 1990s, several cases of physician-assisted death for psychiatric reasons also seemed to exceed the guidelines and raised questions about how far Dutch physicians would go. In one of these cases, a woman in her twenties was killed by a physician at her request after a decade of extremely severe, uncontrollable anorexia; in another, in May 1993, a physician assisted with the suicide of a severely depressed woman who had been traumatized by the death of her two children and the failure of her marriage. Both of these physicians were charged with murder.[16]

American physicians tend to see what they want in the Dutch practices. Opponents of physician-assisted dying are convinced that the Netherlands has "started us on a decline that will take us all the way—to eliminating everyone deemed unfit."[17] The physician Carlos Gomez found that in 26 cases of assisted dying in the Netherlands, the physicians failed to follow one or more of the guidelines, yet there were no legal repercussions.[18] On the other hand, Arthur Caplan, although he is opposed to physician-assisted dying in the United States, concedes that in the Netherlands, "It's impressive that there are so few problems. . . . They feel comfortable with it. They are not afraid the doctor will kill them because they lack insurance."[19]

The Hemlock Society

The Hemlock Society was founded in the United States in 1980 by Derek Humphrey,[20] a former British journalist, to help people with terminal illness die painlessly and with dignity. The society advocates limits on assisted suicide; it believes that laws should be liberalized only to assist dying for people who are both competent and terminally ill—not for chronic invalids, mental patients, or comatose patients.

The Hemlock Society is perhaps best known through its books, which are usually written by Derek Humphrey and give detailed instructions on how to kill oneself quickly and painlessly. No state has tried to ban the sale of these books, which are of course protected under the First Amendment. In 1991, Humphrey's *Final Exit* was a surprise best-seller and sold millions of copies.

The Hemlock Society and its publications have become popular because many Americans are afraid that their physicians will violate their wishes, forcing them to live their final days, months, or even years in pain, tethered to machines. As the writer and journalist Shana Alexander said about dying in a hospital, "When it comes to following my wishes, I trust my lawyer more than my physician."[21]

The Hospice Movement

In the 1960s, two physicians—one working in the United States and the other in England—began a movement to change medicine so that it could accommodate the special needs of dying patients and their families. These two physicians were Elisabeth Kübler-Ross (who was born in Switzerland) and Cicely Saunders (born in Britain); their program is called the *hospice movement*. Some leaders of the hospice movement say that requests for physician-assisted dying arise only when people do not know how modern hospice care works.

Kübler-Ross and Saunders developed special institutions that did not try to fight death or delay it but merely made the dying patient as comfortable as possible. A hospice tries to give dying patients dignity and maximal control over the final months of their lives. Originally, hospices were special separate facilities, but the concept soon evolved to emphasize care in which most treatment is delivered by visiting nurses and physicians, allowing dying patients to stay at home.

As the result of the work of Kübler-Ross and Saunders, physicians are much more attuned today than they were 20 years ago to relief of pain and to the psychological needs of dying patients. In-home medical care, which includes hospice care, is now one of the fastest-growing fields of medicine, accounting for a large percentage of new jobs for nurses and aides. In the United States, Medicare (the program for people over 65) now pays for hospice care for dying patients.

DR. KEVORKIAN AND ASSISTED DYING

In June of 1990, Janet Adkins asked Jack Kevorkian, a retired pathologist, to help her die.[22]

Janet Adkins, who lived in Oregon, was 54 years old. She loved music, sports, and the outdoors; played tennis; and had hiked in the Himalayas—but now she was in the initial stages of Alzheimer's disease. For some time, she had been growing more and more frustrated by her increasing inability to remember things, and she had found that she could no longer read the sheet music for her piano.

Alzheimer's disease, the fourth-largest killer of Americans, is characterized by devastating loss of memory, resulting from irreversible degeneration of neural cells, and it is incurable. On average, people with Alzheimer's disease live 10 years after the onset of symptoms; in the final phase, which can last many years, these patients become vegetative.

According to her husband, Ron Adkins, the diagnosis of Alzheimer's disease hit Janet Adkins "like a bombshell. . . . Her mind was her life"[23] At the urging of her family, she tried THA (Tacrine), an experimental drug. According to her son Neil, "The drug didn't work. From then on, her mind was set. Quality of life was everything with her. She wanted to die with dignity intact." Janet Adkins had been a member of the Hemlock Society and strongly believed in the right to take one's own life.

Since at the time assisted suicide was not illegal in Michigan, where Kevorkian lived, Janet Adkins flew there with her husband and her three sons. Her family was ambivalent about her intention to die, and her husband, hoping that she might change her mind, had bought a round-trip ticket for her. In the end, however, the entire Adkins family supported her decision.

Jack Kevorkian, who was then 63, had grown up in Pontiac, Michigan, the son of Armenian immigrants, and graduated from medical school in 1953. After finishing his residency, he worked from 1969 to 1978 in Detroit at Sarasota Hospital as director of laboratories. Later, he was employed at other hospitals, the last in southern California in 1982. When he retired from hospital work, he began to live on his social security benefits—$550 a month—and on his savings; his home was a tiny, 2-room apartment above a florist's shop in Royal Oak, a suburban town near Detroit.[24] For some years before Janet Adkins contacted him in 1990, Jack Kevorkian had actively publicized his views on physician-assisted death.

When Janet Adkins arrived in Michigan, Kevorkian and his two sisters interviewed her and her family for 2 hours; this was on June 3, a Saturday afternoon. None of the interviewers thought that Janet Adkins was irrational, depressed, or ambivalent about her decision to die; nor did any of them think that she could be helped by medicine. Janet Adkins and her family signed documents and made videotapes to prove that they were competent and understood what they were doing. Then the two families had a meal together to get to know each other better; after that, Janet Adkins and her family spent the night thinking things over.

The next day—Sunday afternoon, June 4, 1990,—Janet Adkins met Kevorkian alone and the two drove in his rusty 1968 Volkswagen van to a public park in north Oakland County, Michigan. Kevorkian had not been able to find any better place where he could help his patient kill herself. He had forthrightly told several clinics, churches, and funeral homes what he intended to do, and none of them would let him use their facilities. In desperation, he had decided on the park and had put a cot and his suicide device in the van.

The simple device in the van that would allow Janet Adkins to kill herself painlessly consisted of three intravenous (IV) bottles hung from an aluminum frame; Kevorkian called it a Mercitron. At the park, he connected an IV line to Janet Adkins and started a saline solution for fluid volume. Then she took over and pushed a switch that stopped the saline and released thiopental, a powerful sedative. The switch also started a 6-second timer which soon activated a drip of potassium chloride. The thiopental rendered Janet Adkins unconscious, and the potassium chloride killed her about 1 minute later. In effect, Kevorkian said, Janet Adkins had "a painless heart attack while in deep sleep."[25] The whole process took less than 6 minutes.

Neither the Adkins family nor Kevorkian had anticipated the landslide of publicity that followed. Kevorkian was prosecuted for murder by the local district attorney. A local judge dismissed the case because there was no law against assisted suicide in Michigan, but he also ordered Kevorkian not to use the Mercitron machine again. (Since assisting suicide was not against the law, the judge's basis for issuing such an order was unclear.)

•

Jack Kevorkian had begun to form his views on euthanasia when, as an intern, he cared for a middle-aged woman whose body was ravaged by cancer.[26] He then became interested in death, and also in obtaining transplantable organs from prisoners and dying patients—long before it was technically feasible to transplant organs.

During his residency at the hospital at the University of Michigan, he decried the waste of the bodies of condemned criminals and proposed that physicians render such prisoners permanently unconscious and then use their bodies for risky medical experiments. "He was forced to leave when [university] officials heard of his proposal";[27] in his career as a pathologist, however, he never had any complaints filed against him by patients.

When he was working as a hospital pathologist, he proposed that blood be transferred directly from bodies of dead soldiers on a battlefield to wounded soldiers lying nearby. In the decade before he became famous, he crusaded to let prisoners on death row become organ donors: "Each condemned prisoner could save five, six, seven lives. They're young, they're in good shape. What a waste."[28]

In 1986, he heard about the decriminalization of physician-assisted dying in the Netherlands. Instead of simply advocating the use of similar guidelines in the United States, he expanded "his death row proposal to include experimentation on willing patients who opt for euthanasia"[29] and—under the mistaken impression that euthanasia had actually been legalized in the Netherlands—he went there to implement his proposal. (He found, of course, that euthanasia was not legal in the Netherlands, and his ideas about allowing dying patients to be used as subjects of medical experiments seem not to have been received warmly there.)

Although Kevorkian has always sought ways to increase the availability of subjects for medical research and organs for transplantation, he has never been a medical researcher or a surgeon; nor has he ever been directly responsible for patients in hospital beds. Thus his proposals about research subjects and organ transplants are perhaps more abstract than those of physicians on the frontiers of medical research who must watch their patients die because of their own inability to help.

In fact, Kevorkian was himself not originally interested in compassionate assistance to the dying. He writes that when he was first contacted in 1989 by a patient with end-stage lung cancer, he felt "it only decent and fair to explain my ultimate aim": not to help patients achieve painless, dignified death, but to get terminal people to volunteer for "invaluable experiments."[30] This aim would have constituted a new medical speciality, which he called "obitiary" or "medicide."

Jack Kevorkian has always been a loner and extremely independent. Except for a brief membership in one society of pathologists, he has scorned membership in medical societies: "Instinctively, as a student, I thought they were corrupt," he says. "I've been independent all my life."[31]

Since 1990, when he assisted at the death of Janet Adkins, Kevorkian has received hundreds of letters a year from people whose suffering is of truly biblical proportions. He is afraid to fly and hates to drive very far, so his patients must come to Royal Oak, the suburban town near Detroit where he lives. Thus he does not help anyone who is too ill to travel, and this has been a source of frustration for those who cannot find a way to get to Michigan. He accepts no money himself for helping patients; any donations go toward building a suicide center, the "Obitorium."[32]

In the fall of 1991, Kevorkian assisted in the double suicide of two women patients: one with multiple sclerosis and another with chronic vaginal-pelvic pain. To comply technically with the order of the judge in the Adkins case, he used not the original Mercitron but a more sophisticated version of it. He was again indicted for murder, but again the charges were dismissed, since he had still not violated any Michigan law. However, his medical license in Michigan was suspended in November 1991.

With his license suspended, he could no longer obtain sodium pentothal and potassium chloride, and so he began using carbon monoxide (CO) with his next patients. In May of 1992, he helped another victim of multiple sclerosis to kill herself; this time the patient put on a mask in order to breath in the CO. Kevorkian came to believe that CO was a good way to commit suicide: the gas "has no color, taste, or smell; and it's toxic enough to cause rapid unconsciousness in relatively low concentration. Furthermore, in light complexioned people it often produces a rosy color that makes the victim look better as a corpse."[33] After some trial and error, he began to teach patients to attach one end of a plastic tube to a canister of CO and the other to the kind of small plastic mask used in hospitals for oxygen therapy. When the gas is turned on and the patient breathes normally, death occurs within 5 minutes.[34]

•

Many laypeople regard Jack Kevorkian as a folk hero, but most physicians and many medical ethicists have denounced him. Asked about criticisms of his actions, he responds, "Why should I care what brainwashed ethicists and non-thinking physicians say?"[35] Nor has he worried about violating the Hippocratic oath: he calls physicians who follow these ancient ideas "hypocritic oafs."

In 3 years after the Adkins case, publicity about his other cases and his own eagerness to speak his mind made him a familiar figure in the American and Canadian media. After Janet Adkins's death, he appeared on television talk shows and news programs to publicize his invention, his ideas, and his services.[36] He regards himself as a Socratic gadfly to the sluggish medical profession and compares himself proudly to the crusader Margaret Sanger, who was attacked by the medical profession for her work in birth control.[37] On occasion, he sees his struggle in heroic, even cosmic terms, comparing himself to Mahatma Gandhi, Martin Luther King Jr., and Albert Einstein; he has even compared his early efforts at assisted dying to the birth of Christianity.[38]

Kevorkian came to be represented by a skilled attorney, Geoffrey Fieger, a highly successful malpractice lawyer who had previously won a $1 million judgment in a case against a hospital involving misuse of antipsychotic drugs. Fieger earned two degrees in theater at the University of Michigan before graduating from law school; his parents had been active in organizing unions and voter registration in Mississippi during the 1960s, and he himself seemed to love a good public fight. Neither Fieger nor Kevorkian will discuss their financial relationship, but Fieger denies that he is representing Kevorkian for money and says that he is doing it because judges and other lawyers have turned against ordinary people. Fieger and Kevorkian disdained the traditional medical forums and took their impassioned arguments directly to the public. Fieger seemed to realize that the blunt-spoken, eccentric Kevorkian would never do well within the medical establishment.[39]

Kevorkian has nothing but scorn for physicians who assist dying only by withdrawing treatment and are too cowardly to stay for the death itself:

> Moreover, in sharp contrast to the timorous, secretive, and even deceitful intentions and actions of other medical euthanists on whom our so-called bioethicists now shower praise, I acted openly, ethically, legally, with complete and uncompromising honesty, and—even more important—I remained in personal attendance during the second most meaningful medical event in a patient's earthly existence.[40]

Kevorkian has sometimes been called a Dr. Frankenstein, but he does not consider himself a dangerous man and actually welcomes that comparison: "Frankenstein was benevolent, a dedicated researcher and doctor. He created this monster because he was interested in life and death. The monster was very loving."[41]

DR. QUILL: ANOTHER APPROACH TO ASSISTED DYING

In 1990, Timothy Quill, an internist in Rochester, New York, was asked by one of his own patients to help her die and consented to do so. The case of Timothy Quill and his patient—known only as "Diane"—is frequently cited as a contrast to Jack Kevorkian's cases.

As a young woman, Diane had survived vaginal cancer and had overcome alcoholism.[42] In 1990 she was 45, was suffering from leukemia, and had been a patient of Quill's for over 3 years. At that point she suddenly developed acute myelomonocytic leukemia—one of the very worst kinds.

Quill explained to Diane that she had a 25 percent chance of long-term survival if she endured treatment. The treatment would consist of 3 weeks of induction chemotherapy (75 percent of patients respond to this and 25 percent die); then consolidation chemotherapy (another 25 percent die after this, so that the net survival rate becomes 50 percent); and finally bone-marrow transplantation (requiring whole-body radiation and 2 months of hospitalization—another 25 percent die of graft-versus-host disease, so that the net survival rate drops to 25 percent). For the last treatment to work well, a well-matched bone-marrow donor would need to be found. All these treatments would almost inevitably cause infections, loss of hair, and nausea. With no treatment at all, death would be certain in days, weeks, or at most several months.[43]

As is customary, the oncologists—who believe that any delay is dangerous in cases like this—began making plans to insert a Hickman catheter into Diane to start chemotherapy "that afternoon." However—also as customary—Diane resisted being rushed in this way (a typical reaction among independent patients). On reflection, she decided that a 25 percent chance of long-term survival was not worth "so toxic a course of therapy," especially because the hospital had no closely matched bone-marrow donor. Quill, who apparently felt more positively about the 25 percent chance of survival, was disturbed by Diane's rejection of treatment; but he had known her for 3 years, considered her mentally acute, and was aware that her family supported her decision.

A few days after she had decided to forgo treatment, Diane began to worry intensely about a lingering death and concluded that she wanted barbiturates so that she could kill herself when the time came. Quill, on his part, was worried that her "preoccupation with her fear of lingering death would interfere with Diane's getting the most out of the time she had left." Having made sure that she was not irrationally depressed, he wrote a prescription for barbiturates and told her how to use them for both sleep and suicide.

Diane then experienced 3 "tumultuous months." Her son stayed home from college, and her husband brought all his work home. Several times she became weak or developed infections but bounced back. Near the end, Diane had 2 weeks of "relative calm," but this was followed by rapid decline.

Because Diane was now faced with what she feared most, "increasing discomfort, dependence, and hard choices," Quill knew that her end had come:

> When we met, it was clear that she knew what she was doing, that she was sad and frightened to be leaving, but that she would be even more terrified to stay and suffer. In our tearful goodbye, she promised a reunion in the future at her favorite spot on the edge of Lake Geneva, with dragons swimming in the sunset.[44]

Quill published an account of Diane's death in a respected medical journal and was prosecuted for murder after his article appeared; however, the grand jury refused to indict him.[45] As noted above, his case is often described as contrasting in several ways with those of Jack Kevorkian: Timothy Quill had known Diane well and had been treating her for a long time; he first offered her a course of treatment that might allow her to survive; he helped her die privately and without publicity at the time; he preserved her anonymity; he presented his account in an established medical forum; and he was not a "specialist" in assisted dying. Some critics who are strongly opposed to Jack Kevorkian have reacted more positively to Timothy Quill.

ETHICAL ISSUES

Patients' Autonomy

One significant issue in physician-assisted dying—as in assisted suicide, discussed in Chapter 2—is patients' autonomy. Autonomy was an important concept for John Stuart Mill, who argued in *On Liberty* that "over his own body and mind, the individual is sovereign." Mill believed that government should not impose on individuals its view of when and how they should die.

One way to put the argument for patients' autonomy with regard to assisted dying is to compare a person's life to a business: if I own a business that is making money, it makes sense for me to keep it open; but if the business is losing money, I would be imprudent to wait until there was no money left at all before closing.[46] Similarly, a terminally ill patient owns his or her body and need not "stay in business" till the very end.

Risk of Error

People who are opposed to physician-assisted dying often point out that there is almost always some risk of error: that is, a patient who is helped to die may in fact have been able to survive, at least for some time. In other words, there is a danger of dying too soon and losing valuable months or years.

The surgeon Christiaan Barnard recalls a young woman with ovarian cancer who repeatedly begged him to kill her painlessly with morphine.[47] Aware that her condition was terminal—and hearing her screams at night—Barnard decided that he should help her die. When he came into her room with a syringe loaded with morphine, she was quiet, and he thought at first that she was in too much pain even to scream. Then he realized that she was in a state of semiconsciousness, apparently beyond pain, and at the last moment he changed his mind. The next morning, the woman felt better; soon she was in remission, and she lived another few months. Stories like this abound in medicine.

In the Netherlands, some critics of the guidelines for assisted dying claim that physicians are often mistaken about what is "intractable and unbearable" suffering and imply that some physicians are sending patients to needlessly premature deaths.[48] In Janet Adkins's case, many people were quick to say that physicians aren't infallible diagnosticians and that patients sometimes defy a dire prognosis.

Let us put this point differently. In bioethics, many discussions begin with a phrase like, "If a patient has a terminal illness . . . ." Notice the word *if*. In presumably terminal illnesses, there are actually few absolute facts until the patient's very last days. Before then, how "terminal"—how close to death—the patient actually is may depend on many factors that are not easy to assess precisely: the patient's attitude, the family's attitude, the attitude of staff members, the quality and level of care, and so on. Moreover, it is true that some supposedly terminal patients have been misdiagnosed altogether and have recovered with different treatment. The fear is that physician-assisted dying will allow mistakes of this kind to pass too easily. Once physician-assisted death has taken place, of course, it is like capital punishment: there is no appeal.

It should be noted that the existence of risk is not in itself a conclusive argument against physician-assisted dying. For one thing, decision making would become impossible if we tried to avoid all risk in all circumstances; in other words, some degree of risk is often inevitable. Moreover, alternatives to assisted dying also carry some risk: a patient who simply does nothing and waits for death risks, for example, intense suffering and loss of dignity; a patient who accepts treatment risks at least pain and undesirable side effects, and possibly a disastrous outcome. The wife of a former secretary of Health, Education, and Welfare "waited" (as some critics contend Janet Adkins should have done) and then spent "much of the last 5 years of her 14-year bout with Alzheimer's in a nursing home as a near vegetable"; her husband wrote that her death at age 80 "was a very delayed blessing."[49]

Risk, however, gives rise to several questions that are important issues in physician-assisted dying: Who is best qualified to assess the danger of dying too soon? What degree of risk is "acceptable"? Who should determine "acceptability"? How does the risk of dying too soon compare with the risks entailed by alternative courses of action?

Physicians, not surprisingly, believe that they are best qualified to assess risk, and they may be right as far as statistical risk is concerned. But *acceptable* risk is evaluative as well as statistical, and many patients want the right to make their own evaluative judgments about what they consider acceptable or unacceptable risk. Throughout life, taking risks is one of our most human activities; at the end, deciding to die rather than live can be seen as no more or less than a continuation of what we have been doing all along. Accepting the risk of assisted dying may represent the last evaluation a patient can make; if so, shouldn't it be the patient, not the physician, who controls that last evaluation?

It is important to realize that when terminal patients make such evaluations, their concern is more than just fear of pain. Derek Humphrey of the Hemlock Society has written, "It isn't just a question of pain. It is a question of dignity, self-control, and distress. If you can't eat, sleep, or read, and the quality of life is so bad, and there is a certainty that you are dying, it is a matter of dignity" to be able to end your life.[50] It is also important to understand why such patients want and need help from physicians: problems of unassisted suicide are discussed in Chapter 2, but Humphrey sums them up more succinctly: "Decent people don't want to shoot themselves or their loved ones—[or] blow their brains out on a bedroom wall."

It is also important to emphasize that in order to make the best decisions about acceptable risk, patients and their families need information. The philosopher Margaret Battin holds that physicians rarely discuss options with dying patients.[51] She believes that patients' informed consent should be sought not only for medical research but also for ways of dying. Especially when experimental drugs and surgery are involved, terminal patients should be informed about different outcomes and different ways of dying so that they can choose the "least worst death." At present, however, adequate information is rare, and thus genuine choice by patients is also rare. For Battin, the right to control the circumstances of one's own death is "the most important civil-rights issue" of the 1990s.[52]

Mercy

One of the most persuasive arguments for physician-assisted dying is the appeal to mercy. Observing another human being in untreatable pain howling like a wounded animal can move even the most callous of us to tears. The most natural response—the virtue that is called *compassion*—is to end such suffering. We do this for dogs, cats, or horses, so why can't we do the same for humans? Moreover, as has been described above (and will be described again later), the suffering of terminal patients is not confined to physical pain, as bad as that is: it also involves helplessness, stress, exhaustion, terror, loss, and other experiences that are wrenching even to imagine.

Mercy means different things to different people, however, and if we intend to be merciful, we will need to understand what each individual patient wants. To some patients, mercy may mean being helped to die. To others, mercy may simply mean relief of pain. To still others, it may mean reassurance—relief from the fear of becoming incompetent, or of living hooked up to machines, or simply of dying in a hospital. (For many people, dying in a hospital is indeed a terrible process; Alex Capron, a law professor, has noted, "The more you talk to people, the clearer it becomes that there is serious concern in this country about how we die. Medicine needs to respond much more clearly to the extended, frightening, and expensive process of death."[53]) And it should be remembered that to some, mercy may mean being supported and encouraged in their efforts to live—being offered treatment as long as there is a chance of survival.

As the medical ethicist K. Danner Clouser has said, "I think suicide can be moral and rational. It is not so in every instance. But one person's therapy is another's torture."[54]

Relief of Pain

One major issue of physician-assisted dying has to do with relief of pain. At first, this may appear to be a factual dispute among physicians about whether complete relief of brute, physical pain is possible. However, the actual issue is broader: what would ability, or inability, to relieve pain imply about physician-assisted death?

Let's begin with the narrower question of relieving pain itself. Joanne Lynn, a physician and hospice director, believes that no patient need die in pain:

> [Lynn] has cared for over 1,000 hospice patients, and only two of these patients seriously and repeatedly requested physician assistance in active euthanasia. Even these two patients did not seek another health care provider when it was explained that their requests could not be honored. New patients to hospice often state they want to "get it over with." At face value, this may seem a request for active euthanasia. However, these requests are often an expression of the patient's concerns regarding pain, suffering, and isolation, and their fears about whether their dying will be prolonged by technology. Furthermore, these requests may be attempts by the patient to see if anyone really cares whether he or she lives. Meeting such a request with ready acceptance could be disastrous for the patient who interprets the response as a confirmation of his or her worthlessness. Future research should systematically document the number of patients who prefer voluntary active euthanasia even in the supportive environment of hospice.[55]

Similarly, the physician Cicely Saunders, who founded St. Christopher's Hospice in London, says that patients there need never suffer pain.[56] She gives these patients a "Brompton cocktail"—a powerful brew of morphine, heroin, alcohol, and cocaine. (Note that British physicians do not worry about making terminally ill patients "drug addicts.")

On the other hand, Derek Humphrey of the Hemlock Society argues that "it is generally agreed that 10 percent of pain cannot be controlled. That is a lot of people."[57] It is also true that not everyone experiences pain in the same way, and a condition which would be acceptable to some patients might be intolerable to others.

A related question is not simply whether or to what extent pain can be relieved but what the cost of relief might be, and what costs are acceptable. In this context, we are not talking about financial costs: the issue is the cost to the patient's well-being. Powerful narcotics like the "Brompton cocktail" numb consciousness and can reduce patients to a vegetative state during their last months of life. In other words, patients must make a tradeoff between consciousness and relief of pain, and not every patient considers that tradeoff acceptable. For some patients, being conscious and able to talk with their families and friends is more important than avoiding pain. Here again, autonomy becomes relevant. What counts as a "benefit" or a "harm" must be defined within the each patient's own value system, and who else but the patients themselves can make judgments about this tradeoff?

A wider question, as noted above, is what relief of pain implies about physician-assisted dying. As we saw earlier in this chapter, leaders of the hospice movement believe that few if any patients would ask for assisted death if they were aware that hospice care could keep them free of pain. However, advocates of physician-assisted dying argue that pain is only one aspect of suffering and therefore that relieving a patient's pain does not necessarily relieve his or her suffering. *Pain* is physical; *suffering* is a broader and more personal matter.

Peter Admiraal, a physician and one of the leaders of assisted dying in the Netherlands, agrees that uncontrollable pain is rarely the only reason for death:

> . . . There is severe dehydration, uncontrolled itching and fatigue. These patients are completely exhausted. Some of them can't turn around in their beds. They become incontinent. All these factors make a kind of suffering from which they only want to escape. . . .
>
> And of course you are suffering because you have a mind. You are thinking about what is happening to you. You have fears and anxiety and sorrow. In the end, it gives a complete loss of human dignity. You cannot stop that feeling with medical treatment.[58]

The Role of Physicians

Physicians as healers   Some critics fear that physician-assisted dying may create a dangerous new role for physicians, conflicting with their traditional role as healers. The law professor and bioethicist George Annas, for one, has said that Jack Kevorkian is "on the lunatic fringe" and that it would be very difficult "to find one other doctor in the country who would support" him.[59] The physician Leon Kass has said of Kevorkian: "I feel the deepest shame for my profession that he should be counted a member."[60] Arthur Caplan testified against Kevorkian in a Michigan court as an expert witness on medical ethics.[61] The philosopher Daniel Callahan, who founded a bioethics think tank (the Hastings Center), said that Kevorkian's assistance was:

. . . a dangerous and wrong thing to do. I can't think of a single way to defend him. [Legalization of euthanasia] would add a whole fourth new category where private individuals would, in effect, be licensed to kill one another to relieve suffering. We don't want to expand the category where one could kill even in the name of mercy. It would change the nature of medicine and open the way to abuse. We are better off without such a law.[62]

The bioethicist Thomas Morawetz argues that "the patient is entitled to believe that the doctor is pursing his or her best interests and does not have divided loyalties."[63] He argues, further, that there is an imbalance of power in the physician-patient relationship, and one way of rectifying it is to insist that the physician's mission be focused on healing and on saving life. However, Morawetz begs the question of what constitutes a patient's "best interests"; he seems to assume that for every patient, the best interest is always "healing," but that of course is the point at dispute. Morawetz also seems to beg another question: why should we assume that forbidding assisted dying will rectify the imbalance of power he describes? If a patient wants to die and a physician forces him or her to live, wouldn't that increase the imbalance of power?

Some critics who support Morawetz see physicians as arrogant and as having too much control over their patients' lives and deaths; they argue that giving physicians the option to kill would vastly increase their power. Some physicians themselves think that medicine as a profession has difficulty controlling excesses by its members and that it would also have difficulty preventing abuses of assisted dying. Such objections are essentially practical rather than theoretical, however: it can be argued in response that, given adequate safeguards, these considerations would not necessarily compromise the role of physicians as healers.

Part of the real debate here is about the question, "What is medicine *for?*" Patients reply, "To help patients as they require help." Physicians may reply, "To heal," and they may add, "To advance the ideals of the profession of medicine and to uphold its professional norms." Patients' and physicians' replies can lead to the same results in some cases, but not all. If one ideal of medicine is the sanctity of life, for example, that might conflict with helping terminal patients die.

Physicians as patient advocates   Why aren't physicians "patient advocates"? Whose side are they on, and why aren't they on the side of their dying patients?

Why can't medicine ensure that patients will die as they want? If a patient cannot die painlessly, who is to blame? If a physician doesn't keep a patient free of pain, isn't that *patient abandonment?*

Why are so many patients afraid to enter a hospital? Why is there no guarantee of continuity of care? Why don't hospitalized patients trust their physicians to help them have a "good death"?

Questions like these arise because every month seems to bring a new case where physicians overrule the expressed wishes of a patient or family, and usually the patient and the family end up traumatized.[64] Let us consider some of the factors involved in the issue of physicians as patient advocates.

With regard to hospital care, for example, even if a patient has signed an advance directive and has designated a proxy, a relative can challenge the patient's decisions. Also, the hospital's risk manager as well as the patient's own physician will be expected to take steps to avoid lawsuits brought by family members. Additionally, a member of the nursing staff may oppose a decision to let a patient die. In many cases, the easiest thing for medical professionals to do is let the process of dying take its course, even though that may be precisely what the patient didn't want.

The general public, of course, wishes that physicians and hospitals would worry less about litigation and allow the patient to make his or her own decisions. In 1990, in a poll conducted by *USA Today,* 67 percent of Americans said that the terminally ill should be allowed to end their lives with assistance by physicians in medical facilities.[65] (These results were almost identical to those of a Roper poll in 1986.[66]) Most people feel that if the patient is a competent adult, the physician should do what the patient wants—no matter what that may be. They would like the physician to say, "After we've discussed these matters, I'll follow your wishes exactly, even if I personally don't agree with your decision and even if one of your family members threatens to sue me. My job is to do what you want and to respect your trust in me and the medical profession. I'll keep you free of pain, in control as much as possible, and if it comes to it, I'll help you die peacefully—even if it means taking somewhat active means. Even if I have to go to court, even if I need to fight my own hospital, and even if I must fight your family's lawyers, I'll be on your side."

These people also argue that physicians do not necessarily know best. Fifteen years ago, almost all physicians were as staunchly opposed to removing respirators as they now are to assisted dying: the medical profession held that removing a respirator would compromise the physician's role and violate "medical ethics." A few years later, the profession said the same thing about withdrawing nutrition and hydration. Could it be that physicians do not understand what their role should be and when they should change it?[67]

On this issue, medical opinion clearly differs from public opinion. Although physicians acknowledge the needs and suffering of dying patients, most of them resist any changes that would expand the physician's role to "patient advocacy" if that entailed killing. Part of their argument is that physicians should "do no harm";[68] but this begs the question of what constitutes "harm." If a patient requests assistance in dying, refusing to give that help may itself be "harm." Another factor in physicians' opposition seems to be reluctance to give up or share control. One review expresses a complaint by physicians that the public wants to "wrest control of the dying process from the healing professions."[69] This is perhaps unfortunately worded; it sounds as if a hypothetical physician is saying something like: "It is better for you, the dying patient, to die according to the natural processes of your disease than for me to change my role, because I am most comfortable with my role as it is now." An argument which would be at least more tactful is that physicians feel *responsible* for their patients and are disturbed by the idea of abdicating that responsibility. Finally, some physicians argue that they are not even needed for assistance in dying (or, to cite two other issues, for capital punishment or abortion); these physicians would permit "designated" technicians to provide assistance in dying.

On the evidence, it seems safe to conclude that most laypeople do not accept any of these arguments by the medical profession and would like to see physicians act more as patient advocates. Public opinion in general seems to be that the professionals who know the most about disease and dying should assist in death, that it is physicians who know most about disease and dying, that it is the job of physicians to help patients, and that therefore physicians should help terminally ill patients die as they wish.

•

With regard to the general debate over the role of physicians as healers or patient advocates, two final points should be noted. First, if the law allowed physician-assisted dying, this wouldn't mean that every physician in the United States would have to assist every patient who wanted to die. As with abortion, only a small percentage of physicians might actually be involved in assisted dying. Indeed, given the tendency toward specialization within American medicine, geriatrics might easily take over this function.

Second, the controversy about the role of physicians has perhaps focused too much on the quirky personality of Jack Kevorkian and not enough on the larger picture. Every year, over 2 million Americans die. Most of us will die of cancer, coronary artery disease, stroke, or one of the degenerative diseases. Despite all the newest drugs and all the medical advances, some of us will have a very bad death that medicine cannot do much to alleviate. On any given day—while people write articles about the pros and cons of physician-assisted dying and AMA resists it—hundreds of people are dying in a way they hate.

Jack Kevorkian may not be everybody's idea of the right physician to lead the movement for physician-assisted dying, and his motives may not always be entirely pure, but at least he is *doing* something. He is willing to think innovatively about the physician's role, he always takes the patient's side, and he is willing to criticize other physicians. Moreover, he doesn't expect anyone else to do the hard part. Other physicians who assist in dying simply write a prescription for a large dose of barbiturates and warn the patient or the family, with a wink, about "not taking the whole thing at once"; or they order a morphine drip to be started by the nursing staff at 3 A.M. If something goes wrong, they're at home asleep, and the patient must suffer until they're available. Kevorkian stays with his patients, making sure that things end as intended. He is not afraid of being called a "quack" by his medical colleagues or by bioethicists; he is undaunted by the accusation that he stays with his patients until the end because he enjoys watching people die; he seems unafraid of going to jail. Is he our medical Socrates?

Active versus Passive Euthanasia

Chapter 1 describes how medical practice in the United States has evolved to a point where most physicians feel ethically comfortable with forgoing or withdrawing treatment—including artificial nutrition—to hasten death in a terminal patient. However, "intentional termination" of a dying patient's life is still considered unethical by AMA and is also, of course, illegal. Homicide is a crime.

According to one bioethicist, Jack Kevorkian's assistance to Janet Adkins raised the question "whether there is any clear distinction between assisted suicide and active euthanasia."[70] In assisted suicide, as the term was being used in that passage, the patient ends his or her own life; in active euthanasia, the physician's action is the immediate cause of death. A leading physician in medical ethics has admitted, "I have had occasion to give a patient pain medication we both knew would shorten her life."[71] Is this much different from killing the patient? Most physicians now respect a patient's request to withdraw nutrition or hydration, but most would still resist doing anything *directly* to cause the death of the patient. This asymmetry assumes a profound difference between acting to withdraw treatment (with the intention of hastening death) and acting to actually cause death (with the same intention). Is there really any difference?—or, to put it another way, is the difference only semantic?

In 1975, in a famous article in the *New England Journal of Medicine,* the philosopher James Rachels attacked the distinction between "active" and "passive" euthanasia.[72] Rachels argued that this distinction, though still dominant in modern medicine and law, has no inherent moral value and that—when it is erroneously taken for anything more than a shorthand pragmatic rule—it leads to decisions about death based on irrelevant factors. Rachels's logic cuts two ways: first, letting a vegetative patient die is just as bad (or good) as killing him or her; second, killing a vegetative patient is just as good (or bad) as allowing him or her to die. There is nothing moral or immoral in the act of passive or active euthanasia itself; rather, morality or immorality is determined by motives and results in the context of that act. Focusing on whether an act is "active" or "passive," he argued, may confuse our judgments, leading us to think that passively "allowing" people to die slowly and horribly is morally superior to "actively" bringing about a quick, painless death.

Rachels's position was controversial. Is intending death by removing a respirator equivalent to suffocating a patient with a pillow? If a patient is "allowed to die," isn't that patient killed by the disease? But if someone acts directly to bring about dying, isn't that human agent the cause of death? One critic argued:

> What is the difference between merely letting a patient die and killing that patient? Does it depend upon activity or passivity? Does it depend on an agent's intentions? I think that neither of these factors is relevant. What is relevant is the cause of death. When the cause of death is the underlying disease process, the patient is simply allowed to die.[73]

In support of Rachels, it can be argued that in practice the line between "active" and "passive" is hard to draw. In some cases, *not* acting can be considered "active"; one example might be not giving antibiotics to Karen Quinlan to treat the pneumonia she developed in her final weeks. The neurologist and medical ethicist Ronald Cranford sees no great difference between letting die and killing and argues that "most medical professionals are just wrong on this issue." Cranford also holds that if the physician's motive is to relieve suffering in a dying patient, it is permissible to "kill."[74] However, this does not imply (as is sometimes feared) that there is no difference between killing and assisted dying; as Jean Davies argues, just as "rape and making love are different, so are killing and assisted suicide."[75]

The "Slippery Slope"

Opponents of physician-assisted dying sometimes argue that if it became an option, patients would feel pressured to choose it, since no one wants to become a burden on his or her family or on society. This concern raises the issue of a possible *slippery slope* in the context of assisted dying. (The slippery slope, introduced in Chapter 1, is also discussed above with regard to "euthanasia" in Nazi Germany.) A slippery-slope argument can refer to predicted, disastrous consequences ensuing from a major change in morality or to a line of reasoning that will follow from acceptance of certain premises. When it takes the form of predicting real-world consequences, a slippery-slope argument is often inductive, purportedly based on (though not always citing) concrete evidence. Both types of slippery-slope argument can be found in the debate on physician-assisted dying.

In 1987, the national columnist Nat Hentoff—a disability-rights advocate who opposes abortion and any kind of euthanasia or assisted suicide—expressed his concerns about the implications of the *Quinlan* decision.[76] Supporters of physician-assisted dying usually say that they are seeking this option only for patients who are adult, rational, dying, and "voluntary"; but Hentoff emphasized that in 1975 Karen Quinlan met none of these criteria. Later, in 1992, he described Jack Kevorkian's actions and the decriminalization of physician-assisted dying in the Netherlands as a "reckless cheapening of life."[77] Hentoff believes that we are now on a slippery slope:

> The September 1991 official government Remmelink Report on euthanasia in that country revealed that at least 1,040 people die every year from involuntary euthanasia. Their physicians were so consumed with compassion that they decided not to disturb the patients by asking their opinion on the matter.[78]

Similarly, some Dutch journalists claim that although assisted dying began with terminally ill patients, it soon expanded to nonterminal adult "voluntary" patients—people whose quality of life was destroyed by uncontrolled, gross swelling from cancer or advanced multiple sclerosis.[79] It also seems to have expanded to patients who are not adults: if children are dying, incurable, and in great pain, the Royal Dutch Medical Association has accepted that they have a right to die, even if their parents oppose it.[80]

Some people base slippery-slope arguments on the "idealization" of physician-assisted suicide in movies such as *Whose Life Is It, Anyway?* and *Dax's Case* (see Chapter 2). These people point out that such accounts show the "easy" cases: an unmarried patient without a family, obviously competent and unambivalent; no complicating factors; intense, unbearable pain. In typical actual situations, the patient's condition may not be definitively "terminal"; the patient may be ambivalent, confused, or unable to express or even identify his or her real needs; the patient's family or friends may have conflicting opinions; there may be financial problems (such as no insurance for long-term care in a nursing home); pain may not be "unbearable." Isn't there a slippery slope from the rare "easy" cases to the more ambiguous ones? In ambiguous cases, should physicians be allowed to assist dying without any opposition or confrontation?

Another slippery-slope argument has to do with motivation and coercion. The law professor Yale Kamisar observes that "not all people are kind, understanding, and loving. Yet they will be making decisions about the elderly and helpless. A lot of pressure may be placed on people to choose euthanasia when they really don't want it."[81] Norman Fost—a pediatrician and medical ethicist who maintains that in every society where physician-assisted suicide was legal it was applied too broadly and "the situation got out of control"[82]—argues that assisted dying "gives a doctor and the patient an easy out."

In this connection, some people fear that physicians will be pressured by skyrocketing medical costs into urging assisted dying on high-cost, low-benefit patients, mostly old and poor patients.[83] One medical historian says, "A good deal of the debate is about whether we could control all of the steps that might coerce or intimidate a patient."[84] These critics note that families can be financially crippled by the cost of supportive services for a dying or vegetative patient. They also note that cost containment has become a driving force in the American health care system;[85] is it wise to institute "managed care" and physician-assisted dying at the same time? Finally, they argue that much of modern-day medical ethics evolved during times of economic prosperity and fear that bad times—such as a worldwide depression—might motivate individuals and communities to accept or demand euthanasia in more and more situations. (Was it not a crumbling economy that presaged the rise of the Nazis in Germany?)

Still another slippery-slope argument is based on the idea that if physicians accede to assisted dying, what reason do we have to suppose that they would not soon *recommend* it? And once physicians began recommending assisted dying, how do we know that they—and others—would not try to make it mandatory? In the past, any number of public health measures that were initially simply recommended were eventually required. A related line of reasoning notes that in the last two decades, society has quickly legalized previously unacceptable ways of aiding death; the argument is that in time, more and more ways will become permissible. For instance, there is a "trickle down" argument that physician-assisted dying will loosen restrictions on nonphysicians.

Considerations of "quality of life" also lead to slippery-slope arguments. If quality of life justifies one kind of decision, it is argued, why not another? A spokesman for Right to Life says that if you "accept quality of life as the standard," then "first you withdraw the respirators, then the food and then you actively kill people. It's a straight line from one place to the others."[86] Daniel Callahan says that the logic of the case for euthanasia will inevitably lead to its extension far beyond terminally ill competent adults. If relief of suffering is critical, Callahan says, "why should that relief be denied to the demented or the incompetent?"[87] Several cases have been reported in the United States of nurses and aides in nursing homes deciding to kill dozens of their clients because of "low quality of life." In Vienna, Austria, in 1989, an aide was found to have killed at least 49 elderly patients in a nursing home by lethal injection or by forcing water into their lungs.[88] The cases of Elizabeth Bouvia and Larry McAfee in Chapter 2 might also make one pause. If quality of life becomes a standard for assisted dying, why wouldn't it also become a permissible standard for assisted *suicide*—applicable, that is, to people who are not dying but have chronic conditions that impair their quality of life? Why wouldn't it become permissible for people whose quality of life is impaired by nonmedical factors such as poverty?

Some critics offer a slippery-slope argument based on the possibility of prejudice. Suppose that physicians accepted or even recommended assisted dying; how do we know that some of them would not have overt or unconscious biases against certain groups of patients who have historically faced discrimination? Might physicians agree to help patients die, or recommend assisted dying, differentially for people of color, women, gay men, lesbians, Muslims, or Jehovah's Witnesses?

Supporters of physician-assisted dying reply that the metaphor of the slippery slope is inappropriate. They argue that assisted dying represents small readjustments which society can make without changing all our values about life and death; they also argue that it is alarmist to assume that physicians and families would be eager to kill patients. Furthermore, they point out that if any state legalized physician-assisted dying and abuses occurred, the law could be repealed; change is not necessarily final. (Remember Prohibition.)

Money

It is odd that in formal discussions of ethical issues in medicine, money rarely plays any but an abstract role. One emergency room physician, Norman Paradis, has bravely raised this issue, however.

Paradis describes the case of his father—a surgeon—who was diagnosed with pancreatic cancer, the most lethal and swift of all cancers.[89] Paradis's father told him that he had seen "physicians torture dying patients" and insisted that he wanted neither surgery nor chemotherapy. Norman Paradis assured his father that, as a physician, he knew what to do. He was sure that his strong, direct, professional-to-professional communication with his father's physicians was unequivocal: Make my father comfortable; do no more.

As soon as he left, however, his father was taken to surgery. Why? Because, Norman Paradis says, "consulting surgeons get paid thousands of dollars an hour when they 'decide' to operate." When the younger Paradis called to refuse his consent for further surgery, he was told that his decision was "mistaken." His father underwent further, massive surgery and died the next day. Medicare paid more than $150,000 for these operations. When Norman Paradis objected to Medicare officials, claiming that his father's physicians had proceeded without consent and had violated proper procedures, he was told that there were so many cases of fraud over $1 million that they could not be bothered with his case. Paradis concludes, "Our health system is structured to meet reimbursement rather than patients' needs."

Perhaps the surgeons in this case were genuinely convinced that surgery was an acceptable risk and in the patient's best interest, but perhaps they were guilty of a conflict of interest. If it is fair to argue against physician-assisted dying by pointing out that some families and institutions may seize the advantage to save money, it is also fair to note that some physicians and institutions make millions by maintaining the status quo. Isn't it possible that some specialists could lose enormous amounts of money if assisted dying were practiced? And if so, might they not have a conflict of interest in opposing assisted dying?

In most areas of life, we assume that people work for money, and we give them monetary incentives to work harder. When it comes to physicians, we assume that they will be moral and will not recommend treatments only to make money. Perhaps most of them don't. However, when a reasonable case can be made for denying treatment, treatment is often administered anyway—and the physician makes more money. Is this just a coincidence, or is there some connection?

UPDATE

In 1991, voters in the state of Washington narrowly defeated a measure that would have allowed physicians to assist in requested suicide of a patient diagnosed as terminally ill by two independent physicians. The Hemlock Society, which had championed the bill, felt that it was defeated partly by an intense campaign by Catholic bishops and partly by a negative reaction among some voters to the methods practiced by Jack Kevorkian. A few years earlier, a similar proposal had been narrowly defeated in California. On December 15, 1992, the governor of Michigan signed a law making assisted suicide illegal there as of March 30, 1993—a date that would soon be moved forward to February 28, 1993.

•

Only a few hours before the Michigan bill was signed into law, Jack Kevorkian had helped his seventh and eighth patients—both women—to die. He vowed to disobey the new law against assisted dying, saying that it was "immoral" and that his actions were "on a higher plane." During 1993, Kevorkian assisted in the death of several more patients, including one physician, bringing his total to 20 (the five cases that took place after the Michigan law went into effect will be described later). Not all these patients were terminally ill, but they all suffered from conditions which they found intolerable and for which medicine could offer little help. For example, Hugh Gale, age 70, was suffering from end-stage emphysema and congestive heart disease. Gale's wife said that he "was in terrible pain, [was] on 100 percent oxygen, could not walk, and could not go out of the house";[90] with Kevorkian's guidance, Gale inhaled carbon monoxide. Kevorkian did take some respites; he sometimes said that he was becoming exhausted from helping so many people die, and that being present as his patients died took too much out of him.

During the spring of 1993, Kevorkian received some especially intense criticism. The physician Timothy Quill said, "Suicide is the sole basis for the relationship he has with his patients, and that is frightening."[91] One politician in Michigan expressed the attitude of the legislature as, "Hit the road, Jack, and don't you come back no more, no more." Some people called him "Dr. Death" and "Jack the Dripper." Kevorkian's bitter foe, the Oak County prosecutor Richard Thompson, called him "Jeffrey Dahmer in a lab coat" and said that his cases "prove the impossibility of ever regulating assisted suicide. Even in the Netherlands, physicians abuse it."[92] Thompson, a conservative Republican, had twice prosecuted

Kevorkian for murder, once in the Adkins case and later in 1991 (though, as we have seen, these charges were dismissed); and it was Thompson who emerged as Kevorkian's most fanatical prosecutor.

However, Kevorkian found allies among many ordinary people. His neighbors in Royal Oak, Michigan, support him ("We all love him at the library," one librarian has said[93]); and one poll suggested that two-thirds of the public might accept well-regulated physician-assisted suicide.[94] Kevorkian had also found a powerful ally in his lawyer, Geoffrey Fieger, who proved himself capable of responding in kind to these attacks when his client could not. Fieger called Governor John Engler, who had attacked Kevorkian, "a truly goofy, stupid man, certifiably evil."[95] He called one judge who tried to stop Kevorkian "a vile malignant legal lunatic." Lawyers who have faced Fieger in court call him, respectfully, "a very dangerous adversary."

Fieger understood that politicians and physicians in Michigan, as anywhere, did not want to be the first to accept physician-assisted dying; they wanted someone else to grapple with the problem, leaving them to get on with their normal lives and work. But Fieger insisted that settling this issue is the responsibility of politicians and physicians, not of dying patients, and so he had devised a strategy that would hold the feet of Michigan politicians to a media "fire." He had counseled Kevorkian to continue assisting deaths as long as he was free (especially in the jurisdiction of the hostile prosecutor Richard Thompson), and to go on a hunger strike if he was imprisoned. Bit by bit, Fieger painted his client's opponents into a corner, forcing a trial: they would have to allow Kevorkian to assist in more and more deaths (some of these deaths took place only two blocks from a police station) or would have to face Fieger and Kevorkian in a trial that would receive national attention. "The gauntlet is down," Fieger said. "It is ending now. Either this immoral law ends or Dr. Kevorkian's life does."[96] Fieger carefully arranged dramatic "media events": later, for instance, when Kevorkian was indeed about to be jailed, a reporter for the *New York Times* watched as Kevorkian ate breakfast at a pancake house (a single scrambled egg, ham, toast, and coffee); "You may well be looking at his last meal," Fieger said ominously.[97]

As noted above, five of Kevorkian's cases—involving his sixteenth through twentieth patients—took place after the Michigan law had gone into effect. The sixteenth patient was Ron Masur, on May 16, 1993, in Wayne County. Charges were brought against Kevorkian for helping Ron Masur die, but Wayne County Judge Cynthia Stephens dismissed them, finding the new law unconstitutional on a technicality. Her decision was appealed; the Michigan Court of Appeals heard the case in January 1994 and reinstated the law until its own ruling, which was not expected for many months. Geoffrey Fieger continued seeking a way to resolve the issue, preferably by a public trial.

On August 4, 1993, Kevorkian assisted in the death of his seventeenth case; where this death actually occurred would become an issue later. This seventeenth patient was Thomas Hyde, a 30-year-old in the last stages of Lou Gehrig's disease, amyotrophic lateral sclerosis. Immediately, Kevorkian explicitly admitted, and described in great detail, his role in Thomas Hyde's death; impatient with criticism by other physicians that he should wait until assisted dying became legal, he said:

[Physicians are] politicians first, businessmen second, and they ought to be ashamed of themselves to [let] human beings like Thomas Hyde suffer immensely. . . . [Hyde is] unable to move any muscle, [he] cannot speak, [he] cannot swallow, [and he has] pain in addition to all that. . . . [Physicians] turn their heads because "we've got to discuss this a little more."[98]

Referring to a widespread belief that the Michigan law was unconstitutional, Geoffrey Fieger said, "This is a deliberate decision on our part to end this equivocation."[99] Kevorkian was charged with assisted suicide, and Fieger, citing his client's right to a speedy trial, pressed for a jury trial in Wayne County. On September 9, 1993, Judge Willie Lipscomb agreed to go to trial in the Hyde case.

That same night—September 9—in Wayne County, Kevorkian assisted in the death of his eighteenth patient, Donald O'Keefe, who was 73 and suffering from bone cancer. He was also charged with assisted suicide in the O'Keefe case.

As Wayne County pushed back the date for his trial in the Hyde case from September 1993 to February 1994 (it eventually opened in April 1994), Kevorkian turned up the heat in another county—Oakland, where his own apartment was. On October 22, 1993, he assisted in the death of his nineteenth patient in his apartment: the patient was Merian Ruth Frederick of Ann Arbor, a prominent state Democrat who was deteriorating badly from amyotrophic lateral sclerosis; her body was found by the police in the apartment that same day.[100] On November 8, 1993, Kevorkian was charged with assisted suicide in Oakland County, in the Frederick case.

Meanwhile, in Wayne County—still in November 1993—Kevorkian refused to post $20,000 bail in the Hyde case, and Judge Thomas Jackson ordered him jailed. Kevorkian fasted for 3 days in the Wayne County jail, but then one of his opponents (Jack DeMoss, a lawyer) posted the bail to reduce the publicity the case was generating. (Kevorkian's opponents were aware of Fieger's strategy and scrambled to prevent Kevorkian from becoming a martyr.)

On November 23, 1993, while out on bail, Kevorkian assisted (in Oakland County) at the death of his twentieth patient—Ali Khali, a physician who specialized in pain control but was now himself suffering uncontrollable pain. Khali had bone cancer, and although he wore a morphine pump his condition was described as like having fractures in 500 different parts of the body, each fracture causing ceaseless pain 24 hours a day. He had already attempted suicide unsuccessfully (by inhaling carbon dioxide in his garage), and didn't trust any of his colleagues on his own medical faculty to help him die.[101]

On November 30, 1993, Kevorkian was arraigned in Oakland County for the assisted suicide of Merian Frederick, refused to post bail of $50,000, and was again jailed—now in Oakland County jail, where he again began fasting. This time, no one else posted bail for him (partly because it was not certain that the man who had posted bail the first time would get his money back).

Meanwhile, in Wayne County, on December 14, 1993—at a hearing requested by Kevorkian's lawyer, and while the ruling by the court of appeals was still pending—Chief Judge Richard Kaufman voided the Michigan law against assisted suicide: "When a person's quality of life is significantly impaired by a medical condition and the medical condition is extremely unlikely to improve," that person has a "constitutionally protected right" to commit suicide, provided the decision is reasonable and not made under duress. Kaufman explicitly dropped the charges against Kevorkian in the O'Keefe case; however, Kevorkian remained in jail in Oakland County until December 17, when his bail was reduced from $50,000 to $100 by a higher-court judge after an appeal by Geoffrey Fieger. Kevorkian now left jail for the second time, having promised not to assist at any more suicides until the court of appeals had ruled.

At about the same time, Oakland County Judge Jessica Cooper also voided the Michigan law (she was the third judge in Michigan to decide against it). Cooper also dismissed the two most recent charges against Kevorkian: those in the Frederick and Khali cases. Thus the only remaining charges were those in the Hyde case—the charges that had been sought by Kevorkian and Fieger to bring about a public trial.

Jack Kevorkian's trial opened in April 1994. Thomas Hyde, as mentioned above, had Lou Gehrig's disease; in its final stages he could barely walk, talk, or feed himself. Several medical experts testified that, without Kevorkian's assistance, Thomas Hyde would have "strangled to death on his own saliva."[102] In his defense, Kevorkian did not admit that he had intended to cause the death of Thomas Hyde; he said that he had intended to end his patient's intolerable suffering. Kevorkian was acquitted, partly because some jurors accepted that defense, partly because other jurors felt that the law has no business forcing terminally ill patients to suffer by forbidding physicians to help them[103]—and partly because there was some doubt about exactly where Hyde had died and thus about whether or not Wayne County actually had jurisdiction in this case.

At the end of this episode, there was probably hardly an adult left in the United States who did not know about Kevorkian and his crusade. Kevorkian had moved the issue of physician-assisted dying from hushed private discussions among physicians, patients, and families to a national debate. There too, however, was the rub: by then, physician-assisted suicide had become firmly associated with the personality of Jack Kevorkian, and some supporters of assisted death were afraid that this would hurt their cause. Kevorkian himself has said, "Because there is no rational argument against physician-assisted dying, my opponents focus on me."[104] On the other hand, many supporters of physician-assisted death believe that the subject has always needed to be discussed, not in whispers at bedsides, but by ordinary people—at work, at lunch, with their families, with their colleagues. These supporters sometimes say that it was precisely by becoming a focus of the media, a thorn in the side of medicine, and even an object of ridicule that Jack Kevorkian helped break the taboo against public discussion.

•

There have been continuing legal developments, of course. In Canada, a famous case was that of Sue Rodriquez, a 43-year-old victim of Lou Gehrig's disease who led a campaign in 1993 to legalize physician-assisted death. Her appeal went to the Canadian supreme court, where she lost narrowly on a 5-4 vote: the court held that the sanctity of life outweighed individual autonomy and freedom from suffering. According to a Gallup poll, however, 77 percent of Canadians supported Sue Rodriquez's right to die. After the decision, she did kill herself, reportedly with a physician's help.[105]

In the spring of 1994, the Michigan Court of Appeals declared the state's ban on assisted suicide unconstitutional on technical grounds; however, it also ruled that there was no constitutional right to suicide or assisted suicide. In a separate decision, the appeals court reinstated the murder charges against Jack Kevorkian for the deaths of two women in 1991. Whether prosecutors would again be willing to try Kevorkian before skeptical juries remained to be seen.

Within a few days of the Michigan decision, a federal district judge, Barbara Rothstein, struck down a law in Washington state banning assisted suicide.[106] Judge Rothstein held that the Fourteenth Amendment to the Constitution, protecting individual liberty, was broad enough to cover not only a woman's right to end a pregnancy but also the right of a terminally ill patient to assisted suicide.

In the Netherlands, there have been two significant developments. First, on June 1, 1994, amendments to the Act for the Disposal of the Dead became law. Essentially, "voluntary notification" by physicians now became mandatory, and criteria for nonprosecution became statutory rather than case law; the practical effect of this legislation is to make physician-assisted death an exception to homicide.[107] There is also now a standard form to be filled out by physicians, including a 28-point checklist.

Second, on June 21, 1994, the Dutch supreme court ruled on the case of the doctor who had been charged with murder (in May 1993) after helping a depressed patient—the woman mentioned earlier, whose two sons had died and whose marriage had failed—commit suicide. The court refused to punish the physician in this case, evidently having concluded that the guidelines had been followed: among other criteria, that the patient had been suffering intolerable pain and had repeatedly asked to die, and that the physician's conscience gave no choice but to end the patient's life. The physician's lawyer said that this ruling had established the principle that mercy killings were allowed in cases of mental suffering.[108]

FURTHER READING

Margaret Pabst Battin, *The Least Worst Death: Essays in Bioethics at the End of Life*, Oxford University Press, New York, 1993.

Lisa Belkin, "There's No Simple Suicide," *New York Times Magazine*, November 14, 1993.

Howard Brody, "Assisted Death—A Compassionate Response to a Medical Failure," *New England Journal of Medicine*, vol. 327, no. 19, November 5, 1992, pp. 1384–1388.

Willard Gaylin, Leon Kass, Edmund Pellegrino, and Mark Seigler, "Commentary: Doctors Must Not Kill," *Journal of the American Medical Association*, vol. 259, no. 14, April 8, 1988, pp. 2139–2140.

James Humber, Robert Almeder, and Gregg Kasting, eds., *Physician-Assisted Death: Biomedical Ethics Reviews, 1993*, Humana, Totowa, N. J., 1994.

G. E. R. Lloyd, "Introduction," *Hippocratic Writings*, J. Chadwick and W. N. Mann, trans., Penguin, New York, 1978 (trans. 1950).

PART TWO

Classic Cases about the Beginning of Life

CHAPTER 4

In Vitro Fertilization

Louise Brown

This chapter discusses the ethical controversies surrounding the birth of Louise Brown in 1978, following a "test tube" conception, and some issues that emerged later. "Test tube" conception is less emotionally called *in vitro*—"in glass"—*fertilization* (IVF). It involves fertilization outside the womb, in a petri dish, and it is part of a new field called *assisted reproduction*. As some wit remarked about IVF, people already knew how to have sex without making babies, and then they discovered how to make babies without having sex.

A few definitions will clarify our discussion in this chapter (and in Chapters 5 and 6). In human embryology, a successful union of sperm and egg is called a *zygote*. After conception, a zygote immediately begins dividing: it first divides into 2 cells, which then divide to form 4 cells, which then divide to form 8 cells, and so on. At the stage when this organism travels down the fallopian tubes to the uterus, it is often called a *preembryo*. When it attaches to the uterine wall and attempts to grow there, it is called an *embryo*. In an *ectopic pregnancy*, the preembryo does not reach the uterus but instead starts to grow in one of the two fallopian tubes; for the mother, this is a life-threatening condition. From 9 weeks of gestation until birth, the organism is called a *fetus*. A newborn human being, alive outside the womb, is by custom and law called a *baby*.

Conception takes place when a sperm fertilizes an egg. A fairly common but mistaken belief is that this happens in the woman's vagina or uterus. In fact, sperm move up the vagina, through the uterus, and into the narrow fallopian tubes. The fallopian tubes, which are the size of a thin lead stick in a mechanical pencil, carry one egg each month from the ovaries to the uterus. Conception occurs in the upper third of a tube, when the first sperm penetrates the egg. Then, the fertilized egg (now called a *zygote* or *preembryo*) descends the last two-thirds of the tube on its way to the uterus. Three days later, it tries to implant itself on the uterine wall. In at least 40 percent of pregnancies (and possibly as many as 70 percent), the preembryo aborts, probably because half or more of all preembryos have some chromosomal (genetic) irregularities.[1]

BACKGROUND: IVF

Infertility and Its Treatment

According to a 1982 government survey, about 1 in 6 American couples are infertile.[2] However, a more accurate estimate is that 1 married couple in 12 cannot conceive a child after 1 year of trying. Infertility stems from many factors, including the woman's age at the first attempt to conceive (older women are more likely to have difficulty conceiving), damage from pelvic inflammatory disease (PID), previous abortions, uterine abnormalities, and (on the part of the man) a low sperm count. Infertility is often blamed on the woman, but men actually account for 50 percent of it.

At one time, infertile couples simply had to resign themselves to being "barren"; essentially, their only alternative was adoption. Today, adopting a healthy baby has become more and more difficult. In 1973, when abortion was first legalized, 82,800 babies were available for adoption; in 1982, the number had dropped to 50,700.[3] Between 1982 and 1986, the number of babies adopted per year decreased by 37,000, partly because more single mothers kept their babies.[4] Two million American couples now seek the 22,000 white babies available for adoption each year.[5] In states with low minority populations and many college students (such as Vermont), signs with offers to adopt babies appear in bars and laundromats in virtually every town.

Fortunately, treatments for infertility have been developed. To begin with, physicians rule out underlying diseases and counselors consider possible sexual dysfunctions. A woman is instructed to take her basal body temperature daily, in order to predict the exact day (even the hour) of ovulation. Couples are told to have timely, rather than frequent, intercourse because frequent sex lowers the sperm count per ejaculate (to maximize sperm count, 24 hours should elapse between ejaculations). In some cases (though these are rare), couples may even have intercourse in a room next door to a physician's office. One woman who became pregnant after 9 years of such measures observed:

> The whole experience is very degrading. . . . Your whole private life is open, you even carry around jars of sperm. The doctors tell you when to have sex and when not to. And then after sex, everyone comes into the examining room to take a peek and see how successful you were.[6]

If these initial techniques do not result in conception, various tests are performed: to see if the woman's ovaries are releasing mature eggs, if the man's sperm count is normal, if the sperm are able to reach the egg, and if the lining of the woman's uterus is hormonally "prepared" for implantation of an embryo. (Artificial insemination by donor, AID, is an option if infertility results from problems with the man's sperm.)

If necessary, the next step is to take x-rays to detect blockages in the fallopian tubes. In a small percentage of cases, microsurgery can repair damaged tubes by removing blockages. If the tubes are found to be healthy, artificial insemination by husband (AIH) will be tried: after masturbation, the man's sperm may be concentrated and then placed well up in the uterus.

The next measure, with most couples who still need help, is for the woman to receive a follicle-stimulating hormone (preferably pergonal), which causes multiple eggs to ripen and thus increases her chance of conceiving; this method will be successful about 60 percent of the time.

For couples who remain unsuccessful, the last hope is some form of IVF—the method that began in 1978, when Louise Brown became the first child conceived in vitro.

The Doctors: Steptoe and Edwards

The obstetrician Patrick Steptoe and the physiologist Robert Edwards helped the Browns conceive Louise.

Edwards, the physiologist, came from a working-class family. In his early twenties, after military service, he went back to college, but he did not excel there. At 26, he found himself in Edinburgh, broke and with not much of an academic future. Luckily, however, he was accepted for a course in genetics, which at that time—the early 1950s—was just beginning to become a robust specialty. When he went on to earn his doctorate in animal genetics at the University of Edinburgh, he worked at the "Mouse House" trying to fertilize mouse eggs. Later, he received an appointment at Cambridge University.

Edwards's contributions to reproductive physiology are especially remarkable because he worked in such crude facilities: in 1980, his lab at Cambridge did not even have running hot water. Moreover, he not only made important new discoveries but also had to disprove several assumptions about fertilization that had been accepted as "facts."

Edwards discovered that successful conception requires delicate, precise timing of interacting hormones. Once he knew this, he studied preovulatory mouse eggs dividing their chromosomes in preparation for fertilization, and he found that chromosomal division is precise and uniform:

> The chromosomes then moved like soldiers through a prepared drill. First they marched to the center of the egg, then out to the periphery. Next they slowly separated into two equal halves as they glided along a spindle. As if to inaudible military music, one half marched out of the egg forever and into a small body known as the first polar body. The other half remained in the egg. The purpose of their maneuvers was to prepare the egg for fertilization and the precision of it all, as we peered through the microscope, was breathtaking.[7]

The first accepted "fact" dethroned by Edwards was the notion that gonadotrophic hormones could not make a mammalian ovary release eggs. Eventually, Edwards became able to predict to the hour when application of hormones would produce ovulation. He could then give infertile women a carefully balanced mixture of the hormones progesterone and estrogen, which the ovaries normally release to thicken the uterine lining to receive a fertilized egg. (If no egg appears, these hormones decrease.)

A second "fact" Edwards disproved had to do with capacitation of sperm. Human sperm must be *capacitated* for conception; that is, chemicals that inhibit penetration of an egg must be removed from the head of a sperm. Most scientists believed that capacitation required exposure to uterine secretions. But one night in 1965, in his lab, Edwards collected his own semen and, on an impulse, added it to a ripe human egg in a dish. The next morning, when he looked through his microscope to see if anything had happened, he saw the characteristic cell division of human embryology: a zygote had been created.

Edwards soon stopped the process, and he was not able to reproduce this accidental success when, later, he repeatedly tried to do so. Nor did he announce his discovery, probably because he had not been able to repeat it, and possibly because he was worried (as later critics of IVF would also be) about such casual creation and termination of human life. Nevertheless, a human life had started to form outside the womb.

Patrick Steptoe, the obstetrician who helped the Browns, had often encountered infertile couples:

> There were men who, fearful that they were sterile, became impotent. There were women who, desperate, tried folk remedies, prayed long hours in a darkened room, or visited special shrines.[8]

Steptoe perfected an instrument called a *laparoscope* to remove eggs for fertilization outside the fallopian tubes. His contribution was based on fiber optics—extremely thin tubes equipped with tiny lights and cameras that can inspect interior body cavities. Fiber optics revolutionized certain fields of medicine (such as gastroenterology), since previously, physicians could only infer from external signs what was going on inside or—worse—operate to have a look; and this new technology was a factor in the development of infertility assistance.

With Lesley Brown, Steptoe slipped a laparoscope through a small slit at her "bikini line" and guided it into her ovaries, where he searched among the hundreds of eggs for the one being primed for ovulation. Searching for it was difficult enough; but when he found it, he had to insert another thin tube and suction it out. Without Steptoe's perfection of this delicate procedure, IVF would have been impossible.

LOUISE BROWN'S BIRTH

Lesley Brown, the mother of the first child conceived in vitro, grew up unhappily, without much of a family. Her father had left when she was born, and her mother placed her in a state home at an early age. She grew up in Bristol, a port on England's western coast with severe unemployment and widespread illiteracy. In 1963, like many other British teenagers, Lesley dropped out of high school and took a job in a factory. She was later laid off, but by then she had met her future husband, John Brown. A few months after that, they were living together; Lesley had a new job in a cheese factory, and John drove a truck.

John was 7 years older than Lesley. His first wife had run off with another man, leaving him with a daughter, and he was reluctant to remarry. Lesley wanted children, however, and when she and John decided to have a child, John said he would "do the right thing" if she became pregnant. Despite some rocky episodes, they were married; but after 9 years of trying, Lesley never became pregnant. The couple tried to adopt a baby, but babies were scarce.

It was later found that Lesley Brown's fallopian tubes had been severely damaged by ectopic pregnancies several years earlier. (The Browns had been unaware of this damage, which was not discovered until an obstetrician eventually injected dye into Lesley's tubes.) When she was told that the condition of her fallopian tubes made conception unlikely, Lesley (like many infertile women) felt that she was to blame: "I might have done something that had caused the trouble with my fallopian tubes."[9] She felt depressed when other women talked about their children, and she saw a future of "years of just weighing and packing cheese and coming back to a quiet, empty flat." John Brown said that her infertility didn't matter to him; but after almost a decade of trying to conceive, Lesley said that she wouldn't blame him if he abandoned her for a fertile woman.

Then Lesley Brown became a patient of Patrick Steptoe. The Browns traveled to Oldham, the small, bleak city in northern England where Steptoe practiced. Oldham was not the kind of place where medical breakthroughs might be envisioned:

> Early the following morning, we walked up the hill that led to Oldham General Hospital. It was winter in a strange, bleak town and no one was about. We passed open spaces, with buildings flattened by bulldozers or bombs, and great empty mills, still standing, with their windows smashed, leaving dark, gaping holes like wounds.[10]

Newsweek would later describe the hospital as a "cluster of Victorian buildings that were originally a Dickensian workhouse."[11]

Steptoe began his treatment of Lesley Brown by removing an egg from her ovaries with a laparoscope as described above. Then John Brown's semen was introduced to her egg in a petri dish containing a culture fluid of salt, potassium chloride, glucose, and a bit of protein. Examination by microscope revealed that a sperm had penetrated the ovum. Next, the resulting preembryo was cultured for $2\frac{1}{2}$ days. Then the preembryo was mixed with a supportive fluid, put in a syringe that looked something like a turkey baster, and squeezed through Lesley's dilated cervix into her uterus.

In late 1977, Steptoe gave the Browns a Christmas present by telling them that Lesley was pregnant. Before this, many women had had eggs successfully fertilized in vitro; a smaller number had had eggs implanted with a resulting pregnancy. But of the few who had become pregnant, each had lost the embryo or (within a few months) the fetus. Now a long wait began to see if Lesley too would lose her fetus. At 5 months, however, amniocentesis showed a normal pregnancy.

Lesley Brown developed some minor problems during pregnancy: she had a mild case of toxemia (a metabolic disturbance caused by absorption of bacteria at the laparoscopy site); also, the baby was slightly small. She spent the last month of her pregnancy at Oldham Hospital, which by then was under siege by the media.

The baby, a girl, was delivered by cesarean section on July 25, 1978. (After the amniocentesis, Steptoe had known that the fetus was female, but the Browns had chosen not to know its sex.) To protect the family's privacy, the delivery took place at night (slightly before midnight), with only a few people present. A BBC film team in Oldham was still negotiating with the hospital when Steptoe announced that the birth would occur in minutes. By this time, Lesley Brown had begun to realize how special her child's birth was going to be. She left her hospital room in darkness; nurses held flashlights as she walked to the delivery room. "Dozens of policemen and security officers lined every corridor as I walked along. It felt as if I was moving in a dream."[12]

The Browns called their baby Louise Joy. She weighed 5 pounds 12 ounces, was entirely normal, and was described as "beautiful, with a marvelous complexion, not red and wrinkly at all."[13] Immediately after her birth, John Brown said, "For a person who's been told he and his wife can never have children, the pregnancy was 'like a miracle.' I felt 12 feet high."[14]

ETHICAL ISSUES

The Media and the Story

The day after Louise Brown's birth, the London newspapers had huge banner headlines—"IT'S A GIRL!" "THE LOVELY LOUISE!" "BABY OF THE CENTURY!" "JOY TO THE WORLD!"—and the *New York Times* gave the story front-page coverage for 3 days. These headlines were exuberant, but media coverage of the Browns' story had some disturbing aspects.

One disturbing development was the intensity of the coverage. Months into Lesley Brown's pregnancy, word had leaked out that a "test tube" baby would be born in Oldham. Interest in the story was to be expected, but during the last weeks of the pregnancy, and as the birth approached, the integrity of some journalists vanished. One American reporter telephoned a fake bomb threat to the hospital, hoping that it would force Lesley Brown outside; in the ensuing evacuation, one pregnant woman went into labor. Another reporter disguised himself as a priest and approached John Brown, asking to be admitted and offering to comfort Lesley. Throngs of Japanese photographers constantly photographed anyone—man or woman—who left Oldham Hospital, on the off chance that someone might be Lesley Brown. When someone at the hospital revealed that the birth was imminent, six reporters for the *National Enquirer* left Florida and within 24 hours were at Oldham Hospital trying to buy worldwide rights to the Browns' story from Steptoe; and a bidding war started among English tabloids. The *Enquirer* also tried to bribe an administrator, offering $100,000 for details about the birth. After the birth, there were daily headlines of rumors ("TEST TUBE BABY ALMOST DIES"). Lesley Brown was urged not to watch television or read newspapers, and—to escape the scrutiny of telescopic lenses—not to go near the windows.

Another disturbing aspect of the coverage was its sensationalism and inaccuracy. Steptoe and Edwards had refused to be interviewed by reporters. (Although everybody wanted to know the Browns' identity and background, Steptoe had initially protected their anonymity. He did not want Lesley Brown to be upset; he also wanted to act as a go-between to get the Browns a trust fund for their baby, as he eventually did—reportedly $100,000 for an exclusive story.) This silence on the part of Steptoe and Edwards frustrated reporters, some of whom took liberties in their stories or simply guessed at the facts. *Newsweek* said, for instance: "Steptoe, 65, is a flamboyant and somewhat mysterious figure; he declines to discuss his origins (reported to be in Eastern Europe)."[15] In fact, Steptoe was born in Witney (near staid Oxford), had been educated in London at King's College and St. George's Medical School, was married, and had two children. The "flamboyant" physician lived the life of an overworked obstetrician at a county hospital in an English industrial city.

Newsweek also wrote that Edwards often commuted "in the company of a rabbit that was serving as traveling receptacle for an egg under study."[16] But Edwards himself writes:

> We transferred some fertilized human eggs into rabbits to see if they would grow there, but they didn't. This brief episode with rabbits led to all sorts of rumours in the press and elsewhere, and to a description of me taking hundreds of embryos to Cambridge, and of Patrick driving his Mercedes through Oldham with a rabbit in the seat next to him![17]

Sensationalistic reporting had harmed Edwards before the Brown story. (One reason why he refused interviews was his belief that he had been harmed by British television when his work was discussed on a documentary which opened with pictures of an atom bomb exploding.) In previous years, Edwards had worked on infertility at the National Institute for Medical Research in London, experimenting with surgically excised ovaries which he bathed in hormones in an attempt to induce the release of eggs. After an alarmist report on a television show, the institute suspended his funding to avoid controversy. Edwards claims that his scientific supervisor, who had herself frozen sperm, flatly told him his work was "unethical";[18] and that when she was asked "Why?" she would say only, "Because it is." Edwards then left for Cambridge University, where he worked partially on a Ford Foundation grant to study population control and fertility. In 1974, the Ford Foundation stopped funding Edwards's work; the official reason was that his work did not promote population control, but Edwards claims that it was also because his work offended some people.

The press incorrectly called Louise Brown a "test tube baby." This term implied to many people that something bizarre had occurred—that a baby had been created without egg or sperm. Later, when Lesley Brown took her baby outside, neighbors who had absorbed this impression of IVF from the media would peer into the carriage, expecting to see something abnormal, a little monster.

In fact, from the beginning of its coverage of the Browns' story, the press had tended to equate any new means of overcoming infertility with "genetic manipulation" and had worried about the creation of mindless slaves and dangerous superhumans. In 1977, in *Who Shall Play God?* the sensationalistic writer Jeremy Rifkin began a decade of self-serving opposition to all new reproductive techniques. Rifkin decried any kind of assisted reproduction as evil, as "genetic engineering," which he defined as "artificial manipulation of life."[19] Rifkin was not alone; the chief editor at the *London Times,* for instance, equated in vitro fertilization with state-controlled eugenics. (In contrast, John Brown saw in vitro fertilization merely as "helping nature along a bit.")

Countless articles and television reports about "genetic manipulation" appeared; and Aldous Huxley's novel *Brave New World,* written in 1932, was constantly cited by journalists as having predicted the kind of results they were now deploring—a future in which governments would use technology to control reproduction. This view of *Brave New World* was somewhat muddled: the controls Huxley had imagined were based mainly on psychological conditioning and need to be seen in the context of behaviorism, a school of psychology which was then as feared and misunderstood as IVF seemed to be in 1978. The extension of Huxley's fictional ideas about psychological manipulation to "genetic manipulation," and then to IVF—which is not genetic manipulation at all—was slipshod and misleading. Moreover, there was an ironic aspect to these citations of *Brave New World,* since Huxley had described the devastating consequences of loss of choice by individuals, and media arguments that IVF should be banned amounted to saying that couples should be denied a choice in this matter.

The media and journalists often consider themselves guardians of the public interest, but in the case of Louise Brown, many of them did not distinguish themselves. *Quis custodiet ipsos custodes?*—Who guards the guardians?

IVF as a Religious Issue

Scientists see infertility as due mainly to problems of mechanics (blocked tubes) and chemistry (hormones). In contrast, some people feel that infertility is a punishment for sin, imposed by God. Abortions and sexually transmitted diseases contribute to infertility; from these facts, some people conclude that infertile women and men are being punished for their past behavior. Similarly, scientists may see IVF as a medical treatment like any other, whereas religious observers may take other viewpoints.

Let us look at some religious—specifically, Christian—views on this issue: those of the Vatican, Augustine, Joseph Fletcher, and Paul Ramsey. These views differ radically on the ethics of assisted reproduction and exemplify the difficulty of discovering "the" Christian position on any issue in medical ethics.

Catholic views: The Vatican and Augustine   In 1978, the year of Louise Brown's birth, the Vatican condemned in vitro fertilization; and one Catholic priest in New York feared that humanity had slipped from "doctoring the patient to doctoring the race." Lest that condemnation be thought of as merely the hasty reaction of just one clergyman, note that after 9 years of study, the Vatican Instructions of 1987 equated IVF with "domination" and "manipulation of nature."[20] One bishop said: "The Christian morality has insisted on the importance of protecting the process by which human life is transmitted. The fact that science now has the ability to alter this process significantly does not mean that, morally speaking, it has the right to do so."[21] The official position of the Vatican is that sexual intercourse between husband and wife is necessary for "moral" conception; IVF is condemned because it takes place without intercourse.

Nevertheless, many American Catholics reject this condemnation. They see nothing immoral in helping infertile couples have the children they want. Ironically, these Catholics may be closer to historical Church doctrine than the modern Vatican is.

For 1,500 years, Christian theology accepted the views of Augustine, a fourth-century philosopher and theologian who taught that the desire for intercourse (or "concupiscence") was evil. To Augustine, marriage was the only context in which this desire could permissibly be fulfilled, and even then, only for the purpose of having children. For Augustine, having children within a marriage was a license to sin; and once a marriage had produced enough children, that license was revoked. Augustine specified that original sin expressed itself in lust, and that sin was transferred through intercourse from generation to generation, and Christian doctrine thereafter followed his views.

So Augustine might have welcomed IVF. With IVF, a man might "sin" sexually only once in his life. He could masturbate once, collect his sperm, freeze it, and allow his wife to be artificially inseminated for each child desired. Indeed, the marriage need never be consummated: the wife could remain a virgin. The descent of original sin to a new generation might thus be stopped.

Two Protestant views: Fletcher and Ramsey   During the 1970s, the Protestant theologian Joseph Fletcher defended IVF as permissible for Christians. Fletcher favors any way of helping infertile couples have children:

> It is depressing, not comforting, to realize that most people are accidents. Their conception was at best unintended, at worst unwanted. There are those who are so bemused and befuddled by a fatalist mystique about nature with a capital N (or "God's will") that they want us to accept passively whatever comes along. Talk of "not tinkering" and "not playing God" and snide remarks about "artificial" and "technological" policies is a vote against both humanness and humaneness.[22]

For Fletcher, each kind of case should be considered on its own merits to see if it would help or hurt humanity; society must not be locked into antiquated religious prohibitions which take no account of consequences to human beings. Religion is best when it is "pro people," not when it worships abstract "thou shall not's":

> The real choice is between accidental or random reproduction and rationally willed or chosen reproduction. . . . Laboratory reproduction is radically human compared to conception by ordinary heterosexual intercourse. It is willed, chosen, purposed and controlled, and surely those are among the traits that distinguish Homo sapiens from others in the animal genus, from the primates down.[23]

Paul Ramsey, on the other hand, was one of the most eloquent Christian critics of IVF. Ramsey, a conservative Protestant theologian at Princeton University, equated IVF with genetic manipulation and predicted that it would lead to societal horrors. In 1970, in *Fabricated Man,* he implied that if physicians could find a tiny egg and fertilize it, why couldn't they alter its genes?[24] He predicted that if they could, they would; and he held that if they did, they would be sinful. Ramsey came up with some provocative phrases suggesting vague but disturbing harms to society: "test tube babies," "dial-a-baby," "playing God." He was especially good at creating neologisms for rhetorical effect: "mercenary gestation," "supermarket of embryos," "spare-parts man" (a hypothetical cloned twin grown for this purpose and kept unconscious), "celebrity seed" (sperm banks), "human species suicide" (eliminating genetic diseases).

When Lesley Brown was several months pregnant, Robert Edwards attended a symposium on the ethics of IVF at Washington's Kennedy Institute for Bioethics, at the invitation of Sargent Shriver. While senators, national columnists, and other scientists listened, Ramsey condemned IVF and Edwards. As Edwards described it:

> He had to be seen and heard to be believed. I had to endure a denunciation of our work as if from some nineteenth-century pulpit. It was delivered with a Gale 8 force, and written in a similar vein a year later in the *Journal of the American Medical Association.* He doubted that our patients had given their fully understanding consent. We ignored the sanctity of life. We carried out immoral experiments on the unborn. Our work was, he thundered, "unethical medical experimentation on possible future human beings and therefore it is subject to absolute moral prohibition." I was as much surprised as made wrathful by this impertinent scorching attack. He abused everything I stood for.[25]

Ramsey's view of IVF was not based on its presumed consequences to the child, to the parents, or even to society. Rather, it was based on his idea of a preembryo as a person. IVF is wrong in itself, he held, because it is "unconsented-to experimentation" on a "person"—the preembryo.[26] (The status of preembryos is discussed later in this chapter.)

IVF versus Adoption

Although adoption has become increasingly difficult, it is often presented as an alternative to IVF (and to other extraordinary treatments for infertility). Let's look at some of the considerations involved in arguments about adoption "versus" IVF.

One point raised by certain critics of IVF has to do with people's desire to have children that are genetically "their own." It is argued that wanting genetic children too much is "irrational,"[27] and that rearing adopted children can provide equal satisfaction. These critics hold that "most people think that rearing their genetic offspring is better than rearing children who are not genetically theirs, but any difference seems to stem solely from this belief."[28] A strong desire for "genetic children" seems to imply that the experience of childrearing cannot be as valuable for adoptive parents as for natural parents, and this implication may be false.

It is also asked, in this regard, whether society should encourage people to care so much about mere genetic relatedness. This emphasis deeply affects, perhaps adversely, the lives of many women and children. Many men, for instance, want their "own" children and refuse to consider marrying a woman who has had children by another man—and this is one reason why so many women are single heads of households. If people thought of parenthood as *raising* a child rather than creating one, wouldn't everyone be better off?

Additionally, it is sometimes argued that allowing infertile couples to use IVF harms babies and children who are waiting to be adopted. Shouldn't these couples be denied access to IVF, in order to encourage them to adopt children who need homes?

Of course, there are counterarguments. To begin with, we can ask at least three questions: On a personal level, are the pleasures of biological and adoptive parenthood the same—and is the answer relevant? On a moral level, are other people (unadopted children) really affected by a couple's decision to use IVF? And on the policy level, should society really discourage IVF in order to encourage adoption?

With regard to the personal level, it can be argued that the relative satisfactions of genetic and adoptive parenthood are entirely subjective, and that individual perceptions of these satisfactions cannot be "correct" or "incorrect." It can also be argued that childbearing and childrearing are intimate matters. In fact, decisions about whether or not to have children, about acceptable risks in childbearing, about how many children to have, and about whether or not to adopt a child are among the most intimate a couple can make. It is one thing to consider a couple's personal preferences irrational, but quite another to consider these preferences *immoral* or to treat them as an appropriate concern of public policy. Mill, for instance, would say that some areas of life should be immune from social criticism.

With regard to the moral level, it can be argued that other people are not significantly affected when a couple decides to use IVF, that no one is harmed when a baby comes into existence in this way. On this argument, choosing IVF might be a moral issue if babies are harmed by not being adopted; but philosophically, it is quite a stretch to claim that babies are harmed because a couple chooses not to benefit them by adopting them. Although some philosophers do defend an "equivalence thesis"—that not benefiting humans in some contexts is equivalent to harming them—few people follow their lead.[29] (More general arguments about harm depend greatly on how *harm* is defined; some of these are discussed later in this chapter.)

With regard to the public level, it can simply be argued that personal decisions about IVF are not a public matter. Must the personal always be political? If government had a right to interfere with such a decision, wouldn't it also have a right to tell us when *not* to conceive or even when to abort?

It can also be held that any public-policy efforts to encourage adoption by discouraging IVF would be shortsighted. There are not enough adoptable children for all infertile couples, and even fewer healthy, white infants are available for adoption. Champions of adoption often argue that if infertile people want so much to become parents, they should seek the older children, babies and children of color, and handicapped babies and children who now are rarely adopted. But this is not always practical: for one thing, some adoption agencies do not let white couples adopt minority babies, believing that children should be reared by people of their own race;[30] for another, not all couples have the resources to meet the needs of handicapped or older children.

IVF and Concepts of Harm

IVF as a medical procedure   Not all medical researchers greeted Louise Brown's birth with jubilation. Two contradictory forms of criticism were, on the one hand, that IVF was trivial; and, on the other hand, that it was harmful or dangerous. There were also some procedural questions.

The director of one fertility program characterized Steptoe's achievement as merely "a cookbook thing." Another critic said that it was mundane and called the birth a "cheap stunt." James Watson (who had won a Nobel prize for his work on DNA) predicted that dangerous events would follow Louise's birth.[31] Richard Blandau, a well-known fertility researcher, criticized Steptoe for not revealing how many failures had preceded this one success and thus for giving "false hope to millions of women."[32] Blandau also said that Steptoe had violated medical ethics by selling his story to the *National Enquirer* instead of publishing it in a medical journal.

There was probably some element of "sour grapes" here, because institutions with enormous budgets had been surpassed by a self-described "county doc" in a small-city hospital with poor research facilities (one critic described Steptoe's work as a "cottage industry"). Moreover, some of the criticism was unfair. For instance, Steptoe had sold the story to the *Enquirer* not for himself but for the Browns; and Blandau seemed to be missing the point that the significance of Louise's birth was not its probability or improbability, but rather that IVF could be done at all.

Still, Blandau's skepticism was understandable in the light of earlier claims. In the 1940s, the physician John Rock had announced a successful IVF but had been unable to prove it. The Italian researcher Petrucci (also in the 1940s) claimed to have fertilized a human egg in vitro, grown it for 29 days, and then destroyed it because it was becoming "monstrous"[33]—a story that fueled later fears about "monsters," though Petrucci had never provided any evidence for it. IVF does seem to carry some potential for fraud; and to counter skepticism, Steptoe needed to prove that Lesley Brown's fallopian tubes had indeed been irreparably damaged: otherwise, many critics were ready to say that an egg could have "sneaked down" them and been fertilized in the normal way. This could explain why Steptoe delivered Louise by cesarean section and why he filmed Lesley Brown's damaged tubes.

Harm to Louise   Many critics predicted that the first baby born after in vitro fertilization might be defective. One obstetrician emphasized that severely defective babies could be created, and that "the potential is there for serious anomalies should an unqualified scientist mishandle an embryo."[34] Another obstetrician said, "What if we got . . . a cyclops? Who is responsible? The parents? Is the government obligated to take care of it?"[35] Leon Kass, a well-known social conservative, argued strenuously that babies created by artificial fertilization might be deformed. "It doesn't matter how many times the baby is tested while in the mother's womb," he averred, "they will never be certain the baby won't be born without defect."[36] James Watson also feared that deformed babies would be born and that they would then have to be raised by the state in custodial homes, or that they might even be victims of infanticide.[37] Max Perutz, who was a colleague of Edwards's at Cambridge—and, like Watson, a Nobel prize-winner—also condemned IVF research:

> I agree entirely with Dr. Watson that this is far too great a risk. Even if only a single abnormal baby is born and has to be kept alive as an invalid for the rest of its life, Dr. Edwards would have a terrible guilt upon his shoulders. The idea that this might happen on a larger scale—a new thalidomide catastrophe—is horrifying.[38]

Jeremy Rifkin revved up the fear that the baby might be psychologically "monstrous":

> What are the psychological implications of growing up as a specimen, sheltered not by a warm womb but by steel and glass, belonging to no one but the lab technician who joined together sperm and egg? In a world already populated with people with identity crises, what's the personal identity of a test-tube baby?[39]

A founder of the Hastings Center argued that the first case of IVF was "probably unethical" because there was no possible guarantee that Louise Brown would be normal, though it would be ethical to proceed with IVF after this first healthy birth;[40] he added that many medical breakthroughs are actually "unethical" because we cannot know that the first patient will not be harmed.

These arguments do not seem very compelling (the comments of the two Nobelists, especially, suggest that moral wisdom does not necessarily accompany scientific talent). What these critics seem to overlook is that no reasonable approach to life can avoid all risks. Moreover, they also demonstrate a psychologically normal but nevertheless illogical tendency to magnify the risk of a harmful but unlikely event. A highly unlikely result—even if that result is very bad—still represents a very small risk.[41] For instance, an anencephalic baby is an extremely bad but unlikely result, and the (small) risk of an anencephalic baby shouldn't deter people from having kids.

Harm to "possible people": The paradox of harm   Even if "harm to Louise" was not a serious issue, IVF could be a moral question if an IVF baby, who otherwise would not exist, could be harmed by being conceived in this way.

Whether *possible* children can or cannot be harmed by in vitro conception is a philosophically interesting consideration. The theologian Hans Tiefel writes, "No one has the moral right to endanger a child while there is yet the option of whether the child shall come into existence"[42]—on the assumption that IVF subjects a baby to greater risks than normal conception does.

Suppose that a mother smokes and drinks during pregnancy, and as result has a retarded son. Later, the son accuses her of having harmed him. She replies, "I'm sorry, but I was under a lot of stress during that time. Sooner than give up smoking and drinking during my pregnancy, I would have aborted you as a fetus. So you can't complain." This is an example of the *paradox of harm:* the seemingly self-contradictory idea that someone can be harmed by being born. This idea appears to be morally paradoxical because, first, it seems queer to say that we can harm a being by bringing it into existence; but second, it seems equally odd to say that a mother who could have prevented but did not prevent some harm to her child did no harm by that omission.

A paradox results when two different meanings of a key term are used simultaneously. Paradoxes can be dissolved by carefully specifying the different meanings in each part of the paradox and deciding which meaning applies best to each. With the paradox of harm, any approach to dissolving it must distinguish between different meanings of *harm.*[43] Like the concept of good, the concept of harm covers a broad range of meanings. In law school, such meanings are covered in one of the major courses—torts. For our purposes here, two very broad ways of thinking about harm can be distinguished.

In the first way of thinking, both a baseline and a temporal (time) component are necessary, so that a change occurs which makes someone worse off. In this *baseline concept,* harm requires an *adverse change* in someone's condition. With the baseline concept, someone who doesn't yet exist cannot be harmed, because there is no baseline from which change can occur. (Consider the old Yiddish joke: 1st— "Life is so terrible! Better to have never existed." 2d—"True, but who is so lucky? Not one in a thousand.")

In the second way of thinking, harm involves comparing a present deficient condition with what normally would have been. In this *normality concept,* someone can be harmed by being brought into existence with some defect that could have been avoided by taking reasonable precautions. With the normality concept, the event or omission that causes the defect is the cause of harm. The normality concept underlies the belief that women should do everything possible to have healthy, unimpaired babies; that anything less than the maximal effort is blameworthy; and that it is wrong for a woman to take risks with a future person's intelligence or health.

To sum up these two concepts of harm:

- *Baseline concept.* Requires a starting point (baseline) from which an adverse change is plotted; i.e., it requires an existing being who is made worse off.
- *Normality concept.* Requires a norm of development which is not met, e.g., because of a woman's actions or omissions while carrying a fetus.

In *wrongful life* cases in the courts, it is claimed that the lives of some children are so miserable that their very existence is a tort. In *wrongful birth* cases, the claim is not that the child's life is totally miserable but simply that the child has been damaged by being born less than normal. Wrongful birth suits appeal to the normality concept. The courts have rejected wrongful life suits by assuming the baseline concept; that is, they have assumed that preventing a birth or killing a baby cannot possibly be a benefit, even to prevent or end a life of total harm. (For more on such cases, see Chapter 7; as described there, the Curlender case of 1986 is a possibly unique example of a successful wrongful life suit.)

These two concepts of harm can be applied to IVF. According to the baseline concept, a person created by IVF cannot thereby be harmed because otherwise that person would not have existed. According to the normality concept, IVF could harm a baby if it caused some defect or deficiency that the baby would not otherwise have had.

Harm to infertile patients   A significant amount of the controversy about evaluative issues in modern medicine involves who is entitled to take risks and what kinds of risks are *acceptable.* With regard to the development of IVF, most of the consequences of risk were borne not by the actual or potential infant but by the parents; and some opposition to the earliest use of IVF amounted to arguing that public policy should never allow people to take this risk.

Some of the critics who argued that attempts at IVF could harm infertile patients based their argument on the improbability that the procedure would be successful: in the early days, it was said that Steptoe's chance of helping an infertile couple to conceive was only 1 in a 100. Tiefel observed (further on in the passage cited above):

> Even if the meager success rate is explained to couples and they consent to the odds, there are moral limits to surgical risk, time, resources, and stress on human relationships. The fact that prospective parents say that they will do anything to have a baby of their own is not necessarily a moral justification.

Tiefel anticipated the obvious objection that individual couples can decide and should be allowed to decide what risk they consider acceptable:

> This is ethical relativism, where individual choice or preference settles moral issues. Medicine should avoid such quicksand, for shifting individual preferences offer no solid support for the objective values undergirding medicine and research. If one lets go of objective and universal values to defer to dubious patient choice, one also relinquishes the heart of medicine, whose life is the objective value of healing and doing no harm.

Tiefel is arguing here that physicians cannot simply accede to their patients' desire for children, and some physicians share his view. They think that the relationship between people and medicine is not that medicine exists to help people implement their own choices about illness and health, but rather that medicine exists to "heal" people, regardless of what people themselves would choose. Notice that for Tiefel, what people choose is "ethical relativism," whereas healing is an "objective and universal value" at the "heart of medicine." This is a very important distinction and defines a sharply drawn division among some physicians as to what medicine is *for.*

Tiefel's position is a good example of how abstract moral language must be carefully analyzed in concrete terms. Most people would unthinkingly agree with Tiefel's statement that "healing" is an objective value of medicine; yet in this context, Tiefel uses the concept of "healing" to *oppose* treating infertility—and many of those same people would find that conclusion unacceptable.

Statements like Tiefel's seem make sense only if "morality" implies some standard beyond possible harm to human beings. In other words, Tiefel's is essentially a religious viewpoint. As such, it can be seen as a holdover from earlier eras when there was no personal life immune from religious control. Such a view can be described as *omnimoralistic:* it disregards or rejects the distinction between personal life and morality, and makes all aspects of personal life a matter of morality. Many moral critics give lip service to the distinction between personal life and public policy, but they do not seem to accept the implications of that distinction.

Harm to society   Critics of IVF also envisioned potential harms to society. *U.S. News and World Report,* for example, described Louise Brown's birth as a "disturbing" and "ominous" event, an indication of how "science wields its growing power to decide who shall be born, how, and to whom."[44] An unstated assumption here was that "science"—not infertile couples—would decide who is born. Many critics used the "slippery slope" metaphor, among them James Watson, who concluded that an international effort was needed to "deemphasize" research that would circumvent "normal sexual reproduction." For Leon Kass (in the passage quoted earlier), IVF was the first step toward the unthinkable:

> At least one good humanitarian reason can be found to justify each step. The first step serves as a precedent for the second and the second for the third, not just technologically but also in moral argument. Perhaps a wise society would say to infertile couples: "We understand your sorrow, but it might be better not to go ahead and do this."

In the context of criticizing IVF, both Paul Ramsey and James Watson attacked cloning ("carbon-copy people"). Watson warned of the dangers of cloning and foresaw a scenario reminiscent of *The Boys from Brazil*—secret projects for creating teams of little Hitlers. Of course, in vitro fertilization has nothing to do with cloning. In vitro fertilization is *sexual* reproduction; cloning is *asexual* reproduction. In vitro fertilization matches two different sets of 23 chromosomes to create a unique individual with 46; cloning reproduces the 46 chromosomes of the donor. Also, if a government or secret society really wanted to duplicate the fictional experiment in *The Boys from Brazil,* neither cloning nor IVF would be needed: some of the millions of existing unwanted, unclaimed children could be screened, and selected teams could be raised in isolated areas for nefarious purposes. Lest silly fears run rampant, consider that an insurmountable problem would remain: the resulting adults—cloned or not—would not be automatons, mindlessly taking orders, but people who could think for themselves.

Harm to women   Another source of criticism of IVF is concern about potential harm to women as patients or as members of societies worldwide.

One such issue has to do with informed consent to assisted reproduction. In medicine, it is well known that only cancer patients are more willing than infertile couples to try any treatment. With desperate patients, informed consent may be questionable; and given the nature of IVF, concerns about informed consent would pertain mostly to women. When Louise Brown was conceived, in 1977, England did not have a law requiring informed consent for experimental procedures. Did Lesley Brown really understand what was going to occur? Steptoe said that he had explained everything to the Browns, but did Lesley Brown understand why Steptoe was performing a cesarean section rather than allowing her to deliver vaginally? Did she realize that the cesarean delivery was necessary not for her benefit or for Louise's benefit but rather as proof for Steptoe's colleagues?

There are also feminist issues related to IVF. (Different meanings of "feminism" in contemporary moral issues are explored in Chapter 5.) In 1988, for instance, the philosopher Mary Anne Warren suggested the possibility that many new reproductive technologies (NRTs) are really devices developed by men to control women.[45] Although Warren would not ban NRTs or prohibit women from using them, she argues that "every government body with responsibility for the regulation of the NRTs, every ethical oversight committee, and every public agency which funds reproductive research [should] be at least 50 percent composed of women."

Warren also argues that, instead of focusing on NRTs, society should focus on preventing infertility in the first place. She emphasizes "what may be the most important feminist objection to IVF," lack of attention to "social causes" of female infertility. According to Warren, we must look at the macroscopic level, not just at individual infertile women. Since pelvic inflammatory disease (PID) causes much infertility and is associated with "hormone-based contraceptives," she advocates condoms to decrease PID. Moreover, she notes that "heterosexual intercourse is much more likely to transmit infection than either oral sex or masturbation (mutual or solitary)"; and she asserts that such "normal" sexual practice is not the "inalterable result of human biology" but merely a "social institution." Therefore, she concludes, heterosexual sex "must be included among the social causes of infertility."

Some feminists are concerned that women who choose assisted reproduction are being manipulated by the men in their lives or by the male values of the larger society, expressed in the mass media. They see the glorification of pregnancy as condemning women to a traditional biological role. The feminist Janice Raymond claims that "IVF clinics exist because they are immensely profitable. They aren't proliferating out of altruistic impulses for so-called desperate women."[46] When asked about women who themselves demand IVF, Raymond replies, "Recognize the political context. Women are submitting to pressure to have children at any cost because their lives are devalued without children."

Feminist analyses like these are controversial, even explosive. The philosopher Christine Sistare, for one, bristles at the implication that women who choose IVF have been manipulated. To her, that argument is itself sexist because it suggests that these women cannot make free, rational choices.[47] Additionally, it can be argued that some feminist critics of IVF beg the question of choice by assuming that choosing to have children represents coercion, whereas other choices do not. If women are generally coerced, then wouldn't the position of female critics of IVF and NRTs also be a product of coercion? Does the nature of a choice itself tell us who is free and who is not? It can also be noted that in criticisms like War-

ren's, there seems to be an underlying tone much like that of religious conservatives who distrust assisted reproduction—an implication that in using techniques
of assisted reproduction, humans are "playing God," "tinkering with Nature,"
and guilty of "technological arrogance" ("because we can do it, we *should* do it").
More specifically, some defenders of IVF emphasize that this technology is capable of many uses; for example, lesbian couples could use sperm donated by a
brother or male friend to have their "own" children through IVF.

IVF and Public Policy: Costs, Coverage, and Restrictions

There are several issues regarding IVF and public policy. One that has already
been mentioned is whether society should ban IVF in order to encourage adoption. In addition to the consideration that this may be simply impractical (since
not enough children are available for adoption), it seems unfair to direct such a
policy specifically at infertile couples: why not require *all* couples to adopt
unwanted children? It can also be pointed out that since IVF is successful for
only about 15 to 20 percent of the couples who attempt it, there will still be many
couples who might eventually choose adoption.

Another issue has to do with paying for IVF, which costs about $6,000 to
$8,000 per attempt. Most couples need financial assistance for IVF; but in the
United States, many insurers do not cover IVF itself, although most of them
cover related procedures, such as sonograms. Since IVF is a benefit to many infertile people, should insurers be required to pay for IVF? Should society pay for it?

The rationality or irrationality of desiring one's own biological children may
not be an appropriate consideration with regard to banning IVF, either to encourage adoption or to protect infertile couples from risk. However, it may be more
relevant when we consider who should pay for IVF.

It can be argued that if the desire for genetic offspring is irrational, neither
private insurers nor public programs should be required to pay for measures like
IVF. If people want to act irrationally in this context and are willing to finance
their efforts themselves, fine, but they should not ask others to pay. In fact, this
reasoning seems to be widely accepted: at present, only a few states require
insurance companies to cover IVF, and Oregon has voted to exclude IVF from
Medicaid coverage.

However, three counterarguments have been advanced. First, there is the
argument that people have a "right" to procreate, and that this right is not for-
feited because of infertility. The right to procreate does indeed seem to be recognized in the United States; it is generally assumed that society should not usually
interfere with individuals' attempts to have children by such means as involuntary sterilization or mandatory contraception (see Chapter 15). It may follow,
then, that society has some obligation to help infertile people meet the costs of
trying to conceive.

Second, infertility is sometimes claimed to be an incapacitating condition. It
may or may not be appropriate to consider infertility as analogous to a "disease";
but in any case, *health*—defined broadly—is not simply an absence of disease but
maximal functioning. On this argument, people who want to conceive but cannot
are not "healthy," and treating infertility is therefore not merely cosmetic; it is

like any other medical treatment for dysfunction. Using IVF for damaged fallopian tubes, it is argued, is no more cosmetic than using physical therapy for limbs impaired by stroke. Furthermore, insurers often cover very expensive microsurgery to repair damaged fallopian tubes—surgery which works in only a small percentage of cases—and whatever makes such surgery eligible for coverage should also make IVF eligible.

Third, it is argued that when private insurers or public programs are not required to pay for IVF, it becomes a prerogative only of the affluent. If, as many people believe, having one's own biological children is a fundamental good, then this good should be widely available. According to the philosopher John Rawls's theory of justice, a just society will minimize the "natural inequalities of fate" and will help redress them by using public funds to assist the unfortunate.[48] Unjust societies, by contrast, allow such natural inequalities to be magnified. If infertility is a "natural inequality," then, a just society will aid infertile people, especially if the costs can be spread out to make the individual burden minimal.

Still another issue of public policy concerns allocation of or restrictions on IVF; in other words, how many people, and which people, should have access to IVF?

It is sometimes proposed, for instance, that IVF should be available, by law, only to married couples; effectively, this would mean restricting IVF to heterosexuals, since homosexuals cannot legally marry. The Australian philosopher Peter Singer is opposed to this idea and holds that IVF should not be restricted in any way.[49] He argues that this would be the *only* kind of medical treatment for which it is necessary to be married (however, in the United States, many urologists refuse to do vasectomies for unmarried men under 40). He also argues that no restrictions are now placed on unmarried *fertile* heterosexual couples, who may use other forms of medical help to conceive. Additionally, he notes that gay men may be sperm donors and that lesbians may become mothers through artificial insemination, and he concludes that "it would be unjust if a particular self-defining group" was denied access to any treatment available to others.

Certainly, legal restrictions on IVF are not easily defensible. The idea of restricting IVF to married people, and therefore to heterosexuals, for example, seems to be based on an assumption that heterosexuals are in general better parents than homosexuals. But empirical evidence would certainly be needed to support that claim, and even if such evidence were found, it would not prove that any *particular* homosexual couple would be less competent than any particular heterosexual couple; long-term commitment to a relationship and to child-rearing would be a more relevant criterion than sexual orientation. Similar reasoning could be used for proposed restrictions on any other group.

However, IVF can also be restricted, in effect, by a legal environment in which private insurers and public programs need not pay for IVF—as we have just discussed. Is this tantamount to *forbidding* certain people to use IVF? In the United States, abortion is legal, but federal funds do not pay for it; and some people believe that this is essentially the same as forbidding poor women to have abortions. Similarly, since the government now permits anyone to purchase IVF but does not fund IVF for the indigent (and does not require insurers to cover it), is the government actually prohibiting IVF for the poor?

Here, it can be argued that there is a big difference between *forbidding* some-one to obtain a certain benefit (owning a house, going to college, having an abor-tion, having a baby) and *not providing* that benefit. It can also be argued that IVF is an expensive technique, and potentially it could be used by millions of people, if insurers or the government paid for it. Medical costs in the United States are very high, and one reason for this is that when collective insurance pays for med-ical care, no one is motivated to forgo care. Moreover, although infertility may be a personal tragedy for people who place a high value on having biological chil-dren, it is not necessarily a public tragedy or even a medical problem. It was noted above that health may be defined broadly as the absence of any sort of dys-function, but when a society must think of controlling medical costs, this defini-tion may become impractical. However distressing infertility may be, it is not really a debilitating disease like lupus, cancer, cystic fibrosis, or congenital arthri-tis: infertile people can still work and flourish.

Perhaps the question of IVF would be answered best by looking at the whole range of medical services offered and deciding whether, in that context, "justice" requires society to "provide" IVF in the sense of subsidizing it by paying for it directly or requiring insurers to pay for it. (This kind of analysis is a topic of Chapter 18.) In a society where the objective is to give people equal opportuni-ties, but not necessarily equal outcomes, IVF might not be subsidized. In the United States, where more than 39 million Americans lacked coverage for basic care as of 1994, requiring insurers to pay for IVF may seem like a luxury.

Status of Preembryos

Giving extra hormones stimulates *superovulation:* maturation of extra eggs during a monthly cycle and thus availability of more than one egg for fertilization. In IVF, six eggs are often fertilized after laparoscopy, three of which are inserted in the uterus and the rest frozen for possible future attempts. (Three preembryos are inserted to increase the chance that one will become implanted. Inserting more than three preembryos further increases the chance that one will implant, but it also increases the chance of a multiple birth—a risk that not all infertile couples want to take.) What is the ethical status of the "extra" preembryos: those that are deliberately frozen and those that simply fail to implant?

In 1981, the issue of preembryos was dramatized by a famous case, that of Mario and Elsa Rios.[50] The Rioses, an American couple worth millions, traveled to Melbourne, Australia, where several of Elsa Rios's eggs were fertilized in vitro with sperm from an anonymous donor. Three preembryos were produced; one was implanted, and the other two were frozen in a tank of liquid nitrogen for later implantation in case the first attempt failed. Ten days later, the first attempt did fail, but the Rioses were unwilling to make a second attempt immediately and returned to the United States. They later went to South America. In the spring of 1983, they were killed in a plane crash. The story made headlines when it was learned that their frozen preembryos still existed. Neither the Rioses nor the infertility clinic had provided for this contingency, and the legal status of the preembryos was doubtful.

Several ethical questions arose. Could the preembryos simply be destroyed?

If they were implanted in surrogate mothers and carried to term, could they later sue in American courts for their inheritance from the Rioses? Should the anonymous sperm donor be consulted about his wishes? An ad hoc committee of the Australian government recommended that the Rios preembryos be destroyed, having concluded that removing their life support would be the same as removing life support of terminal patients. The Australian parliament, however, reasoned differently and required that the preembryos be preserved until each of them could be "adopted." Presumably, they are still frozen.

Somewhat earlier, in 1979, the obstetricians Howard and Georgeanna Jones had established the first American IVF clinic at Eastern Virginia Medical School (EVMS). In October of that year, opponents of IVF jammed the auditorium of the Norfolk Public Health Department for a debate on the proposed program at EVMS, charging that it would inevitably lead to destruction of "tiny human beings" (these protesters also envisioned "mass production of artificially designed humans"). EVMS is a private institution, not subject to federal regulations, and so its program went forward. But the brouhaha resulted in a ban on federal funds for experimentation on preembryos. Since 90 percent of experimentation in the United States is federally funded, this ban effectively stopped most American research on assisted reproduction.

The Rios case and the episode at EVMS illustrate the issue of the "personhood" of preembryos. Let's look briefly at this question.

Some people believe that personhood begins immediately at conception, with the fertilized ovum. Accordingly, they hold that intrauterine devices (IUDs), which prevent implantation of zygotes or preembryos, kill "persons"; they also hold that dislodging an implanted preembryo by dilation of the cervix and curettage, or scraping, of the uterine lining (D and C) is murder.

Other people consider a preembryo not a person but only a *potential person*. These people observe that a human preembryo has no consciousness, let alone intelligence; it does not even have human form. Consider an analogy: If you cut down a neighbor's large oak tree without permission, you can be sued for substantial damages, but you cannot be sued for destroying one of your neighbor's acorns; an acorn is not an oak tree. To draw another analogy, as many an enthusiast has discovered, an idea with the potential to make $1 million is not $1 million in the bank.

The argument over whether or not "personhood" exists at conception takes place most commonly, of course, in the context of abortion; however, consideration of IVF nicely separates the issue of personhood from that of abortion. (Personhood is discussed further, as part of the issue of abortion, in Chapter 6.)

Writing on this issue, David Ozar pointed out that although a preembryo may not be a person, neither is it just an object, like a pebble.[51] Ozar assumes that preembryos are a unique phenomenon because of their potential: given the right support, each preembryo has the potential to develop into a full person. Thus preembryos are not simply the property of an owner, and they deserve at least "respect" (e.g., they should not be eaten). Ozar also noted that the Supreme Court's decision in *Roe v. Wade* in 1973 cited a "compelling" interest in protecting potential personhood at viability; and that in *Danforth* (1976), the court defined *viability* as "that stage of fetal development when the life of the unborn child may be continued indefinitely outside of the womb by natural or artificial life-support systems." It would seem to follow that frozen zygotes were then technically "viable." This may have been a somewhat idiosyncratic interpretation of the Supreme Court's decisions, however. To avoid such implications, the Court specified in *Colautti v. Franklin* (1979) that viability of fetuses—not embryos—was in question (this decision also left assessment of viability up to the physician).

Peter Singer has argued that destroying preembryos in a situation like the Rios case is no different from destroying an individual egg or sperm.[52] Imagine a sperm and an egg on two sides of an IVF slide. Case 1: Just before the sperm and egg are to be joined, the man and woman change their minds, so both sperm and egg are washed down the drain. Case 2: Same as case 1, but the couple change their minds 1 minute after sperm and egg have been joined. Case 3: Same as case 1, but the technicians discover that the drain is blocked; the sperm and egg may thus have united in the drain, and if not retrieved immediately, the resulting preembryo will die of exposure. Singer argues that these three cases do not differ morally, and that none of these preembryos has a right to life.

It might be objected that even if a preembryo is only a potential person, couples—or women—still have an obligation to gestate potential people. Many commentators, however, think that this objection can be refuted by *reductio ad absurdum:* a line of reasoning which shows that some logical implication of an idea is absurd and thus casts doubt on the idea itself. In this instance, consider that if a woman starts procreating (as is often possible) before her teens and continues throughout her fertile years, she may easily produce a dozen or more children. We have here what Derek Parfit calls the "repugnant conclusion":[53] if each potential person is valuable, then we ought to actualize the greatest possible number of potential persons; but given the consequences of overpopulation, this conclusion hardly makes sense. Also, there is clearly a philosophical difficulty in claiming a "right to life" for a frozen preembryo when—as in the Rios case—no particular woman has a duty to have the preembryo implanted and gestate it.

Finally, considering "failed"—nonimplanted—preembryos as "persons" may also lead to a reductio ad absurdum. A Roman Catholic physician, M. V. Viola, wrote in 1968:

> A significant number of fertilized ova (some estimate one in three) never implant in the uterus under normal conditions. If in fact these are lost souls, the Church should be consistent and make efforts to administer baptism to them.[54]

UPDATE

Research on Preembryos

In the United States, as early as 1979, Congress had created an Ethics Advisory Board (EAB) to advise it on experimentation with human preembryos fertilized in vitro. Like a similar committee in England, EAB recommended limited experimentation on such preembryos; but the recommendation was never accepted by Joseph Califano, then secretary of Health and Human Services (HHS). In 1994,

Congress lifted the ban and created a board to decide which embryonic experiments would be allowed.

Technical Developments in Assisted Reproduction

Between 1978 and 1990, over 24,000 babies were born in the United States, and about twice as many worldwide, through forms of IVF.[55] These numbers were boosted by new methods, such as the use of frozen embryos; donor eggs; and gamete intrafallopian transfer—GIFT—which unites sperm and egg not in a petri dish but rather inside a fallopian tube, approximately where normal conception takes place[56] (the Roman Catholic church condones GIFT). These statistics are one of the great success stories of contemporary medicine.

Assisted reproduction has achieved several technical breakthroughs since the mid-1970s. Egg retrieval no longer requires surgery; it can now be done by tubal aspiration using ultrasound imaging. Also, preembryos are now inserted, if at all possible, in one of the fallopian tubes, rather than in the uterus. Researchers are also doing more and more with fewer and fewer sperm: a Belgian group has succeeded in using a single sperm to fertilize an egg.[57]

The number of multiple births worldwide has soared as a result of multiple-embryo implantation after IVF, and as a result of the introduction of Clomid—a drug which induces superovulation—in the late 1970s.

Some medical centers have begun selecting embryos by sex in order to exclude those vulnerable to sex-linked genetic disorders. The most exciting possibility here is *single-cell diagnosis,* in which one cell of an 8-cell preembryo is removed and the DNA is replicated to provide material for genetic testing. (It is thought that removal of this one cell does not harm the preembryo.) In 1994, this technique was first used with prospective parents who carried the gene for Tay Sachs disease, to avoid creating a child with the disease.[58] (However, when some scientists believed that they had discovered a genetic marker for homosexuality, some critics immediately called for a ban on using single-cell diagnosis to screen for homosexuality.[59])

There has also been at least one nondevelopment. In 1993, American journalism was breathless for a few days when the *New York Times* reported, on the first page of its widely read Sunday edition, that a scientist had "cloned" 17 human embryos into 48 as a way of increasing the supply of embryos in fertility clinics.[60] The next day, other newspapers, CNN, and *Good Morning America* took the *Times* story at face value, as did several bioethicists. Jeremy Rifkin, for one, instantly condemned such cloning as "opening the door to the Brave New Worlds . . . of human eugenics."[61] To its credit, however, *Newsweek* ("once bitten, twice shy"?) got the story right:

> It is one of the most sought-after coups of 20th century journalism, along with the identity of Deep Throat and Senator Packwood's diaries—the first story that can plausibly use "human" and "clone" in the same headline. . . . Last week, *The New York Times,* [on the basis of] an apparent misunderstanding of a paper reporting a technical advance in embryology, touched off an echo of the same hysteria with a page-one story whose headline suggested that human embryos

were being cloned in a laboratory. Within days medical ethicists were gravely measuring the slipperiness of the slope on which humanity now teetered, while demonstrators marched outside laboratories insisting that no one would ever clone *their* DNA.[62]

What most people understood by "cloning" was what Woody Allen had imagined in his movie *Sleeper,* reproduction of an identical physical copy of a human being from some cells of the donor's adult body (in *Sleeper,* the cells were from a dictator's nose); or perhaps what was depicted in the more recent movie *Jurassic Park*—recreation of extinct species (in this case, dinosaurs) from preserved DNA. The *Times* had described copying of undifferentiated cells of embryos by a technique that is common in animal husbandry and could easily be applied to human embryos. But what was *not* emphasized was that once human cells specialize into skin cells, blood cells, and so on, they cannot be returned to their undifferentiated state to create a copy of the entire body of their donor. (From the cells of the dictator's nose, you get . . . a nose!) After the *Newsweek* article, the story simply disappeared. *Newsweek* noted that the *Times* "did not respond to numerous requests for comment last week."

IVF Clinics

In 1993, American IVF clinics were facing legal regulation. During the 1980s, there had been serious problems at some clinics, stemming from false advertising about success rates; but the possibility of regulation in the early 1990s was a result of the misdeeds of one physician, Cecil Jacobson. Jacobson—who, ironically, had been a pioneer in IVF—practiced in a Virginia suburb of Washington, D.C. In 1991, he was indicted on 53 counts of fraud and perjury for not telling female patients that had he used his own sperm with their eggs to create zygotes.[63] He may have "fathered" over 75 children in this way. In other cases, he had told patients that they were pregnant when in fact he had given them a drug which merely produced an appearance of pregnancy. In 1992, he was fined $116,000 and sentenced to 5 years in prison.[64]

Assisted reproduction today is characterized by intense competition among IVF clinics.[65] Between 1974 and 1988, the number of physicians specializing in infertility increased from 3,600 to 10,300.[66] In 1987, there were 50 IVF clinics in the United States; in 1992, there were 235.[67]

In the United States, IVF is a $1 billion to $2 billion business, and top IVF physicians make $300,000 a year.[68] A typical couple may pay $20,000 to $30,000 for several attempts at IVF (as compared with intrauterine insemination in conjunction with fertility drugs, which can cost as little as $1,000 per attempt).[69] Some IVF specialists claim that the big infertility-assistance chains offer the treatment that will yield the highest profit, rather than the treatment that would be best or most cost-effective for individual patients.

With some IVF clinics, misleading advertising remains one of the most serious problems. Some clinics cite national success rates but have never themselves brought even one fetus to term. Actually, there is a conceptual problem with advertising of IVF: the fact that there is no standard measure of success. Should success be expressed as pregnancies per applicant? Pregnancies per implanted embryo? Pregnancies per attempted cycle? For most couples, the only measure which counts is taking a baby home, and with IVF this is something that only about 14 percent of couples eventually do.[70] Because many couples try to produce a baby for more than one cycle (the average is perhaps between 2 and 3 cycles), reports have emerged of grueling ordeals in IVF clinics. Repeated attempts were being made through several cycles, until most couples simply gave up.[71] Despite reports in the media of successful IVFs and happy new parents, the fact is that more than 80 percent of couples who try IVF will be unsuccessful.

There is an infertility consumer-rights group, RESOLVE, which helps infertile couples avoid exploitation and claims to have 24,000 members.

Assisted Reproduction and Social Problems

Techniques of assisted reproduction create an assortment of social problems that are of concern to public policy, in addition to the problem (discussed above) of who should pay for procedures like IVF.

Anonymous donation of sperm can be problematic. Even before Cecil Jacobson's conviction, the practice of artificial insemination of sperm from anonymous donors (AID) had been attacked. David James argued that AID "intentionally creates a child alienated from one parent, which is an abdication of parental responsibility and a violation of the child's fundamental interests."[72] A new group, Donors' Offspring, opposes AID on the ground that "sperm is viewed as a 'treatment' or 'cure' like a drug, rather than as the reproductive gametes of another human being."[73]

The multiple pregnancies that frequently result from assisted reproduction have created ethical issues as well. In a multiple pregnancy, nutrients and oxygenated blood in the womb become a scarce resource; and to prevent disabilities resulting from deprivation in utero, physicians recommend "selective reduction" of all but one or two embryos. In 1985, a Mormon couple, Patti and Sam Frustaci, conceived septuplets but refused to have such a reduction performed. Four of their seven babies died, and the three survivors had severe disabilities, including cerebral palsy. The Frustacis sued.[74]

Multiple-birth babies are often premature (they may weigh less than 2 pounds), are three times as likely as single babies to be severely handicapped at birth, and may have to spend many months in neonatal intensive-care units (NICUs). Nevertheless, in France—where pregnancy is sometimes pursued with an almost religious zeal, and where each new baby means a bonus from the government—the number of triplets has increased tenfold since 1982 and the number of quadruplets has increased thirtyfold.[75]

The 1990s increasingly saw women between the ages of 40 and 50 becoming pregnant with donated eggs. Using laparoscopy, surgeons can remove between 4 and 65 ripe eggs from ovaries of young donor women for implantation in older women.[76] This practice has raised a general question about allocation of scarce medical resources. It has also raised some more specific questions. Should eggs be obtained only through altruistic donation, or should they be bought and sold for profit? There was a customary payment of $1,500 to donors; and although this was seen by many women as a token rather than real compensation for the hassles involved, the philosopher Mary Mahowald wondered whether selling eggs wasn't analogous to prostitution.[77] Also, should there should be an age limit for women seeking IVF? (In 1993, a 59-year-old businesswoman in England gave birth to twins gestated by her from eggs, fertilized by her husband's sperm, that had been donated by a woman in her twenties.[78])

Frozen embryos continue to present problems. In one of the most highly publicized cases, Mary Sue Davis and Junior Davis of Tennessee divorced and fought for custody of seven embryos frozen in their IVF clinic. Initially, Mary Sue Davis sought custody so that she could use the embryos to become a mother, whereas Junior Davis wanted custody to prevent her from becoming pregnant with embryos with his gametes. A lower court judge awarded custody to Mary Sue Davis; but in June 1992, the Tennessee Supreme Court decided that Junior Davis did not have to become a father against his will. Junior Davis won in part because both parties had remarried and after her remarriage, Mary Sue Davis wanted the preembryos in order to donate them to some other infertile couple. In 1993, the United States Supreme Court declined to hear an appeal; but a Tennessee court later ruled, in another hearing, that Junior Davis could destroy the preembryos, which he did.[79] In 1992, in California, the girlfriend of Bill Kane, a wealthy man who had died, sought to use his frozen sperm to impregnate herself. Kane's two children contested this in the courts, and as a result Kane's estate was still not settled.

Single-cell diagnosis has also given rise to social concerns, since it can obviously be used for dubious or even ignoble purposes. Determining the sex of an embryo, for instance, can be used to plan for a boy or a girl.[80] In Korea, China, and India, wealthy people reportedly use IVF and preembryo selection frequently to ensure that their first or only child will be male.[81]

There have also been some new developments that were controversial though not easily classifiable. In 1993, a black woman in England was to have a white donor's egg implanted, fertilized by sperm from the black woman's husband, in order to have a mixed-race child; a similar implantation took place in Italy, where an African woman gave birth to a white baby. Early in 1994, newspapers in England erupted over a report that eggs could be retrieved from aborted female fetuses, implanted in infertile women, and artificially ripened for conception. This extreme measure was apparently being considered because in England donated eggs from younger women are scarce: infertile women who need donated eggs now face a 3-year wait.[82]

The Participants

In 1989, James Watson—who at the time of Louise Brown's birth had made alarmist predictions about IVF, cloning, and genetic manipulation—was named head of the Human Genome Project. The irony of this appointment was lost on most people. Watson later quit the project in the midst of a controversy over patent rights.

The obstetrician Patrick Steptoe died in 1988, age 74. Just a few days earlier, the physiologist Robert Edwards had been given one of the highest awards in the English scientific community, induction as a Fellow of the Royal Society.

Louise Brown is growing up in Whitchurch, a suburb of Bristol. She is blue-eyed, blonde, healthy, and strong-willed. At age 5, she often dawdled at candy stores on the way home from school. At 10, she often played outdoors too late.

On June 14, 1982, Lesley Brown became the first woman to have two children successfully fertilized in vitro, giving birth to a second daughter, Natalie Jane.

In the fall of 1993, Louise Brown (then 15) and Natalie (then 11) toured the United States with their mother to advance the cause of assisted reproduction, appearing on *Good Morning America* and elsewhere. Asked if her classmates ever ribbed her about her unusual origin, the pudgy Louise giggled and replied, "When kids want to tease me, they ask, 'How did you ever fit into a test tube?'"[83]

FURTHER READING

Howard Ducharme, "The Vatican's Dilemma: On the Morality of IVF and the Incarnation," *Bioethics,* vol. 5, no. 1, January 1991.

David James, "Ectogenesis: A Reply to Singer and Wells," *Bioethics,* vol. 1, no. 1, January 1987.

Mary Anne Warren, "The Ethics of Sex Preselection," in K. Alpern, ed., *The Ethics of Reproductive Technology,* Oxford University Press, New York, 1992.

CHAPTER 5

Surrogacy

Baby M

This chapter discusses the "Baby M" case, which involved Mary Beth White-head's "surrogate motherhood" with William Stern. Before the Baby M decision, in 1988, no state supreme court had ruled on surrogate contracts.

Surrogate means "substitute," and so a surrogate mother is a woman who bears a child for someone else. To some people, however, the term *surrogate mother* implies that the woman who gestates the child, rather than the woman who actually raises the child, is the real mother—an implication that is open to debate. To avoid begging any question at the outset, we will use simply *surrogate* to refer to a woman who bears a child for someone else.

BACKGROUND: SURROGATE PARENTHOOD

In the Old Testament, Sarah, who has borne no children with her husband Abraham, tells Abraham to "go unto" her handmaiden Hagar, so that "I may obtain children by her" (Genesis 16: 1-4; Hagar's child is named Ishmael). When Sarah became jealous of Hagar, this arrangement causes problems. The book of Genesis also recounts that Jacob's wife Rachel uses her maid Billah to create a son (30: 1-5). Under Hebrew and Babylonian law, surrogates could produce acceptable heirs.

Another story of surrogacy is found in the brothers Grimm. Their fairy tale Rumpelstiltskin tells of an old, ugly dwarf who makes a contract with the beautiful daughter of a poor miller: the dwarf will spin gold out of straw for the girl, in return for her firstborn child. When the child is born, the girl has her gold and the dwarf demands the child, but the girl resists, "I love my child!" The dwarf retorts, "A deal is a deal." In fairy tales, there are happy endings, and in this one the girl keeps her child.

Today, surrogacy can be combined with modern technology (such as in vitro fertilization), to make many new reproductive arrangements possible. A woman surrogate may, for instance, partially *beget* a child by contributing an egg; *bear* a child by gestating another woman's egg fertilized in vitro; or *rear* a child conceived by or borne by another woman. It is theoretically possible for a surrogate to gestate an embryo conceived by one couple for adoption by a second couple. It is also theoretically possible for a child created by surrogacy to have five "parents:" sperm donor (male), egg donor (female), gestator (female), and two adults (male or female) who rear the child.

Various forms of surrogacy should be distinguished. The Baby M case involved *genetic surrogacy:* the surrogate's (Mary Beth Whitehead's) egg was artificially inseminated with a donor's (William Stern's) sperm. In *gestational surrogacy,* by contrast, one woman's egg is fertilized in vitro by a man's sperm and then implanted in another woman's—the surrogate's—womb. Genetic and gestational surrogacy can be either commercial or altruistic. In *commercial surrogacy,* the surrogate is paid for donating the egg, gestating the fetus, or both. In *altruistic surrogacy,* the surrogate's donation (egg, gestation, or both) is a gift; it has been suggested that altruistic surrogacy exemplifies traditional ideals of motherhood. Atruistic donation is, of course, familiar in the context of giving blood, where it is now encouraged because it is believed to work better than a commercial system,[1] since altruistic blood donors do not have any motive to conceal diseases or other health problems, whereas commercial donors might. (Altruistic donation is required for bone marrow and organ transplants.)

One study found that women become surrogates for various motives: for money, for the experience of pregnancy, as atonement for something in their past.[2] So far, the typical applicant for surrogacy has been a 25-year-old white woman with two children and a high school education. Twenty percent of applicants have been divorced; 25 percent have never been married; about half have been Catholic and half Protestant.

Before Baby M, there had been two particularly odd cases of surrogacy in the United States. In one of these, the surrogate—a woman in Tennessee—blackmailed the adoptive parents, demanding more money than had been agreed on; she also took illegal drugs during the pregnancy. In another case, in 1982, Alexander Malahoff, a 46-year-old accountant, signed a surrogate contract for $10,000 with Judy Stiver, who bore a son born lacking most of the brain. Malahoff asked for blood and tissue tests to determine the paternity of this child, and he and the Stivers actually received the results during an appearance on *The Donahue Show.* When it was learned that Judy Stiver's husband, not Malahoff, was the father, the Stivers huddled and Phil Donahue nervously ad-libbed as tense minutes ticked by. Finally, Judy Stiver said that no one had told her not to have intercourse with her husband before she was artificially inseminated with Malahoff's sperm. She then announced that she would keep the baby. As the show ended, she said, "I'm excited."

THE BABY M CASE

The Sterns and the Whiteheads

The Baby M case involved two families in New Jersey: Elizabeth and William Stern and Mary Beth and Richard Whitehead.

The Sterns, William (or Bill) and Elizabeth, were a well-off professional couple. When the events in the case began they were in their late thirties; when the Baby M trial opened in 1987, they were both 41. Both of them had doctorates—he in biochemistry, she in genetics. William Stern was earning about $40,000 a year; Elizabeth Stern, who had just completed medical school and was beginning her teaching career as an assistant professor of pediatrics, was earning about $48,000 a year, plus fees from patients amounting to at least that much. As a pediatrician, she might later expect to earn over $100,000 a year; this figure would be less if she worked part-time but could be much more if she became a partner in a successful pediatric practice.

Most of William Stern's relatives had died in the Nazi Holocaust, and it was at least partly for this reason that he wanted a genetic child. His wife, however, felt that she should not become pregnant. In 1972 and 1978, Elizabeth Stern had experienced numbness of the extremities, weakness of the legs, and optic neuritis; and in 1980, a neuro-ophthalmologist, who may or may not have actually examined her, said that these symptoms "probably" indicated multiple sclerosis (MS). Some "peer counselors" with MS told her that pregnancy would exacerbate the onset of symptoms, which could include blindness, deafness, incontinence, and paralysis; also, a friend with MS had become paralyzed after bearing a child. These considerations had convinced Elizabeth Stern that pregnancy would be an unacceptable risk.

•

Mary Beth Whitehead was in her mid-twenties when the events in the case began; she was 29 when the Baby M trial opened in 1987. She had dropped out of high school at age 16 and had then worked in a pizza parlor. She met Richard Whitehead while she was working there; he was then a veteran just back from Vietnam, where he had served for 1 year. They were married 6 months later; when the trial opened, they had been married for 12 years and had two children, Ryan (then age 10) and Tuesday (then 9).

Richard Whitehead was 8 years older than his wife. When the trial opened, he was 37 and had been a sanitation worker for 4 years; he was making $28,000 a year. Before that, he had been a gravedigger and a driver for an asphalt paving company, but he had lost his driver's license after two convictions for driving while intoxicated. He characterized himself as an alcoholic who could control his problem.

The Whiteheads had often experienced financial difficulties. Because of these financial problems, they had moved twelve times between 1973 and 1981 and had frequently lived with other family members. In 1978, the couple had temporarily separated; during their separation, Mary Beth Whitehead had received public assistance and—in desperate need of money—had worked for 3 months in a bar owned by her sister, as a dancer wearing a bathing suit. In 1983, the Whiteheads filed for bankruptcy; at that time, they had two mortgages on their home, both in default.

Baby M's Conception and Birth

In 1984, a few months after she and her husband had filed for bankruptcy, Mary Beth Whitehead answered a newspaper advertisement offering $10,000 for surrogacy. The money seemed like the answer to their financial problems; besides, she said, pregnancy wasn't bad and a child was the "most loving gift" a woman could give to another couple. Her husband initially opposed her idea but ultimately went along with it. Soon thereafter, although she had been rejected by the Surrogate Mother Program in New York—an agency with rigorous screening procedures[3]—she enrolled at the Infertility Center of New York (ICNY), which rejected applicants only for reasons of health or age.

In an interview with ICNY in April of 1984, Mary Beth Whitehead said that she would have strong feelings against giving up a child, though she would do it. The interviewer noted that these feelings should be explored before fertilization was attempted. They were not. However, Mary Beth and Richard Whitehead were asked to go over ICNY's Surrogate Parenting Agreement for several hours with an independent lawyer and did make several minor changes in it. The contract stipulated that Mary Beth Whitehead would undergo both a psychiatric evaluation and a second-trimester amniocentesis; that she would terminate the pregnancy if fetal defects were found; and that if the baby was born handicapped, the adoptive parents would accept the child. It further stipulated that, as a surrogate, she would not "form or attempt to form a parent-child relationship" with the baby. With regard to relationships between surrogates and adoptive parents, different agencies worked in different ways: Infertility Associates International of Washington, D.C., for instance, forbade surrogates to meet adoptive couples; but at ICNY, everyone met frequently, and some adoptive couples were present in the delivery room to observe the birth.

Over the next 8 months at ICNY, Mary Beth Whitehead first tried to become pregnant with a client who was eventually found to be producing no sperm. She was offered another opportunity with William Stern, who had entered into an agreement with ICNY in August 1984.

The Sterns had chosen Mary Beth Whitehead from several candidates because she looked like Elizabeth Stern (they would later regret this emphasis on "looks"), and in January of 1985 the Whiteheads and the Sterns met. On February 6, 1985, Mary Beth Whitehead signed a contract with William Stern similar to the one she had previously signed. Later, in a book called *A Mother's Story*, she described what happened after that:

> In the months that followed, Bill and I would meet at the Thomas Edison exit on the New Jersey Turnpike and drive to the Infertility Center in New York together. Bill was always nervous about getting to the city on time. If we were late, he would take off his gloves and cover the clock with them so that he wouldn't look at the time. Then he would drive like a maniac.
>
> The arrangement seemed odd and unnatural. We were two strangers who were attempting to achieve the most intimate human connection possible without ever touching each other. We used to sit there together in all those hours of traffic with little or nothing to say.
>
> When we finally got to the Center, Bill would go into a small private room and come out a few minutes later, carrying his sperm. Then I would go into another private room and be inseminated while he waited outside. After that, we'd start the long drive back.[4]

After each insemination (there were nine in all), Mary Beth Whitehead would lie on her back with her legs up for 45 minutes, to maximize the chance of conception. In August 1985, Mary Beth Whitehead learned that she had become pregnant in July.

At first, the two couples had a "honeymoon" period: they called each other "Betsy," "Bill," "Rick," and "Mary Beth"; everything went smoothly; and Mary Beth Whitehead said that she would give the child up and wanted only an annual picture and a letter. Six months later, though, their relationship turned sour.

By that time, the Sterns thought of the fetus as "their" child, but Mary Beth Whitehead, now in her third trimester, began to think of it as "her" child. In addition, she refused to take a drug that had been prescribed to lower her blood pressure: the Sterns saw the prescription as part of good medical care, but she saw it as a risk to the baby. (She also gave up drinking and smoking during the pregnancy—as required by the contract—because she considered them risky to the baby.) Another conflict had arisen over the second-trimester amniocentesis, which is commonly used to screen for Down syndrome and certain other defects when a pregnant women is older than about 35. Mary Beth Whitehead's obstetrician (whom she had selected at random from the telephone directory), did not recommend amniocentesis, considering it an unnecessary expense for a younger woman; but it had been called for by the contract, and William Stern insisted on it (he probably knew about the Malahoff case). Mary Beth Whitehead did have the procedure performed; but though amniocentesis identifies the sex of a fetus—in this case, female—she would not reveal the sex to the Sterns. Toward the end of the pregnancy, her blood pressure rose, and the Sterns tried to get her to lower it by various means. She claimed that they were trying to take over her life.

During this time, Mary Beth Whitehead began to tell Ryan and Tuesday that she didn't want to "sell" their "sister." A month before she gave birth, she delayed signing the paternity papers that would give the baby to the Sterns, although she eventually did sign them.

•

The baby—who would be called "Baby M" by the trial court—was born on Thursday, March 27, 1986, in Monmouth Medical Center in Long Branch, New Jersey. The Whiteheads did not mention the surrogate agreement to the hospital staff and acted as if they were both the baby's parents. On the birth certificate, Richard Whitehead was identified as the father, and the baby was named Sara Elizabeth Whitehead. When William Stern arrived at the hospital, the nurses were unaware of his involvement and would not let him hold the baby.

Mary Beth Whitehead would later testify that she had bonded intensely with the baby immediately, at birth: "Seeing her, holding her. She was my child. It overpowered me. I had no control. I had to keep her."[5] She also thought that the baby looked like her. The next day, she told the Sterns that she was so troubled about giving up the baby that she felt suicidal.

When she took the baby home from the hospital, however, she agreed to meet the Sterns to relinquish the child; they expressed their gratitude and soon, pressed by the Sterns, she reluctantly let them take the baby and leave. Late that same night, she became distraught and woke her husband to ask, "Oh God, what did I do?"[6] The next morning—March 30—still upset, she went to the Sterns' home and asked to visit with the baby. The Sterns let her do so, and she then told them that she felt terrible about giving the baby up; she also claimed that she had almost tried to kill herself the night before by taking an overdose of Valium. She asked to take the baby home for a week until her feelings stabilized. Believing that she was suicidal, the Sterns reluctantly agreed.

The next day, Mary Beth Whitehead said that she was going to visit an aunt and would be unreachable; actually, she took the baby—now 5 days old—to her parents' home in Florida. A few days later, she called the Sterns and told them that she needed more time to think, saying that her husband had threatened to leave her if she kept the baby; she did not reveal that she and the baby were in Florida. When she returned to New Jersey, the Sterns visited the Whitehead home; at that time, she told them that she wanted to keep the baby permanently and that she would take the child out of the country if they went to court. When William Stern asked to hold the baby, she refused and threatened to call the police. A week after this, the Whiteheads listed their house for sale, intending to move to Florida without telling the Sterns.

Baby M's Case in the Courts

The Sterns, of course, did go to court. On May 5, Judge Harvey Sorkow of the family court in Hackensack froze the Whiteheads' assets to prevent them from leaving the state and signed a "show cause" order directing them to surrender the baby.

With this order, William Stern accompanied local police to the Whiteheads' home. The Whiteheads created a delay by telephoning their lawyer, and during some confusion Mary Beth Whitehead took the baby to a bedroom at the rear of the house and passed the infant to Richard Whitehead, who was standing outside. A few minutes later, she returned to the living room and held out her hands, as if for handcuffs. "The baby's gone," she said. "If you want to lock me up, go ahead."[7] Unable to find the baby, the police and William Stern eventually left. The next day, the Whiteheads fled to Florida with the baby. Their location would remain unknown to the Sterns for the next 3 months.

In Florida, as the Sterns' private detective tried to find them, the Whiteheads lived with various relatives, leaving Ryan and Tuesday with Mary Beth's parents. Mary Beth Whitehead tried to hire a lawyer, but every lawyer she contacted wanted a $5,000 retainer—far more than she and her husband, who didn't even have $50 to spare, could afford. (Eventually they did find a lawyer, who agreed to take their case if they signed the mortgage on their house over to him; when he withdrew after the pretrial hearing, another laywer took the case on a *pro bono* basis. This second lawyer, Harold Cassidy, saw the case through to the state supreme court.)

Around July 15, Mary Beth Whitehead called William Stern. He secretly tape-recorded this call, and his recording was later introduced into the trial proceedings at the instigation of the Whiteheads' lawyer (by then Harold Cassidy). The tape was introduced as evidence of Mary Beth Whitehead's anguished mental state during this time, and the Sterns' lawyer objected to it; but it turned out to be the evidence that shifted public opinion from Mary Beth Whitehead's side to the Sterns'. In the following transcript, William Stern (WS) seems calm, rational, and sympathetic (probably because he is taping the call), whereas Mary Beth White-head (MBW) seems distraught.

WS: Mary Beth, what can we do?

MBW: Bill, I'll tell you right now if you don't do something, I am going to do something that I am going to be very sorry for—

WS: What do you mean, you're going to do something you're going to be sorry for?

MBW: [getting upset] I'm telling you right now, Bill, you think you got all the cards. You think you could do this to people. You took my house. I mean we don't even have a car anymore. I can't even afford the car payments. You took everything away from me.

WS: I, I—

MBW: Because I couldn't give up my child?

WS: Mary Beth—

MBW: Because I couldn't give up my flesh and blood, you have the right to do what you did?

WS: I didn't freeze your assets; the judge froze your assets.

MBW: Oh, but oh, come on, Bill your lawyer did it, and you knew about it.

WS: [matter-of-factly] The judge froze your assets. He wants, he wants you in court.

MBW: [accusatory] Uh-huh, sure, Bill, and how about the baby's sake, and how about Ryan and Tuesday? You're ruining a lot of people's lives.

WS: Aren't—don't you think you're ruining their lives, too?

MBW: I have?

WS: Yes.

MBW: Yes. I have. So maybe I should just, me and Sara, vanish off the face of he earth.

WS: No, you shouldn't face—vanish off the face of the earth.

MBW: Well, that's what you're forcing me to do.

. . .

WS: I want my daughter back.

MBW: And I want her, too, so what do we do, cut her in half? [angry]

WS: No, no, we don't cut her in half. [resigned]

MBW: You want me, you want me to kill myself and the baby?

WS: No, that's why I gave her to you in the first place, because I didn't want you to kill yourself.

. . .

MBW: . . . I didn't anticipate any of this. You know that. I'm telling you from the bottom of my heart. I never anticipated any of it. Bill, please, stop it. Please do something to stop this.

WS: What can I do to stop it, Mary Beth?

MBW: Bill, I'll let you see her. You can have her on weekends. As soon as she
        gets a little older, you can have her a couple of weeks. Please stop this.
WS: [anguished] Oh, God!

. . .

MBW: . . . So you want to go to court and get hurt more?
WS: Well, that's a chance I have to take. I can't live with myself letting her go.
MBW: What do you mean, letting her go? I told you you could see her. We
        could, we could be decent about it.
WS: Hah—you mean I would just get her—
MBW: You can't live with that?
WS: I can live with you visiting. I can live with that, but I can't live with her hav-
        ing a split identity between us. That—that'll hurt her.
MBW: What's the difference if I visit or you visit?
WS: The difference is—
MBW: Who do you think she's going to want more? Her own mother? And I've
        been breast-feeding her for 4 months. Don't you think she's bonded to me?
WS: I don't know what she's done, Mary Beth.
MBW: She's bonded to me, Bill. I sleep in the same bed with her. She won't even
        sleep by herself. You tell me, what are you going to do when you get this kid
        that's screaming and carrying on for her mother?
WS: I'll be her father. I'll be a father to her. I am her father.

. . .

MBW: I took care of myself the whole 9 months. I didn't take any drugs. I didn't
        drink alcohol. I ate good. And that's the only reason that she's healthy, Bill.
        Only—because of me, because of me. . . . I gave her life. I did. I had the
        right during the whole pregnancy to terminate, didn't I, Bill?
WS: It was your body.
MBW: That's right. It was my body, and now you're telling me I have no right.

. . .

MBW: You don't want her; you've made, you've made your point quite clear.
WS: No, I want my daughter back.
MBW: Forget it, Bill. I'll tell you right now I'd rather see me and her dead before
        you get her.
WS: Don't, Mary Beth, please don't do—
MBW: I'm going to do it, Bill.
WS: Mary—
MBW: I'm going to do it; you've pushed me to it. Now you're telling me I can't—
        my children can't get their house back? I've done this to everybody's life.
WS: Wait!—
MBW: I gave her life. I can take her life away. If that's what you want, that's
        what I'll do.
WS: No! Mary Beth. No! Mary Beth. Wait! Wait!
MBW: That's what I'm going to do, Bill.
WS: Please—
MBW: You've pushed me.

WS: Please don't—I want—don't want to see you hurt. I don't want to see my daughter hurt. I really—

MBW: My daughter, too. Why don't you quit doing that, Bill, OK?

WS: OK, OK, all right—

MBW: It's our daughter. Why don't you say it, "our daughter"?

WS: All right, our daughter. OK, Mary Beth, our daughter.[8]

In a later portion of the tape, Mary Beth Whitehead says that if William Stern doesn't drop his suit, she will accuse him of sexually abusing her daughter Tuesday. In her book, she explains this behavior by saying, "I struck out blindly and came up with the most horrible thing I could think of. . . . It was another idle threat, made in a moment of desperation."[9]

Two weeks after this call, Mary Beth Whitehead was hospitalized for pyelonephritis with encephalopathy (a severe kidney disorder that would recur a year later during her appeal to the New Jersey Supreme Court) and left the baby at her parents' home in Florida. The baby was discovered there soon afterward (on July 31) by the Sterns' detective, taken back to New Jersey by authorities, and returned to the Sterns.

Judge Sorkow of the Hackensack family court took several unusual actions. He had already issued some rather extreme orders: as noted earlier, the Whiteheads' assets had been frozen; their property was also confiscated, so that when they returned to New Jersey for the trial, they had no access to their bank accounts and were homeless for 3 weeks. Sorkow had also already accepted documents from the Sterns' lawyer stating that Mary Beth Whitehead was suicidal and that the Whiteheads were unfit parents. On the basis of those documents, he now issued an *ex parte* (one-sided) order awarding temporary custody of the baby to the Sterns, without giving the Whiteheads the customary chance to appeal the order immediately. At the urging of her lawyer, Mary Beth Whitehead allowed print and television reporters into her hospital room to counter the Sterns' story in the public's mind.

When the Whiteheads returned to New Jersey, Sorkow referred them to Lorraine Abraham, who had been appointed guardian *ad litem* for "Baby M," as the child was called by the court. Mary Beth Whitehead claims that Abraham was a personal friend of Sorkow's, that Abraham asked her, "Why are you talking to the *press*, Mary Beth?"—and that when her eyes filled with tears, Abraham snapped at her: "Save your tears for television, because you won't get any sympathy here."[10] At another meeting, according to Mary Beth Whitehead, Abraham asked her, "Tell me, Mary Beth, who's going to play your part in the movie?"[11]

•

The trial, which opened in January 1987, in Hackensack, New Jersey, was to determine, first, the legality of surrogate contracts; and second, the custody of Baby M. Judge Sorkow was presiding.

Mary Beth Whitehead testified—among other testimony—that the baby might not be William Stern's, because she and her husband had had sexual relations during the insemination process (this would of course have violated the surrogacy contract); and the judge ordered an HLA antigen test, which was legal in New Jersey. According to the test results, there was a 98 percent probability that William Stern was the genetic father; later, Mary Beth Whitehead revealed that her husband had undergone a vasectomy 9 years before.

William Stern testified that if he lost the case, it would be better for the baby not to see him anymore; he said that having two sets of parents would not be healthy for her. Mary Beth Whitehead, on the other hand, said that if she lost, she would still want to see the baby.

About half a dozen psychologists, psychiatrists, and psychiatric social work-ers—some of whom were receiving consulting fees of as much as $12,000—testi-fied for the Sterns. They all concluded that the Sterns would be the best parents for Baby M, and most of them said that Mary Beth Whitehead could not separate her own needs from those of the baby.

One issue that arose was Mary Beth Whitehead's involvement of Ryan and Tuesday in these events; seemingly, she had made no attempt to shield them from possible harm. One explanation offered was that this was a strategy urged on the Whiteheads by their lawyer; presumably, on this explanation, he had cal-culated that this would make it more difficult for Sorkow to deny custody to the Whiteheads—it would seem as though the other two children would be "losing their sister." Another explanation is that Mary Beth Whitehead herself had manipulated Ryan and Tuesday, for the same purpose. She had placed a crib in Tuesday's room for the baby and had described the baby to Tuesday as the "sis-ter" who was "sold"; she petitioned the court to let Tuesday and Ryan visit the baby; twice she brought Tuesday to court, where newspaper photographers took pictures of the girl crying; and she also allowed Tuesday to be interviewed for television—during the interviews, Tuesday was said to look often at her mother, apparently for directions. Mary Beth Whitehead also attempted to have Tuesday testify about how much she missed the baby, but Sorkow denied the motion and tried to keep the Whitehead children out of the case.

The main character witness for Mary Beth Whitehead was a former neighbor, Susan Herherhan. By the time she testified, however, Sorkow was convinced that Mary Beth Whitehead was a chronic liar. He felt that she had committed fraud by failing to list some assets when the Whiteheads had filed for bankruptcy; that she had deliberately concealed her husband's vasectomy; that she had twice fled ille-gally to Florida with Baby M; that she had threatened Baby M's life; that she had threatened to bring a vicious suit against Bill Stern for sexual assault; and that she had manipulated her children in order to win custody of the baby. Then Sorkow discovered that Susan Herherhan had forged a letter to him, and she admitted that her testimony was perjured and that she had made up the letter to help Mary Beth Whitehead; this was the last straw.

Judge Sorkow was well aware that his decision would be groundbreaking, and also that a lower-court judge rarely sets even a temporary precedent; there-fore, his opinion was exhaustive (it was 120 pages long) and was written with an eye to higher courts.[12]

Sorkow ruled that the surrogacy contract was legal and did not constitute "baby selling"; gave permanent custody to the Sterns; terminated the White-heads' visiting rights; declared William Stern the baby's father; ordered the birth records changed; enjoined the Whiteheads from interfering with the Sterns; and awarded $10,000 to Mary Beth Whitehead. He concluded that litigation was needed to end the controversy for the good of "Melissa Stern" (as the Sterns had named the baby), who needed to have her parentage established, to have a "strong support system," and not to be manipulated any longer. Therefore, immediately after his ruling, he took Elizabeth Stern into his chambers and allowed her to adopt the baby—thus making Elizabeth Stern the legal mother and specifically denying that Mary Beth Whitehead was the mother in any legal sense. Not only was Mary Beth Whitehead given no visiting rights; she was ordered not to see the baby again.

To many observers, Judge Sorkow's objectivity was questionable. Mary Beth Whitehead's lawyer said that Sorkow appeared "to be growling at us; his face was beet red, his jowls were shaking, and he was really worked into a lather. It was wild to watch so much hatred."[13] Supporters of Mary Beth Whitehead were especially incensed by the adoption proceedings. The next day, some "feminist" supporters of Mary Beth Whitehead demonstrated against the decision outside the courtroom; they carried signs reading, "SORKOW THE TERMINATOR" and "A ONE-NIGHT STAND IN A DISH DOESN'T MAKE A MAN A FATHER"; called Noel Keane, the director of ICNY, a "pimp"; and decried any legalization of "reproductive prostitution." Phyllis Chesler, one of the organizers of the demonstrations, blasted the entire trial: "It was a gang rape. A public daily crucifixion of a perfectly good mother."[14]

•

In February 1988, on appeal, the New Jersey Supreme Court unanimously reversed Judge Sorkow's decision and ruled that surrogacy contracts were illegal.[15] Although the supreme court allowed the Sterns to retain custody of the baby because their home life was more "secure" and "nurturing," the justices specifically disallowed Elizabeth Stern's adoption of the baby. They said, "We thus restore the surrogate as the mother of the child. She is not only the natural mother but also the legal mother, and is not to be penalized one iota because of the surrogate contract."

The higher court also found that surrogate contracts constituted baby selling:

> This is the sale of a child, or at the very least, the sale of a mother's right to her child, the only mitigating factor being that one of the purchasers is the father. The surrogate contract creates, it is based upon, principles that are directly contrary to our laws. It guarantees separation of a child from its mother; it looks to adoption regardless of suitability; it totally ignores the child; it takes the child from the mother regardless of her wishes and her maternal fitness, and it does all this, it accomplishes all of its goals, through the use of money.

The court said that surrogacy contracts also violated "public policy" by assigning custody to a father without a hearing that would focus on the best interests of the child, by guaranteeing separation of a child from its natural mother, and by giving the father (in this case William Stern) greater rights than the mother (Mary Beth Whitehead). The court also agreed with an argument that had been advanced by some feminists: "The whole purpose and effect of the surrogate contract was to give the father exclusive rights to the child by destroying the rights of the mother."

The New Jersey Supreme Court disagreed with Judge Sorkow's reasoning on almost every theoretical point: his 120-page opinion was dissected and left in shreds (gratified supporters of the Whiteheads said that Sorkow was now being treated as contemptuously as he had treated Mary Beth Whitehead). Sorkow had held that surrogate contracts transcended the limitations of existing laws governing adoption and custody, but the supreme court implied that even voluntary surrogacy must abide by ordinary laws of adoption and custody. In an important ruling, the supreme court allowed voluntary, unpaid surrogacy provided that the mother could change her mind and keep the baby.

Some of the supreme court justices themselves seem to have had rather strong emotions about the case. Chief Justice Wilentz often referred to William Stern as the "sperm donor," to Elizabeth Stern as the "stepmother," and to Mary Beth Whitehead as "the baby's mother."[16]

The Aftermath

In May of 1987, Mary Beth Whitehead had gone to Puerto Rico, at the invitation of supportive friends who owned a condominium there, to recuperate and await the decision of the New Jersey Supreme Court. She writes that she met Dean Gould—a tall, athletic young accountant from New York City—on a beach in Puerto Rico, soon fell in love with him, and saw him frequently over the next 3 months.[17] At that time, she and Richard Whitehead were still married, but they had separated; in August 1987, her lawyer felt obligated to write to the New Jersey Supreme Court, informing them of this separation. According to the lawyer's prepared statement, "Extraordinary stress placed upon her marriage and the public discussion of private matters rendered Mr. and Mrs. Whitehead's marriage an inevitable casualty of this unusual case."

Some time later, during a supervised visit with Melissa Stern (whom she continued to call "Sara"), Mary Beth Whitehead confided to a female attendant that she was pregnant out of wedlock by Dean Gould. The attendant, an official of the court, called Lorraine Abraham (this action "shocked" Mary Beth Whitehead), who informed the supreme court. Richard Whitehead soon filed for divorce; and in November 1987—2 weeks after the divorce was granted—Mary Beth Whitehead married Dean Gould. To pay her medical bills, she sold pictures of the wedding to a sensationalistic tabloid, *The Star*, for an undisclosed price. In the spring of 1988, she gave birth to a new child, conceived in the traditional way.

After the supreme court decision, as the legal mother of Melissa Stern, Mary Beth Gould returned to a lower court—the New Jersey Superior Court—to petition for visiting rights. Three superior court judges allowed her to visit with the baby 1 day a week for up to 6 hours; this would be increased to 2 days a week with an overnight stay and 2 weeks during the following summer, and the baby would alternate holidays between the two families.[18] The superior court concluded, "Melissa's best interests will be served by unsupervised, uninterrupted liberal visitation by her mother," and by allowing mother and daughter to "develop their own special relationship." The Sterns felt that the child's best interests would be served by keeping the case out of court, and so they said they would not appeal.

In October 1987, appearing before a subcommittee of the United States House of Representatives, Mary Beth Gould had testified against surrogacy; she also expressed her opposition in an appearance on *Good Morning America*. She said, "Your eyes are not open until you hold that baby in your arms and she becomes real."

ETHICAL ISSUES

The Significance of the Case: Major or Minor

Before the Baby M case, hundreds of babies had been born through surrogacy; only four cases had involved any dispute, and all four had been settled out of court. The director of one surrogate agency said, "The Whitehead case is a real aberration. She's one of half a dozen who have changed their mind, out of 800 to 1,000 surrogates who have given birth";[19] and one family court judge said that the case shouldn't have been handled as a contract dispute at all, but "simply as a custody case."[20] Statistically and theoretically, then, it can be argued that the case of Baby M was blown out of proportion—that it was a minor matter which led, perhaps inappropriately, to major decisions.

In ethics, it is a fallacy to put too much weight on very few cases, let alone on a single case. In medicine, this sort of mistake is described as overreliance on "anecdotal evidence"; in statistics, it is expressed as having $N = 1$; in practical reasoning, it is called *hasty generalization*. Prohibiting surrogacy on the basis of the Baby M case might reflect this kind of error.

Custody fights, of course, are not confined to surrogate arrangements; such disputes are not ideal, but marriage is not forbidden because of them—why, then, should surrogacy contracts be banned? Supporters of surrogacy argue that if hundreds of babies have been created, happily, through surrogacy contracts and fewer than 1 percent of surrogate mothers have expressed any regrets, banning such contracts is unwarranted, a hasty generalization. In other words, on this argument, surrogacy contracts have had a success rate of something like 99 percent, which in any public policy would be considered very good; therefore, whatever harms developed in the Baby M should be seen as rare, as representing a low risk, and as far outweighed by the good experiences of most surrogates and the families they help.

Elizabeth Stern's Decision: Rational or Irrational

One issue that arose during the Baby M case was Elizabeth Stern's decision not to bear a child herself. As noted earlier, she had made this decision to avoid the risk of bringing on or aggravating symptoms of multiple sclerosis (MS), and some commentators criticized her for "using" her possible condition to "avoid" pregnancy.[21] The National MS Society, for instance, thought that women with MS should not forgo pregnancy unless they were too disabled to care for a baby; it also said that Elizabeth Stern would be in little danger from a pregnancy. To the National MS Society, her decision to avoid pregnancy was thus irrational.

On the other hand, several experts testified that Elizabeth Stern's decision was in accordance with earlier medical opinion; and that although prevailing medical opinion had since changed, any pregnancy still carried a 5 to 40 percent risk of intensifying MS.[22] These experts held that her decision was medically reasonable.

In retrospect, this seems to have been a somewhat bizarre—or at least irrelevant—controversy: Elizabeth Stern's decision was a personal matter with no clear bearing on the Baby M case. Also, the position of the MS Society seems inappropriate: understandably, the society wanted to empower women with MS, but that aim would hardly be advanced by attacking a specific woman who might have the disorder. General recommendations about MS and pregnancy should probably be a matter of public policy, based on medical and statistical considerations, not an issue of individual "rationality" or "irrationality."

Surrogacy and Motherhood

Defining motherhood   A basic philosophical question underlying the Baby M case was, "What is a mother?" In the context of surrogacy, who is the real mother: the egg donor, the gestator who caries the fetus to term, or the woman who raises the child?   Perhaps the best answer is simply, "Improper question." In other words, perhaps we need not conclude that one woman must be the "real" mother.

Concerns about biological ties   For some people, surrogacy violates basic concepts of motherhood, parenthood, and families—concepts of what a family is and how it is formed. These people often express the fear that children, and society in general, will be hurt by arrangements like surrogacy, and this fear seems to arise from a sense that the family should be based on biological ties. As one theologian urged:

> Clearly, the notions of marriage and parenting must and do go beyond . . . biological beginnings. But these beginnings are the foundation upon which the rest, the complex network of kinship, bonding, and support, is built. If we untie this biological knot, what will happen to the institution that for so many centuries has taken shape around it?[23]

One critic has argued that if commercial contracts for surrogacy are allowed, "our culture will become more fragmented, rootless, and alienated."[24]

Concerns about weakening biological ties are not, of course, directed only at surrogacy; they have also been raised in other contexts, such as in vitro fertilization (see Chapter 4) and "blended" families, and they sometimes get mixed in with indirectly related (or even unrelated) issues: single parenthood, teenage motherhood, welfare families, abortion. In general, the underlying assumption seems to be that in the past there have been genuine norms of "motherhood," "parenthood," and "family" and that these norms are now under attack from too many directions.

People who express such fears are often described as longing for a Norman Rockwell picture of the family—Mom, with a peaches-and-cream complexion, cooking in the kitchen while two happy kids play nearby. It can certainly be argued that the "Norman Rockwell" family was no more than an idealization to begin with and is a totally unrealistic and inappropriate goal in today's world; but that response may be simplistic. A more cogent argument would be, simply, that family ties have never been only biological: a husband and wife, to take the most obvious example, are not biological relatives. It can also be argued that if "the family" is a good thing, then developing more kinds of ways—including nonbiological ways—to create families should also be seen as a good thing.

Predicting the quality of motherhood   Another issue in the Baby M case had to do with predicting and assessing the quality of childrearing.

Expert witnesses overwhelmingly found Mary Beth Whitehead lacking as a mother. One psychiatrist said that she had a mixed-type personality disorder, with impulsiveness, self-importance, exploitativeness, and lack of empathy.[25] The psychologist Lee Salk said that the Whiteheads lacked emotional stability, peaceful home life, capacity to respond to children's needs, commitment to education, and reasonableness in daily judgments and were not sufficiently hostile to drug-dependence.[26] (However, Salk had never examined Mary Beth Whitehead; and he may not have been entirely objective, since he himself had recently been involved in a custody dispute with his ex-wife, which he ultimately won.) A senior social worker found Mary Beth Whitehead narcissistic and manipulative of her children: "Mary Beth Whitehead appears unable to acknowledge Baby M as a person with an identity and needs separate from her own. Her need for having possession of this baby is overwhelming. . . . She feels threatened if her needs are not met. Mary Beth Whitehead is capable of exploiting her children to achieve her goals."[27]

Other commentators, however, saw Mary Beth Whitehead differently. What was so wrong, they argued, with a mother who was totally committed to her baby? What was wrong with being courageous enough to risk running afoul of the law by moving to Florida? Wasn't that better than going out to work and dropping the kid off at Cradle Rock for 10 hours a day? What was wrong with earning money for her children as a dancer?

One philosopher, who was also a mother, wrote sympathetically: "Not surprisingly, she thought of Sara as her child, and she fought with every weapon at her disposal, honorable and dishonorable, to prevent her being taken away. She can hardly be blamed for doing so."[28] Another woman philosopher objected that it was difficult to evaluate good parenting, that richer parents were not necessarily better, and that to characterize Mary Beth Whitehead as "manipulative, impulsive, and exploitative" did not imply bad motherhood: "She sounds like many normal mothers, a person with cares and feelings."[29]

A law professor defended Mary Beth Whitehead vigorously:

> Judge Sorkow's opinion implicitly counsels: hire a mother for your child whom a judge is likely to view as unfit to raise it. Why aren't we all outraged at this suggestion and all the trashing of Baby M's mother? . . . [She] was successfully portrayed as an ogre for fleeing the police, and fighting the child's father with the only weapons she thought available to protect her daughter.[30]

He added that Judge Sorkow "apparently decided to attempt to dehumanize the Whiteheads, to lionize the Sterns, and to pontificate on the devastation of infertility and the joys of parenthood."

Mary Beth Whitehead herself wrote, "I believed that being a mother and taking care of children was my calling in life. [As a child] I eagerly awaited the day I could do it full-time." When her children went to school all day, she missed having a baby around and felt "the old longing return" for pregnancy: "Being a mother was how I had always defined myself."[31]

Donald Klein, a Columbia University psychiatrist and author of the third edition of the definitive *Diagnostic and Statistical Manual of Psychiatric Disorders* (DSM-III), testified for Mary Beth Whitehead. Klein said that borderline personality disorder could not be diagnosed on the basis of behavior during periods of tremendous conflict or stress; he also testified that the other psychological experts had misdiagnosed her because they had applied outdated standards.[32]

Some other observers also attacked the psychological experts who had found Mary Beth Whitehead "unfit." A physician wrote, "Probably the most stressful and anxiety-provoking act in human existence is the separation of a woman from her newborn infant."[33] After such a separation, he said, humans and animals experience panic, rage, and distress. "Who can dare to judge the psychological acts and responses of a woman put to such a test?"

Some of the feminists who supported Mary Beth Whitehead specifically attacked the experts who had called her an unfit mother. (The general issue of feminism in this case is discussed in the next section.) In an article called "Whitehead vs. Sperm" (sic), the periodical *Off Our Backs* blasted Judge Sorkow, citing the Sterns' "six-figure annual salary" and describing the decision as a "condemnation of motherhood and vindication of father-right":

> The manner in which the trial was conducted has starkly revealed the class bias of reproductive health in the U.S., the pervasive negation of women's right to reproductive control. . . . The primary focus of the trial was a harsh concentrated attack on Whitehead's personality and emotional state and the stability of her home and marriage. The evidence presented at the trial brought out that Whitehead was a high school dropout and mother of two at age 19, was facing foreclosure on her house, that her husband had drinking problems, that she had spent three months as a barroom dancer in 1978 when she was 21, that she had been on welfare. In other words, she was facing the problems of a working-class mother.[34]

Off Our Backs also argued that "emotional instability" and "personality disorders" are typical of the "facetious charges made against mothers fighting for custody," and that it was the Sterns, not Mary Beth Whitehead, who lacked empathy for the child.

Surrogacy and Feminism

As we have seen, Mary Beth Whitehead found considerable support among some feminists. Women who identified themselves publicly as feminists and who sided with Mary Beth Whitehead included Meryl Streep, Gloria Steinem, Nora

Ephron, Susan Sontag, Sally Quinn, Margaret Atwood, Andrea Dworkin, and Donna Shalala. Betty Friedan called surrogate agencies "surrogacy pimps." To understand feminist discourse in the Baby M case, it will be helpful to consider briefly some general aspects of feminist philosophy.

•

There is a deep and widespread tension in feminism and feminist ethics over a question concerning women and parenthood: Are women biologically superior parents, or is that belief a culturally conditioned myth? Do women innately possess any "maternal" traits? More important, is it more sexist to believe that they have such innate traits or to deny that they do? These questions underlay some of the controversy and commentary in the Baby M case.

In 1988, in a survey of feminist philosophy, Rosemarie Tong wrote:

> After more reflection on patriarchy's construction of gender, however, many radical feminists concluded that androgyny was not really a liberatory strategy for women; that is, that it was not desirable for women to "masculinize" themselves in any way, shape, or form. Some radical feminists asserted that "femininity" was not a problem in and of itself. Rather, the problem was the low value which patriarchy assigned to nurturance, emotion, gentleness, and the like. All we need to do is value the feminine at least as much as the masculine, and women will be liberated from the social forces that oppress them. Other radical feminists disagreed, insisting that "femininity" had to be a problem, since it had been constructed under patriarchy for patriarchal purposes.[35]

Carol Gilligan and other feminist scholars in the 1980s attacked male norms in science, medicine, psychology, and (most significantly for our discussion) ethics: they argued that women-centered norms such as caring and nurturing had been neglected in ethics.[36] One woman expert who testified in the Baby M trial said that Mary Beth Whitehead exhibited the female ethics of family and relationships rather than the male ethics of analysis and contracts.[37]

Analyses like these give rise to some questions, however. If women's values are naturally "relational" rather than "analytic," is a women with a sharp, analytical mind "masculine"? Is she perverted? If women empathize with children better than men do, because of bonding during gestation and birth, and if mothers rather than fathers should therefore win custody disputes, doesn't it follow that women should stay at home and raise kids while men work?

The "meaning" of *feminism* is relevant here, and it can be clarified by drawing a distinction between *merit feminism* and *social feminism:*

- *Merit feminism*—Defines justice as equal opportunities for women and men to be rewarded for their talents and work, e.g., in admission to professional schools, freedom from sexual harassment on the job, equal wages for equal work, and promotions for achievement.
- *Social feminism*—Defines justice as equal recognition of the unique natural abilities, talents, and values of women and men in society and in public policy.

Merit feminists think that social feminism perpetuates a falsehood: the idea that "biology is destiny." Merit feminists don't think that a woman can have it both ways, choosing to be a social feminist in some situations and a merit feminist in others, depending on which kind of feminism is to her advantage in each situation. Merit feminists also think that social feminists are sometimes themselves sexist, using Orwellian doubletalk to advocate traditional female roles and values under the banner of "feminism." Social feminists maintain that merit feminists side too often with conservative males. Both of these approaches can be seen in feminist comments on the issue of surrogacy in general and the Baby M case in particular.

●

With regard to surrogacy contracts, one merit feminist, Christine Sistare, argued in 1988 that banning commercial surrogacy would *violate the rights of all women to be the depositors of their own reproductive capacities.*[38] She held that right to have control over one's body—a central tenet of merit feminism—includes a woman's right to profit from letting others hire her body to produce children. Referring to all the paid surrogates who gave up their babies and did not renege on their contracts, Sistare asked, "Are all such women *monsters?*"

Merit and social feminists were divided over "bonding," which is sometimes held to occur as a result of pregnancy, childbirth, and breast-feeding; it became an issue in the Baby M trial because Mary Beth Whitehead had breast-fed Baby M moments after birth and claimed that this experience had "bonded" her to the baby. Social feminists maintained that women do have biologically and hormonally determined feelings about their babies, considering such determinism more acceptable than "disembodied" male norms of epistemology. They argued that all knowledge is "body-mediated" and that because men and women have different bodily experiences, they differ in how they know the world.[39] For social feminists, a pregnant woman has a different body, and hence a different set of feelings, experiences, and beliefs; she is "connected" to the world uniquely, and differently from when she is not pregnant. The author Phyllis Chesler (who can fairly be described as the "Jeremy Rifkin" of this case) asked, "How can we deny that children bond with their mothers in utero, and that children suffer terribly in all kind of ways when this bond is prematurely or abruptly terminated?"[40]

Merit feminists, however, rejected the "epiphenomenalist" view that women's mental states—such as moods and beliefs—are by-products of their fluctuating hormonal states. Also, in a review of the literature on bonding, the philosopher Hilary Baber concluded there was little evidence in the social sciences for the existence of bonding in primates.[41] (It is interesting to note that Baber herself was pregnant when she wrote this review.) While there is evidence that infants need *some* maternal figure, she found no evidence of a psychological connection stemming from gestation or breast-feeding. Children who had wet nurses probably loved their own mothers; also, there is no evidence that biological progenitors are better parents than adoptive couples. Baber noted a minority view that, to gain special attention, traditional mothers have exploited the mystique of bearing a child, and that these mothers see surrogacy as a threat to their own roles and values.

Some social feminists attacked surrogacy from a very different perspective: they doubted that the wives in this situation were really choosing it freely. (A similar argument about choices is discussed in Chapter 4, in the context of in vitro fertilization.) Eleanor Smeal, a former president of the National Organization for Women (NOW), was troubled by Elizabeth Stern's passivity and William Stern's dominant role.[42] Smeal saw surrogacy as mainly for men, not really for infertile couples. Some feminists said that William Stern's desire for a genetic child was a typically male impulse, and that he was like the patriarchs who had abused women slaves to produce heirs. Barbara Katz Rothman said that she was opposed to surrogacy because the man was "hiring himself an extra wife."[43] These feminists argued that although women appear to have more freedom today, men still control women's choices in most circumstances, and that most men still want to produce genetic offspring in one way or another.

Social feminists were also concerned about the surrogate. They were unimpressed by the idea that surrogates act lovingly to offer a "gift of life" to lonely, childless couples; instead, they saw surrogacy as a "compassion trap." One merit feminist, Lori Andrews, has replied that if social feminists believe a surrogate is typically "brainwashed" into becoming a contractual mother, what makes them believe that any woman who becomes a mother in the conventional way isn't also "brainwashed"?[44] Are surrogates so emotional and so socialized to act for others, Andrews asks, that they can't decide not to be surrogates?

Surrogacy, Exploitation, and Commercialization

Many critics saw the Baby M case not primarily as a conflict over procreative rights but as a conflict between the rich and the poor, either because the case had essentially been decided in favor of the Sterns, who were rich; or because paid surrogacy itself represents exploitation or commercialization.

George Annas, for instance, felt that the Sterns' wealth had given them an unfair advantage:

> It was primarily the financial ability of the Sterns to hire an expert on family law and successfully obtain an *ex parte* order for temporary custody that determined the ultimate outcome of this case. In this sense, reinforced by the economic bias of the mental health experts and the judge, those critics who have labeled this custody decision a classist opinion favoring the haves over the have nots are correct. Justice seems to have been for sale along with Baby M.[45]

Some observers felt that Mary Beth Whitehead—a poor woman—had been exploited by surrogacy. Sorkow thought otherwise:

> To the contrary. It is the private adoption that has that great potential, if not fact, for the exploitation of the mother. In the private adoption, the woman is already pregnant. The biological father may be unknown or at best uninterested in his obligations. The woman may want to keep the child but cannot do so for financial reasons. There is risk of illegal consideration being paid to the mother. In surrogacy, none of these "downside" elements appear. The arrangement is made when the desire and intention to have a family exists on the couple's part. The surrogate has an opportunity to consult, take advice and consider her act and is not forced into the relationship. She is not yet pregnant.[46]

Not everyone would accept Sorkow's reasoning, however. It can be argued, simply, that surrogacy is exploitative if the surrogate is paid too little: for example, one surrogate (who was Mexican, not an American citizen) was paid only $2,000 by a California couple; Mary Beth Whitehead was paid $10,000, a figure that also seems rather low. (Lori Andrews has argued that if women are exploited by commercial surrogacy, the problem is not to ban such surrogacy but to get better pay for surrogates.[47]) More generally, it might be argued that financial need is in a sense coercive—that a woman may be "forced into the relationship" by poverty—and therefore that surrogacy can be seen as exploitative in its very nature. If Mary Beth Whitehead had been paid $1 million, would she still have been exploited? The philosopher Mary Gibson says "Yes," because the greater the payment, the harder it is for poor women to resist "undue inducements."[48]

The issue of exploitation should be distinguished from that of commercialization. Those who oppose surrogacy because they consider it exploitation feel that the surrogate is not paid *enough* or that women are in effect forced by poverty to become surrogates. Those who oppose surrogacy because they consider it commercialization base their objection on the fact that the surrogate is paid *anything at all.* One columnist who objected to surrogacy as a commercialization of procreation said: "If a mother can legally turn over the rights to her womb, then the ethic of the marketplace has won. Pregnancy becomes a service industry and babies are a product for sale."[49] A woman law professor agreed: "A woman's relation to her baby isn't like a factory worker's to a product. Will you tell the kid, 'We paid $25,000 for you. How do you feel about the biological mother who sold you?'"[50]

Some commentators, on the other hand, have defended commercialization in this context. Michael Kinsley, editor of the *New Republic,* argued:

> The basic moral case for contract law, and indeed for capitalism itself, rests on the voluntary nature of exchange. Commercial trade is good for all parties involved, or else they wouldn't engage in it. And in the vast majority of commercial transactions—including the vast majority of surrogate-motherhood contracts—the deal goes through with no problem, suggesting that both parties do indeed consider themselves better off.[51]

Kinsley also argued that if women are forbidden to enter into surrogacy contracts, why not ban other kinds of services that women contract to perform? If we want only traditional mothers, why not forbid women to work as maids or nannies? Why not forbid women to work at all? Kinsley reasoned that if the product in question was food or telephones rather than babies, a shortage would be seen as a failure of the system: when the Soviet Union forbade market contracts, shortages occurred; similarly, if the United States banned procreative contracts, shortages would occur.

Perhaps Kinsley should not have the last word here, however. Before we leave this section on class conflict, exploitation, and commercialization, let's consider a related hypothetical issue. The Philippines is a poor country, and when the United States Navy pulled out in 1992, there were about 30,000 prostitutes in

Manila, selling their bodies; now these prostitutes have lost most of their customers. However, today there are about 60,000 Americans who have end-stage renal disease and need kidney transplants. A kidney donor has no increased risk of mortality or morbidity. Therefore, why not let Americans buy kidneys from these Filipino prostitutes (and from any other Filipinos who want to volunteer) for, say, $50,000 a kidney? That would be more than a prostitute could have earned in 10 years; if these prostitutes could sell sex, and if now they can no longer make a living selling sex, why couldn't they sell kidneys? The Filipino donors would have the money; the American recipients would live longer; everybody would be better off.[52]

If you have a sense that there is something repellent about this argument, you may be better able to understand why many people who think of surrogacy as exploitation or commercialized reproduction are opposed to it. These critics say that commerce already dominates too many areas of life; extending it to life itself is intolerable. Our society often works by achieving a compromise between conflicting values, they argue, and the incentives of capitalism must be tempered by humane considerations.

Surrogacy and the Paradox of Harm

Could a child be harmed by being conceived in a surrogate arrangement? When we ask this question, the paradox of harm—discussed in Chapter 4—again rears its head, since it must be assumed that for any actual child the alternative to conception by surrogacy would have been nonexistence.

Mary Beth Whitehead's coauthor proudly asserts that without the Baby M case,

> Countless thousands of infants would have been bought before they were conceived, sold at birth, and forcibly separated forever from their mothers, in a country that prides itself on freedom.[53]

Because commercial surrogacy is now in disfavor, though, thousands of infants have neither been brought into existence nor "bought." Are they better off not existing?

Faced with the paradox of harm, some people argue that even if babies can't be harmed by being brought into the world, they can still be *wronged*;[54] according to this argument, some ways of being created are simply fundamentally wrong. But what does this really mean? Unless *fundamentally wrong* is defined, doesn't this argument beg the question?

Another argument is that whenever parents bring a child into existence, they "create a vulnerability."[55] On this argument, parents should make reasonable efforts to minimize a child's vulnerability, but for various reasons surrogacy increases vulnerability. For example, surrogacy means that, deliberately, only one of the parents will assume responsibility for the child: this may be acceptable to the parents, but later it may be unacceptable *per se* to the child; moreover, that arrangement may be inadequate to meet the child's needs. Additionally, couples who have children through surrogacy may be more reluctant than traditional parents to accept babies born with defects (as in the Malahoff case). Another consideration is that it may be traumatic for a child to learn that he or she was created through surrogacy; there is evidence that some people are disturbed to learn that they were adopted or conceived with sperm or an egg from an anonymous donor, and this may also be the case with children in surrogate arrangements.

Some Legal Aspects of Surrogacy

"Baby selling"   Selling babies or children is, of course, illegal in the western world, and this has been a factor in opposition to surrogacy. It is interesting to note, however, that in earlier times these laws were instituted not to prevent women from becoming surrogates but for an entirely different reason: to protect unwed mothers who might be tempted to sell their children.

Whether or not surrogacy amounts to "selling babies" has been a legally controversial point. A Michigan court ruled that it does, and therefore invalidated one surrogate contract. In the Baby M case, Judge Sorkow decided differently:

> The fact is, however, that the money to be paid to the surrogate is not being paid for the surrender of the child to the father. And that is just the point—at birth, mother and father have equal rights to the child absent any other agreement. The biological father pays the surrogate for her willingness to be impregnated and carry his child to term. At birth, the father does not purchase the child. It is his own biological, genetically-related child. He cannot purchase what is already his.

As we have seen, of course, Sorkow was overruled by the New Jersey Supreme Court on this point (as on many others): the higher court decided that surrogacy contracts are "baby selling." Moreover, Sorkow's last statement here—"He cannot purchase what is already his"—made many critics see red. They emphasized that Sorkow had drawn a false analogy between men who are paid for donating sperm and women who are paid for surrogacy: egg donors, not surrogates, are analogous to sperm donors. Sorkow to the contrary, in creating a baby, donating sperm and carrying a fetus to term are not equivalent contributions!

A slippery-slope argument is sometimes offered with regard to surrogacy as "baby selling." If we allow babies to be sold through surrogate contracts, why not allow babies to be sold into slavery? (In the context of the western world, this might be better described as a *reductio ad absurdum*. In a global context, however, the argument is not just fantasy. It is estimated that there are 6 million slaves in the world today, most of whom were sold into lifelong servitude as babies or children.[56])

Consent   Another legal aspect of surrogacy is consent. Under what circumstances, if any, is it possible for a surrogate to give genuine or "informed" consent to surrogacy?

Mary Beth Whitehead's lawyer Harold Cassidy said that surrogate mothers "cannot know, until after that child is born, their true feelings about bearing that child."[57] The psychologist Lee Salk agreed: "There are neurophysiological changes in pregnancy, and surrogacy interrupts these. Any woman agreeing to bear a child under a surrogacy arrangement should have this explained to her and should be made to watch videotapes of mothers' reaction after birth."[58] The columnist Ellen Goodman wrote that surrogates should be forbidden to sign any contract requiring them to give up the child, implying that true consent is impossible.[59] The "sad, human part of this drama is that neither the Whiteheads nor the Sterns could predict [Mary Beth Whitehead's] emotions," Goodman said. It might also be argued, as noted earlier, that poor women who are paid for surrogacy do not really "consent" but are in effect coerced by their poverty.

Some commentators objected to arguments like these, however, considering them patronizing and even insulting, especially with regard to surrogates who have already experienced childbirth. Salk, who had described Mary Beth Whitehead as "a surrogate uterus and not a surrogate mother,"[60] was also assailed because of this choice of words, which some critics found inappropriate for someone who was supposed to be testifying as a professional. Merit feminists were strongly opposed to Goodman's view: they said Goodman was suggesting that bearing a child somehow overpowers a woman's reason. No matter that Mary Beth Whitehead had already borne two children and knew what childbearing was like, these feminist argued sarcastically, no matter that 400 or 500 other surrogates had given up their babies, no matter that contracts can be drawn up to protect surrogates; despite all this, "women are just like that, aren't they?"—emotional creatures who shouldn't be allowed to be surrogates. (And perhaps these emotional creatures shouldn't be surgeons either, or lawyers, or columnists.) Finally, against the argument that poverty is coercive, it can be argued that being poor does not render women incapable of rational decision making (millions of poor women decide not to become prostitutes or thieves, for instance) and that poverty is not tantamount to "duress."

Contracts   A third legal aspect of surrogacy has to do with contracts. Contract law encompasses a much broader area than is understood by most Americans, whose only experience with contracts may be buying a house or getting married. In fact, contracts affect every facet of American life every day—much of American business is covered explicitly or implicitly by contracts; contracts are a crucial part of daily law practice; and in law school, a full-year course is devoted to contracts. One significant area of contract law regards violations of contracts, for which two major forms of redress are available: *compensation* for damages or *specific performance*; in the latter, the party violating the contract is required to carry through on its terms.

In the Baby M case, there were several issues related to the contract. One of the issues that arose between the Sterns and the Whiteheads was a difference in their attitudes toward the surrogacy contract and evidently toward contracts in general. For the Sterns, contracts seemed almost sacrosanct—things to be studied minutely, carefully negotiated, and adhered to. In contrast, the Whiteheads seemed to regard contracts as unimportant, especially when a contract conflicted with their basic values. (The Whiteheads' attitude, it should be noted, is by no means unusual. Football and basketball coaches, professional athletes, entertainers, and speakers on the college lecture circuit routinely break contracts and do not seem to regard contracts as morally binding.)

Another issue was the legality of surrogacy contracts. As a surrogacy contract, the contract signed by William Stern and Mary Beth Whitehead was not recognized by statute. In various previous cases, however, contracts on the "edge of the law" had been recognized as legal; and whether or not the contract in the Baby M case would be considered legal depended partly on reasons for and against using legal contracts in surrogacy arrangements. As we have seen, Judge Sorkow found that the contract was legal and ordered that it should be carried out, but the New Jersey Supreme Court ruled that surrogacy contracts are illegal.

Even if surrogacy contracts as such were legal, however, any specific surrogacy contract—like the one between William Stern and Mary Beth Whitehead—might nevertheless be illegal, in the sense of being void or unenforceable. A contract can be found illegal, for example, if it is wildly unfair or requires someone to relinquish a right that legally cannot be forgone (selling oneself into slavery would void a contract); if one of the parties is making fraudulent representations; or if one of the parties is a juvenile or deranged. In the Baby M case, the last factor was of course not relevant, but during the lower-court proceedings some observers argued that the contract might be illegal for one or more of the other reasons.

There was, for instance, controversy over the fairness of the contract: some commentators held that all the risks of the contract had fallen on Mary Beth Whitehead. The Sterns denied this, arguing that if the child had been born with defects, they would still have had to accept responsibility; William Stern also emphasized that he had paid $25,000 for an arrangement without a guaranteed result. (That was the fee to the agency, of which Mary Beth Whitehead would receive $10,000.)

Some critics argued that the contract required Mary Beth Whitehead to give up rights which, legally, cannot be relinquished. The feminist periodical *Off Our Backs,* for one, said that "the biological mother's rights must be protected and not be considered disposable by virtue of a piece of paper."

Off Our Backs also raised the question of possible fraud: "Was Whitehead led to believe that she could change her mind about giving up the child after conception? If she was, the contract could be declared invalid on the basis of fraud or misrepresentation under ordinary contract law." (In general, Judge Sorkow's concept of a contract as an essentially unbreakable promise to do something—regardless of what one may feel about it later—was seen by feminists as legalistic machismo.)

UPDATE

In 1988, when the New Jersey Supreme Court decided that surrogacy contracts were illegal, Noel Keane's agency had achieved 200 successful surrogate pregnancies, 47 were "on the way," and 150 couples had been matched and had begun insemination. But the tide seemed to have turned against commercial surrogacy. In 1985, Great Britain had banned it, and in the United States it was forbidden in Florida and Michigan (although the Michigan courts kept the door open for altruistic surrogacy, and apparently an adoptive couple there could legally pay for the surrogate's medical expenses). By 1989, as much as is ever possible in the United States, a consensus had emerged that commercial surrogacy should be discouraged by public policy and that surrogacy contracts should not be legally enforceable. In 1992, New York State, which had previously been a center of commercial surrogacy, banned it. As of the end of 1993, 11 of the 17 states with laws covering surrogacy have ruled that surrogacy contracts are unenforceable, and Michigan has made it a criminal act to participate in a surrogacy contract.[61] Only Arkansas and New Hampshire explicitly permit surrogacy contracts.

However, there has also been an emerging consensus that altruistic surrogacy, under careful regulation, should still be allowed.[62] Additionally, there is general agreement that when custody disputes arise, a surrogate—even in altruistic surrogacy—should not be required to give up her child unless the child's best interest is clearly to live with the father and his wife.

Where altruistic surrogacy is regulated, it is treated more like adoption than like artificial insemination by donor (AID). In AID, whether the sperm donor is a friend or an anonymous donor from a "sperm bank," courts and legislatures have gone out of their way to make the "rearing father" the legal father. With regard to adoption, on the other hand, the courts have not done this, probably because "what ultimately changes hands is not a vial of semen but a live baby, taken from a birth mother biologically and sometimes emotionally prepared to nurture it."[63]

According to the Center for Surrogate Parenting in Beverly Hills, California, there have been nearly 4,000 births by genetic surrogacy since the 1970s; and 80 births by gestational surrogacy since 1987–1988.[64] Most surrogates (commercial and altruistic) have given up their babies without incident, though a few have not. One woman, who became a commercial surrogate to pay off $8,000 in debt, died of complications of pregnancy.[65]

One study of gestational surrogacy has reported that surrogates over age 40 are as successful as younger surrogates, so long as the egg donor is young. In South Africa in 1987, a 48-year-old grandmother successfully carried to birth a fetus created from her daughter's eggs and fertilized with her son-in-law's sperm. In the United States in 1991, Arlette Schweitzer (at age 42) carried twins for her daughter, who had been born without a uterus; the implanted embryos were created from her daughter's eggs and her son-in-law's sperm. In 1992, Catherine Toole, then 36, gave birth as a commercial gestational surrogate to triplets for a Venezuelan couple (she was paid $10,000).

At least one custody dispute has arisen in a case of gestational surrogacy. In 1993, the California Supreme Court ruled against Anna Johnson, a nurse from Orange County who had been paid $10,000 to gestate an embryo created from the sperm and egg of Mark and Crispina Calvert.[66] After the birth, Anna Johnson changed her mind and sued for custody of the child. The only female judge on this court dissented on the ground that the majority had not applied the standard of "the child's best interest."

•

In June of 1994, Mary Beth Gould was interviewed on a television show and spoke freely about the case (the Sterns, however, had declined to be interviewed).

She was still married to Dean Gould (the Goulds by then had two children of their own) and was living in eastern Long Island, New York—about 2 hours away from the Sterns' home in New Jersey. She mentioned that "Baby M" is now called Sassy and said that she had told Sassy everything about her origins. Sassy herself (who was then 8 years old) appeared briefly on the videotape, though she was not interviewed. Reportedly, Sassy has looked up stories about her birth on her school computer. Tuesday, now a teenager, considers her mother a "heroine" who made a mistake but then stood up for what was right.

•

The case of Baby M and the bitter dispute between the Sterns and the White-heads was an important influence on American public policy regarding surrogacy. People on both sides of the controversy have acknowledged that this case alone created significant opposition to commercial surrogacy, and that as a result commercial surrogacy has been largely eliminated.

FURTHER READING

Kenneth D. Alpern, *The Ethics of Reproductive Technology*, Oxford University Press, New York, 1992.

Sue Meinke, "Scope Note 6: Surrogate Motherhood: Ethical and Legal Issues," National Reference Center for Bioethics Literature, Kennedy Institute of Ethics, Georgetown University, Washington, D.C.

William Prior, ed., "Manufactured Motherhood: The Ethics of the New Reproductive Technologies," in *Logos: Philosophic Issues in Christian Perspective: 9*, Philosophy Department, Santa Clara University, Calif., 1989.

Bonnie Steinbock, "Surrogate Motherhood as Prenatal Adoption," *Law, Medicine, and Health Care*, vol. 16, nos. 1–2, Spring 1988.

CHAPTER 6

Abortion

Kenneth Edelin

This chapter discusses the case of Kenneth Edelin, a physician who was charged with manslaughter in Boston in 1973 after performing an abortion; it also discusses the major ethical issues of abortion. The following terms should be kept in mind: before 9 weeks of gestation, the growing organism is called an *embryo;* from 9 weeks until birth, it is called a *fetus;* a newborn human being, existing outside the womb, is by custom and law called a *baby.*

BACKGROUND: PERSPECTIVES ON ABORTION

Historical Overview

Many Christians and Jews believe that the Bible or the Torah forbids abortion. In this regard, however, a British professor of church history writes:

> The Bible certainly teaches the value of human life, and forbids the murder of any human being (Psalm 8). But life, in biblical terms, commences only when the breath enters the nostrils and the man or woman becomes a "living being" (Genesis 2:7). . . . Consequently in biblical terms the fetus is not a person. This is brought out clearly in the laws relating to murder. For though the Ten Commandments in Exodus state clearly, "You shall not murder," the text goes on, in the following chapter, to differentiate between causing the death of an adult human being and causing the death of an unborn human fetus. For whereas "whoever hits a man and kills him shall be put to death" (Exodus 21:12), " . . . if some men are fighting and hurt a woman so that she loses her child, but is not injured in any other way, the one who hurt her is to be fined." There is no suggestion in the Old Testament law, as there is in a comparable Assyrian one, that "he who struck her shall compensate for the fetus with a life." Indeed, the biblical text does not ever regard the loss of her fetus as causing the woman "harm," for it goes on to specify what should happen "if any harm follows." At no point is any consideration given to the notion that the fetus itself might have rights. And this absence of concern for the fetus is also implied by the imposition of the death

penalty on women who conceive out of wedlock, without any consideration being given to the fact that this killed both the fetus and the woman (Deuteronomy 22:21, Leviticus 21:9, Genesis 38:24).

. . . Turning to the issue of abortion as such, I am somewhat puzzled that biblical fundamentalists, who oppose abortion so strongly, should pay so little heed to the silence of the Bible on this issue. . . . Whether this silence is significant or not, the fact ought to be faced that whatever views one many hold about abortion, no straightforward appeal can be made to the teaching of the Bible, for the Bible simply does not discuss it.[1]

Moreover, Jesus does not speak against abortion anywhere in the New Testament.

If abortion is not condemned in the Old Testament or in the Gospels, why have so many Christians, in particular, come to believe that it is immoral? An answer to this question can be given in historical stages, focusing on the Catholic church as an example.

The Old Testament took its final form during the fifth century before the Common, or Christian, era (B.C.E.) and the New Testament around the year 200 of the Common era (C.E.)—the time when Christianity began as an organized religion. As a formal, organized religion, Christianity has always opposed abortion, but its view of what constitutes "abortion" has changed significantly over the nearly 2,000 years of its existence.

By the fourth century C.E., Christian teaching about sex was in crisis. Celibacy was the Christian ideal; but there were two problems with that ideal. On the one hand, Christianity would die out if too many Christians took celibacy too seriously (much later, the Shakers held to the ideal and did die out). On the other hand, as a practical matter lifelong celibacy was impossible for most people. Consequently (as discussed in Chapter 4), Augustine revised Christian teaching to allow sexual intercourse in marriage, but only if the intent was to have children.[2] It follows from Augustine's doctrine that abortion must be sinful, because it thwarts the only permissible purpose of sex.

In the twelfth century, Christian doctrine began to separate abortion from homicide by distinguishing between "formed" and "unformed" embryos—a concept that had to do with the soul rather than with physical development. In the thirteenth century, Thomas Aquinas held that God "ensouled" male embryos at 40 days of gestation and female embryos at 90 days. Aborting a male embryo at 40 days was thus punished more severely than aborting a female embryo at the same age, since the male was "formed" by then but the female was still "unformed." Although any abortion at any time was considered sinful, the penalties (penance, etc.) increased when the fetus was "formed."[3]

During the nineteenth century, science and religion began to conflict in many areas, and scientific evidence began to discredit the Thomistic concept of ensoulment. In 1870, Pope Pius IX reacted against the general conflict between religion and science by convening the First Vatican Council, which declared that his edicts and those of future popes would henceforth be "infallible." The meaning of papal infallibility was unclear at the time and is still debated by Catholic theologians today,[4] but the general reaction of the Catholic church was clear: it moved toward faith and away from the claims of science. As the church retreated from science during the period from about 1869 to 1900, it encouraged worship of Mary (which had been neglected), supported "creationism" against geological explanations of the origins of the universe, emphasized miracles (the miracle of Fatima was recognized shortly after the First Vatican Council), and vigorously attacked Darwinism.

Beginning in the mid-nineteenth century, then, the popes denounced abortion in increasingly absolutistic terms. During this time, Catholicism came close to teaching that personhood began at conception, a view it called *immediate animation.*[5] In an earlier era, as we have seen, the church had differentiated between "formed" and "unformed" fetuses, but Pius IX essentially drew no such distinction: the prohibition was the same for almost any woman who had any kind of abortion. This official Catholic denunciation of abortion has, of course, continued throughout the twentieth century.

However, the Catholic doctrine of *double effect* allowed two exceptions: abortion was permissible in cases of ectopic pregnancy (in which an embryo grows in a fallopian tube) and uterine cancer (in which uterus and fetus must be removed together). According to the doctrine of double effect, an action having two effects, one good and the other evil, is morally permissible under four conditions: (1) if the action is good in itself or not evil, (2) if the good follows as immediately from the cause as from the evil effect, (3) if only the good effect is intended, and (4) if there is a proportionately grave cause for performing the action as for allowing the evil effect. Under this doctrine, exceptions to the general prohibition of abortion were made for ectopic pregnancy and uterine cancer because in both cases the purpose of an abortion was to save the life of the mother.

•

Historically, legal restrictions on abortion were far more lenient than Catholic doctrine. During the seventeenth century, European common law did not consider aborting even a "quickened" fetus an indictable offense. In 1803, an English statute made abortion of a quickened fetus a capital crime; however, it continued to use "quickening" as a dividing point, and it imposed lesser penalties for abortions before quickening. From the seventeenth through the nineteenth centuries, American law followed English common law: abortion before quickening was only a misdemeanor or might even be legal if it was done for therapeutic reasons on the recommendation of two physicians. In 1973, in *Roe v. Wade,* the United States Supreme Court reviewed the legal background of abortion and concluded:

> It is thus apparent that at common law, at the time of the adopting of our Constitution, and throughout the major portion of the 19th century, abortion was viewed with less disfavor than under most American statutes currently in effect. Phrasing it another way, a woman enjoyed a substantially broader right to terminate a pregnancy than she does in most States today. At least with respect to the early stage of pregnancy, and very possibly without such a limitation, the opportunity to make this choice was present in this country well into the 19th century. Even later, the law continued for some time to treat less punitively an abortion procured in early pregnancy.[6]

In the United States, this leniency changed after the Civil War, when most states made abortion illegal, stipulated firm cutoff points, and imposed stiff penalties. The American medical profession was also opposed to abortion in the period from 1870 to 1970. Feminist historians argue that this legislative trend and the stance of the medical profession both reflect paternalism and misogyny:

> Anti-abortion legislation was part of an anti-feminist backlash to the growing movement for suffrage, voluntary motherhood, and other women's rights in the nineteenth century. The prevailing public prudery and anti-sexual moralism condemned feminism and considered sex for pleasure evil, with pregnancy as punishment.[7]

These feminists point out that before the Civil War, most babies had been delivered by midwives, who competed with physicians for clients; thereafter, physicians took over, and almost all physicians were men.

Modern Developments

Before abortion was legalized (or perhaps more accurately, relegalized) in the United States, an abortion was likely to be a horrifying experience. Physicians who performed abortions often did so only for the money and sometimes treated their patients badly. Some physicians demanded sex from their patients as part of the price of an abortion. Other physicians accompanied the abortion with a lecture to the woman on her "promiscuity." Some of the specific medical procedures were meant more to protect physicians from the law than to help patients. Though abortion is a painful process, anesthesia wasn't used; and no explanation was given beforehand of what would happen and why. If there were any adverse effects, the woman had no legal recourse. Frequently, the woman did not even know the physician's name and had been forbidden to try to make contact again. Furthermore, as bad as they were, illegal abortions by physicians were also very expensive. Thus such an abortion was beyond the reach not only of poor women but also of teenagers who might be from well-off families but who couldn't or wouldn't tell their parents.

Despite all this, hundreds of thousands of illegal abortions were performed in the United States during the 1950s and 1960s. Many women died as a result of abortions: 193 women died in 1965 alone, and over 1,000 died during the decade of the 1960s.[8] Because what they had done was illegal, victims of botched or unsanitary abortions came into emergency rooms only at the last possible moment, when they were desperate. Many of these women died of widespread abdominal infection, and those who recovered often found themselves sterile or chronically ill. Poor women ran the greatest risks from illegal abortions, and in 1965, 55 percent of abortion-related deaths were among nonwhite women.

1962: Sherri Finkbine   In 1962, Sherri Finkbine was living with her husband and their four children in Phoenix, Arizona,[9] and she was pregnant with a fifth child. During her fifth month of pregnancy, she took thalidomide tranquilizers. Thalidomide is a teratogen ("monster former"), often producing babies with missing arms or legs—a fact that is now well known but in 1962 was just becoming apparent. It had been tested on animals, but it was not tested on the appropriate species of *pregnant* animals until it had already caused numerous human tragedies.

A "therapeutic" abortion was requested, ostensibly for Sherri Finkbine's health, and was scheduled at a local hospital. A local district attorney threatened to prosecute, however, and the Finkbines had to go to Europe at their own expense to seek an abortion. The severely deformed fetus was aborted in Sweden, where therapeutic abortion had been legal since 1940.[10]

1968: *Humanae Vitae*   On July 29, 1968—5 years before *Roe v. Wade*—Pope Paul VI stunned liberal Catholics around the world by emphasizing in an encyclical called *Humanae Vitae* that the Roman Catholic church would not accept any form of artificial birth control. What perhaps made this ruling particularly startling was its timing: it came during a period of enormous worldwide social change, associated significantly with young people (there were student uprisings in the United States and elsewhere—notably Paris—against the Vietnamese war), and marked by increasing tolerance toward sexual relations outside marriage, partly because unwanted pregnancies were increasingly avoidable.

Humanae Vitae drove many American Catholics to open defiance of official church teachings. In 1993—over 25 years later—though Pope John Paul II had by then made the defense of this encyclical a pillar of his own papacy, 90 percent of American Catholics disagreed with the church's position and believed they were free to make their own moral decisions, even if those decisions contradicted church doctrine.[11] The encyclical also had another unintended effect: it drove many Catholics out of the priesthood and out of Catholic universities. Some of these apostates became founders of the new field of bioethics.[12]

1968–1973: Steps toward *Roe v. Wade*   As a result of social changes, and of cases like Sherri Finkbine's, American culture had come to accept the concept of legalized abortion before *Roe v. Wade* in 1973. In the 5 years just preceding *Roe v. Wade*, 18 states, with 41 percent of the American population, liberalized their own abortion laws; 67 percent of Americans, then, lived either in those states or within a 100-mile drive of one of them. The first state to legalize abortion had been Hawaii (in 1970), followed by New York, Colorado, North Carolina, and California. (Ronald Reagan, who was then the governor of California, signed its bill into law!) If *Roe v. Wade* had not eliminated the need, more states would have followed suit. It is noteworthy that if the United States Supreme Court should ever make abortion a "states' rights" issue, most American women could still have abortions because most of these liberalized state laws are still on the books.

In other words, it is not true that *Roe v. Wade* suddenly "occurred" and that thereupon many people suddenly changed their ideas about abortion. Rather, many Americans had already changed their views, and *Roe v. Wade* reflected this new reality.

1973: *Roe v. Wade*   The decision of the United States Supreme Court in *Roe v. Wade* (1973) concerned "Jane Roe," a woman from Dallas, Texas, whose real name is Norma McCorvey. ("Wade" was Henry Wade, district attorney of Dallas County.) In March 1970, when the events in the case began, Texas had a law criminalizing all abortions; Norma McCorvey wanted a safe, legal abortion by a physician and challenged the constitutionality of the Texas law. [13]

The Supreme Court had already decided in *Griswold v. Connecticut* (1965) that a right to "privacy"—the legal equivalent of "personal liberty"—is implied by the Constitution and had therefore allowed couples to receive birth control pills (the point at issue in *Griswold* was whether a state might forbid such contraception). In *Roe v. Wade,* the Court decided that privacy also implies the right to have an abortion.

This right was not unqualified, however: a woman's right to terminate a pregnancy was balanced against the rights of the fetus, which increase as gestation time increases. The Court emphasized that religious and philosophical views about fetal development and "personhood" differ greatly, but for legal purposes it drew the line at *viability*. After viability, states could make abortions illegal; before viability, they could not.

The Court defined *viability* as the point when a fetus is "potentially able to live outside the mother's womb, albeit with artificial aid. Viability is usually placed at about 7 months (28 weeks) but may occur earlier, even at 24 weeks." The Court summarized its trimester system, in which viability divides the second and third trimesters, as follows:

> A state criminal abortion statute of the current Texas type, that excepts from criminality only a *life-saving* procedure on behalf of the mother, without regard to pregnancy stage and without recognition of the other interests involved, is violative of the Due Process Clause of the Fourteenth Amendment.
>
> (a) For the stage prior to approximately the end of the first trimester, the abortion decision and its effectuation must be left to the medical judgment of the pregnant woman's attending physician.
>
> (b) For the stage subsequent to approximately the end of the first trimester, the State, in promoting its interest in the health of the mother, may, if it chooses, regulate the abortion procedure in ways that are reasonably related to maternal health.
>
> (c) For the stage subsequent to viability, the State in promoting its interest in the potentiality of human life may, if it chooses, regulate, and even proscribe, abortion except where it is necessary, in appropriate medical judgment, for the preservation of the life or health of the mother.

This trimester system for allowing states to legalize and regulate abortion became the subject of great discussion over the next two decades. Justice Rehnquist immediately called it a "Procrustean bed," and Justice Sandra Day O'Connor predicted that it would inevitably be revised.

Note that a state "may" forbid ("proscribe") abortion. It need not. A state could legalize abortion at any time up to the actual birth. Note also that a state may pass a law allowing abortions in the third trimester not only to preserve the *life* of a mother but also to protect her *health*. Antiabortionists argue that this constitutes a loophole justifying almost any abortion, because two physicians can almost always be found who will say that continuing the pregnancy would endanger the mother's health. Indeed, *health* is a vague term and can be used in many ways. In the 1960s, for instance, Alabama law permitted abortions only for the health of the mother, but some physicians interpreted the word quite broadly and performed first-trimester abortions on any woman who decided to terminate her pregnancy.

•

After abortion was legalized in the United States in 1973, the number of legal abortions grew to approximately 1.5 million per year, a figure that has remained steady since then.[14] Of women and girls who have abortions, less than 1 percent are under age 15, though older teenage girls account for about 24 percent. Women in their twenties have 55 percent of abortions; women in their thirties, 18 percent. Married women have nearly 20 percent of abortions. Minority women are more than twice as likely as white women to have an abortion,[15] although many minority women today do choose to bring the fetus to term.

It is interesting to note that most African American legislators have supported legalized abortion, and that, historically, legal abortion has been presented as a way to improve the economic status of poor women and couples—many of whom, of course, are minorities. Having too many children, having children while too young, or having children without a stable marriage limits the chances for economic success in life, and the existence of abortion as a legal option is held to reduce the number of unplanned children. In fact, however, legalization of abortion has not decreased the overall number of children born to mothers who end up on welfare or the number of children born out of wedlock.

THE EDELIN CASE

The Legal Environment: Experiments on Aborted Fetuses

The case of Kenneth Edelin began in Boston in October 1973, and to understand the legal environment, it is necessary to look at a key episode that had taken place several months earlier, in the first quarter of 1973—just after the decision in *Roe v. Wade*.

This earlier event involved two experiments that had been performed on aborted fetuses at Boston City Hospital, where Edelin was a resident. Some physicians reasoned this way: since aborted fetuses were going to die anyway, why not use them in experiments to help other fetuses? This particular research was designed partly to prevent cases like Sherri Finkbine's, in which substances ingested by the mother might harm the fetus: to determine which drugs would cross the placenta, the physicians in the study gave antibiotics to women undergoing abortions and then examined the aborted fetuses. One of the findings was that clindamycin crosses the placenta and becomes concentrated in the fetal liver; this showed that syphilis in the fetus could be treated with clindaymycin if the mother was allergic to penicillin.

This study caused a considerable furor. An article describing it appeared in the *New England Journal of Medicine*,[16] and copies were sent to certain Boston Catholics, who were infuriated. When a councilman held a hearing on September

18, 1973, to investigate fetal experimentation at Boston City Hospital, antiabortionists packed the auditorium. One of the witnesses they heard was Mildred Jefferson, an assistant professor of surgery at Boston University who was not only an antiabortion physician but also an African American physician. (Later, Kenneth Edelin's lawyer had no doubt that Jefferson had been asked to testify precisely because she was black and staunchly opposed to abortion.) Jefferson testified, perhaps correctly, that some of the women undergoing abortion who were involved in the study were too young to consent legally and in any case had not given their written consent. If the researchers had indeed failed to obtain genuine consent, they would technically be open to charges of "grave robbing," illegally procuring bodies for medical experimentation.

Kenneth Edelin and "Alice Roe"

In 1973, Kenneth Edelin was 35 years old, and he—like Mildred Jefferson—was African American. (When he became the first physician prosecuted for performing an abortion after *Roe v. Wade,* many observers would wonder if the fact that he was black had something to do with it, though the district attorney, Newman Flanagan, denied any link.) Edelin, the son of a postman, had grown up in a poor section of Washington, D.C. He did his undergraduate work at Columbia University, received his M.D. from Meharry Medical College in 1967, interned in Ohio, and then served for 3 years as a United States Air Force physician (with the rank of captain) in England. In 1971, he began his residency at Boston City Hospital, which Bill Moyers called the "city hospital in the Boston ghetto" in a documentary on the case. (It was also the model for a later television series, *St. Elsewhere.*) Edelin was in his third year as chief resident in obstetrics when he was assigned to perform an abortion on "Alice Roe."

"Alice" was a 17-year-old, black, West Indian student. She remained anonymous throughout the case, and little is known about her personally or as a patient. She had been examined by Edelin's faculty supervisor, Hugh Holtrop, who estimated that she was 22 weeks pregnant. She was also examined by Enrique Giminez, a first-year resident from Mexico, who later testified against Edelin, giving a different estimate of 24 weeks; and a third-year medical student who assisted during the abortion agreed with Giminez's estimate. At the time, the hospital (which was poor) had no ultrasound machine and so could not reach a more precise estimate of gestation. In either case, however, it was a very late, second-trimester abortion.

Even though Holtrop had admitted Alice Roe, and even though a late second-trimester fetus was involved, Kenneth Edelin was assigned to the abortion. It is true that as a third-year resident, Edelin carried out substantial work at the hospital; it is also true that attending obstetricians like Holtrop all had private practices and actually spent little time at Boston City. Moreover, Holtrop later said that he had admitted Alice simply because he was the only obstetrician on duty when she arrived. However, Edelin disagreed, claiming that Alice Roe had originally been Holtrop's patient; and the surgeon William Nolen, who wrote a book reviewing the case (Nolen is also the author of *The Making of a Surgeon*), concluded that Holtrop had dumped the case on Edelin.[17]

To complicate matters, Holtrop had obtained Alice's and her mother's permission for Alice's participation in another preabortion experiment to see if aminoglutethamide would increase the hormone output of the placenta. Accordingly, the substance was given to Alice intravenously and her urine was analyzed over the next 24 hours; this study took place on October 1 and October 2, 1993.

Edelin planned to abort Alice Roe's fetus by injecting saline solution into the amniotic sac, but when he inserted a needle on October 2 to sample the amniotic fluid, he drew blood. This indicated that the patient had an anterior placenta (that is, a placenta attached to the front wall of the uterus); thus a saline solution injected into the placenta could travel from there into her bloodstream, where it could be lethal.

The abortion was therefore rescheduled as a hysterotomy and was performed on the following day, October 3, 1993. A hysterotomy is essentially abortion by caesarean surgery; it involves cutting through the lower abdominal wall. Instead of Giminez (the resident who estimated gestation time as 24 weeks), Edelin chose as his assistant Steven Teich, the third-year medical student mentioned above. However, Giminez watched the hysterotomy anyway (he was uninvited, and where he was when he observed the procedure became a matter of dispute).

What happened next is controversial. Giminez would later testify that Edelin made the cesarean section, reached in, cut the placenta from the abdominal wall, then waited perhaps 3 minutes, and after this interval removed a dead fetus. If such a wait took place, that would be important, because a baby cannot breathe on its own inside the uterus: it begins breathing (if at all) only when it is brought out. Edelin would later be charged with "neglecting" the baby by not removing it immediately, thereby causing it to suffocate.

Afterwards, the fetus was taken to the morgue, where it was preserved in formalin, as required by hospital policy for aborted fetuses weighing more than 600 grams. This later meant that the district attorney had a "body," and photographs of the "body" were eventually shown to the jury.

One fact about this case merits repeating here. Edelin had originally intended to abort the fetus by saline injection, and if the position of the placenta been different, he would have been able to do so legally. It was for the safety of the mother that he performed the abortion by hysterotomy, leaving himself vulnerable to the manslaughter charge.

The Case in the Courts

Edelin's trial and conviction   A grand jury decided that enough evidence existed to indict Edelin. Some legal strategists believe that Edelin seriously erred by testifying at the pretrial hearing and not invoking his Fifth Amendment right against possible self-incrimination. Holtrop, in contrast, invoked his right against self-incrimination and was not indicted. After the hearing, Edelin changed lawyers.

The actual charge against Edelin was manslaughter, defined in Massachusetts as "wanton, reckless" omission or commission of an act which causes death; Massachusetts law further defines "wanton, reckless" conduct as "the legal

equivalent of intentional conduct" and as "disregard of the probable consequences to the rights of others." The trial judge gave the following description:
"The essence of wanton or reckless conduct is the doing of an act or the omission
to act where there is a duty to act, which commission or omission involves a high
degree of likelihood that substantial harm will result to another."[18]

The principal participants in the trial were Newman Flanagan, the prosecut-
ing district attorney (described as "witty, flamboyant, competent, and tough");
Edelin's trial lawyer, William Perkins Homans, Jr., a well-born Boston lawyer
who often defended unpopular causes; and the presiding judge, James McGuire.
The jurors—selected after much wrangling between the lawyers—were mostly
white; 3 of them were women and 13 were men; 10 were Catholic. (A study had
predicted that jurors likely to convict Edelin would be blue-collar Catholics over
50 years old, who had dropped out of Catholic high schools, and who regularly
read Catholic newspapers.)

Massachusetts did not pass an abortion law until August 1974 (22 months
after *Roe v. Wade),* and in the absence of a specific state law, Judge McGuire
instructed the jury that *Roe v. Wade* was "absolutely controlling." Since *Roe v.
Wade* equated personhood with viability, this meant that the jury would have to
determine whether or not this specific fetus had been "viable." Remember that
the Supreme Court had said only that viability is "usually" placed at 24 to 28
weeks, not that viability necessarily falls within that range; more important, the
Supreme Court had not specified how to determine whether or not viability fell
into the range. In the Edelin case, if the fetus was *not* viable, no "person" had
been killed; and if no person had been killed, Edelin could not be guilty of
manslaughter.

Edelin testified that the procedure he performed on Alice Roe had seemed
long to Giminez because at this stage of pregnancy the thick abdominal muscle
wall was not yet stretched enough to be cut easily. Edelin also said that he had
made a Pfannenstiel ("bikini") incision because he considered it safer than a ver-
tical incision and because it would leave less of a scar. The surgeon William
Nolen later agreed that making such an incision would take awhile, especially
for a resident who had never done one before, though he said that it would certainly not take 3 minutes (as Giminez had testified);[19] however, Edelin's testimony implied that Giminez had confused the intial abdominal incision with the
second incision detaching the placenta.

As noted above, the fetus had been preserved, and the prosecution introduced a picture of it ("the deceased") as evidence, over the angry objection of the
defense attorney, Homans, who argued that the picture would be "inflammatory" and would tell laypersons nothing about fetal age or viability. Judge
McGuire allowed one picture to be shown but charged the jury not to view it
"from any emotional point of view."[20]

When the district attorney, Flanagan, summed up, he argued, first, that the
fetus had been a "person" when the placenta was cut; second, that Edelin had
indeed waited 3 minutes and that this delay constituted "wanton, reckless conduct"; third, that legal abortion was intended to end a pregnancy, not to produce
a dead fetus—and therefore that Edelin should have helped the fetus (which
Flanagan said had been live-born) before cutting the placenta.

Judge McGuire specifically instructed the jury that an unborn fetus was not a person and could not be the subject of a manslaughter indictment. Such an indictment could refer only to a "person," defined by Massachusetts law as a being who has been born. Birth was the key event, and the judge instructed the jury: "You must be satisfied beyond a reasonable doubt . . . that the defendant caused the death of a person who had been alive outside the body of his or her mother."

Thus the jury had to decide two points: (1) Had Alice Roe's fetus been alive outside the mother's body? (2) If so, did the fetus (who would then be called a *baby*) die as a result of "wanton, reckless conduct" by Edelin? The jurors said "yes" to both points and convicted Edelin of manslaughter. Edelin was later sentenced by Judge McGuire to 1 year of probation.

The Edelin trial was followed intensely by the media and the public. Proabortion groups supported Edelin, as did some antiabortion physicians who hated prosecution of physicians more than legalization of abortion. Medical journals also strongly supported Edelin. Antiabortion groups saw Flanagan, the prosecutor, as their knight: Edelin had stepped over a legal line, they said, and had to be punished. A few months later, as described in Chapter 1, Karen Quinlan's physicians would take notice.

When the verdict was announced, liberal Boston media implied that a black man in an abortion case in Boston couldn't get a fair trial from white Catholics. Even the conservative William Buckley said, "The case can be presented as the lynching of a black Marcus Welby by a bigoted community."[21] The foreman of the jury, however, retorted passionately that the aborted fetus was also black and that the jury had also been concerned about its life.

Appeal and acquittal: The higher court's decision   If the conviction by the trial court had stuck, Kenneth Edelin could have lost his medical license. He appealed, however, and the Massachusetts Supreme Court agreed to hear the case on direct review. He was also given, almost immediately, a vote of confidence by the trustees of Boston City Hospital, who offered him a permanent position.

In December 1976, more than 3 years after the abortion itself had taken place, the Massachusetts Supreme Judicial Court overturned Edelin's conviction, declaring that no evidence of criminal negligence had been presented at the trial. The higher court said, "In the comparative calm of appellate review, the essential proposition emerges that the defendant had no evil frame of mind, was actuated by no criminal purpose, and committed no wanton or reckless act in carrying out the medical procedures on Oct. 3, 1973."[22] Notice that for its own reasons—possibly because commentaries by its own judges indicated deep divisions and confusion—the higher court did not require a new trial for Edelin but simply acquitted him.

The Aftermath

After the decision, Edelin was described as "jubilant" and said he felt "terrific" about the verdict, saying, "It's great to be able to smile again after 2½ years."[23] He said that the reversal was a victory for all physicians regardless of whether they performed abortions. He also said that the decision upheld the principle of non-prosecution of physicians who acted in good faith and who followed accepted medical standards.

In his television news program on the evening of December 17, 1977, Walter Cronkite triumphantly announced that Edelin had been acquitted of "manslaughter by abortion."[24]

William Nolen, the surgeon who later carefully examined the evidence in the case, argued that the fetus had not been outside the womb, had thus not been technically "born," and was thus not a person;[25] hence, he concluded, there could have been no manslaughter and Edelin could have broken no law. Nolen's conclusion was particularly interesting not only because he himself was a surgeon but also because he was opposed to abortion. Nolen believed that Edelin had intended the abortion to kill a very late second-trimester fetus but had been surprised to find, once the patient was opened, that the fetus was viable. Nolen doesn't say that Edelin actually suffocated the fetus; but he does say that whether a newborn has a will to live ("that spark") can be known only if it is taken out of the womb, slapped, and helped to breathe:

> What is disturbing in the Roe case is that, by his own admission, Edelin made no attempt to see if the child had that spark. As [Jeffrey] Gould [another physician who testified] said, the will to live isn't always immediately apparent; it becomes obvious only if "the physician will try to stimulate, will try to give a little bit of oxygen, and look for a favorable response." . . .
>
> The Roe baby wasn't given this bit of provocation that might—just might— have shown it had the will to live. Why? The answer is distressingly simple. No one wanted the Roe baby to live.[26]

•

In 1993, Newman Flanagan was still Boston's district attorney. Kenneth Edelin was practicing medicine near Boston and was on the college lecture circuit, speaking about AIDS and reproductive rights.

ETHICAL ISSUES

Two Basic Concepts

Before examining specific arguments about abortion, it is important to consider two essential concepts: *personhood* and *viability.*

Personhood   What is a *person?* In the context of abortion, some philosophers, especially woman philosophers, draw a distinction between a person and a human being. They argue that although a fetus is human, it does not meet certain criteria of personhood; and that since a fetus is not a person, it does not have a right to life. In this sense, *human* is a factual term whereas *person* is an evaluative term, implying a right to life.

The most famous and intuitively plausible of these arguments is probably Mary Anne Warren's. Warren offers a *cognitive criterion* of personhood[27] and holds that a fetus does not meet this standard. According to Warren, to be a person is to be able to think, to be capable of "cognition." What separates a normal, adult person from, say, a rat, is certain capacities—for reasoning, reflective self-awareness, communication, agency (motivated action), and consciousness of the external world. Warren does not think that any one of these capacities alone is sufficient for "cognition": rather, these capacities define the core criterion as a group. A being lacking all of these capacities does not meet the cognitive criterion, and hence cannot be a person.

Let us examine some issues concerning this cognitive criterion. To begin with, it can be objected that the criterion does not represent an adequate definition because it both includes some "nonpersons" and excludes some persons. The cognitive criterion does seem to admit to personhood some beings that we don't naturally regard as persons; there is good evidence, for instance, that apes communicate and are conscious, and there is some evidence that they may reason and may be self-aware, yet we don't usually consider them persons. Moreover, the cognitive criterion seems to suggest that there is no reason, morally speaking, to protect vulnerable human beings whose cognitive capacities are absent, have been lost, or are as yet merely potential, such as patients in the late stages of Alzheimer's disease, comatose patients, or newborn babies. If a fetus can be aborted (and thus killed) because it fails to meet the cognitive criterion and therefore is not a person, why wouldn't these others also fail to meet the criterion, and why wouldn't it also be permissible to kill them?

Suppose, moreover, that we accepted the cognitive criterion. In that case, another problem would arise. If what makes people valuable is cognition, then isn't it wrong to deprive beings of *potential cognition?* And wouldn't deprivation of potential cognition make abortion wrong? In this regard, the philosophers Don Marquis and Warren Quinn offer two premises: first, what is wrong about killing a person—a college student, for example—is depriving him or her of future cognitive experiences;[28] second, what is wrong about killing an adult person is also what is wrong about killing a human fetus.

Marquis and Quinn's argument is an interesting one, and indeed many people would accept their first premise, at least after some reflection. Other explanations of why it is wrong to kill a person—that killing violates a person's rights, for instance, or that killing is against God's will—seem to beg the question: it can be argued that phrases such as *violation of rights* and *against the will of God* are simply other ways of saying that an act is wrong.

However, Marquis and Quinn's second premise may be more vulnerable. It can be argued that a being without an already existing self or personal identity cannot have a personal future to be deprived of. Consider an analogy: imagine an omnipotent deity—God—who creates a universe, then considers creating a second parallel universe, but then decides not to create the second world. Now imagine a powerful evil force—Satan—who wants to destroy the existing universe. It seems, intuitively, that destruction of the existing world by Satan would be wrong; but it does *not* seem wrong for God to refrain from creating a second world. Although God has not allowed a second universe, and thus has disallowed a vast amount of cognitive experiences, he has neither done any wrong nor wronged any person.

Another argument against Marquis and Quinn is analogous to a strategy that is used to dissolve the "paradox of harm" (see Chapter 4): the *baseline* concept. This concept requires a starting point (baseline) from which an adverse change is plotted; i.e., it requires an existing being who is made worse off. We could, then, posit a baseline concept of personal identity and argue that without some baseline of existence as a person, one cannot be harmed. On the other hand, though, the *normality* concept of harm would tend to support Marquis and Quinn's reasoning: this concept requires a norm of development which is not met; and on a normality concept of personal identity, one could be harmed by not existing (because nonexistence deprives a being of any chance to obtain normality).

A different type of argument based on potentiality suggests a *genetic criterion* for personhood: to be a person is to have the unique genes of a specific human being. In the Edelin case, for example, even if Alice Roe's fetus wasn't yet a person, it was certainly a potential person; shouldn't it therefore have been treated as a person?

It may seem, at first glance, as if this argument would imply that contraception, or even masturbation, is wrong, since either of these might prevent potential persons from coming into existence; but this kind of reasoning is a *straw man*—a "false opponent," too easily refuted. No antiabortionist wants to produce billions of extra people; antiabortionists merely see each *particular person* as valuable from conception. John Noonan, who advocates a genetic criterion, argues that when sperm and egg meet and merge genes, a genetically unique individual is created (unless, of course, the zygote divides into identical twins):[29] The resulting embryo has all the potential in its DNA to be a full person, provided that it finds a nurturing uterus. However, having the potential to become a person is not being a person, as we realize when we consider the thousands of frozen embryos stored around the world. Another problem with the genetic criterion is that it collapses the distinction between being human and being a person—as we realize when we consider that a dead human has a unique set of genes. These implications seem to constitute a *reductio ad absurdum* of the genetic criterion.

A third possible criterion for personhood (in addition to the cognitive and genetic criteria) might be called the *neurological criterion*. This is actually a minimal version of the cognitive criterion; it defines a *person* as a human being with a detectable brain wave. This simple standard would be applicable across many issues of medical ethics; it would, for instance, recognize as persons both quasi-anencephalic babies and adults in PVS. With regard to abortion, the neurological criterion would consider a fetus a person when it developed brain waves, but not before (a fetus develops brain waves at about 25 weeks of gestation).

It should be noted that criteria of personhood become relevant in many other issues in medical ethics. For example, the cognitive criterion has been proposed in issues involving patients in PVS (see Chapter 1), impaired newborns in so-called "Baby Doe" cases (Chapter 7), and primates in medical experiments (Chapter 8).

Viability   *When* does a human fetus become a person with a right to life? With regard to this question, personhood has become closely linked with *viability*—the ability to survive as an independent entity.

In *Roe v. Wade*, the Supreme Court said that a state could ban abortion after viability, implying that viability is the key event—the development which separates nonperson, nonprotectable second-trimester fetuses from third-trimester fetuses, who are protectable persons. However, the concept of viability is vague, and the Court did nothing to clarify it. (A *vague* concept is one with no sharp boundaries, e.g., "baldness.") When does viability begin? In *Roe v. Wade*, as we have seen, the Court said only that viability is "usually placed" at about 28 weeks but "may occur earlier, even at 24 weeks," leaving the matter otherwise indeterminate.

In Kenneth Edelin's trial, the district attorney, Newman Flanagan, seized on this vagueness to try to establish that Alice Roe's fetus had been viable. One antiabortion physician testified that a baby could live outside the womb after as little as 12 weeks of gestation. But for how long? Only a few minutes, the physician testified, though maybe for longer. However, the defense attorney, William Homans, counterpunched by asking the physician how he defined viability; the physician said that viability was "capacity to survive [outside the womb] even for a second after birth." As Homans questioned several other physicians who were testifying as expert witnesses for the prosecution, he got each of them to admit that he had never known a fetus to survive for even a few days outside the womb after less than 24 weeks of gestation.

In general, Edelin's critics argued that they knew exactly what was meant by viability: ability to survive independently of the mother. In reality, some fetuses who are born early are not viable: they will die no matter how hard physicians try to keep them alive. Others will survive, though, and neonatologists usually know which is which. (Ultrasound tests can often indicate probable viability.) To Edelin's opponents, the point was that he had never tried to find out if the fetus was viable; he just assumed it wasn't. His supporters replied that of course neither he nor anyone else had tried to determine viability, since the point of abortion is to kill a fetus. The point is not to look inside the uterus, see if the fetus is "viable," and save it if it is; the intention is to kill it, regardless.

Arguments about Abortion

Approaching the arguments: Premises, conclusions, and the fact-value gap   In moral reasoning, a conclusion about a moral issue is supposed to follow logically from certain premises. If the premises logically support the conclusion, the argument is said to be *valid*. In practical reasoning, validity should not be confused with "truth": *validity* refers to the form of an argument, whereas *truth* refers to the content of its premises. A *sound* argument is one that has both valid form and true premises.

In any moral argument, the conclusion will of course be evaluative. Such a conclusion can be based entirely on evaluative premises, or it can be based on some combination of evaluative and factual (nonevaluative) premises. But a moral argument can *never* be valid if the evaluative conclusion is derived from solely factual premises. Moral conclusions commonly state that something "ought" or "should" be the case; factual premises, on the other hand, state that something "is" the case. A point made famous by the eighteenth-century philosopher David Hume is that an "ought" conclusion cannot be validly derived from only "is" premises. A valid moral argument, therefore, must have at least one evaluative premise, so that the evaluative element in the conclusion is not pulled out of the air from factual premises but "flows through" the argument from the evaluative premise or premises to the evaluative conclusion.

In addition, if a moral argument includes a factual premise, in order to be valid it must somehow connect the factual and evaluative elements. The connection can take the form of a separate *connecting fact-value premise,* or it can be part of a larger premise.

Drawing an evaluative conclusion from solely factual premises—or omitting the fact-value connection if any premise is factual—is an error, sometimes called the *is-ought problem* or the *naturalistic fallacy;* more simply, it is called *jumping the fact-value gap.*

For example, suppose that someone says, "First, a fetus has a brain wave after 25 weeks of gestation," and "Second, a conscious adult has a brain wave," and then draws the conclusion, "Killing a fetus after 25 weeks gestation is as wrong as killing a conscious adult." The crucial point with regard to ethical reasoning is that, while either the first or the second statement is entirely permissible as a *premise,* the two statements together do not lead to the conclusion: they are both factual, whereas the conclusion is evaluative. In other words, this is not a valid moral *argument,* because it has jumped the fact-value gap; something important is missing.

By contrast, here is a valid argument:

Premise 1 (factual): A human fetus has a brain wave after 25 weeks of gestation.
Premise 2 (connecting fact-value premise): A human with a brain wave is a person.
Premise 3 (evaluative premise): Killing a person is morally wrong.
Conclusion (evaluative): Therefore, killing a fetus with a brain wave is morally wrong.

As noted above, it would be permissible to combine premises 1 and 2 as "A human with a brain wave is a person (connecting fact-value premise)," if the fact about fetal brain waves is understood. The traditional format for such an argument is:

1. A human with a brain wave is a person.
2. Killing a person is morally wrong.

---

3. Therefore, killing a human with a brain wave is morally wrong.

When a moral argument is valid—that is, when its premises are made explicit and lead properly to the conclusion—we can see it clearly, and we can also see exactly where we agree or disagree with it. In this example, for instance, it becomes clear that either the evaluative premise or the connecting fact-value premise could apply not only to abortion but also to euthanasia; this gives us a perspective from which we may or may not accept these premises.

It is helpful to understand that in a valid argument, each key term must be defined in the same way throughout. To define a key term in more than one way is to commit the fallacy of *ambiguity*. Obviously, then, defining a key term factually in a premise but evaluatively in the conclusion commits two fallacies: ambiguity and jumping the fact-value gap.

Jumping the fact-value gap is in essence a special version of begging the question because the evaluative nature of the conclusion (the question) is "begged" by being assumed in the factual premises. This naturalistic fallacy is sometimes inadvertent, but it often appears when people do not want to make the real premises of their argument explicit. When hidden premises (assumptions) are revealed, these premises must be justified, and that can be a difficult job.

The argument from marginal cases   In the Edelin case, one question that arose was, "Where do you draw the line?"—that is, the line between fetuses which may and may not be aborted. Reasoning based on this kind of question is called the *argument from marginal cases*, and it is one of the most widely used ideas in ethics. With regard to an issue like abortion, the argument from marginal cases is as follows: Beings at the "margins" of personhood cannot be nonarbitrarily distinguished from those at the "core," because personhood and nonpersonhood are linked by a continuum. (The argument from marginal cases often appears in other issues as well, including animal rights—where it is based on the continuity of primates and human beings—and individual versus collective responsibility.)

The argument from marginal cases is related to the problem of jumping the fact-value gap, since another way of expressing this argument is to say that when marginal cases exist, there is no factual point or marker which could serve as a nonarbitrary (true) connecting premise between facts and values. That is, the question "Where do you draw the line?" implies that in certain moral issues, any candidate for a fact-value connecting premise will inevitably jump the fact-value gap. Consider the argument about abortion that was used as an example above:

1. A human with a brain wave is a person.
2. Killing a person is morally wrong.

---

3. Therefore, killing a human with a brain wave is morally wrong.

In this argument, premise 1—which combined the evaluative definition of a *person* with a factual statement about fetal brain waves—was offered as the connection between facts and values; but according to the argument from marginal cases, that premise is arbitrary. Why? Because any other factual event in fetal development might equally well be chosen. Moreover, it is held, any other premise we might suggest to serve in this way would also necessarily be arbitrary, because "personhood" and "nonpersonhood" are connected by a smooth continuum.

Antiabortionists who use the argument from marginal cases say that fetal development is smooth and continuous: there are no quantum leaps. Thus there is no specific, identifiable point of "ensoulment" or "personhood" or even "via-bility." No matter what week of gestation is considered, it seems arbitrary to make *that* week the marker of personhood or viability, because the fetus of a week earlier has almost the same qualities. Whatever time or marker is chosen, someone can always plausibly ask: Why not choose some other time or some other marker? For example, why not choose the preceding week?

Is the argument from marginal cases a good one? People who argue for abor-tion rights sometimes draw an analogy with the color spectrum: although each shade in the spectrum does resemble the shades next to it, colors that are more widely separated—and of course the colors on the two ends—are clearly distin-guishable. Another analogy might also be made: a full-grown oak tree, or even a sapling, differs clearly from an acorn, even though the process by which an acorn becomes an oak is smooth and continuous. Similarly, then, we can in fact distin-guish a newborn baby, and even a late-term fetus, from an embryo despite the continuous development from embryo to newborn. In other words, the existence of marginal cases does *not* make all distinctions impossible.

Furthermore, in practice people make such distinctions all the time, despite the fact that many marginal cases exist. Aristotle, for one, recognized that we habitually make these kinds of distinctions, and he observed that people with education, intelligence, and good judgment—not surprisingly—do this best. (He also thought that a special ability, which he called *phronesis,* was involved.)

Thomson: A limited proabortion view   Suppose that the fetus in the Edelin case *was* a person. Does it logically follow, then, that killing this fetus was immoral? The philosopher Judith Jarvis Thomson has argued that it does not.[30]

Thomson asks you to imagine that you have been admitted to a hospital for an operation, and that after the surgery you awaken to find yourself hooked up to a famous violinist whose kidneys have failed and whose blood is entering and leaving your body through tubes; your kidneys are being used without your per-mission to keep the violinist alive. Thomson argues that it is immoral for the hos-pital to force you to keep the violinist alive by using you in this way without your permission (although presumably you might be used *with* your permission, and it might be saintly of you to volunteer).

Thomson grants the antiabortionists one crucial premise: that the fetus is a person with a right to life. She sets up this hypothetical situation, however, to argue that even so, not all abortions are immoral. In her imaginary situation, the violinist cannot demand as a right that you keep him or her alive by allowing your kidneys to be used. Similarly, Thomson argues, a fetus cannot demand as a right (or its champions cannot demand this right for it) that a woman must keep it alive by carrying it to term. For Thomson, the most telling case is rape, because (by definition) a rape victim has not consented to sexual intercourse and there-fore has not consented to conceiving a child; if conception occurs as a result of rape, the rapist's fetus, in particular, has no claim on the woman's body. Similar arguments might apply when a woman has used contraception responsibly but the contraceptive fails.

Thomson's view is relevant in the Edelin case because there was a possibil-ity—a hint—that Alice Roe's pregnancy had resulted from incest. It was rumored that Alice had waited as long as she did before seeking an abortion because she didn't want to acknowledge what had happened to her, or because she didn't want her mother to know. If Alice was in fact a victim of incest, then Thomson's argument would allow the abortion, even if the fetus was by then a person. However, if Alice had simply been careless about contraception, Thomson's argument would not justify an abortion.

Thomson's argument is an example of reasoning *by analogy.* Here, an analogy is being drawn between the patient who is being used involuntarily to keep the violinist alive and a woman who is involuntarily pregnant—for instance, the violinist's dependence on the other patient is said to be analogous to the fetus's dependence on the mother. When anological reasoning is used in this way, the strength of the argument depends on how appropriate the analogy actually is: the closer the "fit" between the two things that are said to be analogous, the more strongly the inferred conclusion is supported.

In this case, critics of Thomson's argument have objected that the analogy breaks down. They argue, for instance, that the patient who is being involuntarily used can simply unhook himself or herself, and that detaching a cannula from one's vein is not really like killing a fetus by abortion. Since something "active" must be done to end a fetus's life, these critics maintain that to to make the analogy exact, the violinist would have to be doing something like blocking the other patient's way out of the room, so that the other patient could escape only by, say, cutting the violinist up.[31] (To grasp the idea of this criticism, try imagining a gigantic baby blocking the way out.)

It is interesting to note that both Thomson's original argument and this critical response suggest a concept of abortion as "self-defense." This concept is by no means new, however; it goes back at least as far as the sixteenth century, when the theologian Thomas Sanchez argued on this basis that an embryo could be aborted in an ectopic pregnancy.[32] Sanchez, using Augustine's doctrine of "just war," identified an embryo growing in a fallopian tube as an "unjust aggressor" against the life of the mother and maintained that a mother could legitimately kill such an embryo in self-defense.

Feminist views   Certain worldviews support certain moral premises, and some feminists believe that most of the premises in arguments about abortion are ultimately determined by whether a worldview embraces or attacks feminism. Here, *feminism* pertains to the right of a woman to make her own choices and lead her own life in equality with, not under the control of, the men in her life. (This is, of course, a broad, rather loose definition.) Many feminists hold that differing moral opinions about abortion involve not the metaphysics of personhood but the roles of women or women's sexual and economic liberation.

One feminist writer argues that the key question about abortion is whether women should be forced to bear children in a way in which men are not. If an embryo is a person who has a right to life at the mother's expense, then women will always be potential slaves of biological reproduction:

> With all the imperfections of our present-day attitudes, I'm still a lot better off in terms of the sexual choices I have than women of my mother's generation. I was

a lot better off after the sixties than I was before them. What sexual freedom I now have has been very hard-won. I wouldn't give it up for anything. . . . There's a larger crisis, one that has to do with the tensions between feminism and the backlash against it. On the one hand, society is encouraging sexual freedom; on the other hand, it's punishing people for indulging in it and not emotionally preparing them for it. Both women in general and teenagers in particular are caught in the middle.[33]

Conservative religious views   We have already noted the religious argument that personhood begins at conception. A related idea is that each human pregnancy happens for a divine reason, and this may be the basis for an argument commonly called the *sanctity of life*. People who believe in the sanctity of life assume that a particular being, which has been conceived, has survived to implant itself in the uterine wall, and has been growing inside a woman since then, was *meant by God to have been created at this place and time*. It follows that any interference with the growth of this being would thwart God's plans. In the language of laypeople, this is sometimes expressed as, "God must have meant for me (you, her) to become pregnant, or else I (you, she) wouldn't be."

Two replies can be made to this kind of conservative religious view. First, such a view is very fatalistic in terms of one's personal relation to God, and it seems reasonable to ask, "*Why* must I (you, she) accept everything that happens? If everything comes from God, doesn't the choice to have or not to have an abortion also come by God? Why make the fatalistic assumption that one can follow God's will only by accepting pregnancy? Why can't a reasoned choice to have an abortion also reflect God's will?"

Second—and this reply is logically prior to the first one—how does a woman (or a couple) know what God's will about a particular pregnancy might be? Unless God speaks to us directly, revealing his wishes, how can we assume that planning whether and when to have children is not best for us? How do we know that God does not want us to do what we reasonably believe will be best for us, now and in the future?

A Final Consideration: Abortion as a Three-Sided Issue

Many of us in North America are so accustomed to living in a tolerant democracy, where individual liberties are respected, that we sometimes fail to understand how we got where we are or what the larger, worldwide picture is. In the United States, we can easily forget that our historical policy of individual rights and liberty represents a hard-won victory which citizens of many other countries have never achieved. Millions of women in China, for instance, are forced to undergo abortions if they become pregnant before their mid-twenties or after they already have a child: the Chinese government has imposed a limit of one child per family. In Rumania under the long (and only recently ended) dictatorship of Nicolae Ceausescu, millions of women were denied contraception or abortions: the Rumanian government wanted to increase the population and forced women to have as many children as possible.

Perhaps it is this kind of forgetfulness that explains why our media sometimes present abortion as an issue with two sides: antiabortion versus pro-choice.

In fact, the global picture of abortion in recent history is most accurately portrayed as a *three-sided* issue involving two extremes and a compromise between them—forced birth versus forced abortion versus individual choice:

- *Forced birth*—Extreme (example, Rumania)
- *Forced abortion*—Extreme (example, China)
- *Individual choice*—Compromise (example, United States)

In other words, the idea of leaving decisions about abortion up to the women affected is, in terms of the world as a whole, not one of two sides but rather a compromise between two extremes.

UPDATE

The Antiabortion Movement

Efforts to overturn *Roe v. Wade* have taken various paths since 1973. Some have, of course, involved legislation, but probably the most prominent antiabortion activities have taken the form of protest.

Some of the protest has been violent, and the violent elements of the movement invoke a higher, special "antiabortion morality." During the 1980s, protesters bombed many abortion clinics. Two men from Texas who attacked several abortion clinics in Florida were sentenced to 30 years in prison; among other crimes, they had kidnapped a physician who performed abortions. In 1984 alone, there were 24 arson or bombing attacks on abortion clinics. One bombing—in Pensacola, Florida—took place on Christmas morning and was described by one of the conspirators as a "birthday present to Jesus."[34] A few weeks earlier, a bomb at a clinic in a suburb of Washington, D.C., had almost killed a guard.

By the end of the 1980s, public opinion had turned dramatically against antiabortion violence. As a result, the vast majority of the antiabortion movement used the kind of nonviolent protest mounted by Operation Rescue, an organization founded by Randall Terry in 1988. Modeling themselves on the nonviolent demonstrations (such as sit-ins) that had taken place in the south during the civil rights movement, these protesters practiced civil disobedience in front of abortion clinics; they hoped, by their example, to prick the conscience of the nation. Some leaders were fined and jailed for blocking traffic and other minor infractions of the law.

During the 1990s, however, the protest movement targeted physicians who performed abortions as the "weak link" in the chain; these physicians sometimes found protesters outside their homes on Saturday mornings. It was such campaigns of harassment that may have led, in March 1993, to the point-blank murder of the physician David Gunn as he was leaving an abortion clinic in Pensacola, Florida. Dr. Gunn had been performing abortions once a week at the clinic, and his picture had been posted across northern Florida by antiabortionists on the kind of "WANTED" sign used by the FBI for fugitives from justice. Spokespersons for Rescue America and Missionaries to the Unborn announced that Dr. Gunn's death had saved numerous babies from abortion; later, one of these spokespersons "rejoiced" when the Pensacola clinic found it difficult to replace Dr. Gunn.

On July 29, 1994, at another abortion clinic in Pensacola, a second physician—John Bayard Britton—was killed by an antiabortion leader and former minister named Paul Hill. Dr. Britton and his volunteer security escort, James Barrett, were both fatally shot, and James Barrett's wife was wounded; Dr. Britton had been wearing a bulletproof vest, but Hill (who would be convicted in November 1994) was said to have aimed the shotgun directly at his head. That same night, an abortion clinic in Virginia was bombed, though there were no injuries.

Attempted Abortions Resulting in Live Births

Attempts to abort late-term fetuses have sometimes resulted in live births. In 1977, a physician, Ronald Cornelson, testified in a California criminal court that after a botched saline abortion resulted in a live-born 2½-pound baby, his colleague William Waddill had choked the infant and had also suggested injecting potassium chloride to kill it. (It can be noted that a 2½-pound baby may well be viable; this was the birthweight of the jockey Willie Shoemaker, who was born prematurely and was kept warm in a shoebox in an oven.) Waddill was tried twice for murder, but both juries were deadlocked.[35] In 1979, at the University of Nebraska Medical Center, another 2½-pound baby was born alive after an attempted abortion, was purposefully left unattended, and died after a few hours.

Because of such cases, physicians today will rarely perform an abortion after 23 weeks of gestation; and there are some newer techniques for preventing abortions that would produce live births. For example, use of prostaglandins to induce abortion is now avoided, since prostaglandins, although safer than suction or surgical techniques, resulted in 30 times more live births. For first-trimester abortions, the most typical technique was formerly injection of hostile fluids (saline or urea), followed by dilatation and curettage (scraping), a technique called *D and C*; but D and C has been replaced by suction curettage or uterine aspiration. For late-term abortions, dilatation and evacuation—*D and E*—is used: the fetus is cut into parts and removed in pieces. To ensure that all the pieces have been removed (since any fragments left behind would produce infection in the mother), the dismembered fetus must be reassembled outside the womb. Late second-trimester abortions use hysterotomy, as in the Edelin case.

Fetal Research and Fetal-Tissue Research

As we have seen, the legal environment of the Edelin case included issues of fetal research; the somewhat earlier research on aborted fetuses at Boston City Hospital was described above, and (as has been noted) Alice Roe and her mother had consented to a preabortion experiment.

In 1973—the same year as the Edelin case—one study, in which the researchers were trying to develop an artificial placenta, used eight fetuses obtained by hysterotomy. These fetuses weighed between 300 and 1,000 grams;

when the largest of them was placed in a warm saline solution mimicking the amniotic sac, it was described by the researchers as making frantic "gasping" efforts and limb-stretching movements as it died.[36] Another experiment studied effects of lack of glucose on the fetal brain (a condition arising when a diabetic pregnant woman goes into shock). The heads of 12 nonviable fetuses were severed after the fetal heart had stopped but before anoxia had damaged the brain. These brains were successfully maintained with artificial replacements for glucose.[37]

The Protestant theologian Paul Ramsey calls such experimentation "unconsented-to research on unborn babies" and sees it as immoral exploitation of a "tragical case of a dying" baby.[38] His reaction is by no means unusual: these experiments outraged many Americans. In 1979, Congress banned all federally funded research involving fetuses or embryos—not only late-term fetuses but even embryos no older than 3 days—and it did not lift the ban until 1993.

A related issue is fetal-tissue research. Tissue from aborted fetuses may help patients with neurological disorders such as Parkinson's disease. The tissue required for such neurological research must be adrenal tissue producing dopamine; and it must be obtained from fetuses whose gestational age is 8 to 11 weeks, since after 12 weeks the tissue begins to differentiate into the normal cells and structures of the brain and thus loses its "elasticity." Treatment consists of a drug (dopamine) delivered as (fetal) cells: in the operation, a small hole is drilled through the patient's skull and fetal cells are dripped directly into the devastated area of the brain. (Note that this is in no sense a "brain transplant" but simply a tissue transplant.)

A panel of the National Institutes of Health (NIH) studied this issue and concluded that even if abortion may be immoral, fetal tissue obtained from abortions can be ethically used for research if the woman's decision to donate tissue is made separately from, and after, her decision to abort.[39] On January 22, 1993—the twentieth anniversary of *Roe v. Wade*—the newly elected President Clinton lifted a 4-year ban on fetal-tissue research.

RU 486

Antiprogestin drugs provide a nonsurgical way to interrupt a pregnancy at a very early stage. One of these drugs is mifepristone, commonly known as RU 486—the RU stands for the manufacturer, Roussel Uclaf, which is owned by the West German pharmaceutical company Hoechst AG.[40]

RU 486 works by binding to progesterone receptors and thus preventing the binding of natural progesterone, a substance in the body that is necessary to support embryonic development in the uterine lining.[41] When RU 486 replaces natural progesterone, it causes the uterine lining to shed as in menstruation, dislodging the embryo.

RU 486 can also be used in conjunction with synthetic prostaglandin, a substance involved in dilating the uterus during labor contractions. In this case, RU 486 breaks up the uterine lining and the synthetic prostaglandin widens and dilates the cervix; uterine contractions expel the lining, and with it the embryo. Bleeding is like a very heavy menstrual period and continues for 10 to 12 days after the embryo is discharged. The success rate for RU and synthetic prostaglandin is 96 percent.[42]

RU 486 was approved for use in France in September 1987, and it began to be used there September 1988, after a tumultuous beginning: initially, protesters had succeeded in getting it withdrawn, but it was reinstated as a result of vehement counterprotests by groups of gynecologists and obstetricians. By the fall of 1992, over 100,000 women had tested RU 486 in France (where the most extensive trials have occurred), and these tests produced important findings. For instance, the initial method of delivering synthetic prostaglandin by injections may have contributed to two nonfatal heart attacks and one fatal one (in a patient who was a heavy smoker and had high blood pressure); since April 1992, prostaglandin has been delivered orally—a safer method—and has been contraindicated for women who are smokers, are older than 35, or have diabetes, heart problems, high cholesterol, or glaucoma.[43]

In France, RU 486 is prescribed within the first 5 weeks of pregnancy. The procedure is as follows. First, a woman comes to a clinic for counseling about alternatives (this is required by law) and returns home for 1 week to reflect (this is also required by law). On her second visit, 1 week later, she is given RU 486 with a physician in attendance; she then stays in the clinic until the expulsion of the embryo. Before she is released, her physical condition is checked; she must then return 1 week later to be checked again—this is to make sure that the procedure has really worked and also to check her overall health. The entire procedure costs about as much as a routine abortion.

Today, many women are using RU 486 as normal therapy in France, Britain, Sweden, and China. In the United States, by contrast, because of the ban on using federal funds for embryonic and fetal research, no federally funded studies of RU 486 have been done, and through the first half of 1994 there had been only one private study.[44] (President Clinton did not remove the federal ban in January 1993—he removed only the ban on using fetal tissue for medical research.) Thus the entry of RU 486 into the American market has been delayed. In May 1994, however, a German pharmaceuticals company donated its RU 486 patents to the U.S. Population Council, a nonprofit group, which announced that it would test the drug on 2,000 American women that fall. If RU 486 is determined to be safe and effective in the United States, it could be available to American women as early as 1996. According to the Rockefeller Foundation, 75 percent of abortions in the United States are performed within the first 5 weeks of pregnancy—the period when RU 486 is prescribed in France—and so the drug could become very popular here.

Misconceptions still abound about RU 486 as a medical procedure. In fact, it is neither painless nor inexpensive; nor is it "private"—that is, it cannot simply be taken at home. However, the existing evidence indicates that it is far safer for women than the typical abortion techniques of the last decade; unlike invasive procedures, RU 486 carries no risk of perforating the uterus.

With regard to RU 486 as an ethical issue, there seem to be two main points of controversy. First, does using RU 486 amount to killing a person? Most people would say that it does not, because the technique is prescribed at a very early stage of embryonic development—5 weeks.

Second, should RU 486 really be considered "abortion" at all, or is it rather a contraceptive? Since RU 486 initiates a natural process of embryonic rejection by causing the uterine lining to shed, it works in much the same manner as an intrauterine device (IUD), which also causes expulsion of an early embryo from the uterine lining;[45] and an IUD is considered a contraceptive device. Critics of RU 486 call it an "abortion pill," but this may be begging the question. If an IUD is appropriately called a contraceptive, it can be argued that RU 486 should be called a "contraceptive pill"; and according to a Scottish study published in 1992, RU 486 could also be called a "morning after" pill. There does seem to be a significant difference between standard abortion procedures and hormonally dislodging an embryo—although some antiabortionists are unimpressed by this reasoning and describe RU 486 as "chemical warfare on the unborn."

Maternal versus Fetal Rights

The issue of maternal versus fetal rights has developed new aspects during the years since the Edelin case. This general issue, of course, includes abortion, but not all cases of conflicting rights actually involve abortion; some have arisen when pregnant women were willing to continue pregnancy.

A famous case that did involve abortion occurred in 1989, when Nancy Klein, who was in her twenties, went into a coma at an early stage of pregnancy. Her physicians wanted to abort the fetus: they believed that an abortion might bring her back to consciousness; they also felt that an abortion would be in her best interest because certain drugs that she should receive could not be given while she was pregnant (these drugs might injure the fetus), and because her cerebral blood volume would increase once she was no longer pregnant. Antiabortionists went to court to try to block the abortion, while Nancy Klein's husband, Martin, pressed for it. Martin Klein prevailed and the abortion was performed (amid protests). Nancy Klein emerged from the coma after 11 months and now lives a normal life.

Two well-known cases have concerned cesarean section. The earlier of these took place in Washington, D.C., in June 1985, when Angela Carder ("Angela C") and her 26-week-old fetus died shortly after undergoing a cesarean section ordered by a judge for the sake of the fetus. Angela Carder was dying of a rare form of cancer and had evidently requested chemotherapy and resisted the operation, although some witnesses said that she was so confused and dulled that her real wishes could not possibly have been known. The baby was delivered alive but died 2 hours later; Angela Carder herself died 2 days later.[46]

The second of these cases took place in Illinois in late 1993, when the physicians of a pregnant woman referred to as "Mother Doe" sued in court to force her to undergo a caesarean section. The fetus in this case was becoming oxygen-starved, and the physicians wanted to deliver it at once by cesarean section because they felt that if they waited for a full-term delivery, the baby would be born retarded or even in PVS. Mother Doe, on the other hand, was a religious woman who believed that God would miraculously protect the fetus until a healthy infant could be delivered through natural childbirth. The basic issues at odds in this case were whether the fetus had a right to normality at birth and whether a competent woman can ever be compelled to undergo surgery in the interest of a fetus. The Illinois Supreme Court upheld the mother's right to refuse surgery.

An unfortunately common issue that has developed in cases involving maternal versus fetal rights has to do with substance abuse by the mother. In cases like these, the mother typically intends to carry the fetus to term, but because of her abuse of drugs or alcohol, it is likely that the baby will be born impaired. Between 1987 and 1992, 160 women in 24 states were charged with injuring a fetus during pregnancy by taking drugs such as cocaine.[47] Such a case often arises in the third trimester, when the fetus is obviously viable and thus would be considered a person, or at least a near-person, by most people. The conflict then is between a vulnerable fetus, whose interests are served by coming into life unimpaired by alcohol or drugs, and a drug-ravaged mother who often can barely cope with her pregnancy, let alone with her life.

It should be noted that the problem of substance abuse during pregnancy affects not only women and fetuses but society as a whole. Fetal alcohol syndrome, for instance, is often cited as the leading cause of mental retardation.[48] Many people are disturbed that government, through the offices of local district attorneys, can intervene in pregnant women's lives for the sake of fetuses; for other people, however, the prospect of babies—and communities—needlessly harmed by preventable retardation or congenital drug dependency is equally disturbing. There may also be an element of class conflict here, since critics opposed to intervention say that almost all the women who are prosecuted are "lower class" drug abusers rather than "middle class" alcoholics; and it is true that far more babies are harmed by alcohol than by cocaine.

Finding a broad, consistent policy about conflicts between maternal and fetal rights is difficult. It is possible, of course, to conclude simply that no interference with competent pregnant women should be allowed. However, such a conclusion would seem incompatible with a consensus that has become clear in medicine regarding an issue raised by Jehovah's Witnesses. The medical profession holds that a pregnant Jehovah's Witness can be forced to accept blood transfusions to save the life of a third-trimester fetus; the rationale for this policy is that while the woman could be allowed to decline a transfusion for herself, she should not be allowed to decline it for a fetus, who as an adult might not choose to become a Jehovah's Witness. It is sometimes argued that this medical policy also justifies intervening with pregnant substance abusers. (On the other hand, though, the Jehovah's Witness in this example is hospitalized, whereas the substance abuser may not be.)

In moral issues, there are sometimes true tragedies—situations in which, no matter what is done, there can be no good outcome. Cases of maternal-child conflict may be among them.

Viability

In 1983, Justice Sandra Day O'Connor predicted that medicine would push viability "further back toward conception" and that the trimester system established in *Roe v. Wade* would be "clearly on a collision course with itself."[49] Her prediction has not come true, however. Although medicine has made intense efforts to treat premature babies more effectively, in 1992 the consensus in neonatology was nevertheless that "before 23 or 24 weeks, [the fetus] simply cannot survive. And nothing that medical science can do will budge that boundary in the foreseeable future."[50] The problems—apparently unsolvable—are that earlier than 23 or 24 weeks of gestation, the fetal lungs are simply too immature to function, even with a respirator; and that certain essential organs, such as the kidneys, do not develop early in pregnancy.

This recently acknowledged fact weakens one argument against abortion. Clearly, the argument from marginal cases must lose some of its force, since *lung viability* now serves (and has served for over 20 years) as a practical indicator of viability and thus, in fetal development, can be offered as a marker of personhood.

A number of legal developments will be discussed in the following section, but there have also been at least two with regard to viability. In 1979, in *Colautti v. Franklin,* the United States Supreme Court gave physicians broad discretion in determining viability. The decision said that "the determination of whether a particular fetus is viable is, and must be, a matter for the judgment of the responsible attending physician," apparently precluding the possibility of another case like Kenneth Edelin's. However, in 1989, in *Webster* (possibly referring to the Edelin case), the Supreme Court allowed a state to require a physician to check after abortion for viability of the fetus.

Legal Trends

In the two decades since *Roe v. Wade,* abortion-rights advocates have pressed for broader protection and antiabortion forces have mounted legal challenges. A culmination came in 1992, with the Court's decision in *Planned Parenthood v. Casey* (widely known as the "Pennsylvania decision"): the Court reaffirmed the "essential holding" of *Roe v. Wade,* including "the right of a woman to choose to have an abortion before viability and to obtain it without undue interference from the State."[51] (Note in particular the phrase *undue interference.*) A few months later, in December 1992 (this was the month before President Clinton's inauguration)—as if to say that it had taken its stand on abortion law and would not budge in the future—the Court turned down a request to review an appellate decision voiding severe antiabortion restrictions that had been legislated in Guam.

During the last two decades, however, the Court has been willing to fine-tune certain details of *Roe v. Wade,* and to these we now turn.

Consent of fathers   The 1976, in *Danforth,* the Court invalidated state laws requiring a woman to get consent for an abortion from either the matrimonial or the biological father. The Court held that such consent amounted to giving these men a veto over the woman's decision, and because the woman "is the more directly and immediately affected by the pregnancy," she should not be subject to any such veto.

Consent or notification of parents   The *Danforth* decision also said that a state cannot pass a law giving parents of teenage girls a veto over the decision to have an abortion. In 1979, however—in *Bellotti v. Blair*—the Supreme Court said that although a state may not give parents an absolute veto over a minor daughter's decision to terminate a pregnancy, the state may require a minor to obtain the consent of one or both parents if it provides her with an alternative to having to consult or inform the parent or parents. Another decision held that a state law was legal if it merely required a clinic to inform or notify a parent before a teenager's abortion. By 1992, 35 states had laws requiring a parent's consent or notification when minors sought abortions, although only 18 states actively enforced such laws.[52]

Informed consent of patients   During the 1980s, the Supreme Court struck down laws in Ohio and Pennsylvania that required, before an abortion, the patient's informed consent, a 24-hour waiting period, or discussion of alternatives by the physician with the patient. The language in these "informed consent" statutes had been, in fact, dissuasive rather than informative. In its "Pennsylvania decision" in 1992, the Court reversed itself on this point, ruling that informed consent and a 24-hour waiting period did not constitute "undue burdens" on women seeking abortions. This change brought abortion into line with informed-consent requirements for other medical procedures of equal risk.

Government support   Several other decisions concerned whether the federal government or state governments could be required to fund abortions for women who are unable to pay for them. In *Harris v. McRae* (1980), the Supreme Court held that although a woman has a right to an abortion, she does not have a right to a free abortion at the expense of federal or state government. Congress passed laws banning use of public funds for abortions for women unable to afford them, and many states followed suit. The *Webster* decision in 1989 also said that states may ban public employees or public hospitals from performing abortions.

FURTHER READING

Francis M. Kamm, *Creation and Abortion,* Oxford University Press, New York, 1992.

Don Marquis, "Why Abortion Is Immoral," *Journal of Philosophy,* vol. 86, 1989, pp. 183–202.

Warren Quinn, "Abortion: Identity and Loss," *Philosophy and Public Affairs,* vol. 13, 1984, pp. 24–54.

Michael Tooley, *Abortion and Infanticide,* Oxford University Press, Oxford, 1983.

Mary Anne Warren, "On the Moral and Legal Status of the Fetus," *The Monist,* vol. 57, 1973, pp. 43–61.

CHAPTER 7

Letting Impaired Newborns Die

Baby Jane Doe

"Baby Doe" cases arise when parents of impaired neonates or physicians charged with the care of these neonates question whether continued treatment is worthwhile and consider forgoing treatment in order to hasten death. This chapter focuses on the case of Baby Jane Doe, which took place at Stony Brook, New York, in 1983. It also discusses the Baby Doe rules and general ethical issues of "Baby Doe" cases.

BACKGROUND: TREATMENT OF IMPAIRED NEWBORNS

Historical Overview

In ancient Athens, both Plato (in *The Republic)* and Aristotle (in *Politics)* advocated killing impaired newborns. In ancient Sparta, a cyclops baby (that is, an infant born with single eye or with the two eyes fused) would be left to die in a country field. Later, in ancient Rome, babies who looked grotesque were discarded in the same way: Roman parents who didn't want impaired babies abandoned them in rural fields to die of exposure. Exposure remained a very common practice during the first four centuries of the Christian, or Common, era (c.e.); such "letting die" was legal and was not considered infanticide. Actual female infanticide was practiced, for most of two millennia, by Bedouin tribes of Arabia, the Chinese, and much of the population of India.[1]

Around the year 300 c.e., the Roman emperor Constantine was converted to Christianity and was persuaded to ban parental infanticide. Christianity strongly condemned both abandonment and infanticide, but the church had neither funds nor people to care for abandoned babies; it did not establish a foundling hospital until the eighth century in Milan. In his *History of European Morals,* William Lecky observes, with regard to the influence of Christianity, that although it was the first religion to value the "castaways of society," its role in protecting infant life "often has been exaggerated."[2]

During the Middle Ages, wet nurses acted as agents for parents wishing to rid themselves of children (a practice that would continue well into the nineteenth century). In the eighteenth century, when the population of Europe was exploding, exposure and infanticide were used as methods of birth control. During the reign of Napoleon, so many babies were abandoned that he established his own foundling hospitals, where parents could deposit a baby on a sort of turntable set into the front entrance, spin it to send the baby inside, and depart unseen. In France in 1833, over 100,000 babies—20 to 30 percent of all newborns that year—were thus abandoned.[3]

A hundred years ago, Thomas Wakley, the founder of the medical journal *Lancet*, campaigned against exposure, infanticide, and abandonment. In 1870, the Infant Life Protection Society was founded to prevent parents from collecting payments for dead babies from multiple life insurance policies.

In the western world in modern times, "letting die" tends to take place in a different kind of context—the hospital. Neonatal intensive care units (NICUs) were developed during the 1960s primarily to keep premature babies alive, and during the 1970s small respirators and feeding tubes began to be used to save such babies and other infants at risk; these new technologies saved some infants who had been born barely alive. However, caring for infants in NICUs is very expensive, and—although this is often impossible to know from external observation—premature babies have frequently suffered neurological hemorrhages or lung damage from respirators. Both the expense of NICU treatment and the low quality of life that can be predicted for many infants receiving such care have raised ethical questions about which babies should be treated and who should make that decision.

Preceding Cases and Controversies

By 1983, when the Baby Jane Doe case took place, a set of rules known as the *Baby Doe rules* had already been developed as a result of several earlier cases. These earlier cases are described below; the rules themselves are discussed in the following section.

The Johns Hopkins cases: 1971   Down syndrome is a chromosomal abnormality discovered by Langdon Down in 1866; a person with Down syndrome has 47 chromosomes in each cell rather than the usual 46. The extra chromosome is on chromosome 21; hence the syndrome is also called *trisomy 21 (trisomy* refers to an extra chromosome). Down syndrome is a genetic condition that always causes retardation and a characteristic facial appearance; it is often accompanied by cardiac or intestinal problems. In the early 1970s—at the time of the Johns Hopkins cases—parents of children with Down syndrome were likely to be told by physicians that although the eventual IQ of a person with Down syndrome could not be predicted at birth, the usual range was between 25 and 60, with some severely impaired individuals below 25.[4] (Whether or not this information was correct will be discussed later.)

In 1971—when NICUs were still relatively new and few impaired newborns were treated aggressively—three babies who had been born with Down syndrome accompanied by life-threatening intestinal defects were patients in an

NICU at Johns Hopkins Hospital in Baltimore, Maryland. Two of them were allowed to die.

One of the babies who was allowed to die had duodenal atresia, a blockage between the higher duodenum and the lower stomach that prevents the passage of food and water. The mother of this baby—a nurse who had worked with children with Down syndrome—was told that the infant would die if she did not consent to surgery to open the atresia. She immediately refused to consent, and her husband, a lawyer, agreed with her decision.[5] Pediatric surgeons at Hopkins honored this decision and did not go to court.

A film based on the case of this first baby was made by the Joseph P. Kennedy Jr. Foundation; it is called *Who Should Survive?* and has been shown to millions of undergraduate and medical students.[6] Although the film was meant to raise and discuss the ethical issues involved, it has a serious flaw: it never gives the parents' reasons for their decision. In a commentary accompanying the film, the sociologist Renée Fox mentions that the couple appeared to be "of modest means," suggesting that they had a middle-class income at best, and the lawyer William Curran implies that they let their baby die for purely selfish reasons.[7]

The mother of the second baby who was allowed to die already had children; and according to one of the commentators on this case, the theologian James Gustafson, she explained the decision to forgo treatment by saying, "It would be unfair to the other children of the household to raise them with a mongoloid."[8] (Because of the facial characteristics associated in Down syndrome, it was at one time called *mongolism.*) Gustafson describes this mother's decision as "anguished" but also notes that when she learned that her baby had Down syndrome, she "immediately indicated she did not want the child."[9]

The two babies whose parents refused treatment were not killed; they were simply allowed to die—a course that was thought to be more acceptable morally and less likely to incur legal prosecution. One of these babies took 15 days to die; ordinarily, the baby would have died in about 4 days, but some staff members surreptitiously hydrated this infant.

The parents of the third baby eventually accepted treatment, and this baby lived. This baby's parents had originally been given a pessimistic prognosis for Down syndrome, by an obstetrician who referred them to Hopkins because Hopkins had been willing to allow the other two babies to die. However—and perhaps significantly—the staff at Hopkins then gave them a more balanced view.

Lorber's criteria for spina bifida In the early 1970s, because of the increasing incidence of cases like the Johns Hopkins babies in NICUs, several well-known pediatricians went public. These included, for example, two pediatricians at the NICU of the Yale-New Haven Medical Center—R. Duff and A. Campbell—who published an article in 1973 in which they admitted frankly that they had accepted parents' decisions to forgo treatment, and that 43 impaired infants had therefore died early.[10] Duff and Campbell's article caused a minor sensation and led to much soul-searching by pediatricians at other NICUs, who were often asking themselves whether they were doing the right thing. Another of the pediatricians who went public was the English physician John Lorber, in 1971—the same year as the Hopkins cases. Lorber wrote an article in which he implied that some babies are so severely impaired or deformed that they are better off being allowed to die without treatment.[11]

Lorber specialized in spina bifida—which, as we will see, was one of the defects afflicting Baby Jane Doe. *Spina bifida* (the term literally means "divided spine") is a hernial protrusion through a defect in the vertebral column, and it is the most common serious neural-tube defect, occurring, statistically, in 1 in 1,000 live births. It may occur in the form of a meningocele, a protrusion of part of the meninges; or it may take the form of a meningomyelocele, a protrusion not only of part of the meninges but also of the substance of the spinal cord.[12] A baby with spina bifida is almost always paralyzed below the level of the opening and thus has bowel and bladder problems; moreover, the opening makes the baby vulnerable to infections such as meningitis. Quality of life depends on two factors: first, the level of the meningomyelocele; and second, the degree of associated problems such as hydrocephalus—a swelling of cranial tissue which commonly accompanies spina bifida and often causes increased intracranial pressure and decreased blood flow to the brain, resulting in mental retardation. However, the probability of mental retardation can be reduced by aggressive surgical treatment involving tubes called *shunts* to decrease this pressure. (Hydrocephalus was present in Baby Jane Doe.)

Lorber developed criteria to predict which spina bifida babies would die if left untreated: the higher the meningomyelocele on the spine and the larger the affected area of the spine and its coverings, the greater the probability of attendant problems and of death. These criteria were meant to be of practical use, because not all infants with spina bifida die if left untreated, and for infants who live, nontreatment makes them worse off. Lorber's criteria seemed to make it possible to identify babies who *would* die: all those in his lowest category. During the 1970s, criteria like Lorber's were apparently used at Oklahoma Children's Hospital, where it was decided not to treat 24 babies with spina bifida who were in the lowest category and who all subsequently died.[13]

The Mueller case: Conjoined twins   On May 5, 1981, conjoined twins, joined at the trunk and sharing three legs, were born in Danville, Illinois, to Pamela Mueller and Robert Mueller.[14] Robert Mueller, a physician, was in the delivery room when their family physician, Petra Warren, delivered the babies, who were named Jeff and Scott. The Muellers and Warren decided together not to treat the twins aggressively, so that they could die. However, other physicians in Danville were deeply divided over the ethics of the Muellers' decision. An anonymous caller alerted Protective Child Services, which obtained a court order for temporary custody of the children.

The Muellers were initially charged with neglect; at a later hearing, that charge was dismissed, but the Muellers were denied custody. In September 1981, they regained custody after pediatric surgeons testified that successful separation was unlikely and the prognosis for the twins was therefore bleak.

It is interesting to note the subsequent events in this case, however. The twins lived, still joined, for about 1 year, at which time they weighed 30 pounds.[15] Shortly thereafter, they were separated in a long operation. Scott, the weaker twin, died; but Jeff, the stronger twin, survived, and later he entered a regular school. (The parents, Pamela and Robert Mueller, eventually divorced.)

The "Infant Doe" case: Tracheosophageal fistula   The "Infant Doe" case in Bloomington, Indiana, took place about 1 year after the case of the Mueller twins, over the course of only a few days—from Infant Doe's birth on April 9, 1982, to the baby's death on April 15. Infant Doe had Down syndrome with tracheosophageal fistula, and once again physicians—and others—were divided over the issue of forgoing treatment.[16]

The prognosis for tracheosophageal fistula, which is more serious than duodenal atresia, tends to depend on the severity of the fistula, or gap. In Infant Doe's case, the gap was fairly small, and an early operation to close it would have had a better than 90 percent chance of success. However, the referring obstetrician, Walter Owens, downplayed this fact in discussing the case with the parents and emphasized his assessment of the problems of Down syndrome itself: he said that some people with Down syndrome are "mere blobs" and that the "lifetime cost" of caring for a child with Down syndrome would "almost surely be close to $1 million." Infant Doe's parents decided not to allow the operation.

In this case, hospital administrators and pediatricians disagreed with the parents' decision and immediately convened an emergency session with a Monroe County judge, John Baker. Testifying at this hearing, Owens repeated his prognosis: that even if surgery was successful, "the possibility of a minimally adequate quality of life was nonexistent" because of "the child's severe and irreversible mental retardation." Infant Doe's father, a public school teacher who had on occasion worked closely with children with Down syndrome, also testified: he agreed with Owens and felt that such children never had a "minimally acceptable quality of life." It is noteworthy that this hearing was held late at night in a room at the hospital where it was not recorded, and that Judge Baker did not appoint a guardian *ad litem* for Infant Doe. Baker ruled that the parents had the right to make the decision about treatment versus nontreatment.[17]

The county district attorney thereupon intervened and appealed the decision to the County Circuit Court—and, after losing there, to the Indiana Supreme Court. Both appeals failed: each time the court ruled for the parents. The prosecutors then appealed to United States Supreme Court Justice Paul Stevens for an emergency intervention, but Infant Doe died before they arrived in Washington, D.C.

The aftermath of the Infant Doe case is of considerable interest. Owens wrote to the U. S. Civil Rights Commission about his role in the case, maintaining that he was "proud to have stood up for what I and a large percentage of people feel is right"; he also said he was glad that after Infant Doe had died, in only a few days and with little suffering, the parents were able to have another baby—a healthy child who almost certainly would not have been born if the couple had been forced to treat Infant Doe. In 1989, however, reviewing the Infant Doe case and other Baby Doe cases, the commission concluded that Owens's evaluation was "strikingly out of touch with the contemporary evidence on the capabilities of people with Down syndrome."[18]

The Baby Doe Rules

The Infant Doe case was followed intensely by the media and prompted President Ronald Reagan to direct the Justice Department and the Department of Health and Human Services (HHS) to mandate treatment in similar future cases. Reagan, who was opposed to abortion, had appointed as his surgeon general C. Everett Koop, an antiabortion pediatrician who was also opposed to nontreatment of impaired newborns.

Because crimes such as homicide and gross negligence are defined by state rather than federal law, Reagan's Justice Department needed to find an indirect route in order to make nontreatment illegal. The executive branch can set social policy by reinterpreting prior congressional legislation (for example, in the 1960s laws against racial discrimination began as executive orders by President Lyndon Johnson), and such orders are enforced by threats from the Justice Department that institutions violating them will lose all federal funds. It was through this route that the Justice Department and HHS developed the so-called *Baby Doe rules* requiring treatment of all impaired newborns.

The first step was taken on May 18, 1982 (1 month after Infant Doe's death), when nontreatment was defined as a violation of Section 504 of the Rehabilitation Act of 1973, which forbade discrimination solely on the basis of handicap. This interpretation by the Justice Department created a new conceptual synthesis: *imperiled newborns were said to be handicapped citizens who could suffer discrimination against their civil rights.*

The Rehabilitaton Act thus became the basis for an HHS Notice to Health Care Providers which was sent to hospitals, and for large posters which were displayed on the outer glass walls of every NICU:

> DISCRIMINATORY FAILURE TO FEED AND CARE FOR HANDICAPPED INFANTS IN THIS FACILITY IS PROHIBITED BY FEDERAL LAW.

A toll-free 800 telephone number was also posted so that anyone around an NICU could report abuses—including concerned nurses, disgruntled parents, ambulance-chasing lawyers, and anonymous cranks. (This "Baby Doe hotline" was despised by pediatricians, who feared it would be used maliciously.) "Baby Doe squads," composed of lawyers, government administrators, and physicians, investigated complaints.

"Interim Final" Baby Doe rules were proposed on March 7, 1983 (about 1 year after Infant Doe had died), and were to take effect in 2 weeks—on March 21. After these interim Baby Doe rules went into effect on March 21, 1983, however, the American Academy of Pediatrics (AAP) sued in a federal district court to stop them. The suit *(Amer. Acad. Ped. v. Heckler)* was decided in favor of AAP on April 14, 1983, partly on the basis of procedural issues. In July 1983, HHS proposed new interim rules designed to remedy the procedural problems: these new interim rules became the "Final" Baby Doe rules, announced on January 12, 1984, to become effective on February 12, 1984. However, 10 days after the final rules were instituted, another federal court—the Second Circuit Court of Appeals—issued a ruling essentially making them unenforceable. That ruling came in the famous Baby Jane Doe case, which had started a few months earlier, in October 1983.

Before we turn to the case of Baby Jane Doe, it will be interesting to consider the Baby Doe hotline and the Baby Doe squads briefly. As long as they existed, the Baby Doe squads were ready on a hour's notice to rush to airports, fly across the country, and suddenly arrive—as a squad arrived one day at Vanderbilt University—like outside accountants doing a surprise bank audit. Records were seized, charts were taken from attending physicians, and all-night investigations took place. The attitude of the squads was that time was of the essence because an innocent baby's life might be at stake. Besides Vanderbilt, the University of Rochester also suffered (in the words used privately by some pediatricians) a "blitzkreig by the Baby Doe Gestapo." Eventually, because of technical objections, smaller signs were placed inside NICUs, where only staff members could read them (the toll-free number remained on the signs, however); and finally, because of the objections by AAP and the national press, the Baby Doe squads were called off.

How were the hotline and the Baby Doe squads able to exist for approximately 19 months (from May 1982 through most of 1983) while the various Baby Doe rules were being contested and struck down? The answer is that they were operated by HHS, probably under its interpretation of the broad authority conferred by Section 504 of the 1973 Rehabilitation Act.

What was the ultimate effect of the hotline and the squads? The answer is probably that although they were widely resented as *methods*, the *concern* they represented found (and has continued to find) a more positive response. In terms of actual numbers, from March 1983 (when the "Interim Final" Baby Doe rules were issued) until the end of that year, the hotline received 1,633 calls; of these, 49 incidents were actually investigated. *Newsday* (a newspaper in Long Island, New York) studied 36 of the investigations and reported the following:

> In some cases, intervention has saved a baby with a fair chance of living a useful life; in others, extraordinary surgical measures have given babies no more than a few extra days of life at enormous financial and emotional costs. In one case, the medical bills mounted to $400,000 for a baby who doctors say "has zero chance for a normal life expectancy." In a few instances, parents had to give up custody of their children to the state after they refused to permit surgery. . . .
>
> Records of 49 cases investigated by the Health and Human Services Department's civil rights office during the last 19 months show that in only six cases has government intervention appeared to have made a difference, with children given operations or treatment they otherwise would not have had. In 14 of the cases, mostly originated by anonymous calls, investigation proved that allegations of insufficient treatment were false or that treatment was medically impossible.[19]

Thus the Baby Doe squads did force more treatment for some infants (such as the six mentioned, who were sick and profoundly retarded), although during their existence the squads discovered no provable violation of federal antidiscrimination laws.[20]

THE BABY JANE DOE CASE

The Medical Situation: Kerri-Lynn

On October 11, 1983, while the Baby Doe rules were being revised, "Baby Jane Doe" was born at St. Charles Hospital of Long Island, New York. Because she had several major defects, she was transferred to an NICU at University Hospital of the State University of New York (SUNY) campus at Stony Brook, for care by its neonatal specialists.

The baby's name was Kerri-Lynn, but she was called Baby Jane Doe by the media and the courts. Her parents—who were known only as Linda and Dan A.—were lower-middle-class people working hard to improve their lives; Linda A. was 23 and Dan A. was 30. They had been married 4 months when Linda became pregnant, and Dan had built two extra rooms onto what has been described as their "modest suburban home" in the "flatlands of eastern Long Island."

Kerri-Lynn weighed 6 pounds and was 20 inches long. According to testimony, she was born with spina bifida, hydrocephalus, a damaged kidney, and microcephaly (small head, implying a very minimal brain or lack of most of the brain). Her defects must have been traumatic for her parents: for one thing, her spine was open with the meningocele protruding prominently.

At Stony Brook, two physicians—the surgeon Arjen Keuskamp and the pediatric neurologist George Newman—disagreed strongly about treatment in a case like Kerri-Lynn's, although it is impossible to say whether their different moral views caused them to see the facts differently or their different prognoses led them to take opposed moral stances. Arjen Keuskamp recommended immediate surgery to minimize retardation by draining the hydrocephalus. When Kerri-Lynn was examined by George Newman, he told Dan A. that Kerri-Lynn could either die soon, without surgery, or undergo surgery which would save her life but would leave her paralyzed, retarded, and vulnerable to continual infections of both bladder and bowels. According to Newman's later court testimony:

> The decision made by the parents is that it would be unkind to have surgery performed on this child. . . . On the basis of the combination of malformations that are present in this child, she is not likely to ever achieve any meaningful interaction with her environment, nor ever achieve any interpersonal relationships, the very qualities which we consider human.[21]

(Keuskamp, who withdrew from the case, did not testify in court.) Newman probably told Dan A. something like this about midnight on October 11, 14 hours after Kerri-Lynn was born.

After a good deal of consultation between themselves and with others, Linda and Dan A. decided not to allow the operation to drain the hydrocephalus. They acted on their understanding of the distinction between extraordinary and ordinary treatment, disallowing surgery but allowing so-called palliative care: food, fluids, and antibiotics. They assumed that Kerri-Lynn would soon die, but 4 days later the baby was still alive. A social worker wrote at this time that Dan A. was in "despair" because Kerri-Lynn had not yet died; she also noted that Linda A.

was determined to give Kerri-Lynn "as much love as possible" while the infant was still alive. "We love her very much," Linda A. said, "and that's why we made the decision we did."[22]

Kathleen Kerr broke the Baby Jane Doe story for *Newsday* on October 18, 1983. Kerr, who had numerous "firsts" on the story, was also the first reporter (perhaps the only one) to interview the parents. She described the interview:

> Each time he began a sentence, Mr. A. let out a deep sigh, as though seeking strength to answer. Mrs. A. continually touched her husband's arm and rubbed it soothingly. Mr. A. shed his tears openly. . . .
>
> Mr. A. said, "We feel the conservative method of treatment is going to do her as much good as if surgery were to be performed. It's not a case of our not caring. We very much want this baby." . . .
>
> "We're not being neglectful, and we're not relying on our religion [Catholicism] to give us the answer to what we're doing here."[23]

Kerri-Lynn continued to survive, and—as occurs naturally in some cases of spina bifida—her open spinal wound closed.

Kerri-Lynn's Case in the Courts

On October 18, 1983 (the same day that Kerr broke the story), Lawrence Washburn, a municipal-bonds lawyer who lived in Vermont and was active in right-to-life organizations, filed suit in a state court on Kerri-Lynn's behalf, to force treatment. Over the following weeks, the case of Baby Jane Doe proceeded through the courts with enormous speed; everyone seemed mindful of the earlier Infant Doe case, in which the child had died while appeals were still continuing.

An emergency lower-court hearing was held on October 20, with Judge Melvyn Tannenbaum presiding. Because Washburn did not have legal standing to sue, Tannenbaum appointed as Kerri-Lynn's guardian *ad litem* ("for this action or proceeding") another attorney, William Weber. Weber was also temporarily empowered to make decisions regarding Kerri-Lynn's medical care.

At first, Weber supported the parents, but then there was an interesting development. Having talked to Newman, Weber abruptly changed his mind when he read that Newman had written on Kerri-Lynn's medical chart that after surgery, she would be able to walk with braces.[24] Weber concluded that what Newman had written on the chart conflicted both with what he had told the parents and with his testimony in court. On another important point, Newman had testified that the baby had microcephaly and would never be able to recognize her parents. Weber said that this was "A lie. The hospital records shows that the initial measurement of the skull was 31 centimeters (cm), which is within normal limits." A measurement of 31 cm would indicate that Kerri-Lynn had a brain, perhaps even a normal brain. On October 20, therefore, Weber authorized surgery.

The parents' lawyer, Paul Gianelli, then applied to the appellate division of the state supreme court, and on October 21 this higher court reversed Tannenbaum's decision. The justices decided that the law left decisions up to parents when a choice was available between two "medically reasonable" options. This judgment seemed to contradict the legal precedent that to be "medically reasonable," a decision must be not only supported by some evidence but, more important, also in the interests of the child (that is, earlier rulings had required a "medically reasonable option" to be an option in the interest of the child).

Weber, in turn, appealed to another court: New York's highest court, the Court of Appeals. On October 28, Weber lost in this court, which upheld the parents' right to decide. The Court of Appeals noted that this case did not belong in court at all; but that even if there had been neglect of the baby, the parents should have been brought to court by state child-protection agencies—not by unrelated individuals such as Washburn. The appeals court also, emotionally, called Washburn's involvement "offensive" and said that Weber should never have been empowered to make decisions for Kerri-Lynn over the wishes of her parents. It can be noted that, in this decision, the Court of Appeals—along with apparently everyone else in the country who was following the developments—had perhaps become too influenced by the immense publicity surrounding the case. The court seemed to have completely forgotten about the traditional doctrine of *parens patria,* according to which the state protects helpless people against those who might neglect them.

After the decision by New York Court of Appeals, Kerri-Lynn's parents thought they had won. Linda A. said:

> I just want [all this] to end. Just to have a baby like this and deal with it is so much to go through right now. Just let us be with our daughter and leave us alone. . . . If there's hell, we've been through it.

However, by this point action was being undertaken at the federal level, by HHS and the Justice Department.

On October 22, the United States government had informed Stony Brook Hospital that federal investigators were coming to see Kerri-Lynn's medical records. Linda and Dan A. were outraged by this: "They're not doctors, they're not the parents, and they have no business in our lives right now."[25] On October 25, Stony Brook's lawyer announced that the hospital would not let the government examine the records. On October 27, HHS turned the case over to the Justice Department. On October 29, the Justice Deparment filed suit against the hospital in federal court, charging possible discrimination against the handicapped; and Attorney General Edwin Meese and Surgeon General Everett Koop personally sent Justice Department lawyers to the federal court.

A month later—in late November 1983—a federal judge, Leonard Wexler, ruled that the Justice Department could not have the medical records; Wexler also ruled that the parents had not decided against surgery for "discriminatory" reasons. (It is not clear whether Judge Wexler had himself examined Kerri-Lynn's hospital chart.) Dan and Linda A. were pleased, but by now they were also exhausted: "I'm drained physically, mentally, and emotionally," Dan A. said; "I believed that you couldn't look at what we were doing and say we were wrong."

The case later reached the federal Court of Appeals for the Second Circuit, which—on February 23, 1984—denied the government access to Kerri-Lynn's records. This decision, which would presumably apply in similar cases, had the practical effect of making the Baby Doe rules useless, since if the government could not obtain medical records, it could not enforce the rules. The Justice Department appealed to the United States Supreme Court, but in 1986, in *Bowen v. American Hospital Association et al.*, the Supreme Court also held that no records needed to be released.

The Aftermath

As noted, the practical effect of the ruling by the federal appellate court for the Second Circuit in February 1984 was to invalidate the Baby Doe rules. On March 12, 1984—evidently seeking a general ruling—the American Hospital Assocation (AHA) brought suit in the United States District Court for the Southern District of New York, challenging Section 504 as a legal basis for the Baby Doe rules. Eventually, this suit by AHA and Stony Brook's case were consolidated in *Bowen*, in which the United States Supreme Court ruled in 1986 that because the parents were not "federally funded recipients," Section 504 did not apply. In 1984, meanwhile, AMA had joined pediatricians in seeking an injunction that would prohibit HHS from implementing its final Baby Doe Rules; and in December 1984, the injunction was granted by the appellate court for the Second Circuit.

•

During the court battles over Kerri-Lynn, Linda and Dan A. changed their minds and permitted surgery to drain her hydrocephalus—a decision that became known only months later.[26] In addition, the baby had already been given antibiotics after contracting pneumonia (without these antibiotics, she might have died). Kerri-Lynn continued to live and was taken home on April 7, 1984, at age 5½ months. At the time she went home, one physician predicted that she would "probably always be bedridden."[27]

Nearly 5 years later, she was still living at home with her parents. According to Kathleen Kerr, whose stories about the case won a Pulitzer Prize for local reporting, and who visited with the family over those years, Kerri-Lynn was:

> . . . doing better than anyone expected—talking, attending school for the handicapped, and learning to mix with her peers. She still can't walk and gets around in a wheelchair but her progress has defied the dire predictions.[28]

ETHICAL ISSUES

Selfishness

The theologian James Gustafson criticized the parents in the Johns Hopkins cases of 1971, arguing that they had been selfish. Living one's life for others, Gustafson said, is the primary ethical requirement of Judaism and Christianity, and the parents didn't want to do that.[29] (C. Everett Koop, who became surgeon general in the Reagan administration, argued similarly in 1979: "Why not let the family find that deeper meaning of life by providing the love and the attention necessary to take care of an infant that has been given to them?"[30])

John Paris, a Jesuit opposed to Gustafson's position, noted:

That concern, as the spate of press commentaries indicates, finds its roots in a fear that the "me" generation is reverting to the ancient practice of exposing impaired newborns to the elements, or worse, that a "consumer" society is demanding the elimination of its less-than-perfect products.[31]

John Fletcher, an Episcopalian priest and medical ethicist (he was at one time the chief consulting medical ethicist for NIH), also disagreed with Gustafson, taking a different view of the religious values involved. Fletcher said that he himself could "stand by the parents" in such cases and "would not want to come down real hard on them" for letting a baby die by forgoing treatment.[32] Others who disagreed with Gustafson asked whether everyone really sees the purpose of life as living for others; it was also asked whether, if living for others is a religious value, nonreligious people should be forced to adhere to it.

With regard to "selfishness," it can also be pointed out that considering what is entailed by raising and caring for a profoundly afflicted child is not necessarily "selfish" but may be simply realistic. For a couple who both work, for instance, raising a severely disabled child usually means that one parent must give up his or her job—and that the couple will lose this income. Also, some disabilities are lifelong; people with Down syndrome, for example, now have an average life-span of 55, and some of them live into their seventies. Is it so "selfish" for parents to decide that they are not "called" to spend their own lives caring for such a child? (Moreover, parents may well consider that their disabled child might out-live them.)

Disability advocates argue that disadvantaged children cannot be allowed to die merely because they don't fit into their parents' plans; but if we do not consider the family's good in some way, aren't we in effect saying that the birth of an impaired child—a random event—must be fatalistically accepted by every family, no matter what hardships it entails? Families today and the family as an institution seem shaky enough; how much more stress can most families reasonably be expected to manage? Although we cannot always make the interests of the majority the determining factor in a decision, surely those interests must be given some weight, and it can be held that how best to consider them depends on each case and each family.

If we think, then, not about what people want to do but about what they *ought* to do, will we conclude that a parent who allows a disabled infant to die lacks morality or is merely following a different morality? Fred Bruning, a writer for *Newsday*, defends the course of leaving parents alone:

> This is a dilemma that transcends politics, or ought to. Who but parents can begin to interpret the meaning of a child born with terrible handicaps? Here is a situation in which "feelings" alone are inadequate. . . . Nor is sweet reason sufficient either. For every argument, there is a counterargument; for every epiphany, a corresponding burst of doubt. Everything is right, everything is wrong. Morality has deceptive moves. . . .
>
> Travelers familiar with Beirut claim it is a city lost to hope because consensus is impossible. Perhaps it can be said that parents of severely damaged children inhabit a Beirut of the spirit, a place where innocence has no armor, where there is no distinction between suffering and survival. The rest of us are

strangers, and we ought to let the parents consult the doctors, reach their decisions, tend to their babies, grapple with their lives. We ought to respect their
heartache and their wishes. We ought to leave them in peace.[33]

Bruning's words are eloquent, but surely there are limits. It would probably seem
more appropriate to leave parents alone within certain parameters—if we can
decide on those paramaters.

Implications of Abortion

Today, many pregnant women undergo amniocentesis or sonograms, and if the
results indicate a fetus with a chromosomal abnormality, many of them terminate
the pregnancy and try again for a healthy baby. Such abortions may take place
legally even late in the second trimester, when the fetus is large and perhaps at a
stage of development where some "preemies" are saved. This practice raises a
significant ethical issue.

When amniocentesis indicates spina bifida, for instance, the fetus will almost
always be aborted. But if spina bifida justifies abortion, why doesn't it also justify
letting a newborn with spina bifida die? Similarly, if an abortion is permissible
because the fetus has Down syndrome, why shouldn't Down syndrome justify
allowing a neonate to die? Birth, after all, does not change the medical condition:
in this sense, it can be argued that the significance of birth is merely symbolic or
emotional. Note that this logic is neutral between opposed moral conclusions
about nontreatment. That is, if there *no* good reason why a neonate with, say,
spina bifida should be allowed to die, then presumably there is no good reason
why a fetus with spina bifida should be aborted.

If parents want to forgo treatment in these cases, then, should they be
required to justify the decision, or should they simply be left alone? When a
woman decides to abort a fetus (even a healthy fetus), she is not asked to give a
"good reason." Why are we so much more concerned when an impaired newborn is involved?

For medical ethicists, neonatal pediatricians, and others who do not oppose
abortion as such but who do oppose letting parents decide to forgo treatment in
Baby Doe cases, the problem is to find a consistent position—a position that
allows them to accept choice with regard to abortion but not with regard to "letting die."

Nontreatment versus Infanticide

An important moral question is whether it would not be more compassionate to
simply kill impaired and imperiled newborns than to let them die slowly by forgoing treatment. Legally, killing such an infant would be homicide, whereas forgoing standard treatment is at worst neglect, and legal experts agree that forgoing entails much less danger of prosecution than killing; but that is not the point
here. Nor is the major issue whether forgoing is actually more humane, since that
question is at least partly factual. In terms of ethics, the essential issue seems to
be whether infanticide and forgoing are really morally different.

In both forgoing and infanticide, the motive—the death of the baby—is the same, and so is the result: in both, the baby dies. If the motive is the same in both decisions, and if both decisions lead to the same result, how can the two decisions differ morally? This might seem to be a matter of simple logic: whatever makes one decision good (or bad) should also make the other decision good (or bad). If so, the kind of action itself, or its active or passive nature, should make no difference.

Nevertheless, some people do draw a distinction between nontreatment and infanticide. One reason offered for such a distinction—based on the realistic assumption that people are not perfect and make mistakes—is that killing is too quick and too final. Allowing an infant to die, on the other hand, leaves the door open for a while, in case (for example) parents have a change of heart or physicians develop a different diagnosis or prognosis. Another argument for forgoing treatment is that it shows more respect for the value of life: a "quick end" cheapens life, it is held; but when treatment is forgone, parents and professionals must themselves suffer through a slow death.

Personhood of Impaired Neonates

Before he became surgeon general, C. Everett Koop wrote that allowing brain-damaged infants to die would create a slippery slope: it would lead to killing other impaired newborns and end with killing "all people with neurological deficit after an automobile accident."[34] He argued that "each newborn infant, perfect or deformed, is a human being with unique preciousness because he or she was created in the image of God."[35] On the other hand, the Catholic theologian Richard McCormick argued that an infant can realize some "good" of its own only if it can *potentially form human relationships*.[36] The issue of *personhood* underlies both Koop's and McCormick's arguments.

With regard to personhood, it would generally be accepted that moral decisions about forgoing treatment are different when "persons" rather than "non-persons" are involved. The vexed question is what factual qualities confer personhood: as is discussed in Chapter 6, the "core" concept of personhood may be well understood, but "marginal cases" are problematic. (This issue is also discussed in Chapter 8, on animal rights.) Many good thinkers have been frustrated by the attempt to find a theory of personhood which would satisfactorily explain all our intuitions—our basic moral beliefs—about cases at the margins.

In the examples cited above, Koop is arguing that "each newborn infant, perfect or deformed" is a person, whereas McCormick is arguing that not every infant is a person and is proposing the capacity to form human relationships as a criterion or standard of personhood. Consider an anenepchalic infant, for instance (an infant born without a higher brain); according to McCormick's standard, such an infant would not be a person. McCormick's "relationships" standard is probably a reasonable attempt to define or delimit personhood; whatever its theoretical merits, however, there are practical objections to it. For one thing, physicians may not agree about the diagnosis of a condition like anencephaly; in the case of Kerri-Lynn, for example, Newman believed that her small head indicated a state similar to anencephaly and concluded that she would never recognize her parents, but Arjen Keuskamp seems to have disagreed. Moreover, it can be difficult to make accurate or dependable predictions about "potential." Associations of parents of babies with spina bifida hold that a person's potential can never be known until his or her life is lived.

Of course, McCormick's standard is by no means the only criterion of personhood that has been offered. For instance, some commentators who are considering impaired newborns in particular have proposed using a *cognitive criterion* of personhood. This cognitive standard is discussed in Chapter 1 and again in Chapter 6: on one formulation, it identifies certain qualities or characteristics having to do with cognition—thought—and assumes that without these qualities, personhood does not exist (the qualities commonly include reason, memory, and self-awareness); another formulation is simply that to be a person is to be able to think. With regard to impaired infants, some people who apply the cognitive standard argue that a newborn is not a person until some time after birth. The philosopher Peter Singer holds that children should not be regarded as persons until "a few months" after birth; the physician and philosopher H. T. Engelhardt holds that they are not persons until they form a self-concept, around the age of 2; the philosopher Michael Tooley holds that they are not persons until they can use language.[37] For Singer, Engelhardt, and Tooley, newborns fail to meet the cognitive criterion.

How good is the cognitive criterion of personhood? As was noted in Chapter 1, in the context of letting adults die (that is, in the context of "brain death"), the cognitive criterion, though not a legal standard, is actually used by many families. However, its application to impaired newborns may be more questionable. Allowing parents to forgo treatment for an imperiled neonate is one thing; claiming that a child is not a person until perhaps age 2 seems to be quite another. Someone might, of course, suggest that evaluating the personhood of an impaired infant could be *deferred* for some months or even a year or two; but leaving aside the moral status of such a course, it does not take much imagination to see that the practical and emotional difficulties would be enormous.

The personhood of impaired newborns presents significant problems, then, and these problems are relevant to the debate—which is prominent in such cases—over whether forgoing treatment should or should not be a "private" decision. Was Kerri-Lynn's case, for instance, a private, personal "family decision," or was it a case of neglect that public policy must not tolerate? One member of a group advocating recognition of the "sanctity of life" in public policy criticized the parents, maintaining that "private individuals and private groups of individuals don't have the right to make life or death decisions in private in an unaccountable manner."[38] On the other hand, many people argued that Kerri-Lynn's parents should be left alone to make their own decisions about her care. Do problems of personhood effectively prevent us from applying Mill's concept of harm in this context—that is, are we in effect unable to distinguish between *private life* and *morality* here? As discussed in Chapter 1, Mill's harm principle calls for government not to interfere with decisions that put no other *person* at risk of harm; but the principle may not help us in these cases, if we cannot agree on whether or not nontreatment will harm a person. In other words, if the issue of personhood remains unsettled, simply applying the principle of harm begs the question.

It seems important to reach some conclusion about personhood, in order to establish limits for public policy. However, if we decide that (as Koop maintained) every impaired newborn is a person, it might follow that no parent could decide to let such a child die, and this would of course severely limit a family's range of choices—a result that many people would consider unacceptable. On the other hand, if we allow the widest possible range of choices, we are in essence allowing each family to decide for itself what personhood is and which "beings" in the family are and are not persons—and this too might have unacceptable consequences. (In fact, it is not hard to find cases in which limiting the range of "family" choices about nontreatment might seem permissible or even essential. In July 1983, to take one example, the state of Tennessee intervened to allow chemotherapy for 12-year-old Pamela Hamilton, over her father's religious objections. Another such case occurred in Boston in 1988, when a young child became ill; the child's parents, who were Christian Scientists, called a practitioner instead of a physician; the child suddenly died 5 days later, after apparently improving for a while; and the Boston district attorney Newman Flanagan charged the parents with manslaughter. Cases of this nature are discussed further below, in the section on the role of religion.)

What *can* we conclude about personhood, then? Following is one suggestion.

In moral discourse, we usually seek answers to the question, "What is right?" Sometimes, however, we must admit that with regard to a certain issue we are hopelessly deadlocked: fundamentally different answers are given. The personhood of impaired newborns may be such an issue: it is possible—perhaps even likely—that in cases like these, involving the margins of personhood, we will never have precise, absolute answers. This does not imply, however, that we must simply give up on morality and resort to arbitrary decisions or force.

When we must acknowledge the existence of fundamentally different answers to a moral question, there is a natural solution: we can shift from *content* to *process.* In other words, rather than thinking of a "solution" as a specific answer, we can seek a process that will result in the fairest solution. (Trials by jury are one example.) A common problem with the concept of process is that the shift from content to process can be made too soon, before it is really certain that a deadlock has developed; but with regard to the personhood of impaired newborns, it seems clear from decades of experience that many people do disagree fundamentally.

We can, therefore, search for the best *process* to resolve disputes about the personhood of impaired newborns and thus about treatment versus nontreatment. For instance, we can think of such cases not in terms of *what* is decided but rather in terms of *who* should decide. Possible answers would then include parents, judges, physicians, bioethicists, the clergy, and ethics committees; and for many people, the first plausible candidates will be the parents. It should be emphasized, however, that shifting from content to process does not solve the problem of personhood with regard to impaired newborns: with this issue—as with many others—the concept of process provides only *guidelines* for reaching reasonable answers.

Prognoses and Ethical Frameworks

Cases of treatment versus nontreatment are often all grouped together, and sometimes even lumped together with cases of assisted suicide and physician-assisted dying, as "euthanasia." This is confusing and possibly dangerous. It is important to differentiate physician-assisted dying, which involves terminally ill competent adults (see Chapter 3), from assisted suicide, which involves nonterminal competent adults (Chapter 2); it is also important to distinguish both of these from nontreatment of incompetent adults in PVS (Chapter 1); and it is important to distinguish all of these from allowing impaired newborns to die.

One reason why such distinctions are important has to do with establishing *criteria* for forgoing treatment. As discussed in Chapter 1, the criteria for nontreatment of "never competent" patients should presumably be much higher than the criteria for competent or formerly competent patients whose own wishes can be known or inferred. With "never competent" patients, it can be argued that the decision to forgo treatment must be based on evidence which is "beyond a reasonable doubt," and this would also be true for patients (such as some infants with spina bifida) who may be "presently incompetent but later to be competent." On this argument, then, the standard of "beyond a reasonable doubt" would apply to forgoing treatment for impaired infants.

In practice, criteria for nontreatment of impaired babies tend to be based on long-term prognoses, and whether such prognoses are "beyond a reasonable doubt" is at least highly questionable. For one thing, medical diagnosis and prognosis are almost always subject to differences of opinion and to outright error. In addition, when impaired babies are involved, physicians' medical judgments seem to be affected by their own ethical outlooks.

Some medical ethicists try to determine permissible nontreatment by considering what kind of neonatal defect is involved, along a spectrum from less to more serious.[39] Babies whose problems are at the "less serious" end of this spectrum should be treated, whereas it would be permissible to let babies at the "most serious" (devastating) end of the spectrum die. However, cases in the middle of the spectrum—cases like spina bifida and Down syndrome with associated defects—become controversial. In such controversial cases, prognosis is far from absolute and may be influenced by moral frameworks.

For example, consider John Lorber's predictive criteria for spina bifida, discussed earlier in this chapter. One very vocal critic of Lorber's approach is a colleague of his at the same hospital, the pediatric surgeon R. B. Zachary. Zachary argues that the only real option for babies with spina bifida is either to kill them or to do everything possible for each one of them; basically, he is saying that there is no category of babies with spina bifida who can be "allowed to die." Lorber and some other pediatricians say that the mortality rate is high for babies they place in the "worst" category of spina bifida, but Zachary maintains that these physicians do not simply withhold treatment; according to Zachary, they "push the infant towards death" by giving:

> . . . eight times the sedative dose of chloral hydrate recommended in the most recent volume of *Nelson's Pediatrics* and four times the hypnotic dose, and it is being administered four times every day. No wonder these babies are sleepy and

demand no feeding, and with this regimen most of them will die within a few weeks, many within the first week.[40]

Differing moral views would seem to be at least one factor in this controversy. It should be pointed out, though, that (as noted earlier) the prognosis for an infant with spina bifida may depend on what kind of treatment is given: particularly, whether hydrocephalus is drained to minimize brain injury. We will return to this point later.

Prognoses about the intelligence of impaired people seem to be especially heavily influenced by ethical views; this may not be surprising, since "intelligence" is an evaluative concept to begin with. Down syndrome is a good example, especially because of the external characteristics associated with it. Let's briefly consider Down syndrome in more detail.

During the last 40 years, there has been a revolution in thinking about IQ in Down syndrome. Most of the earlier studies were probably prejudiced against people with Down syndrome, because these studies focused on people who were institutionalized—a sampling bias that failed to take into account the possibly higher IQs of people with Down syndrome who lived at home, in supportive families. At present, it seems established that although almost all babies with Down syndrome will have IQs below 70, probably less than one-third of them (some studies say only 10 percent) will have IQs lower than 25 and will thus be "profoundly retarded" and untrainable.[41] This indicates that most people with Down syndrome, especially those who receive good early care, will have IQs above 25; some will have IQs above 50; with the maximum stimulation and support, most will probably have IQs between 30 and 70.

What does this imply about "quality of life" for a person with Down syndrome? IQ is a measure of intelligence, of course, and academics and other professional people tend to associate intelligence with happiness. However, it is an unwarranted assumption to think that people with IQs between about 30 and 70 must be unhappy, unless we simply define unhappiness in those terms. Whether one imagines such an existence by thinking of a 6-year-old or a beloved pet, the conclusion must be that, given reasonable stimulation, love, and supervision, most people with Down syndrome will "have a life." To put it another way, they will have a narrative history, and their lives can go better or worse for them. To put it yet another way, most of them would *not* be better off not existing.

Note, however, the mention of early care, stimulation, and support; as with spina bifida, the prognosis for Down syndrome can vary with treatment: early intervention can raise IQ, whereas "custodial care" will lower it. Thus there is no way to predict at birth whether a baby with Down syndrome will be at the low or the high end of the potential IQ range; consequently, the best interest of these babies is served by maximal treatment.

It is interesting to realize that although the ethical frameworks loosely described as "sanctity of life" versus "quality of life" are commonly held to be incompatible, these two standards would agree on the early treatment of most babies with Down syndrome. In fact, a similar conclusion may be possible for most babies with spina bifida. It would seem that a neonate with spina bifida has a good chance of "a life"—that is, neither genetics nor probable IQ predetermines a life of misery. Often, it cannot be predicted at birth whether a child with spina bifida will be in the high, normal, or low range of IQ; but most such children will *not* be profoundly retarded. If we cannot assume that low IQ precludes any happiness in life, it can be argued that such children should live—that an IQ described as "borderline," "trainable," or even "imbecile" does not make life so bad that nonexistence would be better.

However, "quality of life" and "sanctity of life" do seem to diverge when a prognosis suggests a life of almost total misery and pain: in such a case, considerations of "quality of life" or "the good of the child" would indicate nontreatment. If this outcome can be known in advance (a point that not everyone would grant), it would be immoral, from a "quality of life" standpoint, to save the neonate. It is exactly these cases that traumatize pediatric neurologists and families. Because most of these children die, nontreatment is best—but not all of them die, and those who do not die will be worse off.[42]

Before we leave this discussion of prognoses and ethical frameworks, a related matter should be dealt with. Some commentators raise the point that the prognosis for an impaired neonate has implications for the *family's* "quality of life"; and some parents do see nontreatment as benefiting the family, since caring for an impaired child obviously imposes enormous burdens. If the "quality of life" standard is applied to the entire family, rather than to the baby ("the good of the child"), it may indeed imply nontreatment; however, this would be a radically different interpretation of the standard. When we think of "quality of life" in, say, cases of PVS or physician-assisted suicide, we are of course thinking of the *patient's* quality of life. Trying to apply the standard to a neonate's family is analogous to arguing that a patient in PVS should be allowed to die, or a terminally ill patient should be helped to die, not for his or her own good but for *our* good.

The Role of Religion

In 1984, the secular philosopher Peter Singer started a controversy in *Pediatrics* by arguing that society should be more concerned about killing monkeys in dubious experiments than about nontreatment of impaired and imperiled human neonates. In fact, he maintained that society should allow very impaired human babies to die:

> Once the religious mumbo-jumbo surrounding the term "human" has been stripped away, we may continue to see normal members of our species as possessing greater capacities of rationality, self-consciousness, communication, and so on, than members of any other species; but we will not regard as sacrosanct the life of each and every member of our species, no matter how limited its capacity or intelligence or even conscious life may be.[43]

Singer (whose views are discussed in Chapter 8) emphasized what he saw as a dramatic asymmetry between our undervaluation of animals and our overvaluation of humans. His actual point was obscured, however, when *Pediatrics* was inundated with letters from physicians protesting his use of the words "religious mumbo-jumbo."[44]

The pediatricians who wrote these letters of protest proclaimed that religion was at the heart of medicine. For them, medical ethics was a branch of religious ethics; they could make no sense of ethics without religion.

There is an ongoing and often acrimonious debate between religious and nonreligious physicians, but in many ways the issue is a red herring. This can be seen when we distinguish claims about the importance of religious *values* in medicine from claims about the truth of a religion. That is, whether or not the metaphysical beliefs of the Islamic-Judeo-Christian tradition are correct, modern medicine has undeniably been humanized by values associated with this tradition: respect for human life, family integrity, unselfishness, humility, equal moral worth, and compassion. Perhaps especially, *compassion*—which literally means "suffering with"—has always figured prominently in Judaism, Christianity, and Islam. Moreover, one does not have to be religious in order to value compassion or many other presumably "religious" values. Some religious people believe or argue that atheists must lack compassion, respect for human life, and so on; but so long as these values are not actually *defined* as religious, the claim that atheists cannot hold them is empirical: it can be tested, and disproved, by experience and observation.

In Baby Doe cases, some members of the clergy and some religious physicians have found it difficult to accept parents' decisions to forgo treatment. To many commentators, this attitude seems to lack tolerance and is therefore itself intolerable. Furthermore, it should be noted that some of the people who would advocate nontreatment—or who would at least advocate choice in this matter—are also religious; thus it is not clear how much this particular issue is really about religious values. The issue may have more to do with differing ideas about relationships between physicians and society, physicians and patients, physicians and families, and so on.

The point that "religious values" do not necessarily lead to choosing treatment over nontreatment bears repeating. Earlier, two cases were cited in which religious parents of older children objected to treatment, on specifically religious grounds (see the discussion of personhood): one of these was a girl whose father did not want her to have chemotherapy; another was a boy who died when his parents consulted a Christian Science practitioner rather than a physician about his illness. In both these cases, moreover, society intervened; the state of Tennessee stepped in to allow the girl's chemotherapy, and the state of Massachusetts stepped in (after the fact) to charge the boy's parents with manslaughter.

With regard to religion, some principle seems to be needed to guide society when the issue of treatment versus nontreatment arises. If we want to let parents decide that an impaired neonate should remain untreated, does this imply that parents may also decide not to treat an older child? If it is argued that "religious values" demand treatment for impaired, imperiled neonates, what does this imply about "religious values" which lead parents to deny treatment to older children? The parents of the two children just mentioned belonged to "minority religions" whose tenets came into conflict with standard medical procedures; does this imply that "minority" religious values can be overridden? In practice—in cases involving children of Jehovah's Witnesses, for instance—the courts have mandated treatment by reasoning, first, that religious freedom does not extend to imposing parents' beliefs on their children at risk of life; and, second, that these children may later, as adults, have different religious beliefs. However, the issue in general is complex, and finding a consistent public policy is extremely difficult.

The Role of the Media

Some disturbing questions are raised by the reporting of Kerri-Lynn's case in the print and visual media, particularly when we consider that Kerri-Lynn not only survived but was able to live at home and even attend school. All the major media simply accepted George Newman's negative prognosis, and almost all dismissed William Weber, the child's court-appointed guardian, as a fanatic. The media's stance may have unduly influenced not only the general public but even many physicians and medical ethicists, who also took Newman's prognosis as fact.

For example, after Kathleen Kerr's stories on the Baby Jane Doe case had attracted national attention, the veteran medical reporter and columnist B. D. Colen began to cover the case for *Newsday,* and in one of his "sidebar" articles he painted a grim picture of a case that was supposed to be similar. This sidebar described the grueling life and bitter complaints of a mother whose anencephalic or hydrocephalic baby (coincidentally named Cara-Lynn) had been treated, had not died, and was then 2½ years old. In retrospect, what is most interesting is not this other case as such but the way Colen used it as a basis for drawing conclusions about Baby Jane Doe:

> While Cara-Lynn looks far more grotesque than Baby Jane Doe, whose fate is being argued in the courts, the two mistakes of nature have an almost identical prospect for a life filled with pain and devoid of self-knowledge.[45]

Colen's prediction was essentially the same as Newman's: that Kerri-Lynn would never "achieve any meaningful interaction with her environment, never achieve any interpersonal relationships." In fact, this same assumption had already been made by Kathleen Kerr in her earlier stories.

Why did Newman's opinion prevail? That is an interesting question. A year later, a scathing article about the reporting of the Baby Jane Doe case appeared in the *Columbia Journalism Review,* which is often called the "conscience of the news reporting profession."[46] In this article, by Stephen Baer, it was argued that the press had "egregiously failed to meet" its obligation to report the case accurately. Mary Tedeschi, an assistant managing editor of the popular conservative journal *The Public Interest,* wrote an article for another journal—*Commentary*—charging that coverage of *all* the famous Baby Doe cases was biased.[47] With regard to Kerri-Lynn's case in particular, Tedeschi noted that Newman had written on the chart that "the prognosis was for probable . . . walking with bracing" (a point which Weber had also stressed). She also cited a pediatric neurosurgeon who had treated over 1,000 patients with spina bifida and who held that children whose heads measured 31 cm (as Kerri-Lynn's did) are among "the very brightest" of such children, presumably implying that Kerri-Lynn's IQ could be normal or better.

Admittedly, Stephen Baer was a publicity agent for a right-to-life organization, and Tedeschi also had an ax to grind—she concluded, as a conservative, that "the Baby Doe cases served as a pretext for liberal elites to attack a popular Reagan administration." Still, they both made some good points. Many errors of omission occurred in the reporting of the Baby Jane Doe case. For instance, the public was not informed that although hydrocephalus generally accompanies spina bifida, it does not necessarily cause retardation if it is shunted immediately. Nor was the public informed that when Stony Brook Hospital resisted Koop's attempt to see the baby's medical chart, its motives might have been not to protect the privacy of the family but rather to protect itself from a court suit. Moreover, beyond doubt, pediatricians *did* radically disagree about what treatment was best for Kerri-Lynn, but the two sides of this medical controversy were never presented by the media. As a result, the public—and evidently even some professionals—came to believe that the case involved only moral questions, when in fact medical questions were also at issue. It is astounding to note that such serious charges of inaccuracy and incompleteness could be raised about a story for which the journalist (Kerr) had won a Pulitzer Prize. It also seems astounding that neither the *New York Times* nor the *Wall Street Journal* (to name just two newspapers other than *Newsday*) had checked Kerr's story independently.

At the time of this case, the momentum of the media in support of the parents—and with it the momentum of medicine and medical ethics—became so strong that any dissent was perceived as bigoted fanaticism. Eventually, people read and heard reports of the Baby Jane Doe case with their minds already made up. The nadir may have been reached in November 1983, when Koop was grilled on *Face the Nation* by Lesley Stahl, whose tone implied that she was interviewing a fundamentalist, parent-baiting Big Brother. From the perspective of today, Koop's answers seem impressive: he said that there were discrepancies in the medical chart and that he wanted to see the records simply to learn what was best for the child. Ed Bradley on *60 Minutes* also did a piece on the case, strongly antagonistic to Koop.

With regard to the role of the media, one of the important lessons of the Baby Doe cases is that problems of medical ethics rarely take place in well-defined, predictable circumstances and rarely have neat, clear solutions—and that real-life outcomes may embarrass those who are too confident about their own conclusions. However, this lesson is hardly confined to the media alone.

UPDATE

Legal Trends

Legal developments since the Baby Jane Doe case have involved both litigation and legislation.

Litigation   Most district attorneys are reluctant to prosecute parents in Baby Doe cases, and this attitude seems to have widespread backing. (An editorial in the conservative *Wall Street Journal*, for example, argued that the courts are already clogged enough, without local judges being forced by Uncle Sam to second-guess doctors in the nursery.[48]) Still, by state law a baby is a person with rights: to live, to inherit money, not to be abused, and so on. Thus criminal prosecution of parents for neglect does sometimes occur, as in the case of the Mueller twins. Prosecution of physicians is also a possibility in such cases. When neonatologists disconnect respirators to let impaired babies die, they risk being charged with violating criminal laws. Since 1992, another source of potential prosecution is the Americans with Disabilities Act (discussed below).

With regard to civil litigation, parents can sue physicians in civil courts for allegedly causing babies to be impaired. Courts are hearing many such suits, and the possibility of such a suit may be a factor that physicians in Baby Doe cases should consider. In the United States, 3.2 million babies are born per year, of which 42,000 are impaired. Today, few parents simply accept birth defects as "fated" or as "God's will,"[49] standards of health continue to rise, and couples expect healthy—even "perfect"—babies. When a baby has birth defects, then, parents often blame physicians. (As a result, we see malpractice insurance becoming more and more expensive, especially for obstetricians; we also see more and more lawyers advertising to solicit neonatal suits.) Litigation of this nature against doctors can, theoretically, take the form of "wrongful life" suits or "wrongful birth" suits, and it will be helpful to review these briefly here (see also Chapter 4).

Both wrongful life and wrongful birth suits fall into the general classification of tort law, and in both kinds of actions compensation is sought. A *wrongful life suit* is brought solely by a child. In such a suit, it is claimed that the child would never have been born if not for negligence or error on the part of the defendant, and that the resulting life is so miserable as to be a legal tort or harm; the plaintiff—the child—seeks punitive damages as a compensation for suffering and also to prevent or discourage future errors. A *wrongful birth suit* is brought by a parent or parents of a child born with defects or injuries; in a suit like this, it is claimed that a physician has caused the injury or defect and that the harm is abnormal development (rather than life itself), and thus the parent sues for compensation for care of the child. To put this another way, in a wrongful *life* suit, it is argued that the plaintiff (the child) would have been better off not existing; whereas in a wrongful *birth* suit, the plaintiff (the parent) argues that because of a physician's error, the child needs some kind of special care.

To understand how such suits have been decided in the courts, it is useful to think in terms of the *baseline* and *normality* concepts of harm (these too are discussed in Chapter 4). The baseline concept, as the term implies, requires a starting point—a baseline—from which an adverse change is plotted (an existing being who is made worse off); the normality concept requires a norm of development which is not achieved. So far, the courts have rejected almost all wrongful *life* suits, and these rejections have assumed the baseline concept of harm: that is, they have assumed that life is always a benefit, even if it is filled with pain and suffering, and thus that an infant can never "benefit" by not being brought into existence. (The underlying reasoning here has apparently been that if a child could benefit by not being born, it would follow that he or she could also benefit by actually being killed—a conclusion the courts are not willing to draw. Whether or not that conclusion actually does follow is another matter.) Wrongful *birth* suits, on the other hand, appeal to the normality concept and have been more successful in the courts.

A case which had elements (or "counts") of both wrongful life and wrongful birth was that of Jeffrey Gleitman, in 1967. Sandra Gleitman, Jeffrey's mother, had contracted German measles during the pregnancy; Jeffrey was born nearly blind and deaf, and she said that her obstetrician had failed to warn her of this outcome. She was one plaintiff, suing for the expenses of Jeffrey's lifelong care (this was the wrongful birth aspect); in addition, Jeffrey himself was another plaintiff, and the brief for Jeffrey argued that he was so impaired that he would have been better off not existing[50] (this was the wrongful life aspect). The Gleitmans lost, evidently because of the wrongful life element of the case. The judge found that if Sandra Gleitman's physician had warned her about probable fetal defects she would have had an abortion, and concluded that Jeffrey "would almost surely choose life with defects as against no life at all." The rule established by *Gleitman* is that any child who is born impaired as a result of a physician's bad advice, but who would have been aborted had the advice been correct, is therefore unable to recover damages. Since 1982, courts in New Jersey, Washington state, and North Carolina have agreed that, while life itself can never be an injury, parents may recover damages to pay for care that would not have been required if physicians had not made errors.

There does seem to be one example of a successful wrongful life suit, however: the Curlender case, which took place in California in 1986. In *Curlender*, the court recognized a claim against a laboratory which had mistakenly told the parents of child with Tay Sachs disease that they were not at risk, awarding damages even though the child would not have been born if this mistake had not been made.

Legislation   In 1984, Congress amended its Child Abuse Prevention and Treatment Act of 1974 (not the Rehabilitation Act), to count nontreatment in Baby Doe cases as *child abuse*. These amendments (signed into law by Ronald Reagan in October 1984) circumvented the injunction against the Baby Doe rules. They made states, not the federal government, responsible for such cases—getting Uncle Sam out of the neonatal nursery but also leading to problems of their own.

The only exceptions to the regulations under the child abuse act are (1) when an impaired child is "chronically and irreversibly comatose," (2) when a child is inevitably dying, and (3) when treatment would be "futile and inhumane." These exceptions are often interpreted very narrowly, so as to give parents very few choices. Problems resulting from such narrow interpretation were illustrated dramatically in the Linares case, which took place in Chicago in 1989. Dan Linares held an NICU staff at gunpoint while he himself disconnected the respirator of his 16-month-old son Rudy, who had gone into PVS 9 months earlier, after swallowing a balloon at a birthday party; Rudy soon died, and Dan Linares was charged with first-degree murder.[51] (A grand jury refused to indict Linares for homicide; he later received a suspended sentence on a minor charge arising from his use of a gun.) There was no doubt, in this case, that Dan Linares was a caring parent, and some such tragedy might have been expected sooner or later as a consequence of the narrowness and vagueness of the exceptions to the child abuse act.

In 1992, the Americans with Disabilities Act (ADA) went into effect; this act protects Americans with a wide range of disabilities (including HIV infection, it is interesting to note) from discrimination. The application of ADA to newborns with congenital defects—and thus to Baby Doe cases—is so far unresolved; in February 1994, however, a federal court specifically cited ADA in mandating treatment for a 16-month-old anencephalic infant, Baby K, who had been brought to a hospital emergency room (ER) in Virginia in respiratory distress.[52]

Federal regulations, of course, require hospitals to treat all patients needing care who arrive at ERs; it is because ADA was cited that the Baby K case is of particular interest here. Baby K had been on a respirator since birth. When the case was heard, her physicians wanted to disconnect it and let her die; but her mother insisted on continued care, for religious reasons. At its heart, Baby K's case was about whether or not physicians may, without incurring charges of discrimination against the handicapped, overrule parents' decisions about continuing treatment which seems to be medically futile and pointlessly expensive.

Trends in Pediatrics

Within pediatric neurology, opinion about treatment in Baby Doe cases has changed dramatically over the past decades: in the 1960s and early 1970s, the consensus was that many such cases should not be treated; today, all but the most hopeless cases are treated.[53]

For example, Lorber's criteria concerning spinia bifida initially swung the pendulum toward nontreatment in many NICUs; but during the 1980s, right-to-life organizations and disability advocates swung the pendulum back toward treatment. Also, breakthroughs were made in urology, neonatology, neurosurgery, and CAT-scan diagnosis, and these not only increased the accuracy of prognoses but also improved quality of life for such children. These changes have led to a new understanding:

> Mild to moderate degrees of microcephaly are compatible with normal or even exceptional intellect. This is particularly true in cases of untreated meningomyelocele in which loss of cerebrospinal fluid through the unrepaired hole in the back may decrease the total mass of the head. . . .
>
> Essentially all children with severe meningomyelocele have hydrocephalus. . . . Children with hydrocephalus who are treated reasonably early and who do not develop meningitis have a better chance than 50 percent of being intellectually normal.[54]

The Spina Bifida Association has stated:

> Since we have found it virtually impossible to predict at birth which infants with meningomyelocele will become competitive, ambulatory, and intellectually able, we have not relied on arbitrary guidelines to determine which children should or should not be treated. On the contrary, we believe that all such children should be treated, and we feel that our data show this philosophy to be correct.[55]

The outcome in Kerri-Lynn's case—which was chosen for discussion here because of its fame but was otherwise typical of spina bifida—makes this statement seem reasonable, at the very least. Moreover, the unexpected outcome of the Mueller case and the newer prognoses for Down sydrome suggest that similar reasoning may be appropriate with regard to other defects.

Outcomes

After two decades of debate about Baby Doe cases, the results are equivocal. On the one hand, some impaired babies who would once have died as a consequence of nontreatment are now undoubtedly surviving to lead meaningful lives. On the other hand, the right of parents to make choices in cases of Down syndrome with related defects, or in cases of spina bifida, has declined dramatically. As a result of the amendment to the child abuse act, most NICU physicians actually overtreat severely impaired newborns.[56] Ironically, the present federal regulations are more stringent than the guidelines of the Roman Catholic church: the Catholic guidelines allow treatment to be withheld if its results would be "gravely burdensome."[57]

•

In 1994, B. D. Colen was Lecturer in Social Medicine at Harvard University. He provided an update on Kerri-Lynn:

> Now a 10-year-old, . . . Baby Jane Doe is not only a self-aware little girl, who experiences and returns the love of her parents; she also attends a school for developmentally disabled children—once again proving that medicine is an art, not a science, and clinical decision making is best left in the clinic, to those who will have to live with the decisions being made.[58]

FURTHER READING

Fred Frohock, *Special Care: Medical Decisions at the Beginning of Life,* University of Chicago Press, Chicago, Ill., 1986.

Michael F. Goodman, ed., *What Is a Person?* Humana, Clifton, N.J., 1988.

Peggy and Robert Stimson, *The Long Dying of Baby Andrew,* Little, Brown, Boston, Mass., 1983.

U.S. Commission on Civil Rights, "Medical Discrimination against Children with Disabilities," September 1989.

PART THREE

Classic Cases about Research and Experimental Treatments

CHAPTER 8

Animal Subjects

The Philadelphia Head-Injury Study on Primates

This chapter discusses the conflict between animal-rights activists and scientists over the use of animals in research. It gives a historical overview of opposition to using animals in such research and takes up philosophical concepts underlying the recent animal-rights movement. The central case in the chapter is the research of Thomas Gennarelli, who between 1970 and 1985 systematically inflicted brain injuries on monkeys and baboons to mimic the effects of such injuries in humans. Publicity about this case permanently changed the way animal research is conducted in the United States.

BACKGROUND: ANIMALS IN RESEARCH

Animals and Pain: Concepts and Conflicts

Human beings have used animals for many purposes since prehistoric times, but experimentation on animals did not arise as a specific issue until the beginning of modern science. The premises for the modern debate were set in the seventeenth century, by René Descartes.

Descartes was not only a mathematician and philosopher but also a physiologist, and he studied the circulation of blood by dissecting live animals without anesthesia (which was not invented until the early 1900s). To understand why he considered that permissible, it is necessary to understand his basic philosophical approach, which is known as the *Cartesian* worldview and has deeply influenced western science and philosophy. Descartes, of course, was the author of the famous argument *"Cogito, ergo sum"*: "I think, therefore I am" (it appears in his *Meditations*). According to Descartes, what distinguishes human beings from other animals—what is essentially human—is *res cogitans,* or "thinking stuff," a substantial mind or soul. For Descartes, this mental substance held together transient mental states such as perceptions, feelings, thoughts, and dreams and served as a ground for free will, reason, and moral values. Animals other than human beings, Descartes believed, have no *res cogitans,* no mind or soul, and are therefore ultimately only *res extensa,* or "extended, physical stuff." Thus in Cartesian philosophy animals were merely fleshy machines; no "soul" was reflected in their eyes, and similarly no real pain was reflected by their apparent "pain behavior."

Descartes's idea that animals lack a soul was not unique, of course: this was also Christian doctrine, and Descartes had accepted the teaching that humans have souls created by God whereas animals do not. But Descartes assumed, further, that *soul* is identical to *mind,* so that if animals have no soul, neither do they have a mind; and that if animals have no mind, they cannot feel pain. For Descartes, in order to feel pain, a mind is needed, and—to repeat—only human beings have a mind (indeed, for Descartes, "to be human" was at least partly "to be able to feel pain"). In Descartes's view, there is no middle ground between a human being, who has a soul and thus a capacity to experience pain; and an animal (*any* animal), which has no soul and thus no capacity to experience pain.

Cartesianism represents an attempt to deal with the tension between science and religion by demarcating proper areas for each: the province of science is the study of matter, mathematics, animals, and the human body; that of religion and the humanities is mind, art, and ethics. Obviously, however, it has not come to represent a consensus, or even a widely accepted solution—even for Christians, who are still struggling with the concept of how mind and soul are related, how they relate to morality, and whether animals count in the grand scheme of things (Protestant ministers, for instance, are often asked whether pets go to heaven).

Among Descartes's immediate followers during his own century were an infamous group of early physiologists and vivisectionists (researchers operating on animals without anesthesia) at the Jansenist seminary of Port Royal. Here is a description of the Port Royalists by an eighteenth-century writer, Nicholas Fontaine:

> They administered beatings to dogs with perfect indifference, and made fun of those who pitied the creatures as if they felt pain. They said the animals were clocks; that the cries they emitted when struck were only the noise of a little spring that had been touched, but that the whole body was without feeling. They nailed poor animals up on boards by their four paws to vivisect them and see the circulation of the blood which was a great subject of conversation.[1]

To some extent, the Cartesian concept of animals has persisted into modern times. Some behavioral psychologists, for instance, argued against assuming that animals (especially rats) are conscious and drew a distinction between "pain behavior" and the actual experience of pain. Cows, say, could exhibit "pain behavior," but whether they had mental states and thus had the experience of pain was another matter.

Descartes, as noted above, saw no middle ground between human beings, with minds and feelings; and animals, with no minds and no feelings. The twentieth-century Christian writer C. S. Lewis, however, tried to find a middle ground; he rejected the assumption that animals feel nothing and argued that animals are, in some sense, aware. To describe in *what* sense animals might be aware, Lewis distinguished between *sentience* (ability to feel pain) and *self-consciousness* (awareness of feeling pain): all animals are sentient, he argued, but only human beings are also self-conscious.[2] According to Lewis, then, animals can feel pain, but not as humans do. A rat receiving three electric shocks feels the pain of each shock—the rat is sentient—but it does not think, "I have had three shocks." The thought, "I have had three shocks," requires what Lewis calls "consciousness" or "soul" (he runs these together). Lewis agreed with the eighteenth-century philosopher David Hume, who argued that self-identity requires a permanent self or mental substance which unites all of a person's thoughts as "his" or "hers."[3] For Lewis, a primate (for example), would have a "succession of perceptions," but not the human experience of pain as "my pain."

Lewis, then, identified awareness with self-consciousness or soul (for which he also used the term "deep self"). Some critics have disagreed with this idea, particularly since Lewis assumed that memory depends on self-consciousness. These critics observe that if self-consciousness were needed for memory, animals would never remember anything, and studies of learning in animals would be senseless; but everyone knows that animals can and do remember—a dog that has been kicked by a mailman remembers when he returns. In defense of Lewis, though, it can be replied that much behavior and learning, even with humans, is nonconscious: in driving a car, there is often no conscious thought, "I will stop at this red light"; and painful events in the past may be remembered without being perceived as "mine." That is, as Hume himself insisted, "self-consciousness" is more than simply "consciousness" and more than mere "memory," which might be built into the brain by evolution.

How much pain do animals feel? To what extent is their pain like our pain? On the ladder of evolution from, say, an amoeba to a baboon, at what point does an organism become sentient? At what point can an organism react to pain? At what point can pain be anticipated? How much "mental" pain can be experienced by fish, cats, dogs, or pigs? When can an animal remember pain as "my" pain? How can we know that an animal is experiencing pain as "mine"? Is there a difference between being sentient and being conscious? (If so, how can we know this? If we can't know, why should we use two different words?) Is there a difference between being conscious and having a mind? Is there a difference between being aware of the capacity to feel pain and being aware of a "self" as the subject of awareness? These are not simple questions; in fact, questions about pain in animals raise some of the deepest problems in philosophy of mind and lie behind many controversies about animal research.

Clearly, with regard to questions like these, philosophy of mind blends into ethics. As is discussed in Chapters 1, 6, and 7, one standard of "personhood" is the *cognitive criterion*, whereby certain qualities related to thought—cognition—are considered necessary for being a person. How can we apply this criterion to animals? What cognitive capacities might qualify an animal for membership in the moral community? In other words, what qualities does an animal need to count in the moral calculus? (Sentience? Consciousness? A soul?) How can we verify such capacities in a species, especially if those capacities have important ethical implications? As we consider various answers to such questions, do we have, as a species, any conflict of interest? Do we have any bias toward accepting some answers and rejecting others?

Some Trends in Contemporary Animal Research

How many animals are used in biomedical research in the United States? Since there is no federal law requiring such data to be kept, estimates very widely. The Office of Technology Assessment (OTA) estimates 14 million, for example; *Newsweek* estimates 17 million; and one activist, Andrew Rowan (who is dean of a veterinary school), estimates 71 million.[4] Regardless of the exact figure, however, everyone agrees that scientific research uses immense numbers of animals.

According to Rowan, 40 percent of experimental animals are used in basic and applied research, 26 percent in drug development, 20 percent in safety testing, 8 percent in science and medical courses, and 6 percent in other scientific programs. Animal-rights activists have tended to oppose most strongly three types of research in particular: LD-50 tests, Draize tests, and a number of famous psychological experiments on dogs and primates.

LD stands for "lethal dosage," and LD-50 tests (also called simply LD-50s) determine what amount of a substance is necessary to kill 50 of 100 animals. These tests are done routinely across species for substances ranging from soap to chemotherapies. They have been criticized as crude, blunt measures (one wry critic has said that they tell mice how much of something to take for mass suicide). Largely in response to such criticisms from nonscientists, use of LD-50s has declined 96 percent since the early 1970s; many have been replaced by LD-10s.[5]

The Draize test estimates how much certain products will irritate the human eye; the method is to drip a concentration of the product into a rabbit's eye, which is particularly sensitive. Activists have sought alternative tests using cell cultures and computer models.

Psychological experiments that have drawn severe criticism and even scorn from activists include Harlow's study of baby monkeys deprived of their mothers, and Seligman's research on "learned helplessness" in dogs and monkeys subjected to electric shocks. According to activists, not only are experiments like these are extremely painful and stressful, but the results have been trivial. Many psychologists, on the other hand, regard Harlow's and Seligman's work as landmarks.

In the past 20 years, some famous philosophers who defend animal rights have been joined by a number of celebrities, including Loretta Swit, Lindsay Wagner, Clint Eastwood, and Johnny Carson. A former game show host, Bob Barker, fought the University of Southern California Medical School over its primate research program. Filmmakers have also become involved: animal-rights issues have been taken up in movies such as *Star Trek IV* and *Project X*. As a result of the activities of such "high profile" people, treatment of laboratory animals—which was once a concern of only a few small groups—has become a national issue.

ALF VERSUS UNIVERSITY OF PENNSYLVANIA:
THE HEAD-INJURY STUDY

On Memorial Day in 1984, five members of the Animal Liberation Front (ALF) quietly entered a building of the University of Pennsylvania Medical School in Philadelphia while the school was deserted for the holiday. They went down to a subbasement and broke into a laboratory where they found—and stole—32 audiovisual tapes covering years of experiments on primates.

Everyone agrees that in stealing the tapes, these ALF members broke the law, but there is disagreement over how much other damage, if any, they did. One university official claimed that they had done $2 million worth of damage; but although *American Medical News* reported this figure prominently, no evidence was offered for the exact dollar amount. Subsequent newspaper reports omitted that claim, and it is not mentioned in the final report to the National Institutes of Health (NIH).

The stolen tapes had been made over the course of 5 years by the neurologist Thomas Gennarelli, who was conducting research that involved trying to produce exact brain damage in primates—adult monkeys and baboons. For this purpose, a device had been developed to make a reproducible model of brain injury: a live monkey or baboon, wearing a helmet, would be strapped down, and the animal's head would be subjected to terrific force at a 45-degree angle. Gennarelli had initially used monkeys in these experiments, but the studies with monkeys failed to simulate human head injuries, and as of 1980 he used baboons. All together, Gennarelli's laboratory studied this topic for over 15 years: 1970 to 1985.

There were about 60 to 80 hours of tape in all; ALF heavily edited them to produce a 25-minute segment that showed only abuses. This edited version, called *Unnecessary Fuss* (a quotation from a defender of the project who had thus described the protests), was distributed widely to television stations. It was wrenching and emotionally persuasive; as a reporter for the *New York Times* said:

> One sequence showed a monkey strapped to a table pulling against its bonds. The animal's head was encased in a steel cylinder [attached] to a pneumatic machine called an accelerator. Suddenly, a piston drove the cylinder upward, thrusting the animal's head sharply through an arc of about 60 degrees.
>
>   . . . In another sequence, as an animal lay in a coma, a researcher's recorded voice was heard saying, "You'd better have some axonal damage, monkey," and calling him "sucker."[6]

As shown on the edited tape, the researchers made derogatory and taunting remarks about the animals; these comments sounded adolescent or macho and were particularly damaging to the researchers' position. There was also a lot of profanity, unsterile surgery, and horribly sloppy care of animals. Moreover, the researchers claimed that the baboons were sedated and thus felt no pain; but, as the quotation above describes, several segments showed baboons twisting and struggling to free themselves just before the pneumatic hammer smashed their heads—another damaging point. (Thomas Langfitt, the principal investigator of the overall head-injury program and chairman of the university hospital's neurosurgery department, maintained that even though the animals moved before the tests, they had been anesthetized; his claim is hard to believe when watching the videotape.) Perhaps most repugnant to many nonscientists were several segments which showed the researchers making fun of injured baboons, holding the animals up by broken arms or laughing at conscious but brain-injured baboons. In fact, the effect of these tapes, which the researchers themselves had prepared, was more devastating than any ALF documentary could have been.

Previously, in 1983, several key members of Congress had opposed a bill to strengthen regulation of animal experiments. In September 1984, an organization called People for Ethical Treatment of Animals (PETA) showed the edited tape in two briefings on Capitol Hill; that same evening, the tape was to be shown on ABC's *20/20*. During the briefings, the tape was seen by staffers of Senator Weicker and Congressman Natcher, the chairs, respectively, of the Senate and House committees responsible for the NIH budget.[7] The two chairmen and sixteen other members of Congress decided that the public would not like what it was going to see on television that night, and they sent letters to NIH demanding suspension of Gennarelli's studies.

The broadcast of the tape on *20/20* and on major television networks did indeed create a public outcry which forced Margaret Heckler, Secretary of Health and Human Services (HHS), to review the studies. Officials in Pennsylvania, however, denied that animals were being abused "gratuitously" in Gennarelli's laboratory.

In April 1985, PETA turned the stolen tapes over to NIH for review. This took place, however, only after months of negotiation between PETA and NIH. PETA had feared that NIH, which is the primary funding institute for medical research, would be biased and might suppress damaging material; NIH, for its part, had said that it would be objective but that it would not investigate the charges until it received copies of the tapes.

Meanwhile, in early 1985, the Office for Protection of Research Risks (OPRR), a branch of HHS, had appointed a committee to consider the merits of Gennarelli's research. This committee—which consisted of a neurosurgeon, a veterinary anesthesiologist, and a veterinary pathologist, all of whom used animals in research—issued its report on July 18, 1985. The members assumed that there was nothing intrinsically wrong with injuring baboons in order to study head injuries in humans and did not find fault with the scientific integrity of the experiments: "The research, as proposed, is likely to yield fruitful results for the good of society."[8] However, the committee found Gennarelli guilty of nine (of ten) charges. It noted lack of anesthesia, inadequate supervision, poor training, inferior veterinary care, unnecessary multiple injuries to the same animals, humor, smoking, "statements in poor taste" around animals, and improper clothing: "Taken collectively, these conclusions constitute material failure to comply with the Public Heath Service Animal Welfare Policy." In short, Gennarelli's lab had virtually ignored all the rules designed to protect animals, and the university had developed no mechanism at all to ensure that such rules were followed.

On the same day as the committee's report was released, Margaret Heckler (who had presumably obtained a preview of its conclusions) suspended Gennarelli's research. This was the first time a lab had been closed because of abuse of animals. To Carolyn Compton—a physician, pediatric researcher, and spokeswoman for scientists using animals—the closing was a "tragedy."[9] To ALF, on the other hand, Heckler's decision, and the break-in that led to it, represented a momentous victory. Much of the public and the press, including even the conservative columnist James Kilpatrick,[10] had reacted indignantly to the tapes. As one member of the break-in team (identified only as "Lauren") said at the outset:

> We may seem like radicals to you. But we are like the Abolitionists, who were regarded as radicals, too. And we hope that 100 years from now, people will look back on the way animals are treated now with the same horror as we do when we look back on the slave trade.[11]

OTHER ALF TARGETS

Six weeks after its Memorial Day raid, ALF struck again at the University of Pennsylvania, this time "liberating" three cats, two dogs, and eight pigeons from the veterinary school. The dean of the veterinary school said that the raid "would set back research efforts, including a study to determine the cause of sudden infant death syndrome."[12] An associate dean said that the stolen cats were being used in studies of breathing during sleep, that one missing dog had a steel plate inserted to study osteoarthritis, that another was being studied for ear-canal infections, and that the pigeons were part of a study of broken bones intended to benefit all birds.[13] With regard to the dogs, he also said that the work would benefit other dogs, adding that it had to be done and that more dogs would end up having to be used as subjects.

In December 1984, ALF struck in California. Two rabbits injected with oral herpes and numerous dogs with cancer were taken, along with 100 other animals, from City of Hope National Medical Center in Duarte. ALF members painted a sign in the lab there: "ALF IS WATCHING AND THERE'S NO PLACE TO HIDE!" Ingrid Newkirk of PETA called City of Hope a "concentration camp" where animals were "being used for painful experiments."[14] The associate director of City of Hope said that the theft of these animals had disrupted $500,000 worth of research on emphysema, cancer, and herpes. In this case, ALF had targeted a study testing tobacco carcinogens in dogs. The associate director refused to comment on whether the abducted animals had been treated cruelly but did say that 36 cancerous dogs, 12 cats, 12 rabbits, 28 mice, and 18 rats had been stolen and added, "We're concerned that very important research work may not now be completed."[15]

In April 1985, in what was its largest animal raid to date, ALF hit the biology and psychology laboratories of the University of California, Riverside. In this raid, 467 animals were taken, including a stump-tailed macaque whose eyes had been sewn shut to study a device to help the blind navigate. PETA charged that these animals had been used in painful, unnecessary experiments, some involving starvation; NIH investigated the charges but found no evidence of abuse. The university claimed that $683,000 in damages had occurred, as well as lost research.

In April 1987, an arson fire gutted the $2.5 million veterinary research animal lab at the University of California, Davis; ALF claimed responsibility.

ETHICAL ISSUES

Ethical Theory

Before 1975, "animal welfare" groups focused simply on humane treatment of research animals. Until recently, however, most scientists dismissed such groups as "little old ladies" and portrayed them as antiprogress; and such dismissals have pushed reformers toward more radical theoretical positions.

Singer: Speciesism and utilitarianism   In 1975, the Australian philosopher Peter Singer published *Animal Liberation,* in which he argued that animals must morally count for something.[16] To say that animals do not count because they are somehow inferior, Singer held, is like saying that slaves or women do not count; and just as racism and sexism are evil, so is *speciesism.* According to Singer, every argument that supports equal rights for minorities and women—without begging any questions—also supports animals rights. If our moral concern for children, women, and minorities is based on their sensitivity to pain, family ties, and ability to reason, why wouldn't these factors also be a basis for concern for animals? Such arguments put "speciesists" on the defensive: if the principle of equality applies to all people, despite their obvious differences in ability and intelligence, why shouldn't it also apply to animals?

Singer also argued that a medical experiment using animal subjects must be speciesist unless humans would be willing to substitute irreversibly comatose human subjects. This is an interesting approach. Most people who accept the idea of using, say, a chimpanzee in medical research would cringe at the idea of using an anencephalic baby (an infant born lacking most of the brain). But if the chimpanzee is active, gregarious, sensitive, and responsive whereas the anencephalic baby is hopelessly mute, comatose, and unresponsive, why should the chimp be the victim? If the answer is simply that the baby is human and the chimp nonhuman, Singer would consider the answer speciesist.

In addition to his argument about speciesism, Singer also used *utilitarian* reasoning—the same kind of secular, results-oriented moral premises that scientists use to defend their research. According to utilitarian ethical theory, "right" acts produce the greatest good for the greatest number; for instance, research on presently sick patients would be "right" if it would help a greater number of future patients. Stipulating that the "greatest number" must refer only to humans begs the key question, Singer maintained; and once animals count for something, however small, in utilitarian reasoning, radical conclusions follow: experiments that inflict horrible pain on many animals cannot be justified on the ground that they save a few human lives. Actually, the founder of utilitarianism, Jeremy Bentham, argued during the nineteenth century that animals' suffering should count in the moral calculus; he held that the important question was not whether animals could reason, but whether they could *suffer.* Ingrid Newkirk, the British-born leader of PETA, reasons similarly: "When it comes to suffering, a rat is a pig is a dog is a boy."[17]

Singer's position is open to some of the theoretical and practical objections to utilitarianism in general. For instance, consistent application of utilitarianism would apparently obligate individuals to make great sacrifices to help victims of famine, improve the lives of future generations, and relieve the suffering of animals. It would require a parent, for instance, to donate money for famine relief rather than use that money to send a son or daughter to college: since many lives can be saved by giving $100,000 to CARE, and since $100,000 would pay for the college education of only one child—who does not, moreover, need college to survive or even to be happy—a utilitarian parent could not consider paying for a college education justifiable. Philosophers such as Susan Wolf have therefore argued that although utilitarianism may be a model of moral perfection, it "does not constitute a model of personal well-being toward which it would be particularly good or desirable for a rational human being to strive."[18] To put this another way, consistent utilitarianism requires saintly conduct and total devotion to a higher moral goal, but that would conflict with lesser goals, some of which are outside the sphere of morality—goals like mastering medicine or tennis, reading the great novels, or sending a child to college. To put it still another way, should morality ever require us to choose between family and humanity?

In a sense, this kind of argument against utilitarianism is a *reductio ad absurdum:* the premise "We should act to achieve the greatest good for the greatest number" is said to lead to the absurd or unacceptable conclusion "It is wrong for parents to pay for their children's college education." In the context of animal rights, such an argument would take a premise like "Animals should count in calculations of the greatest good for the greatest number" to an absurd conclusion, such as "A few human lives must be sacrificed to save the lives of many dogs." These conclusions, it is held, are absurd or unacceptable because of what they imply about the scope of utilitarianism. For people who argue this way, utilitarianism does not satisfactorily answer the question, "What is morality *for?*" For them, morality must first consider obligations to an "inner circle"—family, colleagues, friends, etc.—even if fulfilling obligations to those in the inner circle does not contribute to "the greatest good for the greatest number." In the context of animal rights, then, the human species might be represented in the "inner circle."

However, not everyone accepts reductios as conclusive arguments against utilitarianism, for at least two reasons. First, it may be contended that a given utilitarian premise does not necessarily lead to a particular absurd conclusion; second, people may disagree on whether or not a particular conclusion is indeed "absurd" or "unacceptable." For instance, it can be argued, in defense of utilitarianism, that an ethical theory which requires a very high standard of conduct may seem to lead to certain absurd or unacceptable conclusions, but that this result is only apparent: the standard may in practice be unattainable, or virtually unattainable, but it is still valuable as a standard. To take one example, early Christianity defined right conduct in a way that essentially required saintliness—"Turn the other cheek," "Go and sell that thou hast, and give to the poor," and so on—but these precepts are nevertheless valued as ideals.

It can be seen that this debate is partly about hypocrisy. Is it hypocritical to profess an ideal such as utilitarianism or early Christianity but not to practice it consistently in actual life? Probably, most people would agree that professing an ideal and not acting on it at all, or not even trying to act on it, is hypocritical. But is it really hypocritical to act on a professed ideal to some extent while taking practical considerations into account—considerations such as the formation of family ties, the inevitability of human weaknesses, and the existence of personal or nonmoral areas of life? Many people would not call that compromise *hypocrisy,* and probably many people do in fact make such a practical compromise in their general approach to living. Still, to a purist a compromise like this is awkward: it seems to amount to saying that starving people or suffering animals are important only intermittently or fractionally—that they are "worth" only one morning a week, for instance, or only 10 percent of one's income. (Hypocrisy is discussed again below, with regard to ad hominem arguments and testimonials.)

Regan: Animal rights   Underlying the controversy over Gennarelli's experimentation on primates is a more basic issue: whether scientific research on animals is ever justified. Tom Regan, an American philosopher and animal-rights activist, thinks not:

> I argue that the whole system of animal experimentation [and] the whole system of commercial and sport trapping and hunting are morally bankrupt institutions. The only way you change these things fundamentally is by eliminating them—in much the same way as with slavery and child labor.[19]

Regan argues that human beings have rights because they *have a life*. That is, humans have lives that can go better or worse for them, and this is true for each human being independently of whether or not others value him or her. In other words, people have inherent, not instrumental, value. Peter Singer, as we have just seen, applies utilitarianism to animals as well as to humans; Regan, analogously, applies to animals as well as humans the rights-based idea of treating each life as an "end in itself." Regan maintains that many species of animals, like humans, have lives that can go better or worse for them, and he draws this crucial inference: "They too have a distinctive kind of value in their own right, if we do; therefore, they too have a right not to be treated in ways that fail to respect this value."[20] Regan reasons that if humans "count" in the moral calculus because they possess a certain quality, and if animals possess the same quality, then it is inconsistent not to count animals equally. Anyone who wants to argue that there is some difference here must bear the onus of proving why.

Regan's critics say that his argument runs several unjustified inferences together. First, they ask, if any being (human or nonhuman) has a life that can go better or worse, does that fact give every life a distinctive value? Second, and more important, does "having a life" really give animals a value equal to that of humans? Can't human lives go "better or worse" in more complex ways than lives of cows and rabbits? Note, however, that Regan is careful to include a qualification: he says that animals (like humans) have lives which can go better or worse *for them.* His reasoning is that with this qualification, no real comparison is possible between human and animal lives. If fish in an aquarium "have a life" that can go better or worse *for them,* from that standpoint the fishes' lives become as important as human lives.

Of course, simply being clear about the terms or conditions of Regan's argument does not settle the matter, since his position is in fact extremely controversial. Many animal-rights activists agree with him, and some are even more radical; Ingrid Newkirk of PETA, for instance, holds that any experiment which does not treat animals and humans equally is speciesist; thus sacrificing an animal to save a human would not be justifiable. Charles McArdle, a scientist, also agrees. Suppose that either a dog or a man but not both can remain in a lifeboat: Regan implies that because "animals aren't there to be used as our resources," it is morally wrong to kill the dog to save the man, and McArdle concurs—"I would seriously have to question whether I would allow an animal to die just to protect me."[21] On the other hand, the pediatric researcher Carolyn Compton disagrees: "I love animals, but there's no question in my mind that if I were able to sacrifice an animal life to save a human being, I would do it."[22]

Cohen and Frey: A pro-human approach   Some opponents of the animal-rights movement take the position that the scope of morality should not be expanded to animals. Their reasoning is somewhat similar to the argument that abortion is permissible because the scope of morality cannot be expanded to embryos or early fetuses.

The philosopher Carl Cohen, who teaches at a medical school, defends the use of animals in biomedical research by arguing that animals cannot share in the human community. In an article in *New England Journal of Medicine,* Cohen said:

> Notwithstanding all such complications, this much is clear about rights in general: they are in every case claims, or potential claims, within a community of moral agents. Rights arise, and can be intelligently defended, only among beings who actually do, or can, make moral claims against one another.[23]

For Cohen, animals cannot make moral claims and thus have no rights. He rejects the analogy between racism, sexism, and speciesism: although racism and sexism are indeed bad, he maintains, speciesism is not. "I am a speciesist," he declares, and he adds, "Speciesism is not merely plausible; it is essential for right conduct, because those who will not make the morally relevant distinctions among species are almost certain, in consequence, to misapprehend their true obligations."

Another philosopher, Raymond Frey, argues that the concept of "animal rights" uselessly adds to the confusion in a moral terrain which is already muddled enough. Tom Regan, as we've seen, holds that animals possess rights simply by coming into existence and being the sort of creatures they are. Frey, however, argues that:

> In the case of intrinsic or fundamental, unacquired moral rights . . . what grip we had on rights has, I think, been lost. Rather, we are at sea in a tide of theoretical claims and counter-claims, with no fixed point by which to steer.[24]

What are the appropriate boundaries of the "moral community"? This is a difficult question, especially if we are trying to develop and apply consistently a reasonable interpretation of the cognitive criterion of personhood. It is interesting to note that many advocates of animal rights are also advocates of parental choice with regard to abortion (Chapter 6) and forgoing treatment in "Baby Doe" cases (Chapter 7); for this reason, people who oppose abortion and nontreatment of impaired newborns charge that animal-rights advocates value animals more than humans. (One student wrote a paper comparing the views of an animal-rights philosopher on abortion and animal research, entitling it, "I'd Rather Be His Pet.") It is also argued that expanding the circle of moral concern to include animals while contracting it to exclude human fetuses and impaired neonates is rather odd. In response to this charge, though, it can be said (as Singer would point out) that whether moral concern should expand or contract with regard to a particular issue depends on the characteristics of the beings in question (sensitivity to pain, awareness, sociability, etc.); it does not depend on membership in a species.

Testimonials and Ad Hominem Arguments

In informal logic, one common fallacy is what is called an *ad hominem* appeal. *Ad hominem* literally means "to the man"; in an argument, the term means an inappropriate personal reference. For example, in a debate during the presidential campaign of 1988, a reporter made an ad hominem attack on Michael Dukakis, asking whether Dukakis (who was opposed to capital punishment) would want a man who had raped and killed his wife to be executed. Dukakis tried to respond logically, but since the question was based on emotion rather than reason, he was not very successful. In a formal debate, which is a purely intellectual exercise (unlike a presidential debate, which is supposed to be informational), one effective reply would be to point out that the question was not pertinent and had been asked to elicit an inappropriate response; another appropriate and effective counterthrust would itself be emotional, an expression of outrage—"I'd kill the bastard with my own hands." The point here, however, is not how a member of a debating team might deal with an ad hominem argument: for our purposes, the important point is that such an argument is a logical error. Thus it can be held that our position on a moral issue should be affected only by the strength of the arguments, not by the emotional impact of answers to personal questions.

In fact, the debate on experimentation with animals has been characterized by ad hominem appeals, which sometimes take the form of *testimonials:* the personal behavior of commentators is often cited, and the specific issue of experimentation is often placed in a wider context. Many animal-rights activists, for instance, mention that they themselves are vegetarians; and both Peter Singer and Tom Regan criticize circuses, factory farming, eating meat, hunting for sport, and wearing furs, and urge others to avoid these practices.

Intuitively, it may seem that an argument by a philosopher—or anyone else—gains greater force when he or she not only argues for acting in a certain way but also does act that way. On reflection, however, it is unclear why ad hominem appeals and testimonials should carry much, if any, weight. In popular culture, of course, such appeals do influence behavior, but their role in rational argument is more questionable.

Consider that once the door is opened for appeals to personal life, many things can walk through. At one conference about animal rights, the English philosopher Stephen Clark chided his audience for feeding meat to pet cats and dogs. At this same conference, some animal-rights activists followed Albert Schweitzer in revering all life and killing nothing, and some emphasized ecological purity, opposing extinction of any species; they themselves, of course, did not hunt. Some people at the conference were vegetarians; some were "vegans"—eating no animal products, not even eggs (from "captive" chickens). Some refused to buy any animal products at all. Some regarded zoos as demeaning to animals and refused to take their children to such places. The most radical people at the conference condemned even pet ownership; Ingrid Newkirk of PETA described the life of pets as an "absolutely abysmal situation brought about by human manipulation."[25]

Leaving aside the personal danger of developing a "holier than thou" attitude—and the practical consideration that such an attitude is unlikely to win many friends for one's moral position—how legitimate are such testimonials? If they are offered, is it legitimate to argue that they are irrelevant? And on the other hand, is it legitimate for opponents of animal rights to demand them? Scientists, for instance, often ask whether critics of animal experiments are vegetarians; if those critics turn out to be meat eaters, the scientists stand ready to accuse them of hypocrisy.

In this regard, it seems useful to distinguish between our evaluation of *arguments* and our evaluation of *people*. In an argument, it is not always correct or appropriate to ask about personal behavior; when we make ethical judgments about people, however, it is certainly relevant to consider their actual behavior as well as their arguments. If we hear someone decry exploitation of the poor and then discover that this person is a slumlord, we will probably decide that he or she is a hypocrite; on the other hand, this does *not* mean that we ourselves must decide to advocate exploiting poor people. In other words, an argument offered by a hypocrite is not for that reason alone necessarily a poor argument. By the same token, it is true that most activists for animals do not eat "animal flesh," and this may make us respect these advocates as sincere—but respecting someone's sincerity need not necessarily lead us to accept his or her conclusion. When we evaluate *individuals*, then, inquiries into personal behavior are sometimes appropriate; and it soon becomes obvious that because espousing morality is far easier than practicing it, hypocrisy abounds in life. But whether we encounter hypocrisy or sincerity, we need to be able to disregard it in considering an *argument*.

Scientific Merit

Assessing basic research   The scientific merit of Thomas Gennarelli's research with primates—a specific issue that will be discussed below—can be put into perspective by considering the extent of *basic research* and why it is valuable. Scientific research might be compared to an iceberg. The results or findings that will be applicable to humans are the tip of the iceberg, visible above the water. This small tip is supported by the much larger part of the iceberg, the part that is invisible under the water; that large invisible portion consists of basic research which goes on quietly in labs and is rarely discussed in national media.

Many animals are used in basic research—far more than most people could possibly guess. For every practical success in human medicine, such as cyclosporin or knee replacement, there are perhaps a dozen failures in studies with human subjects and a hundred failures in studies with animal subjects. To arrive at each success, then, hundreds or thousands of animals are used as "guinea pigs." In the United States alone, there are nearly 130 medical schools and a dozen or so pharmaceutical and research institutions using millions of animals each year—mostly rats and mice, but also dogs, pigs, cats, rabbits, and primates. (Worldwide, of course—in Germany, France, Switzerland, Japan, Canada, and Australia, for instance—scientists also use great numbers of animals.) In one year, 1983, a single institution, the Charles River Breeding Laboratories (called the "General Motors" of the American animal breeding industry), produced 10 million animals destined to be research subjects.

At what point, if anywhere, can we draw a line between basic experimentation on animals that is "useful" or "necessary" (and thus, arguably, acceptable) and "useless" or "unnecessary" experimentation? This is a difficult problem. Few people would advocate stopping basic research that offers direct clinical benefits to humans, and few would even recommend stopping research that offers indirect benefits. What most critics want to stop is "trivial" or "repetitive" research, but when these critics cite specific examples (Harlow's research on maternal deprivation in monkeys, say, or Seligman's research on "learned helplessness" in dogs), the researchers often staunchly defend the importance of the work. If all basic research were stopped, medical progress would also stop. On the other hand, if no basic research can be stopped, animal experimentation would simply proceed as it has always proceeded.

"Stopping" research typically takes the form of cutting off funding, and one suggestion has been that only "worthwhile" research should be funded. This sounds reasonable, but actually deciding what is "worthwhile" is very difficult.[26] In practice, this decision is the job of NIH committees of peer reviewers who consider applications for grants. These reviewers are experts, and if they knew in advance exactly which projects were "worthwhile," they would fund only those—but of course they don't know in advance. Sometimes an apparently insignificant project can yield important results, and sometimes an apparently important project can yield little or nothing of value.

At bottom, researchers have faith that the costs of basic studies—in terms of money, effort, time, and the suffering of animals—will one day be outweighed by benefits. At bottom, animal activists are skeptics who doubt or deny that the benefits to humans outweigh the costs to animals.

Assessing the Philadelphia study   Assessment of Gennarelli's research with primates has involved not only the scientific merit of the project itself but also the treatment of animals by the researchers. These are separate issues, though it can be argued that they are related.

Let's first consider some commentary on the value of this research as such. A peer committee reviewing Gennarelli's grant said that his research would contribute information about the effectiveness of drug called *mannitol* in reducing brain swelling after trauma, and about management of metabolic balance in comatose patients. Later, the university's own investigator, Thomas Langfitt, claimed that Gennarelli's research had provided the first evidence that regeneration of damaged nerve cells (the great hope of patients paralyzed by spinal cord injuries) may be possible.[27]

On the other hand, critics called these justifications *ad hoc*—simply a way to paper over a lack of real findings. Nedim Buyukmichi, an activist and veterinarian, argued that Gennarelli's studies were too inconsistent to result in a reproducible model of head injuries and too limited in scope to adequately mimic injuries sustained by human victims of accidents: "After 15 years and $11 million to $13 million, essentially nothing has come out of this research that hasn't already been known from studies of human head trauma."[28] Other critics were unimpressed by the purported findings about regeneration of nerve cells, comparing that claim to the ubiquitous trumpeting of "possible" cures for cancer and AIDS.

Interestingly—even amazingly—in all the commentary on Gennarelli's studies, no one on either side has specifically attacked or defended the hypothesis of his research. The explanation may be that it is unclear whether Gennarelli actually had a hypothesis; he seems to have had no goal other than creating one exact injury in one baboon after another.

Lack of a hypothesis might not necessarily imply that Gennarelli's research was valueless, however. Gennarelli can be described as working at the bottom of a pyramid of basic research on head injury. To him, it may have seemed obvious that the first step in such research would be to produce one head injury precisely and reliably, so that it could be replicated and studied by others. Scientists point out, for example, that knowing how to produce different kinds of burns in animals is the first step in studying the physiology of burns and the metabolism of healing. On the other side, animal activists held that Gennarelli had merely bashed primates' heads for a decade without getting anywhere. They argued that even if he had succeeded in devising a reproducible model of head injuries, such a model would offer little help in actually treating such injuries (an argument that scientists have denied).

A separate issue, as noted above, has to do with Gennarelli's treatment of his animal subjects. In turn, this issue itself has two aspects. First, there is the question of how badly or insensitively the animals were treated. Some of Gennarelli's defenders have said that the apparently insensitive comments and behavior of researchers on the tapes were comparable to the type of cynical humor typical among medical residents; also, as noted above, the university's investigator, Langfitt, said that the animals had been anesthetized. Both of these arguments, of course, have been attacked; and neither of them seems very convincing in light of what the tapes show. Activists argue, further, that the researchers were pursing lucrative grants and professional prestige and may therefore have been blinded to their own insensitivity, and to their subjects' plight, by a conflict of interest.

The second question is this: if the animals were indeed mistreated and the researchers were insensitive, does that necessarily affect the scientific value of the research? In other words, could researchers conduct an excellent project even though they mistreated their subjects? For animal activists, Gennarelli's treatment of his animal subjects in itself proved that his project was immoral and thus unjustifiable. Were they right? Can the scientific value or merit of a study be assessed independently of the researchers' behavior?

Before we leave this question, it is relevant to note that many animal researchers say they treat animal subjects with great respect. Since laboratories are now closed to the public, this is hard to verify. However, reports from some students who work as aides in such labs—and some videotapes like Gennarelli's—indicate that these researchers' claim is at least sometimes false.

Ends and Means: Civil Disobedience and Other Tactics

Tactics for stopping experimentation on animals are often debated by opponents of such experimentation. One question in this debate is whether illegal, unsavory, or even immoral tactics should be used to attain a higher goal. Does the end justify the means?

In discussions of the strategies of animal-rights activists, the terms *civil disobedience* and *terrorism* are often used. It seems important to distinguish between these two concepts. Civil disobedience—as associated with figures like Ghandi in India and organizations like the Southern Christian Leadership Conference in the United States—involves public but nonviolent violations of the law, for the purpose of protesting policies regarded as evil. According to the philosopher John Rawls (who has developed a famous theory of justice), civil disobedience is *not* terrorism if three conditions are met: (1) It must be public, with the protesters clearly identified (the protesters do not conceal themselves under white sheets). (2) It must be nonviolent (the protesters hurt no one; no innocent bystanders are injured or killed). (3) The protesters must accept the legal consequences of their actions (for instance, children actually went to jail in Birmingham, Alabama, during the "children's crusade"). (4) Protesters break a law only after trying to change the law by all possible legal means. The other side of this coin is that activities which do not meet these criteria *are* considered terrorism; and the point of the distinction is that civil disobedience is justified whereas terrorism is not. According to Rawls's criteria, then, many acts of the antiabortion group Operation Rescue would be justified civil disobedience, and some acts of animal-rights activists—especially in England—would be unjustified terrorism.

Let's consider a few examples of specific tactics involving illegality. In England, the Animals Rights Militia planted bombs outside the homes of four animal researchers as a warning and then alerted the police by telephone; no one was injured. Hunt Saboteur, the most radical English group, has bombed meat-packing factories and butcher shops and has strung metal wires as booby traps for fox hunters; Marley Jones, one of the leaders of Hunt Saboteur, has said:

> In Britain we [animal activists] tend to think that most types of actions [which prevent cruelty to animals], short of killing someone, are morally justified. Physical violence, in my opinion, is justified as a last resort, if all appeals to reason fail and there is no other way to save the animals.[29]

In late 1988, four bombs were set off outside English department stores, including Harrods, to protest the sale of furs; a columnist for the *Times* of London commented vehemently:

> Of all the Single Issue fanatics who increasingly infest our society, with their conviction that nothing matters beside their particular cause and that any action, however violent, dangerous, or criminal, is justified in the pursuit of it, the most monomaniacal are those who claim to defend "animal rights."[30]

Here are some examples from the United States. In California in 1988, ALF destroyed a new building for animal research at the medical school in San Diego and burned down a veal-packing plant in Oakland; masked ALF spokespersons took credit for these attacks in televised interviews, vowing to continue them "until the killing of the innocent animals stops." That same year, in Connecticut, a bomb was planted by Stephanie Trutt outside a company which made surgical staples and used animals to train surgeons in handling them; she was arrested for attempted murder.[31] (Access to American medical schools at night and on weekends was once fairly easy, but as a result of such activities, that has changed: new security systems have been installed, allowing entry only to people with specific authorization.)

Some tactics of animal-rights activists, though legal, are ignoble; like the illegal tactics, these are held to be justified by higher ends. In the controversy over abortion, a former priest named Joseph Scheidler at one time urged antiabortionists to infiltrate and spy on pro-choice groups; Alex Pacheco, the president of PETA, used a similar strategy. In May 1981, Pacheco volunteered to work in the primate lab of the psychologist Edward Taub in Silver Spring, Maryland. Pacheco told Taub that he wanted to become a research scientist and needed experience, but his actual intention was to videotape Taub's research on animals for PETA.[32] Taub was studying "somato-sensory deafferentation" in monkeys by surgically cutting all the nerves in one limb and then trying to stimulate regrowth. His hypothesis was that some of the damage was due to "learned helplessness," and the research was intended to benefit the half-million Americans who are disabled by strokes each year. Pacheco entered the lab late one night with an accomplice and succeeded in photographing experiments; as a result, Taub was tried in Maryland on charges of cruelty to animals and was convicted on one charge (failing to provide adequate veterinary care).

Tactics similar to Pacheco's were also advocated by Donald Barnes, a former Air Force psychologist whose radiation experiments on primates were portrayed in the movie *Project X*.[33] Barnes is an example of a leader who has abruptly switched sides on a moral issue.[34]

Another legal but ignoble strategy is deliberately shoddy or unfair argumentation. Barnes, for example, recommends tricks such as monopolizing all the time in a debate, working up an audience's passions before actually appearing, refusing to talk to researchers in private, and flattering reporters. He urges animal-rights activists not to discuss whether a particular experiment is good science or offers benefits: "As much as possible, avoid getting caught up in 'scientific' arguments which you can't win. Beat a hasty retreat to philosophy and brandish your weapons: Tom Regan's *The Case for Animal Rights* and Peter Singer's *Animal Liberation*." He also says, "Bear in mind that the only rationale for using nonhuman animals in research is that, 'The end justifies the means'" (an especially interesting comment when we consider that he presumably considers his own ends as justifying his own means). Tactics like Barnes's, of course, are not confined to the issue of animal rights: many leaders of many causes resort to unfair arguments and appeal to our emotions instead of using logic and solid evidence.

The Enemy and the "Algeria Syndrome"

One question about animal rights is, "Who is the enemy?" Answers to that question lead us to some significant considerations, including a phenomenon which can be called the *Algeria syndrome.*

To animal-rights activists, of course, animal researchers are the "enemy"—and vice versa. In this regard, however, it is interesting to realize that the activists and the scientists actually have much in common. For instance, subscribers to leading animal-rights magazines are overwhelmingly white, are mostly nonreligious (65 percent are agnostics or atheists), and tend to hold managerial and professional positions; 84 percent are college-educated; 25 percent have M.A. and Ph.D. degrees.[35] Subscribers to *Physiologist* are overwhelmingly white, are not very religious, and hold academic and professional positions; most of them have Ph.D.s.[36]

Though science and scientists have been condemned by officialdom or the public at various times in the past (Galileo and Darwin are famous examples), modern researchers have not been accustomed to being seen as an "enemy"; in fact, until quite recently they occupied rather high moral ground, at least among educated people. Today, scientists find themselves accused of irrationality, bias, conflicts of interest, money-grubbing, and even ignorance; with regard to animal rights, they are accused of inflicting pain on animals without guiding hypotheses or controls and for trivial purposes, such as proving what is already obvious. Moreover, it is true that until the mid-1980s, most scientists adopted a siege mentality and resisted reforms.

It should be noted, though, that with respect to animals in research today, television and the print media present some contradictory images. On the one hand, there are accounts of "miraculous" research breakthroughs which would have been impossible without using animals; on the other hand, there are also accounts of researchers who abuse animals, and in these stories a stereotype of the "mad scientist"—a Frankenstein or a callous torturer—is frequently implied.

Are scientists really *"the* enemy"? Are they the only problem or even the primary problem in the issue of animal rights? Scientists are rather remote from nonscientists, and "science" is a rather abstract concept for most of us; and it is often easier to attack what is far away and abstract than to confront what is nearby and concrete. We might call this the *Algeria syndrome.* It is somehow easier to take a position against the specter of "research on animals" than to take a position against, say, our own neighbors who do not spay or neuter their pets. This point is worth considering here.

In the United States alone, 22 million dogs and cats are abandoned, killed, or lost each year by owners who fail to make adequate provisions for their care.[37] Many of these owners will simply replace the lost animal with a new pet, as if it were no big deal. At the same time, only about 180,000 dogs and 50,000 cats were used in medical research, and almost all of the dogs would have died anyway in pounds. In fact, for every dog used in medical experiments, perhaps 100 dogs kept as pets will die because of neglect by their owners. Who is the "enemy": a scientist who uses five dogs in 7 years, or our own neighbor whose cat gives birth to unwanted litters of kittens? For utilitarians—and for anyone even slightly sympathetic to utilitarianism—numbers like these should count for something. We fall victim to the Algeria syndrome when we attack the abstract target of "Frankensteins" but do nothing to change the situation next door.

UPDATE

Organizational Responses:
IACUCs, Foundation for Biomedical Research, PETA

Several experiments reviewed by NIH in the 1980s fared poorly. Among these were studies at City of Hope Medical Center in Duarte, California, which was find $25,000, lost $1 million in grants, and also lost its Animal Care Assurance, a semilegal document in which an institution promises to abide by federal regulations. Columbia University lost all its grants involving vertebrates after ALF released pictures of poor lab conditions and inspectors made an unannounced visit.

In 1986, as a result of such abuses—and Gennarelli's—Congress established Institutional Animal Care and Use Committees (IACUCs) for all institutions receiving federal funds for research on animals. These committees try to reduce the number of animals involved in experiments and the amount of pain to which research animals will be subjected; they also try to have lower species used rather than higher species. Although IACUCs are composed mostly of researchers themselves (not laypeople), they do force experimenters at least to justify their projects to fellow scientists—some of whom can be critical at times. Since the existence of IACUCs is directly attributable to the exposure of Gennarelli's experiments, his work can be called the "Tuskegee study" of animal research (see Chapter 9).

Animal activists see IACUCs as "window dressing" and insist that the committees do little real good. They also say that the Department of Agriculture, which is responsible for inspecting labs, has had a traditionally cozy relationship with animal-abusing agribusiness. They emphasize that veterinarians on IACUCs are caught in the middle, charged with protecting animals but salaried by the researchers.

During the 1980s, faced with what they perceived as devastating losses in public confidence, scientists decided that they could no longer ignore animal-rights activists. Accordingly, they established the Foundation for Biomedical Research, which lobbies for 350 universities, drug companies, manufacturers of medical devices, and commercial animal-supply companies. The foundation has a paid staff member in most states that have research institutions; it also maintains many lobbyists in Washington, D.C., to counter the equally numerous lobbyists of PETA.

People for the Ethical Treatment of Animals (PETA) is estimated to have 350,000 members and $5 million in annual income. It supported Bill Clinton during his campaign for President and was allowed to sponsor one of his inaugural balls, at which naked bartenders of both sexes wore signs proclaiming, "I'd rather wear nothing than fur."

Today, scientists are vying with animal-rights activists for young minds through extensive educational outreach programs. The Foundation for Biomedical Research sponsors talks by scientists for science majors, medical students, and graduate students about the necessity of using animals in research. A group called Putting People First was started by Kathleen Marquardt in 1992 after a one-sided presentation by a PETA spokesperson in her daughter's elementary school;[38] Marquardt says that her organization has 35,000 members, 100 chapters in the United States, and a paid staff of six.

The Taub Case

The tactics used by PETA in the Taub case were controversial. To obtain evidence for the trial, Alex Pacheco invited activists such as Donald Barnes, John McArdle (both discussed above), and Michael W. Fox to search Taub's lab at night; when warrants were served on Taub shortly thereafter, several television stations recorded the event while PETA leaders distributed press releases outside. During the trial itself, each element seemed to have been orchestrated for the maximum emotional impact in the media—with the predictable result that the media portrayed Taub as another Josef Mengele and PETA as the animals' Robin Hood.

As noted earlier, Taub was convicted of one charge—failing to provide proper veterinary care—which had been based on the fact that he did not bandage the animals' wounds. Taub testified that it was better to leave the wounds unbandaged because many years of experience had showed him that the monkeys would only bite and claw the bandages off, making their wounds worse. Veterinarians could not agree on whether or not Taub was right about this; but eventually Taub was exonerated of any failure to provide adequate veterinary care by the American Psychological Association's Ethics Committee, by the NIH (after his appeal), and by an ad hoc committee of the American Physiological Society. After their own investigation of the charges, the medical school and psychology department at the University of Alabama at Birmingham hired him as a full professor.

In 1991, according to the "story of the year" for ethics in *Discover*, four of Taub's monkeys showed:

> . . . dramatic new evidence of the adult brain's capacity to "rewire" itself, something previously thought to be impossible. And ironically, it was PETA's success at keeping the monkeys away from research for a decade that made the discovery possible.[39]

The 15 surviving monkeys had been transferred in 1986 to the federally funded Tulane Regional Primate Center in Covington, Louisiana. In 1990, in an experiment which PETA opposed, a brain researcher—Timothy Pons—tested Taub's hypothesis by examining the brain of a dying monkey before euthanization. Pons was "flabbergasted" to discover that "the entire patch of the cortex corresponding to the arm—about half an inch wide—had been rewired to receive input from the face." Pons concluded, excitedly, "The results offer hope that the brain can be coaxed into rewiring itself after injury." Data from other monkeys in the study later supported this finding; to date, however, the exact significance of these results appears uncertain.

Animal Research Facilities Protection Act

In 1992, Senator Howell Heflin (Democrat, Alabama) proposed the Farm and Animal Research Facilities Protection Act, which was signed into law by President Bush in August of that year. The act makes it a federal crime to break into a research facility or the premises of a company that breeds research animals; violators face prison sentences of up to 1 year for illegal entry and fines up to $5,000. A vice-president at UAB Medical Center, which had originated the bill, said that this legislation would protect scientists against "activists who use terrorist techniques to interfere with potentially life-saving research."[40]

The 1993 Federal Decision

In February 1993, animal-rights activists won a significant victory for dogs and primates used in laboratory research. Judge Charles Richey of the Federal District Court in Washington, D.C., ordered the Agriculture Department to improve the rules that Congress had asked it to write in the Improved Standards for Laboratory Animals Act of 1985—the act creating the IACUCs.[41] Judge Richey concluded that the Agriculture Department had violated the act by giving all power to interpret it to local IACUCs: he implied that members of such committees, including veterinarians, were almost always employed by the institutions they were supposed to regulate and hence had a conflict of interest; and he ordered the rules to be rewritten in order to give someone else the final say about them. The Foundation for Biomedical Research called the ruling "very disappointing" and planned to appeal it. According to the foundation, the decision would make obsolete the retooling which many labs had undergone during the previous 5 years to comply with the original interpretation of the act; and implementing the new decision would cost institutions as much as $2 billion.

Richey also criticized the government for taking 9 years to implement some of its own rules, and he implied that some of the rules were intended more to increase profitability than to ensure the welfare of research animals.

On the other hand, Richey apparently rejected the argument of activists that "a rat is a pig is a dog is a boy": he dismissed claims that detailed records should be required for the 21 million rats and mice used in American research. That is, researchers can treat rats and mice differently from dogs and primates.

FURTHER READING

Carl Cohen, "The Case for Animal Rights," *New England Journal of Medicine*, vol. 315, no. 14, October 4, 1986, pp. 865–870.

Caroline Fraser, "The Raid at Silver Spring," *New Yorker*, March 30, 1993, pp. 66–84.

R. G. Frey, *Rights, Killing, and Suffering*, Basil Blackwell, Oxford, England, 1983.

James Rachels, *Created from Animals,* Oxford University Press, New York, 1990.

Tom Regan, *The Case for Animal Rights,* University of California Press, Berkeley, 1983.

Peter Singer, *Animal Liberation,* New York Review of Books, New York, 1975. (This book is an expansion of an earlier article of the same title which appeared in *New York Review of Books*.)

Susan Sperling, *Animal Liberators,* University of California Press, Berkeley, 1988.

CHAPTER 9

Human Subjects

The Tuskegee Syphilis Study

The Tuskegee study of untreated syphilis in hundreds of poor African American men is one of the most condemned experiments in American medicine. A true understanding of the issues involved requires some historical perspective; but because the study was investigated behind closed doors, its details never became widely known, and it is usually discussed in only simplistic, emotional terms.

BACKGROUND: ABUSE OF HUMAN SUBJECTS

For centuries, the craft of medicine used trial-and-error methods to develop drugs and remedies, but it was not until the *science* of medicine actually began that experimentation became a major part of it.

In the nineteenth century, some "gentleman physicians" experimented in their leisure time, and some of them became famous. One was William Beaumont, whose experimental subject was a patient named Alexis St. Martin. In 1822, Beaumont treated St. Martin for a bullet wound in the stomach; the patient survived, but the wound healed strangely, leaving a hole. Beaumont then employed St. Martin as a servant in order to observe him, and was able to prove that stomach juices digest food. Even this very early relationship between researcher and subject had its problems: eventually St. Martin refused to continue and ran away, and Beaumont had him sought by the police.

During the early twentieth century, the work of Koch and Pasteur inspired other physicians to experiment. The germ theory of disease opened a new door in medicine, and some physicians eagerly went through it.

In the middle of the century, during World War II, some medical experimentation took disturbing or even horrifying forms. Some questionable wartime research in the United States will be described later. On a far more serious level, Japanese physicians carried out deadly experiments on Chinese prisoners of war, killing over 3,000 of them, mostly at unit 731 in Harbin. These Chinese prisoners were injected with dozens of diseases to study the natural course of anthrax, syphilis, plague, cholera, and so on; in one study of plague, 700 Chinese died.[1] It was Nazi Germany, though, which became—and remained—a symbol of the perversion of medical research.

The Nazis and Mengele: Symbols of Medical Evil

Indeed, medicine in Nazi Germany has come to be almost synonymous with evildoing in the name of science. "Euthanasia" under the Nazis is discussed in Chapter 3: physicians sympathetic to Nazi ideology participated in programs in which disabled, insane, and comatose patients were involuntarily killed; and even some of the most prestigious German professors of medicine supported extermination of racially "inferior" people. In addition to "euthanasia," there was also a great deal of experimentation on human subjects, much of which was at least irregular and at worst almost unimaginably savage and brutal.

Research on typhus is one example. From 1943 to 1945, experimental vaccines against typhus were given to prisoners on ward 46 of the concentration camp at Buchenwald: gay men, convicted criminals, Russian officers, Polish dissidents, Jews, and Gypsies. In one experiment, a medical professor from the Robert Koch Institute injected blood infected with typhus into 40 involuntary subjects, who then served as a treatment group. All in all, about 1,000 prisoners were used, and 158 died (high morbidity occurred in unimmunized controls, almost all of whom died). No thresholds of infection were established.[2]

Deliberate harm to subjects also took place in other studies. In experiments at Buchenwald, hormones were implanted to "cure" homosexuality, inmates were shot to study gunshot wounds, inmates were starved to study the physiology of nutrition, and women's bones and limbs were surgically removed to study regeneration. In research on malaria, anopheles mosquitoes were flown in from swamps across the world to transmit malaria to subjects. Ernst Grawitz, Reich Physician of the SS (*Schutzstaffel,* or secret police), infected the lower legs of women subjects with staphylococci, gas, and tetanus bacilli. In some subjects, particles of glass and stone were rubbed into wounds to test the efficacy of sulfa drugs.

Experiments at Ravensbrück by Sigmund Rascher—"the Captain"—a doctor for the Luftwaffe (the German air force), were described later by a ward clerk named Eugene Kogon. To study human survival during rapid changes of altitude, Rascher devised something called a "sky ride wagon" which purportedly simulated such changes: an enclosed box on wheels with monitoring equipment inside. He reported that "the blood does not yet boil at an altitude of 70,000 feet."[3] Rascher also experimented with revival after freezing; in this research, he killed about 70 of 200 involuntary subjects—Jewish and Russian prisoners. These subjects were forced to strip and were then exposed to icy water or blizzards. Kogon wrote, "When their screams created too much of a disturbance, Rascher finally used anesthesia." In the next phase of the experiment, nude Jewish women were used to revive the subjects, and Rascher reported "in detail how revived subjects practiced sexual intercourse at 86 to 90 degrees Fahrenheit." The rationale of this study was supposed to be its application to Luftwaffe pilots downed in icy seas; but since nude women would hardly be available to revive such pilots, the actual point seems to have been little more than degradation of the subjects.

At the concentration camp at Auschwitz, Josef Mengele, a physician who came to be known as the "angel of death," participated in the death of 400,000 victims. Since Mengele is the most infamous of the Nazi physicians, we should consider his career briefly here.

Mengele was the oldest of three sons of a successful manufacturer of farm equipment and was raised as a conservative Catholic. He was above average in intelligence but seems to have achieved success in school more by hard work than by intellectual facility. Because he considered the family business too limiting, he chose medicine. Like many pioneering physicians, the young Josef Mengele was ambitious and sought fame. He studied in Munich between 1930 and 1936, with a special concentration in anthropological genetics; in the 1930s, this was a fashionable field and was part of a eugenics movement that had become influential in Germany and in the United States.

In 1931, Munich was the center of the Nazi party and, as such, a center of the Nazi program of "racial purity." To advance himself with his politically conservative medical professors (in the German context, these were professors who simply accepted whatever power controlled political life), Mengele became a Brownshirt, that is, a Nazi storm trooper. Academically, he cultivated professors favored by the Nazis and oriented his own research to their interests; his doctoral thesis, which was published, was on racial jaw morphologies. His aim in research was to secure a full professorship—a rare, highly prestigious appointment. In 1934, Mengele made another astute move by marrying a professor's daughter. Two of his biographers say, "They made a dashing young pair: Irene—tall, blonde, and good-looking; Mengele—handsome in a Mediterranean way, dapper, and with a passion for fast cars."[4]

In May 1943, Mengele began a 20-month appointment as women's physician at Birkenau. His appalling experiments were conducted at nearby Auschwitz, though he was never officially assigned there. He began by clearing the camp of typhus, an accomplishment he achieved by "triaging" sick prisoners and gassing about 1,000 Gypsies; his superiors admired his methodical efficiency and unsentimental attitude toward the sick. Thereafter, he was able to focus on research that was part of his plan for his future professorship. This work was meant to find a way to overcome the effects of genetics by modifying the environment: more technically, to influence a genotype to obtain a desired phenotype. He wanted to find ways to produce traits such as blue eyes, blonde hair, and a healthy body free of genetic disease. As subjects, he needed identical twins, who would be "natural controls" for environmental differences.

Eventually, Mengele would greet incoming trains of boxcars filled with Jews destined for execution. He would examine them, looking for twins and other usable subjects and signaling his choices by a flick of the wrist. The people he chose would live while they participated in his experiments; the rest would be killed at once.

Mengele's experiments are painful even to describe. He experimented with six children to see if blue eyes could be obtained by injecting blue dye; when this study was finished, he cut out the twelve eyes and hung them on a wall of his laboratory, along with some other human organs. He forced female twins to engage in coitus with male twins to see if twin children would be produced. He interchanged blood of identical twins, to see what would happen; then he interchanged blood between pairs of twins. One pair of fraternal (nonidentical) twins—children—consisted of a hunchback and a normal child; Mengele surgically grafted the hunchback to the other child's back, creating the effect of conjoined twins, and accentuated this effect by also sewing their wrists back to back. A witness, Vera Alexander, reported that when the children came back to the barracks: "There was a terrible smell of gangrene. The cuts were dirty and the children cried every night."[5] Mengele had many of his twins (between 150 and 200) killed; some of them he killed himself. Here is a description by another physician who was present at a series of executions:

> After that, the first twin was brought in, a fourteen-year old girl. Dr. Mengele ordered me to undress the girl and put her head on the dissecting table. Then he injected the Epival into her right arm intravenously. After the child had fallen asleep, he felt for the left ventricle of the heart and injected 10 cc of chloroform. After one little twitch the child was dead, whereupon Dr. Mengele had her taken to the corpse chamber. In this manner, all fourteen twins were killed during the night.[6]

In other research, Mengele tried to establish limits of human endurance by subjecting 75 male and female prisoners to electric shock; 25 of them died immediately. To study sterility, he subjected a group of Polish nuns to high dosages of radiation, burning them severely. At one time, he found a hunchback and the hunchback's son; he had both of them killed, their bodies boiled, their flesh stripped, and their skeletons dipped in gasoline for preservation for his anthropological studies of body types. When he came upon seven dwarfs from a Rumanian circus family, however, he kept them alive in order to exhibit them to visiting German physicians.

Although his temper occasionally flared when anyone subverted his plans, Mengele was noted for being cool, impersonal, and detached. When, because of an oversight, 300 Jewish children managed to escape a gas chamber and fled to a nearby field, Mengele had them recaptured, then had a gasoline fire set in a large pit and had the children thrown in. Some of the children, on fire and screaming for their lives, clawed their way over dead bodies to the top, where Mengele and SS men kicked them back in.

As the Russian army approached Auschwitz in 1945, Mengele fled. Almost immediately, he was listed as a major war criminal; but even though he used his real name, he managed to escape to Brazil and Paraguay, where he lived in relative freedom for 40 years, several times eluding Simon Wiesenthal and other Israelis who tried to catch him. Later, in conversations with his grown son Rolf, Mengele never expressed any regret for his actions or even any consciousness of having done wrong. He reasoned that it was not his fault that Jews were to be killed at Auschwitz, and since they were to die anyway, why not use them first to advance medical knowledge, Nazi programs, and his own chance of a professorship? Mengele died in Brazil in the summer of 1985 (the identity of his body was confirmed by matching his DNA with DNA donated by his son).[7]

Mengele's actions are often attributed to a pathological personality, but it must be noted that he did not appear to be a psychopath. Of course, we could define his behavior as pathological: that is, we could say that anyone who behaves this way must be a psychopath. However, this would probably be simplistic, and it would fail to allow for what the philosopher Hannah Arendt calls the "banality of evil"—the possibility that ordinary people, in relatively normal circumstances, can do terrible things.[8] That the "banality of evil" may indeed be a reality seems to be strongly indicated by Stanley Milgram's research on obedience to authority.[9]

The Nuremberg Code

After World War II, at the Nuremberg trials in 1946, German physicians defended themselves against charges of war crimes by saying that they had merely been following orders, that their experiments had been properly related to solving medical problems of war, and that what they had done was not substantially different from research done on captives by American physicians.

Although such a defense would be ludicrous for anyone like Mengele, it might have some credence for minor figures who may have conducted morally dubious research or mistreated their subjects without committing actual atrocities. However, a problem faced by the judges at Nuremberg in evaluating defenses, charges, and evidence was lack of a code of ethics for experimentation on captive populations. The judges therefore referred to 10 principles for permissible experimentation, which afterward came to be known as the *Nuremberg code*. The most important principle of the Nuremberg code was that captives should freely consent to participation in any experiment.

It is noteworthy that one of the observers at the Nuremberg trials was a young physician named Leo Alexander. Later, in an article in *New England Journal of Medicine*, Alexander gave shocking details of Nazi experimentation and "euthanasia" and advanced a now famous "slippery slope" explanation,[10] which is discussed in Chapter 3.

American Military Research in World War II

As noted above, some research in the United States during World War II was ethically questionable. In 1941, for example, American researchers experimented on orphans at the Ohio Soldiers and Sailors Orphanage, on retarded inmates at New Jersey State Colony for the Feeble-Minded, and on patients at a mental institution in Dixon, Illinois.[11] One purpose of this research was to develop a vaccine against shigella (a bacterial disease causing dysentery), and researchers injected deadened forms of shigella bacteria into their subjects. No one died as a direct result, but many of the subjects got very sick.

Some questionable research used military personnel as subjects. Cornelius ("Dusty") Rhoads, director of the leading American cancer hospital—Memorial Sloan Kettering in New York City—became head of the military's secret chemical warfare service. As Robert Bazell, a science reporter for NBC, writes, Rhoads:

> . . . supervised the long secret and now infamous tests where thousands of American troops were intentionally exposed to mustard and other poisonous gases. Rhoads discovered that the mustard gas killed white blood cells and other

cells that divided rapidly. After the war he and others began to experiment with mustard gas as a cancer treatment and also to search for other systemic poisons that kill dividing cells.[12]

According to a report by the Institute of Medicine in 1993, in most of the research conducted by the armed forces on the acute effects of these poisonous agents, the subjects were "volunteers" who did not know what they were volunteering for; there was no attempt at informed consent.[13] The testing involved 60,000 subjects, of whom 4,000 to 5,000 were used in tests on mustard gas in gas chambers.

Wartime research in the United States had some significant consequences. One later development was that when subjects of the chemical research applied for treatment at veterans' hospitals, the Veterans Administration (VA) denied that they had been exposed to toxic agents (this scenario would be repeated after the war in Vietnam and again after "Operation Desert Storm"). Another development was that these same toxic agents would later be used as "chemotherapies" against cancer—an outgrowth of the use of military personnel as "guinea pigs" in World War II.

A third long-term consequence was that World War II institutionalized medical experimentation, including some doubtful practices. The Americans (like their opponents) sought cures for dysentery, malaria, and venereal diseases; and when the war itself came to an end, the fight against diseases in the United States did not. In fact, "the prospect of winning the war against contagious and degenerative illness gave researchers in the 1950s and 1960s a sense of both mission and urgency that kept the spirit of the wartime laboratories alive."[14]

During the war, for instance, Franklin Roosevelt established the Committee on Medical Research, which approached its work with a wartime mentality that carried over into researchers' attitudes after the war: disease was the enemy, researchers were the soldiers, and victory could be won—with enough resources and enough will. Also, while the war was still in process, considerations of ethics and informed consent had carried little weight:

> A wartime environment also undercut the protection of human subjects, because of the power of the example of the draft. Every day thousands of men were compelled to risk death, however limited their understanding of the aims of the war or the immediate campaign might be. By extension, researchers doing laboratory work were also engaged in a military activity, and they did not need to seek the permission of their subjects any more than the selective service or field commanders did of draftees. . . .
>
> In a society mobilized for war, these arguments carried great weight. Some people were ordered to face bullets and storm a hill; others were told to take an injection and test a vaccine. In philosophical terms, wartime inevitably promoted utilitarian over absolutistic positions.[15]

Postwar Criticisms

After the war, it became apparent that some researchers had gone too far in their zeal for results; moreover, by the 1970s, the wartime sense of urgency had begun to be tempered by other voices. Faith in the inevitability of scientific progress was waning, and with it faith in medical research. Rachel Carson's *Silent Spring* described the ravages of pesticides; the Cuban missile crisis showed how close we could come to nuclear destruction; drugs hailed as "miraculous" were found to have dramatically harmful side effects, such as the severe birth defects caused by thalidomide. Thus the use of human subjects in medical research began to be considered more critically.

In 1966, in *New England Journal of Medicine*, Henry Beecher—a medical professor at Harvard—criticized 22 specific medical experiments involving human subjects.[16] All of these studies had been published in medical journals, but none of them had obtained informed consent from subjects, and several of them bordered on abuse. Beecher claimed that these 22 studies were not exceptions but rather represented the norm of medical experimentation. At about the same time, another physician, Henry Pappworth, criticized 500 medical experiments on similar grounds.[17]

In considering such criticism, we need to keep a sense of proportion about abuse of subjects in American research, which of course is nothing like what went on in Nazi Germany. Moreover, the Nazi atrocities stemmed from systematic contempt for "undesirables," whereas abuses in American studies have arisen in a basically different way. In American medical research, mistreatment of subjects has tended to arise from conflicts of three types of goals: helping future patients, advancing the researchers' careers, and protecting the interests of subjects. That is, abuses typically arise when researchers fail to keep their subjects' welfare in balance with their other goals.

THE TUSKEGEE STUDY

The Tuskegee study of syphilis began during the great depression—around 1930—and lasted for 42 years. Because of its long time span (as noted at the beginning of this chapter), some historical background is important for understanding the many issues raised by the Tuskegee research.

The Medical Environment: Syphilis

Syphilis is a chronic, contagious bacterial disease, often venereal and sometimes congenital. Its first symptom is a chancre; after this chancre subsides, the disease spreads silently for a time but then produces an outbreak of secondary symptoms such as fever, rash, and swollen lymph glands. Then the disease becomes latent for many years, after which it may reappear with a variety of symptoms in the nervous or circulatory systems. Today, syphilis is treated with penicillin or other antibiotics; but this treatment has been possible only since about 1946, when penicillin first became widely available.

Until relatively recently, then, the common fate of victims of syphilis—kings and queens, peasants and slaves—was simply to suffer the sequelae once the first symptoms had appeared. Victims who suffered this inevitable progress included Cleopatra, King Herod of Judea, Charlemagne, Henry VIII of England, Napoleon Bonaparte, Frederick the Great, Pope Sixtus IV, Pope Alexander VI, Pope Julius II,

Catherine the Great, Christopher Columbus, Paul Gauguin, Franz Schubert, Albrecht Dürer, Johann Wolfgang von Goethe, Friedrich Nietzsche, John Keats, and James Joyce.[18]

•

It is generally believed that syphilis was brought to Europe from the new world during the 1490s, by Christopher Columbus's crews, but the disease may have appeared in Europe before that time. In any case, advances in transportation contributed greatly to the spread of syphilis (similarly, much later, transportation would be a factor in the spread of AIDS). For hundreds of years, syphilis was attributed to sin and was associated with prostitutes, though attempts to check its spread by expelling prostitutes failed because their customers were disregarded. Efforts to eradicate it by quarantine also failed.

In the eighteenth century, standing professional armies began to be established, and with them came a general acceptance of high rates of venereal disease. It is estimated, for instance, that around the year 1900, one-fifth of the British army had syphilis or gonorrhea.

Between 1900 and 1948, and especially during the two world wars, American reformers mounted what was called a *syphilophobia* campaign: the Social Hygiene Movement or Purity Crusade. Members of the campaign emphasized that syphilis was spread by prostitutes, and held that it was rapidly fatal; as an alternative to visiting a prostitute, they advocated clean, active sports (in today's terms, "Just say no"). According to the medical historian Alan Brandt, there were two splits resulting from disagreements within this reform movement: once during World War I, when giving out condoms was controversial; and later during World War II, when giving out penicillin was at issue. In each of these conflicts, reformers whose basic intention was to reduce the physical harm of syphilis were on one side, whereas those who wanted to reduce illicit behavior were on the other side.[19]

The armed services during the world wars took a pragmatic position. Commanders who needed healthy troops overruled the moralists and ordered the release of condoms in the first war and penicillin in the second—and these continued to be used by returning troops after each war.

•

The spirochete (bacterium) which causes syphilis was discovered by Fritz Schaudinn in 1906. Syphilis is, classically, described in three stages:

- *Primary syphilis*—In this first stage, spirochetes mass and produce a primary lesion causing a *chancre* (pronounced "SHANK-er"). During the primary stage, syphilis is highly infectious.
- *Secondary syphilis*—In the second stage, spirochetes disseminate from the primary lesion throughout the body, producing systemic and widespread lesions, usually in internal organs and other internal sites. Externally, however—after the initial chancre subsides—syphilis spreads silently during a "latent" period lasting from 1 to 30 years, although secondary symptoms such as fever, rash, and swollen glands may appear. During the secondary stage, the symptoms of syphilis vary so widely that it is known as the "great imitator."

- *Tertiary syphilis*—In the third stage, chronic destructive lesions cause major damage to the cardiac system, the neurological system, or both, partly because immune responses decrease with age. During the tertiary stage, syphilis may produce paresis (slight or incomplete paralysis), gummas (gummy or rubbery tumors), altered gait, blindness, or lethal narrowing of the aorta.

Beginning in the sixteenth century, mercury—a heavy metal—was the common treatment for syphilis; it was applied to the back as a paste and absorbed through the skin. During the nineteenth century, this treatment alternated with bismuth, another heavy metal administered the same way. Neither mercury nor bismuth killed the spirochetes, though either could ameliorate symptoms.

In 1909, after the spirochete of syphilis had been identified, two researchers— a German, Paul Erlich; and a Japanese, S. Hata—tried 605 forms of arsenic and finally discovered what seemed to be a "magic bullet" against it: combination 606 of heavy metals including arsenic. Erlich called this *salvarsan* and patented it; the generic name is arsphenamine.[20] Salvarsan was administered as an intramuscular injection. After finding that it cured syphilis in rabbits, Erlich injected it into men with syphilis. (According to common practice, none of the men was asked to consent.)

At first, salvarsan seemed to work wonders, and during 1910 Erlich was receiving standing ovations at medical meetings. Later, however, syphilis recurred, fatally, in some patients who had been treated with salvarsan; furthermore, salvarsan itself apparently killed some patients. Erlich maintained that the drug had not been given correctly, but he also developed another form, neosalvarsan, which was less toxic and could be given more easily. Neosalvarsan also was injected intramuscularly—ideally, in 20 to 40 dosages given over 1 year.

Though better than salvarsan, neosalvarsan was (as described by a physician of the time) used erratically, and "generally without rhyme or reason—an injection now and then, possibly for a symptom, [for] some skin lesion, or when the patient had a ten-dollar bill."[21] It was also expensive. Moreover, neither salvarsan nor neosalvarsan was a "magic bullet" for patients with tertiary syphilis.

Another researcher, Caesar Boeck in Norway, took a different approach: from 1891 to 1910, he studied the natural course of untreated syphilis in 1,978 subjects. Boeck, a professor of dermatology at the University of Oslo, believed that heavy metals removed only the symptoms of syphilis rather than its underlying cause; he also thought that these metals suppressed what is today recognized as the immune system. He therefore decided that not treating patients at all might be an improvement over treatment with heavy metals.

In 1929, Boeck's student and successor, J. E. Bruusgaard, selected 473 of Boeck's subjects for further evaluation, in many cases examining their hospital charts.[22] This method had an obvious bias, since the more severely affected of Boeck's subjects would be most likely to have hospital records. Despite this bias, however, Bruusgaard was surprised to find that in 65 percent of these cases, either the subjects were externally symptom-free or there was no mention in their charts of the classic symptoms of syphilis. Of the subjects who had had syphilis for more than 20 years, 73 percent were asymptomatic.

Bruusgaard's findings contradicted the message of the syphilophobia campaign: they indicated that syphilis was not universally fatal, much less rapidly so. These results also suggested the possibility that some people with syphilis spirochetes would never develop any symptoms of the disease.

When the Tuskegee study began in 1932, Boeck's and Bruusgaard's work was the only existing study of the natural course of untreated syphilis.

The Racial Environment

In the 1930s, American medicine was, and had long been, widely racist—certainly by our present standards and to some extent even by the standards of the time. For at least a century before the Tuskegee study began, most physicians condescended to African American patients, held stereotypes about them, and sometimes used them as subjects of nontherapeutic experiments.

The historian Todd Savitt, for example, has described how in the 1800s, J. Marion Sims, a pioneer in American gynecology, practiced techniques for closing vesical-vaginal fistulas on slave women.[23] John Brown, a former slave who wrote a book about his life under slavery, described how a physician in Georgia kept him in an open-pit oven to produce sunburns and to try out different remedies.

The best-known account of the racial background of the Tuskegee study is James Jones's *Bad Blood* (1981; the significance of the title will become apparent below).[24] In the late nineteenth century, the United States was swept by social Darwinism, a popular corruption of Darwin's theory of evolution by natural selection (see Chapter 16). Some whites predicted on this basis that the Negro race (to use the term then current) would be extinct by 1900: their idea was that Darwin's "survival of the fittest" implied a competition which Negroes would lose. (It bears repeating that this is a misconception and misapplication of Darwin's actual theory.) According to Jones, this popular belief was shared by white physicians, who thought that it was confirmed by defects in African Americans' anatomy and therefore became obsessed with the details of such presumed defects. Although comparable defects in white patients went unreported, defects in black patients were described in great detail in medical journals and became the basis for sweeping conclusions; to take one example, genital development and brain development were said to vary inversely.

In addition to social Darwinism, physicians shared many of the popular stereotypes of African Americans; well into the twentieth century, physicians often simply advanced such stereotypes as "facts." The following example appeared in *Journal of the American Medical Association* in 1914:

> The negro springs from a southern race, and as such his sexual appetite is strong; all of his environments stimulate this appetite, and as a general rule his emotional type of religion certainly does not decrease it.[25]

African Americans were also seen as dirty, shiftless, promiscuous, and incapable of practicing personal hygiene. Around the turn of the century, a physician in rural Georgia wrote, "Virtue in the negro race is like 'angels' visits'—few and far between. In a practice of sixteen years in the South, I have never examined a virgin over fourteen years of age."[26] In 1919, a medical professor in Chicago wrote that African American men were like bulls or elephants in *furor sexualis,* unable to refrain from copulation when in the presence of females.[27]

Ideas about syphilis reflected this racial environment. For white physicians at the time when the Tuskegee study began, syphilis was a natural consequence of the innately low character of African Americans, who were described by one white physician as a "notoriously syphilis-soaked race."[28] Moreover, it was simply assumed that African American men would not seek treatment for venereal disease.

The historian Alan Brandt has suggested that in the United States during the early 1900s, it was a rare white physician who was not a racist—and that this would have remained the case throughout many years of the Tuskegee study. He writes, "There can be little doubt that the Tuskegee researchers regarded their subjects as less than human."[29]

Development of the Tuskegee Case

A "study in nature" begins   Studies in nature were distinguished from experiments in 1865 by a famous experimenter and physiologist, Claude Bernard: in an experiment, some factor is manipulated, whereas a *study in nature* merely observes what would happen anyway. For a century before the Tuskegee study, medicine considered it crucially important to discover the natural history of a disease and therefore relied extensively on studies in nature.

The great physician William Osler had said, "Know syphilis in all its manifestations and relations, and all other things clinical will be added unto you."[30] As late as 1932, however, the natural history of syphilis had not been conclusively documented (the only existing study, as noted above, was that of Boeck and Bruusgaard), and there was uncertainty about the inexorability of its course. The United States Public Health Service (USPHS) believed that a study in nature of syphilis was necessary because physicians needed to know its natural sequence of symptoms and final outcomes in order to recognize key changes during its course. This perceived need was one factor in the Tuskegee research.

A second factor was simply that USPHS found what it considered an opportunity for such a study. Around 1929, there were several counties in the United States where venereal disease was extraordinarily prevalent, and a philanthropical organization—the Julius Rosenwald Foundation in Philadelphia—started a project to eradicate it. With help from USPHS, the foundation originally intended to treat with neosalvarsan all syphilitics in six counties with rates of syphilis above 20 percent. In 1930, the foundation surveyed African American men in Macon County, Alabama, which was then 82 percent black; this was the home of the famous Tuskegee Institute. The survey found the highest rate of syphilis in the nation: 36 percent. The foundation planned a demonstration study in which these African American syphilitics would be treated with neosalvarsan, and it did treat or partially treat some of the 3,694 men who had been identified as having syphilis (estimates of how many received treatment or partial treatment range from less than half to 95 percent). However, 1929 was the year when the great depression began; as it ground on, funds for philanthropy plummeted, and the Rosenwald Foundation pulled out of Tuskegee, hoping that USPHS would continue the treatment program. (Funds available for public health were also dropping, though: USPHS would soon see its budget lowered from over $1 million before the depression to less than $60,000 in 1935.)

In 1931, USPHS repeated the foundation's survey in Macon County, testing 4,400 African American residents; USPHS found a 22 percent rate of syphilis in men, and a 62 percent rate of congenital syphilis. In this survey, 399 African American men were identified who had syphilis of several years' duration but had never been treated by the Rosenwald Foundation or in any other way. It was the identification of these 399 untreated men that USPHS saw as an ideal opportunity for a study in nature of syphilis. The surgeon general suggested that they should be merely observed rather than treated: this decision would become a moral crux of the study.

It is important to reemphasize that the USPHS research—it was undertaken in cooperation with the Tuskegee Institute and is called the *Tuskegee study* for that reason—was a study in nature. The Tuskegee physicians saw themselves as ecological biologists, simply observing what occurred regularly and naturally. In 1936, a paper in *Journal of the American Medical Association* by the surgeon general and his top assistants described the 1932–1933 phase of the Tuskegee study as "an unusual opportunity to study the untreated syphilitic patient from the beginning of the disease to the death of the infected person." It noted specifically that the study consisted of "399 syphilitic Negro males who had never received treatment."[31]

There are also two important points to emphasize about the subjects of the Tuskegee study. First, at the outset the 399 syphilitic subjects had *latent syphilis,* that is, secondary syphilis; most of them were probably in the early latent stage. During this stage, syphilis is largely noninfectious during sexual intercourse, although it can be passed easily through a blood transfusion (or, in a pregnant woman, through the placenta). However, latent or secondary syphilis (as noted above) has extremely variable symptoms and outcomes; and external lesions, which can be a source of infection during sex, do sometimes appear.

Second, these 399 syphilitic subjects were not divided into the typical experimental and control or "treatment" and "no treatment" groups: they were all simply to be observed. There was, however, another group of "controls," consisting of about 200 age-matched men who did not have syphilis. (Originally, there was also a third group, consisting of 275 syphilitic men who had been treated with small amounts of arsphenamine; these subjects were followed for a while but were dropped from the study in 1936—perhaps because funds were lacking, or perhaps because the researchers were by then interested only in the "study in nature" group.)

The middle phase: "Bad blood"   The Tuskegee study was hardly a model of scientific research or scientific method; and even on its own terms, as a study in nature, it was carried out rather haphazardly. Except for an African American nurse, Eunice Rivers, who was permanently assigned to the study, there was no continuity of medical personnel. There was no central supervision; there were no written protocols; no physician was in charge. Names of the subjects in the study group of 399 were often mixed up with the "controls." The subjects were not housed at any one location or facility. Most worked as sharecroppers or as small farmers and simply came into the town of Tuskegee when Eunice Rivers told them to do so (she would drive them into town in her car, a ride that several sub-jects described as making them feel important).

There were large gaps in the study. The "federal doctors," as the subjects called them, returned only every few years. Visits are documented in 1939 and then not again until 1948; 7 years passed between visits in 1963 and 1970. Only the nurse, Eunice Rivers, remained to hold the shaky study together. When the physicians did return to Tuskegee after a gap, they found it difficult to answer their own questions because the records were so poor.

Still, there were some rudimentary procedures. The physicians wanted to know, first, if they had a subject in the study group; and second, if so, how far his syphilis had progressed. To determine the progress of the disease, spinal punc-tures (called *taps*) were given to 271 of the 399 syphilitic subjects. In a spinal tap, a 10-inch needle is inserted between two vertebrae into the cerebrospinal fluid and a small amount of fluid is withdrawn—a delicate and uncomfortable process. The subjects were warned to lie very still, lest the needle swerve and puncture the fluid sac, causing infection and other complications.

Subjects were understandably reluctant to leave their farms, travel for miles over back roads to meet the physicians, and then undergo these painful taps, especially when they had no pressing medical problem. For this reason, the physicians offered inducements: free transportation, free hot lunches, free medi-cine for any disease other than syphilis, and free burials. (The free burials were important to poor subjects, who often died without enough money for even a pauper's grave; but USPHS couldn't keep this promise itself after its budget was reduced and had to be rescued by the Milbank Memorial Fund.) In return for these "benefits," the physicians got not only the spinal taps but, later, autopsies to see what damage syphilis had or had not done.

There seems no doubt that the researchers also resorted to deception. Sub-jects were told that they had "bad blood" and that the spinal taps were "treat-ment" for it; moreover, the researchers sensationalized the effects of untreated "bad blood." USPHS sent the subjects the following letter, under the imposing letterhead "Macon County Health Department," with the subheading "Alabama State Board of Health and U.S. Public Health Service Cooperating with Tuskegee Institute" (all of which participated in the study):

> Dear Sir:
> Some time ago you were given a thorough examination and since that time we hope you have gotten a great deal of treatment for bad blood. You will now be given your last chance to get a second examination. This examination is a very special one and after it is finished you will be given a special treatment if it is believed you are in a condition to stand it.[32]

The "special treatment" mentioned was simply the spinal tap for neurosyphilis, a diagnostic test. The subjects were instructed to meet the public health nurse for transportation to "Tuskegee Institute Hospital for this free treatment." The letter closed, in capitals:

> REMEMBER THIS IS YOUR LAST CHANCE FOR SPECIAL FREE TREATMENT.
> BE SURE TO MEET THE NURSE.

To repeat, the researchers never treated the subjects for syphilis. In fact, during World War II, the researchers contacted the local draft board and prevented any eligible subject from being drafted—and hence from being treated for syphilis by the armed services. Although penicillin was developed around 1941–1943 and was widely available by 1946, the subjects in the Tuskegee study never received it, even during the 1960s or 1970s. However, as will be discussed below, it is not clear how much the subjects with late noninfectious syphilis were harmed by not getting penicillin.

The first investigations   In 1966, Peter Buxtun, a recent college graduate, had just been hired by USPHS as a venereal disease investigator in San Francisco. After a few months, he learned of the Tuskegee study and began to question and criticize the USPHS officials who were still running it.[33] By this time, the physicians supervising the study and its data collection had been moved to the newly created Centers for Disease Control (CDC) in Atlanta. CDC officials were annoyed by Buxtun's questions about the morality of the study; later in 1966, having invited him to Atlanta for a conference on syphilis, they harangued him and tried to get him to be silent. He expected to be fired from USPHS; he was not, though, and he continued to press CDC for 2 more years.

By 1969, Buxtun's inquiries and protests led to a meeting of a small group of physicians at CDC to consider the Tuskegee study. The group consisted of William J. Brown (Director of Venereal Diseases at CDC), David Sencer (Director of CDC), Ira Meyers (Alabama's State Health Officer from 1951 to 1986), Sidney Olansky (a physician at Emory Hospital who was knowledgeable about the early years of the study and had been in charge of it in 1951), Lawton Smith (an ophthalmologist from the University of Miami), and Gene Stollerman (chairman of medicine at the University of Tennessee). In general, this group avoided Buxtun's questions about the morality of the study and focused on whether continuing the study would harm the subjects. Meyers said of the Tuskegee subjects, "I haven't seen this group, but I don't think they would submit to treatment" if they were told what was going on.[34] Smith (the ophthalmologist) pressed hardest for continuing the study; only Stollerman repeatedly opposed continuing it, on both moral and therapeutic grounds. At the end, the committee overrode Stollerman and voted to continue the study.

Also in 1969, Ira Meyers told the physicians in the Macon County Medical Society about the Tuskegee study. These physicians did not object to the study; in fact, they were given a list of all the subjects and agreed not to give antibiotics to any subject for any condition, if a subject came to one of their offices. It should be noted that although this medical society had been all-white in the 1930s, during the 1960s its membership was almost entirely African American.

In 1970, a monograph on syphilis was published, sponsored by the American Public Health Association, to give useful information to public health officers and venereal disease (VD) control officers. This monograph stated that treatment for late benign syphilis should consist of "6.0 to 9.0 million units of benzathine penicillin G given 3.0 million units at sessions seven days apart."[35] The first author listed on the monograph is William J. Brown, head of CDC's Tuskegee section from 1957 to 1971. Brown had been on the CDC panel in 1969 (when the monograph was probably written) and had argued for continuing the Tuskegee study, in which, of course, subjects with late benign syphilis received *no* penicillin.

The story breaks   In July of 1972, Peter Buxtun, who had then been criticizing the Tuskegee research for 6 years and was disappointed by CDC's refusal to stop it, mentioned the Tuskegee study to a friend who was a reporter for the Associated Press (AP) on the west coast. Another AP reporter—Jean Heller, on the east coast—was assigned to the story, and on the morning of July 26, 1972, her report appeared on front pages of newspapers nationwide.[36]

Heller's story described a medical study run by the federal government in Tuskegee, Alabama, in which poor, uneducated African American men had been used as "guinea pigs." After noting the terrible effects of tertiary syphilis, the story said that in 1969 a CDC study of 276 of the untreated subjects had proved that at least 7 subjects died "as a direct result of syphilis."

Heller's story had an immediate effect. (It might have made even more of an impact, but it was competing with a political story which broke the same day—a report that the Democratic candidate for vice president, Thomas Eagleton, had received shock therapy for depression.) Some members of Congress were amazed to learn of the Tuskegee study, and Senator William Proxmire called it a "moral and ethical nightmare."

CDC, of course, responded. J. D. Millar, chief of Venereal Disease Control, said that the study "was never clandestine," pointing to 15 published articles in medical and scientific journals over a 30-year span. Millar also maintained that the subjects had been informed that they could get treatment for syphilis at any time. "Patients were not denied drugs," he said; "rather, they were not offered drugs." He also tried to emphasize that "the study began when attitudes were much different on treatment and experimentation."[37]

The public and the press, however, scorned Millar's explanations. One political cartoon, for instance, showed a frail African American man being studied under a huge microscope by a white man in a white coat with a sign in the background: "This is a NO-TREATMENT study by your Public Heath Service."[38] Another cartoon showed ragged African American men walking past tombstones; the caption read: "Secret Tuskegee Study—free autopsy, free burial, plus $100 bonus." Another showed a white physician standing near the body of an African American man, partially covered by a sheet; the chart at the foot of the hospital bed on which the body lay read "Ignore this syphilis patient (experiment in progress)"; in the background, a skeptical nurse holding a syringe asked, "*Now* can we give him penicillin?"

CDC and USPHS had always feared a "public relations problem" if the Tuskegee study became generally known, and now they had one. So did the Macon County Medical Society: when its president told the *Montgomery Advertiser* that the members had voted to identify remaining subjects and give them "appropriate therapy," USPHS in Atlanta flatly contradicted him, retorting that the local physicians—African American physicians—had accepted the Tuskegee study. The society then acknowledged that it had agreed to continuation of the study but had not agreed to withhold treatment from subjects who came to the offices of its members, whereupon USPHS documented the physicians' agreement to do exactly that.

The aftermath   Almost immediately after Heller's story appeared, Congress commissioned a special panel to investigate the Tuskegee study and issue a report. (The report was supposed to be ready by December 31, 1972; as we will see, however, it was late.)

Also almost at once, senators Sparkman and Allen of Alabama (both Democrats) sponsored a federal bill to give each of the Tuskegee subjects $25,000 in compensation. The southern African American electorate had been instrumental in electing these two senators and many southern members of Congress in the 1960s and 1970s, as well as presidents Kennedy and Johnson.

On November 16, 1972, Casper Weinberger, Secretary of Health, Education, and Welfare (HEW), officially terminated the Tuskegee study. At that time, CDC estimated that 28 of the original syphilitic group had died of syphilis during the study; after the study was ended, the remaining syphilitic subjects received penicillin.

In February and March 1973, Senator Edward Kennedy's Subcommittee on Health of the Committee on Labor and Public Welfare held hearings on the Tuskegee study. Two of the Tuskegee subjects, Charles Pollard and Lester Scott, testified; one of them appeared to have been blinded by late-stage syphilis. These two men revealed more about the study: Pollard said they had not been told that they had syphilis; both said they thought "bad blood" meant something like low energy. Kennedy strongly condemned the study and proposed new regulations for medical experimentation.

In April 1973, the investigatory panel that had been commissioned when the Tuskegee story broke finally issued its report, which did not prove to be very useful. Moreover, for some reason this panel had met behind closed doors, and thus reporters had not been able to cover it.[39]

On July 23, 1973, Fred Gray, representing some of the Tuskegee subjects, filed a class-action suit against the federal government. Gray, a former Alabama legislator (in 1970, he had become the first African American Democrat elected in Alabama since Reconstruction), had been threatening to sue for compensation since Heller's story first broke, hoping for a settlement. He presented the suit as an issue of race, suing only the federal government and omitting the Tuskegee Institute, Rivers, the Tuskegee hospitals, and the Macon County Medical Society.

Eventually, the Justice Department decided that it couldn't win the suit in federal court, since the trial would have been held in nearby Montgomery, in the court of Frank Johnson, a liberal Alabama judge who had desegregated southern schools and upgraded mental institutions. Therefore, in December 1974 the government settled out of court.

According to the settlement, "living syphilitics" (subjects alive on July 23, 1973) received $37,500 each; "heirs of deceased syphilitics," $15,000 (since some children might have congenital syphilis); "living controls," $16,000; heirs of "deceased controls," $5,000. (Controls and their descendants were compensated because they had been prevented from getting antibiotics during the years of the study.) Also, the federal government agreed to provide free lifetime medical care for Tuskegee subjects, their wives, and their children. By September 1988, the government had paid $7.5 million for medical care for the Tuskegee subjects. At that time, 21 of the original syphilitic subjects were still alive—each of whom had had syphilis for at least 57 years.[40] In addition, 41 wives and 19 children had evidence of syphilis and were receiving free medical care.

By the time this settlement was reached, more than 18 months had passed since Jean Heller's first story, and the Tuskegee issue was no longer front-page news: even the *New York Times* was giving it only an occasional short paragraph or two on inside pages. The issue was, after all, complicated; ethical standards had changed over the long course of the Tuskegee research; and, as noted above, the special panel commissioned to evaluate the study had met in secret. The public, therefore, had more or less forgotten about the Tuskegee study.

ETHICAL ISSUES

Deception and Informed Consent

Two related ethical issues in the Tuskegee study are deception and informed consent. As has already been noted, the researchers undoubtedly deceived the subjects about "bad blood" and the spinal taps. Moreover, according to J. D. Williams, an African American physician who was an intern at Tuskegee Institute Hospital when the study began (he was 73 when the story broke in 1972), the subjects did not know that they were part of a study, did not even know what syphilis was, and did not know that they weren't being treated with available drugs.[41] Assuming that such deception did take place, was it justified? What does it imply about informed consent?

The federal panel established in 1972 faulted the Tuskegee researchers for deceiving subjects and for failing to obtain subjects' informed consent. A counterargument has been advanced, however, by one apologist for the Tuskegee study: R. H. Kampmeier, an emeritus professor of medicine at Vanderbilt Medical School who worked as a syphilologist during the decades of the study.[42] Kampmeier considers it unfair to condemn a study undertaken in the 1930s on the basis of lack of informed consent—a legal notion which first appeared in court decisions in the 1960s. He argues that this amounts to judging earlier research by modern standards. He also describes such criticism as "tilting at windmills" because it would presumably apply to most of the great researchers of the past, who never bothered with consent: does it really make sense to call someone like Pasteur unethical? Furthermore, Kampmeier cites a study by USPHS in 1943 involving use of penicillin with 35,000 syphilitics; this study is considered a landmark, but it did not obtain informed consent from its subjects. He notes, in addition, that during the early years of the Tuskegee study, it was accepted practice for physicians to walk into a patient's room and simply announce that they were taking out the patient's gallbladder.

The medical historian and physician Thomas Benedek also dismisses the issue of informed consent as "anachronistic" with regard to the Tuskegee study, noting that USPHS did not require informed consent until 1966.[43]

It is true that informed consent in medical experiments was mandated by court decisions during the late 1960s, and that before then it had not been a legal requirement. Still, the accepted presumption was always that physicians would neither harm patients nor allow harm to occur ("First, do no harm"), and this presumption would also seem applicable to physicians who were doing research with human subjects. Advocates of patients' rights argue that failure to adhere to this presumption—leading to situations like the "landmark" USPHS study of penicillin and syphilis—is what created the need for laws about informed consent in the first place.

Moreover, it can be argued that we need to distinguish between obtaining consent for procedures which might benefit subjects (*therapeutic* procedures) and *not* obtaining consent for procedures which might harm subjects (*experimental* procedures). On this argument, informed consent would always be required for experimental (potentially harmful) procedures and thus would represent a legitimate criticism of the Tuskegee study.

Finally, we can ask some rather simple questions. Granted that telling patients or subjects the truth was not legally required before 1960, and granted that this was not always a medical norm, was it really *not* wrong for the Tuskegee researchers to lie to their subjects, even in the 1930s? Did the researchers really believe they were doing *no* wrong?

Racism

Another issue in the Tuskegee study is racism. The study, of course, began long before the civil rights movement; it took place in the deep south—in Alabama—and all its subjects were African American. Under such circumstances, was it only a coincidence that the subjects were deceived and left untreated? Would white subjects have been used in the same way?

In *Bad Blood*, James Jones sees the Tuskegee study as a result of pervasive racism in American medicine during the 1930s and earlier, and Kampmeier acknowledges that few whites of the time transcended this racism. It is important to realize exactly how bad the 1930s were for African Americans: to take just one example, black students at Tuskegee Institute lived in fear of rural white toughs just outside the campus. In such a racial climate, it seems very probable that the researchers in the Tuskegee study would be willing to withhold the truth—and treatment—from African American subjects.

Also, although "studies in nature" were still important in medicine of the early 1930s, there was no reason why a study in nature of syphilis should have used only African American subjects. On the contrary: some physicians believed then that syphilis ran a different course in different races, and this would imply the need for a parallel study of untreated white syphilitics. There was no parallel study of white subjects, however, and it is hard to imagine that an analogous study of whites could have been undertaken or even contemplated.

On the other hand, the Tuskegee study continued for 40 years, during which the American racial environment changed significantly. In 1969, when CDC decided to continue the Tuskegee study, all of the following events had already taken place: the bus boycott in Montgomery led by Rosa Parks (1955); integration of Rich's department store in Atlanta by students (1960); the Freedom Riders (1961); integration of the University of Alabama in Tuscaloosa, despite Governor Wallace's posturing at the "schoolhouse door" (1963); discovery of the bodies of Cheney, Schwerner, and Goodman (1964); the Voting Rights Act (1965); the assassination of Martin Luther King, Jr. (1968); and riots in Watts and Washington, D.C. (1967 and 1968). In this different climate, it may not be clear to what extent the decision by CDC was influenced by racism. Another point to consider in this regard is that in 1969 the Macon County Medical Society, whose membership was mostly African American, did not object to the Tuskegee study and indeed cooperated with it.

Research Design

As has already been seen, the Tuskegee study was certainly not an example of good research design.

For instance, Kampmeier's justification of the Tuskegee research was based on a claim that untreated syphilitics fared no worse than syphilitics who were treated. A claim like this could be tested only through careful use of controls: that is, by comparing untreated subjects (an experimental group) with treated subjects (a control group). As noted earlier, the Tuskegee study originally started to follow 275 men with syphilis who had received a small number of arsphenamine injections and who might have served as a control group, but they were not reported on after 1936. Thus in the Tuskegee study the "controls" were actually the approximately 200 men who initially did *not* have syphilis at all. This means that the Tuskegee study could not compare treated and untreated syphilitics, and thus that it never learned—and never could have learned—anything about the effectiveness of treatment versus nontreatment.

It can be argued that, as a "study in nature," the Tuskegee research was not supposed to learn anything about treatment versus nontreatment but was simply intended to discover what happens as untreated syphilis runs its course. Even on these terms, though, it is not clear how the study can be justified. In studies in nature, controls of some kind are still needed, so that the researchers can be reasonably sure that what they observe over time in, say, untreated syphilitics would not also be found in treated syphilitics or in nonsyphilitics. Since after 1936 the Tuskegee study had no control group of treated subjects, it could learn nothing about the course of untreated syphilis as opposed to treated syphilis. And although it did have a "control group," of sorts, of people without syphilis, its handling of these "controls" seems to have been so questionable that it could not even have learned anything useful about untreated syphilitics as opposed to nonsyphilitics.

To begin with, recordkeeping was poor, records were often lost, and—as was mentioned earlier—the names of the syphilitic subjects were often confused with the "controls." Furthermore, the researchers assumed (naively, given the high rate of syphilis in Macon County) that the "controls" would remain unaffected; as it happened, though, many "controls" eventually contracted syphilis and had to be switched to the "subject" group. (Note that "controls" who became subjects in the "study in nature" group were also given no treatment by the researchers.)

Even the handling of the syphilitic subjects themselves was careless enough to cast any findings into doubt. During the course of the research, many of the 399 syphilitic subjects, who were supposed to remain untreated, actually did get some treatment—neosalvarsan or, later, penicillin—outside the study or outside Macon County. James Lucas, a CDC physician, said later that "effective and undocumented treatment had been given to the vast majority of patients in the syphilitic group,"[44] and that the value of the study was thus undermined. The researchers could not be sure which subjects had received such treatment and therefore could not drop them from the "study in nature" group. As a result, no one could know whether what was observed really represented the consequences of untreated syphilis.

In short, even as a "study in nature" the Tuskegee study proved nothing. Before the study began, it was already known that morbidity and mortality were higher for syphilitics than for nonsyphilitics and (from Boeck and Bruusgaard's research) that not all people with late latent syphilis would die of syphilis; the Tuskegee research added nothing to this existing knowledge.

As Lucas remarked, the Tuskegee study was "bad science." Anyone who wanted to argue that its subjects had been inadvertently "sacrificed to science" would have to acknowledge that the sacrifice was in vain: nothing of scientific value was gained.

Media Coverage

In defending the Tuskegee study, Kampmeier criticized the news media: in October 1972, he objected to the "great hue and cry" in the media a few months earlier, and to the journalists' claim that "treatment was purposefully withheld to evaluate the course of untreated disease." He said about *Time* and *AMA News* (later *American Medical News*): "In complete disregard of their abysmal ignorance, members of the fourth estate bang out anything on their typewriters that will make headlines."[45] Neither of Kampmeier's objections seems well-founded. Interestingly, though, the answer to his second objection suggests that the media did a better job than he said, while the answer to his first objection suggests that the media did a worse job.

To begin with the second objection, Kampmeier attacked the media for reporting the damaging aspects of the study, such as the withholding of treatment; but withholding treatment was indeed, and precisely, the intention of the study. Here it seems undeniable that the media reported the situation accurately.

With regard to the first objection, Kampmeier's description of a "hue and cry" seems exaggerated. Actually, in terms of how much of a hue and cry journalists did raise in 1972, how much they should have raised, and how much they would raise today, the media seem to have botched the story. Coverage shrank within days—in newspapers, the story moved to back pages, where it was covered in only short paragraphs—yet the Tuskegee study surely deserved more attention and analysis. The issues were complicated and involved racism, at a time when the United States was undergoing racial turmoil; today, such a story might receive weeks of nationwide scrutiny in print and on television.

The role of the professional media can also be questioned. Before Heller's story broke, the Tuskegee study had been reported routinely and repeatedly in medical journals: there were at least 17 articles between 1936 and 1972. In 1964, for instance, an article in *Archives of Internal Medicine* was titled, "The Tuskegee Study of Untreated Syphilis: The Thirtieth Year of Observation."[46] In other words, no attempt was made to conceal the study within the medical profession. Despite this, no professional publication or editor, and no physician, ever alerted the general media to the story.

Harm to Subjects

One of the most important ethical issues of the Tuskegee case has to do with whether the subjects were harmed. When we discuss whether, or how, the subjects of the Tuskegee study were harmed, it is important to be clear about counterfactual conditionals in philosophical discourse. A *counterfactual conditional* is a deceptively simple statement of the form "If X had not happened, then Y would not have happened," and it is *not* permissible in a logical argument.

For example, Kampmeier argued that if the Tuskegee "study in nature" had never been conducted at all, its subjects would still have received no treatment and therefore would have been no worse off. It is apparent why such a claim cannot be proved. In this case, an infinite number of other things might have happened if the Tuskegee study had not taken place as it did. Some local organization might have provided neosalvarsan (as the Rosenwald Foundation had originally intended). Somebody like John Steinbeck might have written a novel about Macon County, arousing national concern, as *The Grapes of Wrath* did about migrant workers; then, the pressure of public opinion might have led to a federal program to provide neosalvarsan or, later, penicillin—ironically, such treatment might well have been provided through USPHS.

The problem of counterfactual conditionals cuts both ways, however: we cannot say that if the Tuskegee study had *not* been conducted, the subjects would have received treatment and therefore would have been better off. Again, many other things might have happened: the subjects might not have received treatment from another source (this was Kampmeier's supposition); they might have failed to benefit if they did receive treatment; they might have been killed or disabled in combat during World War II (recall that the researchers prevented the subjects from being drafted); and so on.

Keeping the problem of counterfactuals in mind will be helpful as we consider harm in the context of the Tuskegee research.

Are spinal taps traumatic?   One issue of harm arises with regard to the spinal taps which many of the Tuskegee subjects were given. Some physicians regard spinal taps as an insignificant "harm," justified by the need to prove that neurosyphilis is present or absent; some of them would argue, further, that lying about such an insignificant procedure is not an enormous concern. It is understandable that from the perspective of physicians who constantly see devastating diseases and injuries, a spinal tap is not tremendously significant; physicians and researchers who deal continually with life-threatening heart attacks, terminal cancer, kidney failure, and psychotic self-mutilation may feel that only laypeople, who lack this kind of experience, would protest vehemently about spinal taps.

Patient advocates, on the other hand, emphasize that most physicians and researchers have never undergone a spinal tap themselves: that is, professionals who describe a spinal tap as "insignificant" are thinking in terms of administering a tap rather than receiving one. A spinal tap is not simply a minor procedure like taking a blood sample. Some patients, though admittedly only a small minority, will experience bad side effects, such as being unable to stand for a week without a severe headache; 1 in 1 million will become paralyzed. In December 1988, a malpractice suit brought against Medical Center Hospital of Vermont in behalf of a 28-year old woman who had gone into a coma after being incompetently "tapped" by a resident was settled out of court for $2.7 million.[47] "Tapping" someone involuntarily—i.e., without obtaining informed consent—is legally battery; and researchers who need healthy volunteers for spinal taps now offer as much as $500.

It is interesting to note, moreover, that paid volunteers may not be representative of the general population: many people would not undergo a nontherapeutic tap for $5,000 or even $10,000, and some would not do it for any amount. There is no reason to believe that people would have been any more likely to consent to a nontherapeutic tap at the time of the Tuskegee study in the 1930s.

Fundamentally, defenders of the Tuskegee study say that the spinal taps were not traumatic and that lack of consent was therefore not a serious issue. Its critics say that such an attitude was at the heart of the problem. Today, patient advocates argue that physicians can become blind to the needs and rights of people outside medicine. Physicians who are also researchers may be especially likely to develop such a blind spot, since they have a conflict of interest—they are torn between serving science and preserving the rights of patients and subjects.

Withholding treatment: Can "studies in nature" injure subjects?   A more general and more crucial ethical issue arises from the fact that the subjects in the Tuskegee study were not treated for syphilis: what harm, if any, resulted from nontreatment? This question might seem odd or even absurd; that is, it might seem obvious that since the subjects were left untreated, they must have been harmed. However, the issue may not be that simple, and according to some commentators—especially some physicians—there is no proof that the Tuskegee subjects were harmed by nontreatment.

At the outset of the study, when penicillin was not yet available, what was withheld from the subjects was heavy-metals treatment, particularly neosalvarsan. Neosalvarsan was expensive and cumbersome to administer; thus the subjects might not have received it even if they had not become part of a study based on nontreatment. (For one thing, as noted earlier, it required 20 to 40 injections over the course of 1 year; these cost $1 each, and during the depression, few Alabama sharecroppers could afford them.) Moreover, as we have seen with regard to Boeck and Bruusgaard's research, the benefits of heavy metals were controversial. Benedek, for instance, has reviewed the medical evidence available in 1940 and concluded that in 1937 untreated syphilitics had actually lived longer and in better condition than those who were partially treated with heavy metals.[48]

On the other hand, Benjamin Friedman points out, with regard to heavy metals:

In the 1940s it was known that patients receiving as few as 20 injections of arseni-
cals rarely developed symptomatic aortic disease. Since we could not determine
in advance which of the latent syphilitics would, after 20 or 30 years, develop
symptomatic aortic disease, it was necessary to treat all of them. One cannot
maintain that some small number of syphilitics deprived of treatment did not
therefore suffer injury.[49]

Furthermore, as early as 1934 the major professional organization of physicians
treating syphilis, the Cooperating Clinical Group, had demonstrated that use of
heavy metals improved Bruusgaard's statistics and had therefore recommended
neosalvarsan, mercury, and bismuth as therapy for all syphilitics.[50] Thus even if
many patients might not be able to afford such therapy—and even though many
might be expected to fail to complete the lengthy course of treatment—it would
certainly seem that all patients should at least have been informed about the recommended procedure.

Later in the study, of course, penicillin became available. An early form of
penicillin had been discovered by Alexander Fleming in 1929, though its value
was not appreciated until it was tested in 1941; as a result of wartime production, penicillin became generally available by 1946.[51] The implications of this
development with regard to harm in the Tuskegee study are disputed, however.

Kampmeier—who has argued in public what many physicians argue in private—believed that withholding penicillin had not been harmful, for several reasons. First, he called latent syphilis a "chronic, granulomatous, self-limiting disease," which would imply (as Boeck and Bruusgaard thought possible) that it
may not be devastating or fatal without treatment. Second (perhaps on the basis
of later or better information), he held that according to "incontrovertible evidence," the late manifestations of latent syphilis have occurred within 20 years
"in almost all instances": that is, with or without treatment. Third, he argued that
definitive proof of the effectiveness of penicillin was not published until 1948—
and this proof was only for primary syphilis, not for the secondary or tertiary
phase. What his second and third arguments would imply is that by the time
penicillin became available as a proven therapy, the Tuskegee subjects (who originally had latent, or secondary, syphilis) could no longer have been helped by it;
the damage of syphilis had already been done.[52]

Benedek argues similarly with regard to aortic disease (which, interestingly,
is more frequent among African American than white syphilitics). According to
Benedek, aortic disease occurs in only 10 percent of untreated syphilitics and
begins 15 to 20 years after the initial infection—after which it does its permanent
structural damage. He cites as an example 70 syphilitic subjects who were examined in 1948, when all of them had had syphilis for at least 18 years, and implies
that penicillin would most likely have been ineffective for them, since it would
not have reversed such damage. Benedek maintains that giving penicillin to
latent syphilitics in the 1940s "might have exerted a definitely beneficial effect on
the prognosis of only 12.5 percent of the subjects." He notes, further, that virtually all the syphilitic subjects of the Tuskegee study who were alive in 1973 had
outlived the nonsyphilitic "controls." Benedek concludes:

The Tuskegee study had been in progress for 12 years when the possibility of dramatic improvement of treatment appeared, for 16 years when new insights into the ethical implications of research began to be advocated, and was 39 years old when it abruptly became the subject of severe criticism for ethical deficiencies. . . . The righteousness of the ethical critics fails to take into account that in the context of the 1930s thoughtful physicians could detect no ethical dilemma in an investigation such as the Tuskegee study, and also refuses to accept the evidence that very little would have been accomplished therapeutically by initiating penicillin treatment in the 1950s.

Some defenders of the Tuskegee study have pointed to Erlich's experience in 1910, when the hoped-for "magic bullet" had turned out to be unreliable, sometimes simply missing its target and sometimes hitting the wrong target and killing the patient. In the early 1940s, who could be sure that penicillin might not be another disappointment? Benedek emphasizes that physicians in the 1940s did not know optimal dosages of penicillin and had no way to determine at that point whether or not penicillin would have any effect on long-term syphilis. (Kampmeier went further; in 1974, he said, dramatically, "Today—26 years later—we know no more about the effectiveness or ineffectiveness of penicillin in late latent syphilis than in 1948."[53]) These commentators are saying, in effect, that hindsight is always 20/20: at the time, the picture was less clear.

However, as regards penicillin most physicians disagree with claims such as Kampmeier's. His argument that it was not proven effective until 1948 is especially weak. As Friedman notes, "Penicillin replaced all the [heavy-metal treatments] and was available in adequate doses after 1946. . . . After Mohoney's studies in 1943 it became apparent that penicillin in adequate dosages was effective" for early syphilis. Also, the prophylactic effect of penicillin on latent syphilis was expected and has been proven: "The progressive decline in syphilitic heart disease since 1930 from the fourth highest cause of heart disease to almost total disappearance is strong indirect evidence that penicillin has a preventive effect." It can also be added that Benedek's estimate of how many subjects might have been helped by penicillin in the 1940s—12.5 percent—is hardly a negligible figure.

Practically speaking, though, it would be difficult or even impossible to prove conclusively that syphilitics are harmed by not getting penicillin and thus that the Tuskegee subjects were harmed. The reason why such proof is lacking is that since the introduction of penicillin, everyone with syphilis has been treated with it. To obtain proof *now* that withholding penicillin is harmful, it would be necessary to set up a study comparing an experimental group and a control group—that is, comparing treated and untreated syphilitics. In other words, to *prove* that the Tuskegee study was harmful or unethical, another harmful, unethical study would have to be done.

What can we conclude, then, about harm in this case? First, from a moral standpoint it may not be necessary to prove absolutely that the Tuskegee subjects were harmed by being left untreated (this point is discussed further below). In other words, the study cannot be excused simply by saying—as CDC tried to say—that it can't be proved to have harmed anyone. It may have been only a matter of luck for the researchers that the study caused no more harm than it did.

Second, a crucial point about harm is that when penicillin became available, *it should have been hypothesized that penicillin might help subjects with latent syphilis.* For all anyone knew at the time, penicillin could have prevented lethal aortic heart disease. At the very least, therefore, the originally untreated latent syphilitics should have been divided into two groups, one of which would receive penicillin. After penicillin became available—and everyone else with syphilis was getting it—continuing to withhold it from the Tuskegee subjects was tantamount to using them as involuntary, unknowing "controls" for the rest of the nation.

Effects on subjects' families   To critics of the Tuskegee study, one especially troubling aspect of the issue of harm is that no effort was made to survey syphilis in the subjects' families—their wives and children. Benedek read correspondence in the National Library of Medicine and discovered that "virtually all subjects were or had been married" and that the subjects had an average of 5.2 children. Keep in mind, moreover, that the researchers' disregard of families took place in a county where the rate of congenital syphilis was 62 percent.

When we consider the subjects' families, another disturbing issue is the fact that the 399 subjects were not told they had syphilis. Wouldn't the husbands in the study want to know that they had syphilis? Even if they were originally in the latent stage, wouldn't they need to know that they might become infectious again—that they might then infect their wives and thus give future children congenital syphilis? Did the researchers withhold the truth because they accepted the racist myth that African American men couldn't refrain from sex?

Today, we know that late syphilis is almost never reinfectious; but when the Tuskegee researchers began their study, over 60 years ago, they did not know this. These researchers thus simply took a chance with the wives and children of their subjects. Either the researchers failed to consider possible harm to the subjects' families, or they decided that possible harm didn't matter compared with the goal of the "study in nature."

Motives of Researchers

When the Tuskegee study was debated within USPHS and CDC, many physicians and administrators assumed that if no harm could be proved, nothing immoral had been done; this is also one basis of Kampmeier's argument. Focusing on consequences, however, is only one way of judging morality. Another way—and in this case perhaps a more appropriate way—is to focus on *motives* or *intentions.*

It is important to understand that in medical research, "provable harm" is a very self-serving standard. To see why this is so, consider that physicians and medical researchers seldom want to be held to the analogous standard of "provable benefit": they typically argue that "benefit" needs to be no more than "likely," "probable," or even "possible." This argument, moreover, is perfectly reasonable. Suppose, for instance, that no treatment were reimbursable unless its benefit to patients had been conclusively proved. Since it is estimated that as much as one-third of all medical practices are scientifically unproven, much of medicine would then have to be free. (Here is one example: though the cost of hospital care is much higher in ICUs than in normal rooms, there is no proof that patients do better in ICUs.) But this reasonable argument about benefits would seem to apply equally to harm—and if it does, "provable" harm would not be a necessary or fair criterion.

As with benefit, then, a better criterion may be likely, probable, or possible harm. If we adopt such a standard, we do not ultimately need to prove that harm has been done; instead, we may consider motives or intentions in light of whether harm was likely. From this point of view, it should be emphasized that people do not exist to serve medical science. Human beings—of any race, rich or poor, sick or well, educated or uneducated—have a right to control their bodies and their medical treatment without risk of harm from researchers.

To argue that the Tuskegee researchers acted immorally in terms of motivation, then, we do not necessarily have to claim that they were motivated by racism or malice or even self-interest. They may have been motivated, primarily, simply to conduct a study in nature and thereby learn something. The point is that, given a likelihood of harm, they should also have been motivated to protect their subjects. In other words, since harm was possible, their motivations should have included an intention not to do harm. Instead, through systematic deceit and nontreatment, these researchers put their subjects at risk of harm, depriving them of their rights.

UPDATE

IRBs

In 1972, the federal government required all institutions that conducted human medical experimentation and received federal funds to have Institutional Review Boards (IRBs). The original function of IRBs was to review proposals for medical research before these experiments were evaluated for funding; later on, IRB reviews were expanded to cover research on humans in the social sciences. Today, IRBs—which scrutinize written proposals—are the formal line of defense against abuses in medical research.

Before the criticisms by Beecher and Pappworth in the 1960s and the revelation of the Tuskegee study in 1972, support for outside review of medical research (IRBs), or for peer review, was lukewarm. Afterward, however, medical research was forced to operate under quasi regulation in a multistage process. (As discussed in Chapter 8, after Gennarelli's animal studies were revealed similar quasi regulation came to animal research.)

Later Analyses of Tuskegee

James Jones, the author of *Bad Blood*, later found many documents that had been filed by the Tuskegee researchers. *Bad Blood* was published in 1981, 9 years after Heller's first story and 49 years after the Tuskegee study had begun.

In the 1990s, the Tuskegee study attracted renewed interest. In 1992, Sidney Olansky, then age 78 and practicing in Atlanta as a dermatologist, was interviewed on the television show *Prime Time Live*. Olansky had been in charge of the

Tuskegee study in 1951 and had been at the CDC meeting which decided to continue the Tuskegee research in 1969. He supported Kampmeier's defense of the study and—like Kampmeier—did not believe that anyone could be proved to have been harmed by the study. In fact, like almost all the physicians who have ever been interviewed about the study, even in 1992 he did not believe that anything unethical was done. After the interview was broadcast, Olansky was upset by the reaction. "They made me look like a mad scientist and a bigot," he said.[54] Leaflets were distributed around his office building, urging his patients to "stop Olansky"; he received hate mail and a telephone call from a woman in California calling him a "murderer." Olansky's son David, also a physician (the two were in practice together), observed about his father, "These are very proud men. They know their intentions were good and they can't accept people questioning that. There's so much ego involved in medicine. They just can't admit that their methods, in retrospect, might have been wrong."[55]

Also in 1992, on a special *Nova* broadcast devoted to the Tuskegee study, some of the other Tuskegee physicians echoed Olansky's sentiments.[56] They did admit that nothing was learned from the study, but they refused to admit that they had done anything wrong. Among the people quoted by *Nova* in defense of the study were John Cutler, who had harangued Peter Buxtun at the CDC syphilis conference in 1966; and David Sencer, who had been a director of CDC and had convened the 1969 meeting.

During the early 1990s, *Miss Ever's Boys*, a play about the Tuskegee study written by the physician David Feldshuh, became popular around the country. Feldshuh's drama placed the study in its historical context and emphasized the deliberate omission of penicillin, the nontherapeutic spinal taps, and the "benign" deception. In 1992, *Miss Ever's Boys* was produced at the Alabama Shakespeare Festival in Montgomery and was given a special one-night performance in nearby Tuskegee, at which four survivors of the Tuskegee study were present.

Some months after Olansky had been interviewed on *Prime Time Live*, a replay was seen by the most famous of the Tuskegee survivors, Charles Pollard, who remarked: "I don't think I'd have anything to say to that man. I think I'd hit him in the face."

Secret Nuclear Medical Experiments: A Parallel Episode?

In 1994, Hazel O'Leary, Secretary of the Department of Energy, began to declassify 32 million pages of secret documents about research on nuclear energy by the federal government during World War II and through the "cold war." Among the initial findings was the revelation that physicians working for the government had used many Americans as human guinea pigs in radiation experiments.

The purpose of these experiments was to study effects of exposure to radiation in order to determine safe levels of exposure for workers in programs such as the Manhattan Project (which developed the first atom bomb). In one experiment, about 130 male prisoners, most of whom were African American, were paid $200 to undergo x-ray radiation of their testicles; afterward, these men got vasectomies. In another, an indigent 36-year-old Texan who had injured a leg was given a shot of plutonium in the injured leg, which was then amputated. In 1945,

Eda Charlton, a woman who had entered Strong Memorial Hospital in Rochester, New York, with a mild case of hepatitis, was secretly injected with plutonium-239 to study how the body eliminates radiation and then was followed for years so that the effects could be observed (she died of a heart attack in 1983).

During the 1940s, many researchers seemed to have been enthralled with radiation. Joseph Hamilton of the University of California at Berkeley, for example, injected plutonium into 18 unsuspecting patients diagnosed with cancer (3 of these patients were at the University of California–San Francisco). According to Kenneth Scott, a scientist who later investigated abuses, two patients had actually been mistakenly diagnosed but nevertheless were given "many times the so-called lethal textbook dose of plutonium."[57]

From the 1940s until the 1960s, as many as 1,500 military aviators and members of submarine crews were given radium "treatments" like the procedure used with three former aviators, who were exposed to encapsulated radium on the end of wires inserted high into their nostrils for several minutes and who were not told why they had been selected or what the purpose of the experiment was. At the time, some of these men complained of developing intense headaches immediately after exposure: "I went out of my mind," one subject said.[58]

There were also studies of radioactive isotopes used in diagnosis and research. (The Veterans Administration was a pioneer in using such radioisotopes to diagnose thyroid disease, brain tumors, and leukemia.) In the late 1940s, at Vanderbilt University, 819 pregnant women were injected with radioactive iron as part of a nutritional study; a follow-up study in 1960 found that 3 of their children had died of rare forms of cancer.[59]

Another disturbing study was the Green Run experiment, which took place around 1950: federal scientists deliberately released a cloud of radioactive iodine-131 in eastern Washington state to see how far downwind it would get. The cloud reached Spokane and the California-Oregon border, carrying hundreds (perhaps thousands) of times more radiation than was emitted by the accident in 1979 at the Three Mile Island nuclear reactor.

It was also revealed that the Department of Energy had conducted about 200 more secret underground nuclear tests from about 1945 to 1969 than it had acknowledged, probably subjecting people in surrounding areas to much higher levels of radiation than the government had previously admitted.

Physicists who had worked on nuclear energy at the time would later defend the experiments, arguing that such research was justified by necessities of the world war and the postwar period.[60] However, after studying 31 experiments dating back to 1945, Representative Edward Markey of Massachusetts wrote that American citizens had become "nuclear calibration devices for experimenters run amok."[61]

FURTHER READING

Thomas Benedek, "The 'Tuskegee Study' of Untreated Syphilis: Analysis of Moral Aspects versus Methodological Aspects," *Journal of Chronic Diseases*, vol. 31, 1978.
James Jones, *Bad Blood*, Free Press, New York, 1981.

CHAPTER 10

Organ Transplants

Christiaan Barnard and the First Heart Transplant

When Christiaan Barnard performed the first heart transplant in 1967, new ethical questions arose—questions about whether a heart donor was really dead, about whether transplant surgeons had conflicts of interest, about quality of life, and about burdens on families. This chapter discusses this pioneering case in surgery and the ethical issues it raised.

BACKGROUND: THE PATH TOWARD TRANSPLANTS

Early attempts to transplant human organs involved the skin (which is technically an organ), and Indian doctors transplanted skin as early as the year 600 before the Common Era (B.C.E.)[1] In the sixteenth century of the Common Era (C.E), Tagliacozzi, an Italian, transplanted skin tissue and recognized that the body rejected tissue from other bodies. In the same century, physicians successfully reattached noses and ears severed in duels, but only onto the original victim—never successfully onto another person. Lamb blood was also transfused into humans in the sixteenth century, but with miserable results; during the nineteenth century, England and several other countries banned blood transfusion.

In 1900, an Austrian physiologist, Karl Lansteiner, found that human red blood cells exist as distinct types, and this discovery explained in part why most early attempts at transplants had failed. Lansteiner used letters of the alphabet arbitrarily to designate blood groups: A, B, AB, and O. Type B blood contains antibodies that attack protein markers in A blood, and type A blood contains antibodies that attack protein markers in B blood. However, type AB blood is compatible with either A or B (because it "recognizes" itself in either). Curiously, A, B, and AB all accept type O blood, though O accepts only O; people with type O blood are thus universal donors. Landsteiner's monumental discovery went unappreciated for 30 years, until he finally received the Nobel prize in 1930.

In 1953, Peter Medawar discovered protein markers, or *antigens*, on the surface of cells and found that white blood cells (called *T-lymphocytes*) recognize foreign antigens and then signal antibodies to attack. (In AIDS, a virus burrows inside T-lymphocytes and takes them over, destroying the body's ability to recognize foreign substances.) Highly specific antibodies develop against highly specific antigens. Medawar's work stimulated research on how the immune system works, and on how to suppress it so that transplanted organs would not be rejected. Progress in this direction was difficult, however. Medawar's work can be seen as the base of a pyramid whose apex, today, is routine organ transplantation. In building that pyramid, perhaps the most difficult part was overturning perceived or accepted "truths" (this was also true of in vitro fertilization, discussed in Chapter 4). For example, antibodies had been thought to mediate the immune system, but they do not; most important, research eventually showed that rejection was not a progressive, unstoppable process.

The technological key to the first transplant was the heart-lung machine, developed between 1931 and 1953 by the surgeon John Gibbon and further improved in the early 1960s. (In fact, the heart-lung machine opened a door not only for heart surgery but also for actual replacement of the "pump.") Before the heart-lung machine was devised, the few operations that could be done at all had to be done in 1 minute, while the heart was stopped and the brain was without oxygenated blood. Early versions of heart-lung machines were problematic because blood clots formed on their surfaces (which were made of a synthetic substance, Mylar). In a later version, air bubbles supplied the blood with oxygen and were removed by a greasy foam; but if the bubbles were not removed, or if the debubbling mixture returned to the blood, the patient would die. The slightest mishap with the heart-lung machine—an electrical failure, a leak, contamination—turned the machine into a killer.[2]

An important figure on the path toward heart transplants was the surgeon Owen Wangansteen, under whom Christiaan Barnard would study. Wangansteen was the mentor of most American transplant surgeons; three modern pioneers of heart surgery—Michael DeBakey, Norman Shumway, and John Kirklin—also studied with him. As a medical student, DeBakey devised a booster pump which became the essence of the heart-lung machine and which made open-heart surgery possible in the 1960s. Shumway was to discover that cardiac nerve connections, which are severed during transplantation but are too numerous and too fine to be reconnected, didn't actually matter because the heart has an independent electrical "ignition" that triggers its beats and rate. He would also find that it was better not to transplant a whole heart but instead to leave the upper walls (atrium or auricles) intact, thereby reducing operating time by half. Kirklin would later perfect cardiac surgery for congenital defects and would found the Kirklin Clinic in Birmingham, Alabama.

THE FIRST HEART TRANSPLANT

The Surgeon: Christiaan Barnard

Christiaan Barnard, a South African surgeon, was 44 years old on December 3, 1967, when he achieved international fame by transplanting the heart of a 25-year-old woman into the body of a dying 55-year-old man.

In many ways, Barnard was a stereotypical surgeon: brusque, driven, and given to offending nurses, colleagues, and staff members. He has been described as cold and moody, and—by Phillip Blaiberg, the recipient of his second heart transplant—as having the "personality of a genius"[3] (though, interestingly, Blaiberg said that the cardiologist Velva Shrire was the "brains behind the transplant team"). Owen Wangansteen, with whom Barnard studied in the United States, remembers him as lean, nervous, hardworking, intense, and constantly smoking other people's cigarettes. Barnard's first wife, Louwtjie, said that he was a perfectionist at home, unable even to watch meat being cut sloppily at dinner. His relationship with his daughter Deirdre seems to have typified his personality: she was a good water-skier, and Barnard expected nothing less of her than a world championship; he relates in his autobiography, *One Life,* that he drove her ruthlessly and spent all his free time with her.[4] Deirdre did become a South African champion, but after she had several accidents it became clear that she would never be a world champion; Barnard then forced himself to stop living through her and seek fame for himself.

•

Barnard was born in 1923 and grew up in a rural sheep-farming area of South Africa. In the town where his family lived, two Dutch Reformed churches stood side by side, one for whites and the other for "coloreds"; his father was the minister of the "colored" church. The Barnards were therefore of low social status, and also poor: his father was paid only one-third as much as the minister of the white church. Young Chris is said to have played football barefoot when his teammates all had shoes.

Barnard was able to attend college, however, and to obtain European-style medical training. He then joined a practice in Ceres, a wine-growing area, from 1948 to 1951, as the second junior partner of an elderly family physician. According to his own account, he was forced out because patients began to favor him over the older man. He next went to City Hospital in Cape Town as senior surgical resident from 1951 to 1953. He received his M.D. in 1953.

In Cape Town, Barnard began to study bowel obstructions, operating experimentally on 49 dogs before he was successful with the fiftieth. He applied for a prestigious scholarship, but he did not win, and the winner privately gave him a troubling analysis: Barnard, the winner said, hadn't had a real chance at the scholarship because his children (he had been married in 1948 and had two daughters) went to an English-language rather than an Afrikaans school; the theory was that this gave the family more of an option to leave South Africa. As it happened, losing this scholarship did leave Barnard free, in 1955, to accept an offer to study at the University of Minnesota Medical School under the pioneering surgeon Owen Wangansteen. Barnard, ambitious and dedicated, jumped at the chance, despite the opposition of his family.

Barnard's 2 years with Wangansteen in Minnesota (in Minneapolis–St. Paul) were not easy. For one thing, he lived in poverty there—South African physicians did not have anything like the income of American physicians. He shocked his colleagues by working as a night nurse and doing menial jobs for people in his neighborhood to earn enough to bring his family to the United States. Then, when he did succeed in bringing his family over, his wife hated the United

States: she found American racial attitudes puzzling and hypocritical, feared violence, and (like Barnard himself) detested the cold winters. She and their children soon returned home. Also, Barnard had a heavy work load: he had to work under Wangansteen during the day while serving as an attending assistant physician and studying pathology and German at night. Moreover, in South Africa he had already been a surgeon, so he resented being treated as a medical student, though he swallowed his pride. During this time, too, he developed arthritis, a devastating occupational handicap for a surgeon; other physicians might have switched to another specialty, but Barnard persevered.

During his studies in Minnesota, Barnard and two other surgeons-in-training would drive on Saturdays to the Mayo Clinic in Rochester, where Barnard learned from John Kirklin how to close a defect in a ventricle without causing a heart blockage. Barnard also studied hard to learn how to operate a heart-lung machine; and he spent a week with the cardiac surgeons Michael DeBakey and Denton Cooley in Texas. (Cooley impressed Barnard. Where Kirklin and DeBakey were methodical, quantitative, and cognitive, Cooley was brash and intuitive; other surgeons would open a femoral artery by slicing away piece by piece, whereas Cooley would confidently make one decisive cut; others took 3 hours for a cardiac operation, but Cooley took only 1.)

In his autobiography, Barnard describes a professional disaster during his time in Minnesota, a cognitive mistake which illustrates the frailty of heart technology at that time and which actually took place while the patient's father was watching. Operating on a 7-year-old boy to repair a heart defect, Barnard ordered an assistant to cut a bit of tissue protruding from the vena cava.[5] When it was cut, a hole ripped open in the heart wall and blood gushed up. Barnard panicked and, rather than simply putting his finger in the hole to stem the loss of blood (the correct procedure, as he learned later), he tried to clamp the hole shut. This only enlarged the hole even more; the boy's blood pressure dropped rapidly from 85, to 65, . . . to 42; then his heart stopped. The surgeons immediately connected the heart-lung machine and repaired the damaged wall, but they could not restart the boy's heart.

Barnard completed a 6-year course of study at the University of Minnesota in 2 years, earning a doctorate in surgery. In 1958, when the doctorate was awarded, he returned to South Africa as director of surgical research at University of Cape Town Medical School. There, from 1958 to 1967, he did research on diseased heart valves and on replacing them with artificial valves; in 1960, he attracted international attention by transplanting a second head onto a dog. Over several years, he made six more trips abroad, and by 1965 he had obtained the best and most advanced training available in surgical research. (He always said that he had learned most from American surgeons.)

By 1966, everyone realized that the real difficulty in performing a heart transplant lay not in the surgery but in getting the new heart to be accepted, so in late 1966 and early 1967 Barnard spent 3 months training under the transplant surgeon David Hume in Richmond, Virginia; there he learned what little was then known about immunosuppressive agents.

•

In 1967, Barnard returned to South Africa with a new heart-lung machine; the $6,000 grant for its purchase had been arranged by Owen Wangansteen through contacts in Washington, D.C. Did Wangansteen expect Barnard to perform the first heart transplant? It seems not. As Barnard himself said, Wangansteen treated him as a student, not as a surgical colleague. Another transplant surgeon, Thomas Starzl, says in his own memoirs that everyone expected Barnard to start doing kidney transplants rather than a heart transplant.[6] (Barnard did perform a kidney transplant in 1967 and wanted to do another, but then became intrigued by the possibility of a heart transplant.) On the other hand, the transplant surgeon Donald Kahn of Birmingham, Alabama, a friend of Barnard's, believes that Norman Shumway and others implicitly gave Barnard permission to attempt the first heart transplant.[7] Most probably, though, no one really thought that a heart transplant would be attempted until the problem of immune rejection had been solved.

The Patient and the Donor

This first heart transplant was not performed, as might have been expected, at a prestigious center of medical research; it took place at an obscure hospital in Cape Town, South Africa, called Groote Schuur—"big barn" in Afrikaans. Groote Schuur was associated with the University of Cape Town Medical School; set deep into the slope of a mountain above Cape Town, the hospital was a landmark visible from all over the city. It looked like a resort hotel, with even-spaced windows and double wings and an ancient forest on both sides. Ambulances brought patients from the city to either of two entrances—one for whites, one for nonwhites. Barnard had quietly begun to assemble a team at Groote Schuur to perform the first human heart transplant. He did set up the best organ-transplant team outside the United States; even so, however, facilities at Groote Schuur were much more primitive than at American transplant centers. Other physicians at Groote Schuur were close-mouthed about Barnard's plans, and no American hospitals were informed.

•

Barnard had asked the cardiologists at Groote Schuur to refer to him a possible candidate for a heart transplant. He approached Velva Shrire (his superior, the chief cardiologist at Groote Schuur) and obtained permission for the transplant; Shrire also gave him the name of a patient—Louis Washkansky, 55 years old and dying. Louis Washkansky was white, a salesman with a fondness for playing cards, drinking, eating, smoking, and in general living life fully. As a young man, he had been athletic (a weightlifter and an amateur boxer); during World War II, he had served in the army. He was a big, intelligent man with a ferocious desire to live, exuberant, extroverted, and well-liked. He was married and was a macho type, pretending to his wife that everything was fine, snitching cigarettes, never slowing down, flirting with nurses.

Louis Washkansky was about as sick as a cardiac patient can be and still live. He had diabetes, coronary artery disease, and congestive heart failure; his flabby heart was so swollen that it extended across the entire inside of his large chest, from wall to wall. Washkansky had first been hospitalized in 1965: he felt an attack coming on, got to the hospital an hour later, and climbed the stairs to the cardiac unit—where his heart collapsed. He could not breathe at night and was kept breathing with drugs. In April 1966, he was diagnosed as in terminal cardiac failure and given only a month or two to live.

In October 1967, amazingly, he was still alive. He was deteriorating, though: he needed to take 15 pills a day; and at one point, in September 1967, he had developed so much edema (swelling from fluids) in his legs that drainage holes had to be opened. He then spent 5 days without sleep, sitting in a chair with water running down his legs into basins. His skin was almost black from lack of epidermal circulation. It was about at this point that he was referred to Christiaan Barnard.

When he was approached about the transplant, Louis Washkansky did not hesitate. He knew he was dying, and his life had been hellish for 2 years. Barnard said that he told his patient, "We can put a normal heart into you, after taking out your heart that's no longer good, and there's a chance you can get back to normal life"—and that Louis Washkansky replied, "So they told me. So I'm ready to go ahead."[8]

After obtaining this consent, Barnard waited 3 weeks for a donor. Meanwhile, the patient developed fulminant pulmonary edema—a sign of imminent death—and Barnard was afraid that his chance to perform the first heart transplant would pass. This had happened to other surgeons: two patients of James Hardy in Mississippi, for instance, had died before donors could be found.

•

On the afternoon of December 2, 1967—a Saturday—25-year-old Denise Ann Darvall left her home, driving in a car with her brother, father, and mother. After parking the car, Denise and her mother walked a few blocks to a bakery, which was half a mile below Groote Schuur Hospital. A few minutes later, Ann Washkansky, Louis's wife, on the way up the mountain to visit him at the hospital, saw a crowd gathered at the scene of an automobile accident.

The accident had occurred without warning, when Denise Darvall and her mother left the bakery. A speeding car smashed into the mother, killing her instantly and throwing her against her daughter. Denise herself had been thrown through the air and killed on impact, but she was rushed up to Groote Schuur Hospital; though she was brain-dead, her heart was still healthy.

Shortly after Denise's arrival at the hospital, Barnard spoke to her shocked father, Edward Darvall. At a moment like this, everything depends on people's trust in the medical profession: Edward Darvall, who had just learned of the death of his wife and daughter, also had to accept Barnard's right to ask a very delicate, sensitive question. When Barnard approached Edward Darvall, he said, "We have a man in the hospital here, and we can save his life if you give us permission to use your daughter's heart. . . ." According to Barnard, Edward Darvall replied simply, "If you can't save my daughter, try and save this man."[9]

The Operation

The operation took place during the early hours of December 3, 1967. As we've seen, Louis Washkansky had already been told about, and consented to, a possible transplant. Within 2 minutes of being informed that a donor had become available, he reaffirmed his consent. Blood typing was done (Denise Darvall was type O, a universal donor; Washkansky was type A). Calls went out to the transplant team; as the story is told, some of the team members arrived at the hospital in pajamas, and some were breathless because their car had broken down and they had run up the mountain to Groote Schuur.

As he was rolled into surgery, Louis Washkansky was still awake. For the first time, he felt "kind of shaky," like a person "going into the ring when you don't know who you're up against." He said that Barnard, as his surgeon, was his manager, but now he wanted to know what his opponent looked like. Barnard says that, though he told his patient nothing, he thought to himself, "I knew what [his opponent] looked like. He was the Skoppensboer—the wild Jack of Spades. He was death and against him I had only the King of Hearts."[10]

Denise Darvall was declared dead after her heart had actually stopped beating; surgeons then opened her body, preparing it for Barnard's excision of the heart. Meanwhile, in an adjacent room, in preparation of the excision of *his* heart, Washkansky was anesthetized, given drugs to produce paralysis and prevent spontaneous breathing, and placed on the heart-lung machine. The two operations that were about to take place had to be precisely coordinated.

At this point, everything almost failed. Washkansky's femoral artery, where a tube was attached, was so narrow from buildup of cholesterol that the machine couldn't force blood into his heart. The pressure on the tube climbed to 290, just below the point where the lines would blow, spilling gallons of blood over the room. Frantically, Barnard and other surgeons reattached the line directly to Washkansky's aorta, and gradually the pressure dropped.

Barnard then walked to the next room and excised Denise Darvall's heart, leaving part of the wall attached to it like the lid of a jack-o-lantern. He put her heart into a basin of chilled fluid and walked 31 steps back to Washkansky's operating room, where he gave it to a nurse to hold.

Then, Barnard cut out Washkansky's flabby heart. (As he peered down into Washkansky's huge, empty chest cavity and looked at the two hearts, he said, "This really is the point of no return."[11]) Next, he sewed the Denise Darvall's heart (with the attached wall) into Louis Washkansky's chest, where it looked quite small.

The two operations had taken 5 hours, but cardiac surgeons regarded the surgery itself—the cutting out of the patient's own heart and the transplantation of the donated heart—as relatively simple. The interesting questions were, first, whether the transplanted heart would start beating in a foreign body; and if it did start beating, whether it would then be rejected.

The operation team therefore watched expectantly, hoping that the transplanted heart would simply start beating spontaneously as the patient's blood temperature rose to normal. This did not happen in Washkansky's case (though it would happen, later, with the second transplant patient); and reports differ about what took place next. According to United Press International (UPI), the transplanted heart began to beat after Barnard shocked it slightly, whereupon Barnard gasped, "Christ, it's going to work!"[12]—one surgeon at the operation described this effect as "like turning the ignition switch of a car."[13] But according to Barnard's own account, things were not so easy. A human heart does not always start beating when shocked; and Barnard says that although Louis Washkansky's new heart did start and continue to beat after the first shock, it then stopped. Moreover, at first the new heart didn't take over from the heart-lung machine. Thus it was only after another attempt that the new heart began to beat regularly, whereupon the patient was quickly weaned from the heart-lung machine, which was then turned off.[14]

The Postoperative Period

After working all night, the surgeons had finished the operation at 7 A.M. on December 3. An hour later, Louis Washkansky regained consciousness and tried to talk. Thirty-six hours later, a hungry Washkansky ate a soft-boiled egg and toast.

Louis Washkansky was encouraged to eat—to get protein into his system— but his recovery progressed slowly. He had 5 rough days immediately after surgery, when his urine output, enzymes, and heart rate were problematic. Also, worried about immunological rejection of the heart, Barnard's team flooded Washkansky with gamma ray radiation from a cobalt unit and administered both prednisone and Immuran (azathoprine), and the patient did not tolerate these treatments well. By day 5, he said, the constant tests were "killing me. I can't sleep. I can't do anything. They're at me all the time with pins and needles. . . . It's driving me crazy."[15]

On the sixth day, though, Louis Washkansky received steroids to prevent rejection of the heart; this began 5 very good, happy days when he laughed, visited with his family, and wanted to go home. At this time, Barnard told a press conference that if his patient's progress held, he would "have him home in 3 weeks."[16]

In retrospect, however, these 5 good days were the eye of the hurricane, merely a brief period before Louis Washkansky's body really began to reject his new heart. As this rejection process went on, he began to feel, as he said, "terrible": he suffered from constant pain in the shoulders; dark circles formed under his eyes; his heart and breathing rates climbed; on the thirteenth day, a shadow of unknown origin could be seen on his lung x-ray. Moreover, his personality changed: this vibrant, forceful man became sullen and irritable. In addition to the threat of rejection, there was also a danger of infection. Unfortunately, most post-transplant symptoms can indicate either rejection or infection, and treatment of one problem can exacerbate the other. It was therefore necessary to wait for a definitive diagnosis, even if the delay entailed a risk of death.

By the fourteenth day after the operation, Louis Washkansky felt that he was dying. He couldn't force himself to eat. He had lost bowel control. He had such severe pain in his chest that he preferred to lie in his own feces rather than try to move. Barnard said that he was "constrained" to insert a nasogastric tube in order to feed his patient, but Washkansky didn't want it. To Washkansky, it didn't look as though he would ever be normal again; he had lost his dignity and hence his will to live.

By day 15—December 18—there were spotty, mottled patches on Louis Washkansy's legs, indicating circulatory failure. He was breathing with difficulty, and x-rays showed that the patches on his lung had grown ominously larger. As

Washkansky gasped desperately for each breath, Barnard decided that he should be placed on a respirator. Washkansky resisted this: he had been on the respirator when he first woke up after the operation, and he knew that reconnecting it would mean giving up speech; and in any case he continued to feel that he was near his end. Barnard disagreed; on December 18, he told Washkansky that there was "a chance" to be home by Christmas. Washkansky replied, "No, not now." His bed was in a sterile tent, and despite his extreme weakness, he grabbed the sides of the tent in an attempt to prevent Barnard from entering to reopen his tracheotomy hole.

As Barnard entered, Washkansky persisted in refusing, saying, "No, Doc."

Barnard replied, "Yes, Louis,"[17] and put him on the respirator. Washkansky would never speak again.

On December 19 or 20—day 16 or 17—Ann Washkansky called, telling Barnard that reporters were saying Louis was dying. Barnard lied to her and said that the reporters were lying. (Both Barnard and Washkansky saw Ann Washkansky as weak and unable to bear the truth.) New x-rays now showed that bilateral pneumonia, klebsiella, and pseudomonas had infiltrated Washkansky's lungs. Penicillin had been administered earlier, but though it had killed one organism, it had allowed others to grow. The anti-immune drugs given to suppress rejection had also allowed all these organisms to flourish.

On December 20—day 17—Ann Washkansky was allowed to see Louis, but she wasn't told it might be the last time. Barnard urged her to encourage her husband to keep fighting. Louis Washkansky, now on the respirator, couldn't speak, and his wife didn't understand why. She was told not to touch him because of germs. All Louis Washkansky himself could do at this last visit was, with enormous effort, open his eyes and move his arm a bit.

After his wife had left, the patient received 40 percent oxygen; then, as his breathing continued to worsen, this was increased to 100 percent. Between midnight of day 17 and 1 A.M. of day 18, the physicians gave him drugs to help his breathing, but it was too late: germs had overrun his lungs. Louis Washkansky began to suffocate.

After 2 hours of Louis Washkansky's dying gasps, Denise Darvall's heart went into wild fibrillation from lack of oxygen and stopped beating. Even then, Barnard was not ready to give up; he rushed a team together to put Washkansky on a heart-lung machine. At this point, another physician challenged him, arguing passionately that it was "madness" to continue and that Washkansky was "clinically lost." Reluctantly, Barnard agreed. At 6:30 A.M. on December 21, after having lived 18 days with a transplanted heart, Louis Washkansky died.

The next morning, Barnard watched the postmortem, which showed that lobar pneumonia had destroyed the lungs; thus the heart-lung machine would ultimately have been useless. The heart itself and Barnard's surgery were perfect.

The Aftermath

This first heart transplant made Christiaan Barnard a celebrity. In the days after Washkansky's death, Barnard flew to the United States to appear on CBS's *Face the Nation* and NBC's *Today Show*. In the United States, he also recorded an episode for a television show called *The Twenty-First Century,* met with President Lyndon Johnson at the LBJ ranch, and filmed another, full-hour television show for NBC. When he arrived in San Francisco, he received as much fanfare as the Beatles. He appeared on the cover of *Time* magazine, which called the heart transplant the "ultimate operation." Barnard enjoyed his fame. He became the first surgeon to make a record album (it discussed his operation); perhaps not surprisingly, though, it didn't sell well, and one wit suggested that it might be improved with a soundtrack by the rock group the Grateful Dead.

As we will see in the section on ethical issues, reactions to the first heart transplant were mixed. Newspaper reports at the time, for instance, ranged from concerns about "harvesting the dead" to hopes that human immortality was at hand. In South Africa, Barnard's feat was hailed as a national triumph. The prevailing medical opinion was that the operation had been premature, because the problem of rejection was not yet solved; but Barnard did have some defenders within the profession—the heart surgeon Michael DeBakey, for example, said that Barnard had broken through a medical barrier and had made a great achievement. In January 1968, Barnard himself predicted that in 20 years animal hearts would be successfully transplanted into humans. (He thought that if large pigs could be grown on special farms, their hearts could be easily transplanted into humans, and he considered primate hearts the next best possibility.[18])

On January 2, 1968, Barnard performed his second heart transplant. The recipient of this second heart was Phillip Blaiberg, a 58-year-old retired dentist; the donor was a 25-year-old man, Clive Haupt, who had died of a cerebral hemorrhage. Phillip Blaiberg (whose physical condition was much better than Louis Washkansky's and who was therefore a better candidate for the operation) had been identified as a potential recipient before Washkansky died and reaffirmed his consent afterward. Blaiberg was discharged from Groote Schuur on March 16 and would live 20 months after his transplant. (He would eventually die of hepatitis, which emerged when his immune system was suppressed, and of rejection of the donor heart.)

Magazines called 1968 the "year of the transplant." During 1968, 105 hearts were transplanted. After 1 year, of the 105 heart-transplant patients, 19 had died on the operating table, 24 had lived for 3 months, 2 had lived for 6 to 11 months, and 1 had lived for almost a year. Of 55 liver transplants in 1968 and early 1969 (the 15 months after Barnard's landmark operation), 50 patients failed to live as long as 6 months. Clearly, most of these early transplants were failures; the immune system was simply too powerful.[19]

ETHICAL ISSUES

First-Time Surgery: Pressures and Publicity

Although Barnard's heart-transplant team had expected surgeons and physicians to notice the operation, neither they nor anyone else had anticipated the enormous worldwide publicity that resulted. The issue of publicity is closely linked to another problem—"pressure to be first."

To begin with, there is the question *who* should "be first." Some American surgeons privately complained that Barnard should not have been first to transplant a heart, since his training in transplants and in the use of the heart-lung machine had occurred through the generosity of American medicine. They argued that it was a mistake to have given Barnard such a machine when other surgeons had worked longer and harder in the hope of being first to do a transplant. In the opinion of many of these physicians, the first surgeon to implant a heart should have been Norman Shumway at Stanford in California, who did transplant the first adult human heart in the United States shortly after Barnard's original operation. Shumway, who had been gearing up for the operation since 1961 and could easily have done what Barnard did, had announced in November 1967 that he was ready to perform a human heart transplant; this was about the time Barnard was looking for a recipient. (As noted above, though, some of Barnard's defenders believed that he had Norman Shumway's tacit permission to go ahead—and that this was because Shumway himself had been stymied by Stanford's research-ethics committee.[20]) At the time, in fact, perhaps a dozen surgical teams at as many hospitals around the world could have done a heart transplant, if they hadn't worried about how long the patient would live.[21]

Another question is *when* "the first" attempt should be made. Almost all the other surgeons who might have performed the first heart transplant had been more cautious than Barnard and had chosen to wait until better immunosuppressive drugs were available before going ahead. Since Barnard did not wait, we might ask whether there wasn't there too much pressure to be first. (In this regard, it can be noted that a few surgeons seem to have waited only because they were forced to wait by lack of a donor.) It may be that the rewards for being "first" are both good and bad for the patient, motivating physicians to scale new heights but also motivating them to compromise on what is best for their patients. However, in 1987, on the twentieth anniversary of the first heart transplant, Barnard himself denied that he had felt involved in any "race" to be first; he also said there had been no sense of urgency in planning to perform heart transplants.[22]

Still another question is *why* we consider it so important to be "first." There is something inherently arbitrary in remembering only those who first did something. Adrian Kantrowitz, for example, performed a heart transplant on a newborn very soon after Barnard's operation on Louis Washkansky. Kantrowitz needed an anencephalic infant as a heart donor for his patient and found one 2 days after Barnard's "first"; if it had taken him less time to find the donor, Kantrowitz would have been "first" and it would have been his name that was famous today,[23] even though the baby who received the heart died after only a few hours.

One factor in the issue of publicity and "being first" is, of course, the media. The media tend to feed the public's hunger for medical breakthroughs; and this tendency can lead to journalistic inaccuracy and sensationalism, and to medical haste and imprudence. (One Brazilian patient first learned of the possibility of a heart transplant when he woke up with another heart inside him.[24])

In the case of the first heart transplant, it is probably true that Barnard both wanted media attention and did not know how to handle it. He allowed the first conversation between Louis Washkansky and his son after the operation to be filmed by a television crew. Allowing reporters and cameras into Washkansky's hospital room, even in sterile gowns, can hardly have been best for the patient (it also seems inconsistent, since later the patient's wife was not allowed to touch him because of the danger of infection). Barnard seemed to relish publicity even while complaining about it. He held daily, candid briefings until doing so became overwhelming and the government information office took over. He favored American journalists and was criticized for taking payments from them for access to himself and Washkansky.[25] (Barnard justified this by saying that the money would benefit his program and therefore future patients.)

It is also true that the realities of Louis Washkansky's death were under-reported, though it is unclear why this should have been so. Perhaps reporters didn't seek out other transplant surgeons and other surgeons didn't seek out reporters. Perhaps the other surgeons were simply inured to such deaths. Certainly most reporters had too little medical background to understand what was occurring. Possibly more important, the public was certainly more interested in what seemed to be a medical miracle than in the clinical details of the patient's death.

Concerns about Donors: Criteria of Death

Although Barnard did not discuss this with Edward Darvall, he must have had some concern about whether Denise Darvall's "brain death" would be generally accepted as such. His criteria were certain to be scrutinized for any sign of conflict of interest or Frankensteinian overeagerness.

Louis Washkansky needed a heart in the best possible condition; and if Barnard had waited too long before excising the donor heart, he might have lost it. Barnard's brother Marius, who was also a surgeon on the transplant team, described a disagreement between them over when Denise Darvall's heart should be removed.[26] Marius Barnard wanted to remove it before it stopped beating (to ensure the best possible conditions for Washkansky); instead, Christiaan Barnard waited until the donor heart had stopped beating (which would have taken several minutes—a long time in heart surgery), and then waited another 3 minutes to be certain it wouldn't resume beating spontaneously. One ethical question here concerned who the patient was, Louis Washkansky or Denise Darvall. In this regard, did Marius Barnard have a conflict of interest? Did Christiaan Barnard have such a conflict? In such a conflict, whose interests should have come first?

A noteworthy point is why the donor's heart stopped at all, since Denise Darvall had a healthy heart. Actually, the surgeons had placed her on a respirator, and they had to cause her heart to stop by turning the respirator off; this damaged the heart slightly and was done only to deflect anticipated criticism. As the surgeon Thomas Starzl explained much later:

> [Standards of brain death] were not in effect during the first trials . . . and would not be until 1968. Rather than trying to maintain a strong heartbeat and good circulation in the cadaver donors, the legal requirement before the end of 1968 was the opposite. Because all such donors were incapable of breathing if the brain

actually had been destroyed, they were supported by ventilators. The steps to donation began with disconnection of the ventilator, which the public called "pulling the plug." During the 5 to 10 minutes before the heart stopped and death was pronounced, the organs to be transplanted were variably damaged by oxygen starvation and the gradually failing and ultimately absent circulation.[27]

Because of ethical considerations, then, recipients like Louis Washkansky received damaged hearts that could have been supplied in better condition.

On the other hand, most transplant surgeons at the time realized that they had little choice in this matter. For one thing, moral caution coincided with their professional interests. Transplant surgery depended entirely on altruistic, voluntary donations, and any suspicious or doubtful procedures would sabotage donations. Even as late as 1985, a Gallup poll showed that 44 percent of Americans hadn't signed organ-donor cards because they feared being declared dead prematurely.

Another consideration at the time was that some influential conservative critics were claiming that a heart should be transplanted only when it had stopped beating. To these commentators, taking a beating heart from a body, even a brain-dead body, was ghoulish. In 1968, for example, one pioneering cardiac surgeon, Werner Forssmann, publicly criticized Barnard.[28] Forssmann had developed cardiac catheterization and had experimentally put tubes into his own heart nine times; in 1956, he had won the Nobel Prize for medicine. He was troubled by the "macabre scene" of two surgical teams at work in adjoining rooms, one team waiting, knives in hand, for a young donor to die; the other placing a patient on a heart-lung machine. (Partly because of such concerns, Japanese surgeons do not perform heart transplants even now.)

In the United States today, by law in all states, the physicians who declare a potential organ donor "brain-dead" may not be members of the surgical transplant team; and several sets of criteria for "brain death" have been developed. The highly conservative "Harvard criteria" (which, however, do not require a heart to stop beating before removal) appeared the year after the first heart transplant, probably not by coincidence.

Criteria for death are discussed in Chapter 1; but it is worth noting here that although a person can be defined as "dead" when breathing and heartbeat have ceased, this is a fairly crude, undefinitive criterion. In the Washkansky case, for instance, Denise Darvall's heart could probably have been restarted easily with a small electric shock and (with supportive treatment) could have kept on beating in her brain-dead body; countless patients have been resuscitated in this way. Louis Washkansky himself could have been maintained for a while on a heart-lung machine; but of course he would have been dependent on it, and when it eventually became contaminated, sprang a leak, or broke down, he would have "died" again.

Concerns about Patients

Quality of life   Perhaps the most important ethical issue raised by the first heart transplant concerned quality of life—an issue that would reappear in the cases of Barney Clark (Chapter 11) and Baby Fae (Chapter 13).

One aspect of this issue was what constituted "success." Transplant surgeons equivocated about this; Barnard was asked about it, for example, and replied that he couldn't really say when he would be certain of success. In the first operations, the criterion of "success" was simply making a transplanted organ work for a few days; but patients, many physicians, and society wanted a higher criterion: return to normal life. Another aspect of the issue of quality of life is informed consent.

Louis Washkansky's case vividly illustrates how dramatic surgery can turn a patient's last weeks into a living hell. Did Washkansky know, at the beginning, how bad it might be? If not, was his consent really informed?

The case also illustrates the question of what chance a patient has to survive and be well. Was it ethical of Barnard to say that Louis Washkansky had a chance to return to normal life, when in fact the likelihood was extremely small? Did Barnard paint an overly positive picture only to gain Washkansky's consent? It should be recognized that in 1967, transplanting a heart was like transplanting a head—a spectacular symbol, but with no real value to the patient. Without better immune-suppressing drugs, there was no real chance that Washkansky would live. André Cournand of Columbia University, who worked on cardiac circulation (and had won a Nobel Prize in 1954), lashed out at Barnard for jumping the gun. "Merely demonstrating that it is technically feasible" to transplant a human heart, Courman said, was unethical.[29] The physiologist Norman Staub said that Barnard's operation was "grandstanding" and that physicians should concentrate on preventing disease rather than on transplanting organs.[30]

In the Washkansky case, the patient's chance of recovery—or even survival—undeniably depended far more on postoperative technology than on the surgery itself. The public erroneously assumed that Barnard's skill as a surgeon had allowed him to do the first heart transplant, but many surgeons had already emphasized that the surgery was relatively simple, despite its emotional symbolism. As Norman Shumway said, "It's not *who* does the operation, but *how*";[31] he emphasized that medicine rather than surgery would be critical. No surgeon knew of any way to keep heart transplant patients alive in the postoperative period, and this was why almost no one except Barnard would attempt such a transplant.

With regard to the patient's chance of survival, though, not everyone within surgery considered Barnard's operation premature; that is, not everyone would have agreed that the probability of survival was vanishingly small. A number of surgeons thought very well of Barnard and of some of the operations he had developed. In particular, they were impressed by the surgical unit and support teams he put together; they also pointed out that when he had experimented with heart transplants on dogs, one-third of the recipients lived more than 1 year. In fact, even in the earliest years of transplants, enthusiasm was widespread. Furthermore, one spectacular success was all that was needed for every cardiac surgeon around the world to start doing transplants—and that success came very soon, with Barnard's second heart-transplant patient, Phillip Blaiberg.

However, this general enthusiasm obscured the issue of quality of life. The truth was that recipients generally didn't do well and only rarely returned to normal living. In 1968, as many as 25 percent of transplant recipients became temporarily psychotic, though few reporters got this story (most reporters practiced press-release journalism and felt that the public disliked bad news). The massive doses of immunosuppressive drugs produced initial euphoria (Louis Washkansky's 5 good days are an example), followed by severe symptoms such as catatonia, depression, hysterical crying, and—as noted—sometimes temporary psychosis. Reporters tended to give these the misnomer "side effects."

"Courage"   Reporters hailed the bravery of the first two transplant patients, Louis Washkansky and Phillip Blaiberg, but neither Washkansky nor Blaiberg considered himself particularly brave. Both of them said that a transplant was their only chance to live, that they wanted to live, and that it took no courage to grasp at this straw.

What is courage? Many people would define courage as fearlessness, but Socrates argued, in his dialogue *Laches*, that courage involves overcoming fear and thus is not possible if no fear exists. He also held that courage is more than just overcoming fear: courage differs from rashness or daring in that it has a worthy goal.[32] Fools overcome fear, but for silly goals; thieves overcome fear, but for immoral goals—thus fools and thieves are not really courageous. According to Socrates' definition, a patient who underwent a heart transplant just to postpone dying would not have overcome the fear of death and therefore would not really be showing courage.

Nevertheless, in certain circumstances a patient like Louis Washkansky or Phillip Blaiberg might still be described, accurately, as courageous. Declining a transplant and accepting death—despite the fear of death—might be courageous, for instance (assuming that the patient was overcoming the fear of death rather than succumbing to an even greater fear of surgery or pain). Accepting a transplant could also be courageous, if a patient in, say, Louis Washkansky's situation was informed completely before consenting. In this regard, note that Socrates' definition of courage requires overcoming fear on the basis of genuine knowledge. Thus if heart-transplant patients like Louis Washkansky and Phillip Blaiberg understood the worst outcomes (including their own probable powerlessness to affect the outcomes), and if they feared those possibilities, and if they still went ahead with the operation, then they would be truly brave. On this argument, if a transplant surgeon underwent a heart transplant in 1967, that might have been genuine courage.

Patients' families   In the first year after heart transplants began, attention was always focused on the recipient; effects on the recipient's family often went unnoticed. Families could not object to transplants, and their role was to support the recipient. Whatever problems existed between the recipient and the family had to be suppressed.

In both the Washkansky case and the Blaiberg case, the patient's wife had to ride an emotional roller-coaster. Louis Washkansky's wife, Ann, seems to have been a victim of paternalism: she was never told the truth and continued to expect her husband to return home. For the 18 days that he survived after the transplant, her life was a constant vigil at the telephone.

Although Phillip Blaiberg did much better than Louis Washkansky, whenever he suffered a setback everyone feared it was the end. His first sore throat was a major agony for his wife and physicians; and during his 20 months of life after his operation, all care and attention focused on him. His daughter Jill, who was living on a kibbutz in Israel, became famous involuntarily and was unhappy at her loss of privacy. (Interestingly, in Blaiberg's case he himself was an object of paternalism: he had suffered a major heart attack 12 years before his transplant and had not been told that he could die any day; only his wife and his cardiologist knew the truth. In retrospect, Blaiberg agreed with this decision.)

The relationship between the recipient or the recipient's family and the donor's family is also an issue. Should the donor be identified or anonymous? Public policy, of course, encourages people to become donors themselves and to allow their dead to be used as donors. In the Washkansky case, the identity of the donor was known, and the donor's family became famous. One South African journalist, however, reported that Ann Washkansky would have preferred the donor to remain anonymous. Apparently, she felt indebted to Edward Darvall, felt obligated to repay the debt, but also felt that it would be impossible to repay him. After 18 days, her husband was dead, but she felt a continuing sense of great obligation to the Darvalls. Eileen Blaiberg—Phillip Blaiberg's wife—attended the funeral of his donor, Clive Haupt, and thanked Haupt's wife.

Interracial Transplants

One specific ethical issue for Christiaan Barnard concerned race and interracial transplantation. To begin with, Barnard had been told by Groote Schuur's governing physicians that the first heart recipient had to be white—otherwise, world opinion would charge them with exploiting a nonwhite patient. (Christiaan Barnard's brother Marius said that the first recipient could have been a nonwhite, but he was mistaken; the realities of South African politics, and the world's view of South Africa, dictated otherwise.) This same consideration applied to the first heart donor: using a nonwhite as the first donor would also have been construed as exploitation. In addition, there was a more general question about transplanting an organ from a donor of one race to a recipient of another race.

In fact, though, the racial issue was not clear-cut, even in South Africa's climate of apartheid. Barnard had feared that apartheid might make his first heart transplant impossible; when he received the call informing him that Denise Darvall was a potential donor, he immediately had to ask, "Is she colored?"—and if she had been colored, her heart could not have been used. After the transplant, the first question from many reporters who called long-distance was whether Washkansky was white. (When they learned that he was Jewish and that Denise Darvall had been Protestant, some journalists asked him how he felt about having a "Gentile heart.") In South Africa at that time, moreover, the race of blood donors was recorded, and recipients of transfusions were usually allowed to choose the race of the donor.

On the other hand, interracial kidney transplants were taking place in South Africa. Earlier, a kidney had been transplanted from a white donor to a black recipient (the world press reported this as "racial-physiological integration"); and

Denise Darvall's kidneys went to a black child. Furthermore, the *second* heart transplant was interracial: the recipient, Phillip Blaiberg, was white; the donor, Clive Haupt, was "colored." Little fuss was raised about these interracial transplants.

Some questions asked at the time faded away or turned out to be nonissues. If Edward Darvall had known that his daughter's kidneys would be given to a black child, would he have consented to donate them? (He later said he would have.) Would the average white South African have consented? How many transplants to "coloreds" would be paid for by the South African government? What would happen with transplants in India, with its rigid caste system? Would a Brahman accept a heart from a lower-caste donor?

According to one well-informed source, today "there is no consideration of race in transplantation in South Africa. . . . At Groote Schuur Hospital and the University of Cape Town, all patients are considered on the basis of medical criteria and the likely success of the procedure."[33] The South African Department of Medicine spearheaded the integration of all patient care in the early 1980s, when integration was still illegal; and long before the official end of apartheid policies in 1990, the University of Cape Town Medical School and its hospital were fully integrated.

UPDATE

By 1968, Jean Dausset had identified different kinds of human leukocytes (white blood cells) and suggested that they might be typed as Landsteiner had previously typed red blood cells. Dausset also advanced extremely important ideas about tissue typing and matching for transplants. *Tissue typing* has to do with antigens, which dictate the immune response (the term *tissue* is rather misleading here; "antigen typing" would be more accurate). There are many types of antigens, and so the process of typing them is long; but Dausset argued that they could be matched. He also argued that since the posttransplant immune response is controlled by antigens in cells of donor tissues, the closer the match between donor and recipient, the less the immune response would be. Further, he believed that specific donor antigens provoking rejection could be identified, and thus that an inappropriate donor could be screened out. It was soon verified that antigens can be typed and matched, and analysis of past operations indicated that this would significantly improve transplants. (Dausset won a Nobel Prize in 1980 for his research.)

With most new medical discoveries come new ethical issues, and tissue typing was no different. For one thing, a transplant surgeon at one hospital might have to decide whether to use an available but poorly matched organ for one of his or her own patients or relinquish it to another hospital for a patient who was a better match. In July 1968, at a "summit meeting" on heart transplantation by Christiaan Barnard, Adrian Kantrowitz, and Denton Cooley, Cooley said that he was reluctant to use tissue-typing at all; he argued that if he had a relationship with a dying patient, how could he give up an available donor heart to a someone else's patient—a stranger—simply because the other patient was a better tissue match? Even if his patient might live only 6 months with the donor heart, Cooley would be reluctant to deny the patient that brief time. He also said, "I would not want my immunologists to stay my hand simply because we did not have an adequate tissue match." As subsequent developments with the artificial heart would show (see Chapter 11), it was indeed difficult for anyone—even his colleague DeBakey—to "stay" Cooley's hand. Cooley's desire to do the "big operation" for his own patients conflicted with evidence about how best to make transplants work.

Another issue was that it was unlikely that any one transplant surgeon could match donors and recipients adequately; clearly, surgeons would need a system—a network—for identifying and matching donor organs and patients. Such a system would involve not only donors, patients, and surgeons but also procurers, transporters, administrators, and so on; and it would obviously depend on cooperation rather than competition. This issue would not be resolved until the 1980s, when the United Network for Organ Sharing (UNOS) was established.

•

In addition to general questions about tissue typing and transplants, there was serious questioning of heart transplants as such. Many cardiac surgeons were critical of heart transplants, and they were not alone. Over the 10 years after the first heart transplant, results of subsequent transplants were disappointing. A survival rate of 50 percent after 1 year was often quoted; but after 3 years the survival rate was reduced to 17 percent. Actually, in animals or humans, organ transplants were rarely successful for more than 1 month, let alone years; and to knowledgeable observers, the death rate in early heart transplants was appalling. As we've seen, 1968 had been called the "year of the transplant"; but the following years were by no means the "decade of the transplant"—they seem to have been the "decade of the high-tech last gasp."

In January 1969, the Montreal Heart Institute suspended heart transplants because of poor results, and this suspension provoked widespread discussion about whether a general moratorium should be called. For example, the surgeon Thomas Starzl (who specialized in liver transplants) and several other surgeons declared that they would observe a moratorium until more was learned; and three prominent cardiologists suggested a 3-month moratorium on heart transplants until further evaluation could be done.

For the rest of 1969, almost everyone cooled off on transplants; the number of transplants fell dramatically. In that year, Senator Walter Mondale of Minnesota suggested a presidential commission to evaluate transplants and related research. Many surgeons (not surprisingly) disliked the idea of a commission and said that surgeons should do the evaluating. The surgeon Walton Lillhei, for one, attacked "self-appointed critics" who "are better versed in the art of criticism than in the field under study . . . [and are] frustrated by their own inability to create."[34]

At the end of 1969 and the beginning of 1970, Massachusetts General Hospital, which is associated with Harvard Medical School and had a famous department of surgery under Francis Moore, rejected a heart transplant program because of concerns about poor outcomes (and also about costs). This was a significant and influential decision, and throughout 1970 a moratorium on heart transplants was generally acknowledged to be in existence. Norman Shumway, who had been the first American surgeon to transplant a heart, did not observe the moratorium: he argued that very carefully selected patients could benefit from such transplants. Most surgeons did observe it, however, and most transplant programs withered.

•

In the early 1980s, cyclosporin, a drug that blocks immune rejection of foreign tissue, was introduced. Thereafter, the number of transplants soared dramatically. Dirk van Zyl, who died on July 7, 1994, had lived longest with a heart transplant—23 years. He had been Christiaan Barnard's sixth heart-transplant patient.

•

Christiaan Barnard remained in the news over the next decades, but in different ways. He became a jet-setter, traveling in international social circles. He was divorced from his first wife in 1970; his second marriage also ended in divorce, and in 1987 he married his third wife, a well-known model. His arthritis worsened, and after several years he could no longer operate. During the 1980s, his name became associated with a cosmetics firm that was making dubious claims about collagen facial creams. He became a vocal opponent of keeping hopeless patients alive and criticized Karen Quinlan's physicians. Although he was one of the best-known physicians in the world, he was not as well respected within academic medicine as many heart surgeons at other centers.

FURTHER READING

Christiaan Barnard and Curtiss Bill Pepper, *One Life,* Macmillan, New York, 1969.
Renée Fox and Judith Swazey, *The Courage to Fail: A Social View of Organ Transplants and Dialysis,* 2d ed. rev., University of Chicago Press, Ill., 1978.
Thomas Starzl, *The Puzzle People: Memoirs of a Transplant Surgeon,* University of Pittsburgh Press, Pa., 1992.

CHAPTER 11

Artificial Hearts

Barney Clark

Barney Clark was the first patient to have an artificial heart implanted and live to tell about it. Whether his life was shortened by the implant of this artificial organ, whether his quality of life with the implant was good enough to justify the operation, and whether the costs of developing the artificial heart were justified by the outcome are among the issues discussed in this chapter.

The case of Barney Clark and his artificial heart (which he received on December 1, 1982) is unique in contemporary medicine and medical ethics. As one medical historian observed, "The artificial heart is at once a metaphor of concern about unduly sustaining an aging population, the cost of medical care, plunging into technologic creation without adequate thought to consequences, and . . . accumulation of means as an end in itself."[1] For many laypeople, this case symbolized other things—some good, some not. Perhaps the two most dominant images at the time were Barney Clark as the Tin Man and Barney Clark as part man, part machine, created by a Dr. Frankenstein.

BACKGROUND: STEPS TOWARD ARTIFICIAL HEARTS

After World War II, the federal government—led by Senator Lister Hill of Alabama, who was the son of a surgeon; and Congressman John Fogarty, who was a victim of heart disease—aggressively supported medical research on the heart. Michael DeBakey (see Chapter 10), a professor at Baylor College of Medicine and one of the world's greatest experts on heart surgery, had for years been developing an external "left ventricle assist device" (LVAD); and in 1963 he testified to Hill and Fogarty that if work like his was funded, a larger artificial heart could be created.[2] (An *artificial heart* is defined as a device totally implanted under the chest wall; an LVAD, by contrast, is partly or wholly outside the chest wall.)

LVADs, which would become popular again in the 1990s, are called a *halfway technology:* an LVAD was better than death, since it could keep a heart patient alive in a state of semisickness, but it was not a cure.[3] Thus attempts continued to develop a true artificial heart. National Institutes of Health (NIH) committed

$500,000 for an artificial heart in 1964 and $8.5 million in 1967, hoping to test one by 1972. During the early 1970s, NIH became pessimistic about artificial hearts and switched most of its grants to LVADs; but in general between 1965 and 1982, NIH continued to support LVADs, mechanical assist devices, and artificial hearts, all together pouring $200 million into them.

•

One researcher's work on developing an artificial heart led to a scandal in cardiac surgery. In 1969, a dying heart donor was flown to the Texas Heart Institute in Houston; his healthy heart was to be transplanted by the surgeon Denton Cooley into a patient named Haskell Karp, who was in terminal heart failure.[4] Cooley (who is discussed in Chapter 10) worked not only at the Texas Heart Institute but also at Baylor Hospital and thus was a colleague of Michael DeBakey's. Some of DeBakey's NIH-funded research on artificial heart components was available to Cooley, and Cooley had secretly hired some of DeBakey's staff to develop his own artificial heart.

Before the transplant operation could be performed, Haskell Karp's heart deteriorated even further. On April 4, 1969, Cooley implanted his version of an artificial heart in Haskell Karp. As required by the United States Public Health Service (USPHS), there was a committee to review medical experiments; its chairman was DeBakey, who was away on business in Washington, D.C. However, Cooley had not obtained permission from this committee; he later argued that no review was necessary, because the implant had been therapeutic rather than experimental. (In a subsequent paper, though, he revealed that when he had previously implanted his device in calves, all of them had rapidly died.)

In Washington, a furious DeBakey learned from the front page of the *Washington Post* that Cooley had secretly developed an artificial heart similar to his LVAD. DeBakey was sure that the operation had been done not to help the patient but rather so that Cooley would be the first to implant an artificial heart.

Haskell Karp survived for only 3 days after the operation, and he was comatose for much of that time. After he died, his wife learned that the operation was considered experimental and therefore filed a suit against Cooley for medical malpractice (which in Texas falls under tort law). According to her testimony, neither she nor her husband had understood that the main intent was to see if the device was clinically feasible in a human being; she had not understood that her husband had little hope of returning to normal life; and although both of them had signed consent forms, neither had realized that he would almost certainly die in pain, nausea, and stupor.

DeBakey had indicated that he would testify against Cooley, but at the last moment he did not; this weakened the plaintiff's case, and the suit was dismissed. Cooley resigned from Baylor College of Medicine, though DeBakey continued to teach there. Two years later, Cooley implanted a second artificial heart—again at the Texas Heart Institute in Houston, again without permission from his Institutional Review Board (IRB), and again claiming that it was an emergency. The patient, who was Dutch, died after 2 days. (*Life* magazine praised Cooley, apparently overlooking the fact that he had broken the law.[5])

One of the issues in this episode is a legal doctrine called *therapeutic privilege,* according to which a physician may lie for a patient's good in extreme situations.

Cooley invoked therapeutic privilege when he did not inform the Karps of any-thing that might disturb them or might lead them to withhold consent. The gen-eral opinion in the medical profession, however, was that it is incorrect to extend therapeutic privilege from normal medicine to risky experimentation. (The Tuskegee syphilis study, discussed in Chapter 9, seems to have been an abuse of this concept.)

•

Meanwhile, an unknown surgeon in Utah was working on artificial hearts within the regulations; his name was William DeVries. In early 1982, the Food and Drug Administration (FDA) gave DeVries permission to implant an artificial heart into a patient in the future.

BARNEY CLARK'S ARTIFICIAL HEART

The Patient: Barney Clark

In December 1982, Barney Clark, age 61, was clearly dying. Why he was dying is important to this case, though it was not emphasized in the media coverage at the time.

Barney Clark had been a heavy smoker. He had started smoking cigarettes at age 24 and had continued for years, smoking one to two packs a day. As a dentist, he was well aware of the harmful effects of smoking cigarettes, and—like many other smokers—he had often tried, unsuccessfully, to quit. Perhaps—also like many other smokers—he was planning to quit permanently before any damage was done; if so, he waited too long. He did finally quit at age 49 (he said that quitting was "the hardest thing I've ever done," and there is no reason to think he was exaggerating); but by then he had been smoking for 25 years and had developed the chronic bronchitis, shortness of breath, and fatigue indicative of early emphysema. By the time he was 56, these symptoms forced him into early retirement and were making him unable to enjoy life; he espe-cially missed playing golf, and he told his wife many times, "I wish I hadn't smoked."[6] Eventually, he suffered from two of the worst effects of smoking: heart failure and emphysema.

Barney Clark thus had not only heart disease but also chronic lung disease. Therefore, he was not an ideal candidate for an artificial heart: the operation stood its greatest chance of success if the patient had strong lungs.

•

When Barney Clark was 12 years old—in 1933—his father died. An only child, Barney supported his mother (she was still alive, age 85, when her son died). He grew up in Provo, Utah, and life there in the 1930s must have been hard for a half-grown boy and a widow with a mortgage to pay. Barney sold hot dogs and worked at odd jobs. Later, he worked his way through Brigham Young University and the University of Washington Dental School. He had met his future wife, Una Loy, in seventh grade; they were married in 1944, when he was 23.

Barney Clark set up his practice in Washington state, where he remained until he retired in 1977. Barney and Una Loy Clark had three children, one of whom, Stephen, became a surgeon. Barney socialized mainly with a group of men his own age who played golf at a country club, of which he was twice president. He was 6 feet 2 inches tall; he liked to arm-wrestle and play cards in the men's locker room; he also liked to drink. He was a Mormon.

•

In 1970, Barney Clark began to feel unwell (this was when he finally gave up cigarettes—perhaps he sensed how sick he was and hoped for a reprieve). By 1978, he could no longer keep up with his friends on the golf course; in fact, the slightest exertion left him breathless. Physicians diagnosed emphysema, an incurable, obstructive lung disease; accompanied by congestive heart failure and cardiomyopathy, an incurable disease of unknown origin in which the muscles of the heart degenerate until they are unable to pump blood to the lungs or arteries. In June 1980, he had been sent home from a local hospital with a poor prognosis. At that time, he was described by his cardiologist in Seattle, Terrence Block, as "all huddled up in a ball and icy cold."[7]

Over the next 2 years, Block kept his patient alive with several newly released, powerful drugs (including captopril and hydrazaline) which dilated his blood vessels and made it easier for his heart to pump blood. By March 1982, however, Block knew that Barney Clark was terminally ill.

Block had considered a heart transplant—ideally, Clark would have received a heart-lung transplant—to be performed by Norman Shumway at Stanford (Shumway is discussed in Chapter 10). Unfortunately, Stanford's criteria for heart-transplant patients had an age cutoff: 50 years.

Block then referred his patient to the University of Utah for treatment with an experimental drug in the summer of 1982. There, Barney Clark learned about the university's artificial heart program, was evaluated by William DeVries, and visited the barn where sheep and calves with artificial hearts were kept. One calf, named Lord Tennyson, had survived for 268 days with a Jarvik-7, but Clark also learned that many of the calves and sheep had died.

•

At the University of Utah, a screening committee had been set up to choose the first candidate for its artificial heart, which was called the Jarvik-7 (after the inventor, Robert Jarvik). The committee had decided that the first recipient must be so sick that death was imminent; since the artificial heart might itself kill the recipient, the committee thought it would unethical to choose anyone who might otherwise live for, say, another year.

Barney Clark seemed to be a possible candidate; but according to Block, he initially scoffed at the idea of the Jarvik-7 and said that he couldn't think of anything worse than being tied to such a device. At home, though, as his condition continued to deteriorate, he began to talk about the artificial heart with his son and with Block. Then his condition became still worse: he couldn't get enough oxygen, he was bedridden with fatigue, and—as dying people often do—he changed his mind. On November 29, 1982, he was brought back to the University of Utah by helicopter.

Clark was given an 11-page consent form, which he signed at 8:30 P.M. on November 29. The next day, November 30, he was interviewed by the IRB; also, a group of physicians, testing his determination to see the operation through, tried to get him to change his mind. He held firm, however, and signed the consent form again.

The Researchers: Kolff, Jarvik, and DeVries

The physician Willem Kolff was born in 1911[8] in the Netherlands and invented the hemodialysis machine there in 1943 (see Chapter 12). He had emigrated to the United States after World War II; worked for a decade at the Cleveland Clinic; and then, in the 1960s, joined the University of Utah. The university gave him a free hand to set up a laboratory to make artificial organs, and he worked on such organs there for the next 20 years. Both Jarvik and DeVries were closely associated with Kolff and his lab.

•

To the public, Robert Jarvik, the inventor of the Jarvik-7, seemed to be a much more important figure than Kolff in the story of Barney Clark's artificial heart. Jarvik, who was not involved in the care of patients, was more accessible to reporters, and his portrayal in the media bordered on adulation.

Jarvik was then 36 years old (he was born in 1946). He was the son of a surgeon, and according to the story widely accepted and reported by the media, he had invented an automatic surgical stapler as a young man, while watching his father operate. According to Jarvik himself, at that time he had no interest in medicine, but after his father died of an aortic aneurysm, he decided to dedicate his own life to cardiac care. It might be supposed that American medical schools would have welcomed the "inventor of a surgical stapler" with open arms, but 15 American medical schools rejected Jarvik (his grades in college had been mediocre, and he has described himself as "not a conventional thinker"). He therefore went to Italy and entered the University of Bologna in the late 1960s. Like most European medical schools, the University of Bologna had open admissions and separated future physicians from a mass of self-selected students only at the end of the second year, by rigorous examinations. After 2 years at Bologna, Jarvik dropped out and returned to the United States; he did not pursue a degree at any medical school but earned a master's degree in occupational biomechanics at New York University in 1971.

Jarvik then joined a company called Ethicon, Inc., which was interested in Kolff's work and offered to continue his salary if he would go to work for Kolff; according to Jarvik, Kolff at first said no but then changed his mind when he found that he and Jarvik both drove a Volvo. Kolff helped Jarvik get admitted to the medical school at the University of Utah in 1972; as soon as he received his medical degree in 1976, Jarvik immediately went to work in Kolff's lab—he did no internship or residency. He remained in the lab until 1979, when he was appointed research assistant professor of surgery and bioengineering at Utah (evidently a specially created position, but in any case one which involved no contact with patients).

•

The surgeon William DeVries had also gotten his start in Kolff's lab; after graduating from college in Utah, he worked there during his first year as a medical student.

DeVries was born in 1943; he was 38 when he operated on Barney Clark. The surgeon was a striking figure—he was 6 feet 5 inches tall and lanky, an athlete (in high school, he had excelled in basketball and high jumping), with a boyish mop of blond hair and a tanned, Nordic face. Because of his rugged good looks, some people saw him as an American archetype, like John Wayne or Jimmy Stewart. DeVries claimed that he slept only 5 hours a night and spent 16 hours a day at the hospital. Any time remaining after commuting and skiing was spent with his wife and their seven children. Like Barney Clark, DeVries was a Mormon.

•

Kolff, Jarvik, and DeVries were all of the "crude mechanics" school of organ transplantation—nothing of the elegance of cyclosporin for them. Various kinds of artificial hearts were constructed in Kolff's laboratory, and critics called it a "tinker toy" lab, but Kolff pointed out that similar naysayers had also dismissed his dialysis machines.

It was not without reason that some sociologists saw the whole story of these researchers and their artificial heart as uniquely American, especially when DeVries incorporated into the first consent form a quotation from Theodore Roosevelt which would later serve as his parting word to his critics:

> It is not the critic who counts; not the man who points out how the strong man stumbled or where the doer of deeds could have done better. The credit belongs to the man who is actually in the arena, whose face is marred by dust and sweat and blood; who strives valiantly; who errs and comes short again and again because there is no effort without error and shortcoming; but he who does actually strive to do the deeds; who knows the great enthusiasm, the great devotion, who spends himself in a worthy cause, who at the best knows in the end the triumph of high achievement and who at the worst, if he fails, at least failed while daring greatly, so that his place shall never be with those cold and timid souls who neither experience victory nor defeat.[9]

The Implant

In a biological heart, blood is pumped by the powerful lower part—the two ventricles. The device called the Jarvik-7 was in effect a replacement for the ventricles. It was made basically of molded polyurethane with two chambers of plastic and aluminum holding an inner diaphragm; the two chambers were separated by a wall of thin membrane through which blood could pass. The diaphragm in the Jarvik-7 was a substitute for the membrane and muscles of the ventricles. The source of power for this diaphragm was air from a compressor (the kind used by auto mechanics), brought up by 6-foot tubes inserted through the patient's stomach. The compressor itself weighed 375 pounds and was carried around on what physicians at Utah called a "grocery cart."

The Jarvik-7 worked as follows: the compressed air inflated the diaphragm, which compressed the right ventricle, which in turn pushed blood into the lungs for oxygenation and then back to the left ventricle; the left ventricle then pushed the oxygenated blood to the body. The Jarvik-7 also contained synthetic valves; these were the same commercial valves routinely implanted by heart surgeons, and as in a natural heart, there were four of them (analogous to mitral, tricuspid, etc.). The opening and closing of these valves against the walls of the Jarvik-7 produced clicks that were audible when an ear was pressed to the patient's chest.

•

DeVries had scheduled Barney Clark's surgery for December 2, 1982—almost 15 years to the day after Christiaan Barnard's first heart transplant. Outside the hospital, snow began to fall on the mountains; television news teams reported that a history-making operation was about to take place; and a thief ransacked the Clarks' home and stole photographs of the patient, perhaps hoping to sell them to reporters. (There would be another theft in this story: after the operation, two Jarvik-7s were stolen from DeVries's office.)

Meanwhile, Barney Clark—who already had chronic atrial fibrillation—began to experience ventricular tachycardia ("V-tach"), a potentially fatal condition. During the evening of December 1, according to DeVries, Clark's heart had weakened to a point where his life was in immediate danger,[10] and so the operation began that night at 11 P.M. rather than the next morning as planned. On his way to the operating room, Clark joked, "There would be a lot of long faces around here if I backed out now."[11]

As the surgery began, at DeVries's request, the sounds of Ravel's *Bolero* filled the operating room. Upon opening the chest, DeVries found a flabby, enlarged heart: it was twice the size of a normal heart and was merely quivering rather than contracting; one physician who was present described it as looking like "a soft, overripe zucchini squash."[12] DeVries first cut away the lower part of the heart, the two ventricles; then he stitched two Dacron cuffs to the intact upper part, the atria. He then had to connect to these Dacron cuffs—with Velcro fasteners—the two plastic ventricles of the Jarvik-7. However, the patient's atrial walls were paper-thin (this was an effect of the steroids Barney Clark had been taking), and when the Velcro fasteners were snapped, the pressure ripped the atrial stitches; the cuffs therefore had to be restitched into a new section of heart wall and the fasteners gently snapped into place.

The cuffs then held; but when the Jarvik-7 was turned on, it didn't work—it was not pumping blood out of its left ventricle. DeVries, increasingly frustrated, tried for 1 hour to get it to work correctly. He opened the ventricle by hand three times, each time running the risk of introducing air into the blood and causing a stroke. (Until the patient awakened, DeVries would not know if he had managed to avoid this.) At one point, DeVries reportedly exclaimed, "Please, please, please, work this time!"[13] Finally, he replaced the faulty ventricle altogether with parts from another Jarvik-7 and got the machine working, 2 hours after it was supposed to have started. Jarvik, who had scrubbed and entered the operating theater when his machine was implanted, helped DeVries to get it working; throughout this ordeal, he was very nervous.

The operation, having taken all night, concluded about 7:00 A.M. on December 2.

Postoperative Developments

A few hours after the surgery, when the anesthesia wore off, DeVries watched anxiously as Barney Clark opened his eyes. If the patient had missed a bad stroke, he would be able to respond to requests to move his extremities; he was therefore asked (without explanation) to move each arm and his toes. He did so, and everyone felt relieved, though his surgeons would now watch to see if his immune system would rebel against the Jarvik-7.

Later that day, at a press conference, university physicians enthusiastically described the operation as a "dazzling technical achievement," something "as exciting and thrilling as has ever been accomplished in medicine";[14] it would also be called "one of the most dramatic stories in medical history."[15]

•

People are often shocked when they visit an intensive care unit or see a patient after major heart surgery; certainly Una Loy Clark was when she saw her husband.[16] Barney Clark had a hole in his throat through which a breathing tube ran, a feeding tube running into his stomach, a bladder catheter, and of course the two hoses connecting the Jarvik-7 through his upper abdomen to the 375-pound air compressor at his bedside.

Like Louis Washkansky, Clark felt horrible after the operation. Also, though he had not suffered a massive stroke, he experienced what is called *intensive care psychosis* (or *acute brain syndrome*), which involves confusion, delirium, massive loss of memory, and periods of semiconsciousness. On December 4, more surgery was required to repair ruptured alveoli (air sacs in the lungs).

On December 6, he felt somewhat better and asked DeVries how he was doing. DeVries replied, "Just fine"; but seconds later, Barney Clark began to have seizures—involuntary shuddering from head to toe—perhaps caused by the dramatic increase in blood flow after the Jarvik-7 implant. A muscle tranquilizer (Valium) and an anticonvulsant (Dilantin) were injected. For the next several hours, the patient was unconscious and the seizures continued, though gradually the quivering became confined to his left leg and left arm. Throughout the next months, he would have continuing periods of confusion.

The following days were bad. DeVries later said that during this period, there were times when Barney Clark wanted to die and one time when he asked directly, "Why don't you just let me die?"[17] This reaction, however, is not uncommon after traumatic surgery, and it often passes. Still, Barney Clark was depressed by his lack of energy, his difficulty in breathing, and his stupor. Several times, he told a psychiatrist, "My mind is shot."

On December 14, things got worse when one of the $800 welded commercial valves inside the Jarvik-7 broke. The patient's blood pressure dropped dramatically, threatening his life, and DeVries had to operate again to replace the valve.

Nineteen days after implantation of the Jarvik-7, Barney Clark was doing much better, and DeVries said there was a good chance that he would eventually go home. Instead, though, complication after complication began to develop. Drugs were being administered to prevent clots by keeping the blood thin, but this medication also caused severe bleeding (from normal sores and cuts that didn't clot and therefore didn't heal). On January 18, a persistent, severe nosebleed had to be surgically sealed.

More serious was the patient's underlying emphysema: it created pneumothorax (escape of air from the lungs into the chest cavity), requiring another operation to relieve pressure on Barney Clark's weak, smoke-damaged lungs. From January to March, Clark complained of conditions caused by his emphysema: he constantly complained that he was never able to get a good breath. In fact, he was suffocating—a situation unrelated to the Jarvik-7. On February 14, Barney Clark left the surgical ICU for a private room, but on February 15 he went back to the ICU because he needed a respirator; he spent the next 9 days in the ICU, presumably on the respirator.

On February 24, however, he was able to return to the private room, and his best week was at the end of February. On March 1, Barney Clark made several videotaped interviews with DeVries. One of these was edited, and parts of it were released to the public on March 2; two others, in which Clark had nothing positive to say, were not released at all. According to the cardiologist Thomas Preston, the final short segment of the material that was released "came from an extensive interview in which, encouraged by Dr. DeVries, Clark issued a semblance of a positive statement."[18] This clip showed what was the best moment to be found in the interviews: Barney Clark—tethered to a huge machine, in some pain, and apparently not fully conscious—was not a happy man; but he claimed that he was glad to be alive and was not sorry he had undergone the operation. Moreover, it seemed possible that he might improve.

The next day, however—March 3—Barney Clark developed severe nausea and vomiting; some vomit was aspirated, and this led to pneumonia. On March 21 he developed reduced renal function and a high fever. This was the beginning of the end.

On March 23, 1983, at 10:02 P.M., having lived 112 days with his artificial heart, Barney Clark died of multiple organ collapse. Large doses of antibiotics had killed most of the useful, benign bacteria in his colon; thus necrosis of the colon developed and produced toxins that entered his blood. This was accompanied by increasing expansion of his extremely fragile veins, to the point where they could no longer transmit blood. Degeneration of the colon and veins in turn led to the death of the kidneys, brain, and lungs, since little blood was reaching these organs, and the blood that did reach them was increasingly septic.

The Jarvik-7, of course, continued pumping. Una Loy Clark was asked if she wanted to be present when it was turned off; she said that her husband was already dead and left the room.[19] Someone (it was not revealed who) stopped the machine after a few hours. It had beaten 12,912,499 times.

•

The media had been following all this intently—during the initial surgery, hundreds of reporters had swarmed around the University of Utah Medical Center in Salt Lake City—but on the whole journalists were dissatisfied with the conditions under which they covered the story.

For one thing, the Clark family signed an exclusive contract with a magazine, and other reporters felt left out. Also, DeVries's attitude toward his patient was protective, and reporters resented this (as described in Chapter 4, the same kind of conflict had arisen when the first baby was born through in vitro fertilization). For their part, DeVries and the university officials said that they did want a "media circus," though it should be noted that they themselves had invited the media.[20] During the postsurgery period, the physician-administrator Chase Peterson, the university's vice president for health affairs, ran interference with the media and functioned as a public-relations professional. At one point, reporters exploded when Peterson said there would be no further news. The hospital later changed this policy, but reporters became angrier and angrier as weeks went by and the hospital kept trying to put the best "spin" on the facts about Clark's condition.

The Aftermath

Following Barney Clark's death, public and professional reactions were mixed. Some people called the operation "one of the boldest human experiments ever attempted"; others concluded that it had failed to prove its worth, and that even if it had been worthwhile, it would represent one of the most expensive therapies in existence. The university's IRB and the FDA postponed any further implants until more data could be studied (though, as we will see, DeVries was allowed to perform three more implants). A few months later, predictably, Kolff defended the artificial heart: "A number of doctors were opposed to the artificial kidney and wrote articles against it. I decided not to respond at all. . . . I still have the same policy now [for] people [who] tell us that the artificial heart has no future. . . ." DeVries made a surprising comment: "After the first two days, 95 percent of the issues we were dealing with concerned ethics, moral value judgments, communications with the press—problems I had never thought about."[21]

A few weeks after Barney Clark died, the hospital corrected an "oversight": it revealed to irritated reporters that it had not informed them about another valve failure. Within days after Barney Clark's death, a valve had broken and killed Ted E. Baer, a 220-pound ram that had lived 297 days with an artificial heart—the world's record for survival by a mammal.[22] (Ted E. Baer was the model for "Flash" and his "Craig 2000" artificial heart on the television series *St. Elsewhere*.)

DeVries's referrals from physicians in Utah dropped to almost zero; claiming that he was unhappy with "red tape," he moved in 1984 to Humana Hospital in Louisville, Kentucky, a for-profit center where he would be given a freer hand and (reportedly) three times his former salary.[23]

As has been noted, after Barney Clark died FDA allowed DeVries three more such operations. At Humana, DeVries implanted a second Jarvik-7 into William Schroeder on November 25, 1984 (nearly 2 years after Barney Clark's operation). "Bionic Bill" was 51; he was not only younger than Barney Clark but also much healthier (he had no emphysema), and he lived much longer—21 months. However, he had suffered a stroke only 19 days after his operation (probably from a clot formed where the Velcro connectors attached to what was left of his natural heart wall); thereafter he had a cascade of strokes, repeated bouts of endocarditis, and numerous other problems. Eventually he underwent a tracheostomy, a surgically created hole in the neck to the trachea, usually performed to insert a breathing tube. On August 6, 1986, he died of suffocation.

On February 17, 1985, Murray Haydon had become DeVries's third recipient of a Jarvik-7. He started to suffocate on the seventeenth day after the implant, and he too had a tracheostomy. Murray Haydon soon became dependent on a breathing tube connected to a respirator, and he also experienced various infections; he lived for 10 months and 2 days, however, with his infections and on the respirator. After he died (on Deccember 19, 1986), an autopsy revealed that a hole from a catheter in part of his natural heart wall had not healed, and so blood had poured into his lungs.

It was the case of the fourth recipient, Jack Burcham, that caused the real downfall of the artificial heart in the public mind. Going into surgery, Jack Burcham thought there was little risk; but he lived only 10 days (April 16 to 25, 1985) after a disastrous operation: DeVries found that the Jarvik-7 wouldn't fit inside his chest. When Jack Burcham left the operating room, "his chest, draped with sterile dressing, . . . [was] only partly closed around the device."[24] The autopsy showed that large blood clots had clogged the valve openings in his artificial heart. Afterwards, DeVries admitted that the surgery had probably shortened the patient's life.[25]

Eventually, DeVries's referrals in Louisville dropped (as they had in Utah), and he was forced out of the artificial-heart business. Referring physicians were afraid that he was more absorbed with the Jarvik-7 than with patients; some patients were afraid that after what was supposed to be routine cardiac surgery, they might "wake up . . . with an artificial heart."[26] Privately, also, many physicians didn't refer patients to DeVries because they saw only miserable outcomes, grandstanding, and obliviousness to clinical realities; they simply didn't trust him to do what was best for patients—given his desire for success and his financial conflicts of interest, his patients seemed to come in third. For some time, DeVries continued to claim that the Jarvik-7 could be successful, but he was a voice in the wilderness.

ETHICAL ISSUES

Criteria for Success: Quality of Life

Some medical ethicists criticized DeVries because he did not state his criteria for success; they wondered what DeVries would count as a good result.[27] Michael DeBakey, for one, said that success should be defined as being restored to normal life, though Christiaan Barnard cheered DeVries on, urging him to ignore his critics and not to give up.[28]

DeVries countered in two ways. First, he argued that the operation had been successful "from a research standpoint."[29] On these terms, he found considerable support. Most commentators agreed that the operation had proved that an artificial heart could keep a patient alive much longer than had been expected; and some pointed out that radical medical experiments had seldom, if ever, been more successful with the first patient.[30] After all, the machine had circulated the blood, and initially it had not formed clots.

Second, DeVries argued that it was up to Barney Clark and his family, not to others, to decide if the patient's quality of life was high enough. On these terms, the issue was much less clear-cut. Barney Clark himself said that the operation was "worth it if the alternative is that . . . [you] either die or have it done";[31] but Una Loy Clark later said that the operation was only a "partial" success because there had been no full recovery. Moreover, it could be argued that quality of life can appropriately be evaluated by others—for example, by potential recipients,

referring physicians, cardiac surgeons, researchers, hospitals, IRBs, funding institutions, and insurers.

Chase Peterson, the spokesperson for the University of Utah hospital, called
the operation a "modified success," but he predicted that the public would put
up with only a few more such partial successes before insisting on a real success.[32] What was needed, Peterson said, was a case (like Christiaan Barnard's second heart transplant) where the patient would go home and enjoy a reasonable
quality of life.

The general public agreed with Peterson; in the public view, the whole point
of the artificial-heart program should be to restore normal life. In fact, to the public, Barney Clark (like Karen Quinlan) became a symbol of how not to die: he
illustrated how mechanical technology can cruelly reduce a life to painful gasps
for the next breath. In the videotaped interview that was released, Barney Clark
had seemed to be on the brink of suffocation—his attention seemed to be so
focused on breathing that he hardly noticed the cameras. The *New York Times*
thought that DeVries had given Clark not an extra 112 days of good life, but an
extra 112 days of dying.[33] For the general public, then, the question whether it is
a "success" to live tethered to a huge machine and gasping for breath hadn't
been answered, or had been answered only too clearly.

Referring to experimental cardiac surgery in general, P. M. Park has elo-
quently expressed concerns about quality of life:

> It is sometimes hard to meet the eyes of patients who have improved enough to
> have been moved to the regular postop floor and finally become alert enough to
> communicate their despair and disappointment. . . . Often, after entering the
> experience with great hope, patients for whom transplantation has been series of
> setbacks clearly articulate their feelings of betrayal: "No one ever told me it could
> be like this."
>
> Certainly they were told that there would be no guarantees, and that it
> would be hard, and that there would be setbacks—but probably not how hard, or
> what some of the worst-case scenarios could be. When they were told, "You have
> to have a transplant or you're going to die," they were left a very slim margin for
> decision making. These people need to know not only what it will be like not to
> be dying any more, but what it may be like to not live so well.[34]

Park emphasizes an important point: like Barney Clark, most patients at the end
of their lives are not completely aware of the likely outcomes of various interventions.[35]

This consideration and the fact that Clark's mental life deteriorated both
raise an issue closely related to quality of life—informed consent. Stephen Clark
said that his father "was never the same mentally" following the violent convul-
sions he experienced a week after his implant. In that condition, could Barney
Clark have given his informed consent to continue the experiment? If not, was
his family ever asked to consent?

Before we leave the subject of "success" and quality of life, it is worth noting
that surgeons often define success as survival for 30 days, by which time most
patients are out of the hospital with their incisions healed. Simply being able to
leave the hospital is, however, a very minimal criterion. Most people, as we have

seen, want far more before they would consider surgery successful; what most of us want is a return to some semblance of normal life, without great pain or suffering, and with the ability to do most or much of what we have always done and to remain the same kind of person. In this everyday sense, Barney Clark's surgery was not successful.

Technical Problems

Technological difficulties were obviously a factor affecting quality of life.

For one thing, something about the case seemed fishy. Cardiologists around the country were saying privately that the whole project was "erector set medicine" because a serious physiological problem hadn't been solved—how to keep blood from clotting while in contact with artificial surfaces. For a recipient of an artificial heart, the most serious problem was the tradeoff between potentially fatal clots and potentially fatal internal bleeding. Sooner or later—especially after several months—blood clots formed on the heart or its plastic connections; when a clot broke free, it might travel to the small vessels of the brain and lodge there, blocking the blood flow and thereby causing brain damage (a stroke). But when a blood-thinning medication (such as Heparin) was given to prevent such clots from forming, internal cuts would be unable to heal and the patient would bleed to death.

Another problem was infection. All the recipients of the artificial heart contracted infections where the drive lines entered the body. Antibiotics, of course, are used against infection, but continued use of antibiotics will result in resistant infections.

Still another problem was mechanical. It is very, very difficult to make replacements for the heart or its components that will last for years without breaking or failing. At the same time, with an artificial heart there is almost no margin for error. Early dialysis machines broke down frequently and were sometimes unsuccessful, and cardiac pacemakers often failed, but the patients didn't die. By contrast, when a Jarvik-7 failed, loss of blood to the brain would produce irreversible damage within minutes. (It can be noted that in 1986, the Shiley company of Irvine, California, stopped making its Bjork-Shiley heart valves after repeated experience had shown that the struts on the valves eventually cracked, causing the valves to fail and thereby causing heart failure, and in some cases death; the valve whose failure caused the death of Ted E. Baer was probably also a Bjork-Shiley. Between 1979 and 1986, Bjork-Shiley valves had been implanted in more than 55,000 patients; in 1992, the manufacturer paid $215 million in legal settlements to families of 300 patients who had died after these valves failed.[36])

With regard to technological problems, many critics felt that DeVries waited too long to publish his results. In early 1988, *Journal of the American Medical Association* carried three signed editorial reviews, in which the reviewers concluded that doing further implants would only document greater problems. These reviewers, who were surgeons, implied that further implants would be unethical—that they might build the ego of the implant surgeon but would harm the patient. What is more, at least one of the reviewers implicated the Jarvik-7 as a specific cause of fatal complications:

At the time of device implantation or at autopsy, thrombi have frequently been identified on components of the mechanical heart. Prolonged, although temporary, use of prosthesis, similar to a permanent heart substitution, only provides time to increase the number of thromboembolic events and to allow further establishment of infection.[37]

Patients' Self-Determination: Barney Clark's "Key"

During the first few days after the operation on Barney Clark, Willem Kolff and Robert Jarvik both said that the patient had a "key" with which he could turn off his artificial heart if he decided to die.[38] His consent form did stipulate that he could withdraw from the project, even if withdrawal entailed his death; but as soon as Kolff and Jarvik mentioned this "key," Chase Peterson issued a press release softening their statement. Dispelling the notion that Clark himself could shut off the Jarvik-7, Peterson said that the "key" was only a metaphor, not an actual physical instrument. Undoubtedly, DeVries had told Peterson to downplay the "key," lest the media get the idea that Clark could really kill himself. Later, as Clark's breathing became forced and his consciousness became murky, nothing more was said about the key.

The truth is that a physical key did exist: the air compressor was locked "on" with a key. However, this key was not meant to give Barney Clark the option to die; it was meant only to prevent anyone from turning the compressor off inadvertently. Jarvik and Kolff seem to have interpreted it erroneously; furthermore, if their intention was somehow to give Barney Clark control of such a key, that would surely have been unwise. Neither Jarvik nor Kolff seems to have appreciated the usual postoperative mental problems; as has been noted, temporary mental confusion after major traumatic surgery is so common among patients in ICUs that it has been given a common (if loose) name: *intensive care psychosis.*

Jarvik also remarked—when he was pressed on whether a key actually existed—that whether or not Barney Clark did have a key, no key was necessary; according to Jarvik, it would be easy for a patient such as Clark to kill himself: "People can die in many ways, and they are amazingly creative about it."[39] Here again, Jarvik seemed not to grasp postoperative realities. By the time Barney Clark became miserable enough to want to die, he would be too weak to do anything; he would probably be barely able to lift an arm. Also, at this point he would probably be mentally incompetent.

Therapy versus Research

An important issue in the case of Barney Clark was whether implanting an artificial heart was therapy or research. In general, there are two ways in which a procedure that is not well established may be used ethically with a human patient. An *experimental* procedure (research) is permissible if the patient is dying (and has given informed consent); though such an experimental procedure should be based on good research design and supported by animal studies, no therapeutic benefit needs to be claimed. If the patient is not dying, however, the procedure must be *therapeutic* (therapy): that is, it must be expected to have a definite benefit for the patient. The difference between therapy and experimental procedures is important; although some researchers try to get around the entire issue by talking about "therapeutic research," this blurs a useful distinction.

When FDA gave DeVries permission to implant an artificial heart in a future patient, it exempted him from having to prove any therapeutic benefit.[40] This would imply that the surgery was experimental; and that also seems to have been Barney Clark's understanding: he did not really expect the Jarvik-7 to be therapeutic for him but simply hoped that it might be, and that if it was not, it might make some contribution to scientific progress. If the artificial heart was experimental, the patient would have to be dying; we need to consider, then, whether Barney Clark's death was actually imminent. If death was *not* imminent in his case, an experimental procedure would not be appropriate; we would then need to ask whether the artificial heart could have been considered therapeutic for him.

Was Barney Clark dying?   As we've seen, DeVries originally scheduled Barney Clark's implant surgery for the morning of December 2, 1982, but then moved it forward to 11 P.M. on December 1. A few hours after the surgery, DeVries claimed that he had made this decision because without the operation, the patient would have been dead "at midnight."

The cardiologist Thomas Preston, however, argued later that death had not been imminent, and that DeVries had made this claim only to justify trying an artificial heart (Preston also disputed that Clark benefited from the Jarvik-7).[41] According to DeVries, Barney Clark had been experiencing a potentially fatal arrhythmia; according to Preston, on the other hand, the arrhythmia was probably caused by the medications Clark was on, and during the preceding 18 months Clark had had identical arrhythmias which had been reversed.

In the nature of things, of course, it is impossible to resolve this issue factually: there is no way to reconstruct the situation to see how soon the patient would have died without surgery. Nor is it easy to resolve the issue in terms of some general criterion or criteria of "imminent death." For Preston, the only patient who is truly at death's door is one who has stopped breathing and is being resuscitated; and if Barney Clark was not in such a condition, he was an experimental subject rather than a patient receiving a new therapy. But Preston's standard might be too strict, since not everyone would want to delay an operation until a patient is that far gone; in the Clark case, for instance, the screening committee considered the artificial heart "therapeutic" for a patient who still had a few days to live. Preston's standard might also be considered too lenient, though, since thousands of patients in such a state have been revived.

In brief, then, it is difficult to decide whether death is actually "imminent" in a given case and difficult to arrive at a general, useful definition of "imminent death."

When is surgery therapeutic?   If a patient's death is probably not imminent, the crucial question changes. To decide in such a situation whether a procedure is ethical, we need to ask whether it is therapeutic.

In this regard, it is relevant to consider what, in general, makes a surgical intervention (such as the Jarvik-7) therapeutic. Outcomes of interventions—in terms simply of how many patients live how long—can be graphed: the two axes are time (x) and morbidity, or percent of patients alive (y). On such a graph, a

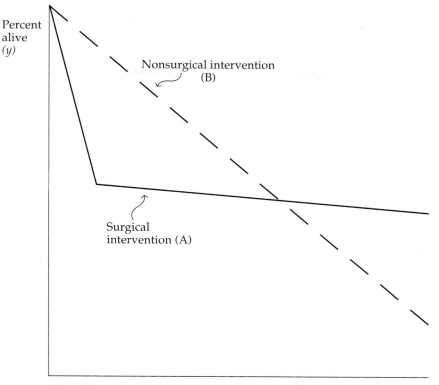

surgical intervention can be represented by one line (call this line A) and a non-surgical approach by a second line (B). Plotting begins, of course, at the left of the *x*-axis (time 0) and the top of the *y*-axis (100 percent of patients alive).

For patients with terminal cardiac disease, line B (no surgery) will slope downward steadily. Line A (surgery) will at first fall downward very sharply—more sharply than B—since the assault of the surgery itself will cause some patients to die immediately or very soon; thereafter, however, *if the surgery is therapeutic,* line A will slope much less steeply and may even level off, as the patients who survive surgery start to do better as a result of it. Initially, then, line A will be behind line B, but later it will meet, cross, and move ahead of line B. With successful therapeutic surgery, in other words, although mortality will initially be higher than in a nonsurgical approach, it will later be significantly lower.[42]

A graph like this is routinely used by surgeons to assess probable outcomes (note also that such a graph could be helpful in illustrating and explaining anticipated benefits and problems to patients, and thus in obtaining their genuine informed consent). In deciding to implant the Jarvik-7, though, DeVries did not use this kind of analysis, and many critics felt that he was irresponsible.

In fact, what chance did this particular procedure have with this particular heart- and lung-impaired patient? Although opinions differed, the predominant evaluation seemed to be that the chance was extremely slight and therefore that the implant was not therapeutic. NIH, which had funded the artificial heart for 20 years, considered DeVries's operation experimental rather than therapeutic and opposed it.[43] FDA, as we have seen, exempted DeVries from having to demonstrate therapeutic benefit; but some commentators, such as the law professor George Annas, criticized FDA for violating its own rules and felt that it had exceeded its authority.[44] The physician Pierre Galetti carefully noted that Clark's case demonstrated only the "clinical feasibility" of the artificial heart, not its "clinical usefulness"—a more important standard.[45]

Selection of Recipients

If the artificial heart was successful, who would receive it? There were at least two issues related to selection of recipients for artificial hearts. For one thing, some critics argued that the recipients would be largely white men over age 50; another question arose over whether or not standards for selection should include the patient's family.

After Barney Clark died, the team at the University of Utah said that one of the things it had learned was the value of strong support from the family and announced that such support would be a criterion in its selection of future candidates; in April 1983, one potential recipient was rejected because of lack of "familial support."[46] This decision, however, was criticized as subjective and therefore unscientific; it was argued that since Clark's family had supported the team at Utah, the team simply liked having families around. One of the critics was Robert Jarvik, who objected, "I have never seen an adult bull visit one of our calves and yet the calves do very well."[47] On the other hand, nurses, social workers, and many physicians agreed with the decision by the Utah team, citing their own long experience with dialysis and coronary patients and maintaining that "everyone knows" such patients do better with support from their families.

Costs

Two separate basic issues about costs arose in this case: the cost for the individual patient and the cost for society.

With regard to the individual patient, how much did this artificial heart cost, who would pay for it, and would it be cost-effective? Barney Clark's total bill was more than $250,000, and although the Clarks had contracted to pay for his treatment, they were released as the costs zoomed. Hospital administrators at the University of Utah had not initially expected this—according to Chase Peterson, they expected that the patient would die in a few days or be discharged in a few weeks[48]—and later the hospital decided not to allow a second implant unless funding was provided in advance. The editor of *Journal of the American Medical Association* questioned the cost-effectiveness of the treatment: "How much is one more day of longer life worth? Is every life worth the same amount and if not, why not?"[49]

The second basic issue was the cost to society. NIH invested over $8 million in research leading up to the Utah project and over $200 million nationally in similar projects between 1964 and 1982. Was this the best way to spend limited funds? Should such expenditures be continued? Moreover, if the artificial heart was successful, could society afford to pay for it? The Office of Technology Assessment estimated that 60,000 Americans might use artificial hearts, at a cost to Medicare of $5.5 billion a year.[50] If that happened, artificial hearts could easily become an exorbitantly expensive program.

There was also a more subtle issue involving costs: this had to do with what economists call *opportunity costs* of funds. If funds were not spent on artificial hearts, what opportunities would exist for funding other programs? For instance, if $5 billion was spent on Jarvik-7s, that $5 billion might otherwise have been spent on, say, medical care for indigent patients. Opportunity costs are often disregarded because once a dramatic and potentially life-saving breakthrough occurs, its momentum becomes virtually impossible to stop. Early on, DeVries said, "I think the snowball's started and I don't think anybody can stop it now";[51] but as one commentator observed, "In our medical system, . . . what physicians establish is what we get, with indifference to relative social or medical value."[52]

Conflicts of Interest

A significant issue in this case had to do with actual or potential conflicts of interest, and this in turn had to do with the profit motive. As we have seen, NIH was supplying public funding for the development of artificial hearts; nevertheless, private profitmaking became an important factor.

For one thing, Robert Jarvik was allowed to patent his machines. For another, the Jarvik-7 was made by a private corporation—Symbion, Inc.—which had been formed in 1976 by Willem Kolff and four others, including Jarvik and Jarvik's secretary.[53] A for-profit hospital chain, Humana (which then owned 91 hospitals nationwide), was also involved. Moreover, DeVries had stock in Symbion; and though the University of Utah forced him to divest himself of his holdings, Humana saw no conflict of interest.

Originally, Symbion simply owned prototypes of artificial hearts; its research and salaries were paid for by the University of Utah, and in return the university would receive 5 percent of sales of any Jarvik hearts and a small amount of stock. On this basis, Symbion limped along for 5 years; then, in late 1981, Kolff went public, looking for venture capitalists to underwrite its expansion. A struggle for power ensued between Jarvik and Kolff (Kolff later characterized this as a son rebelling against a father figure), and Jarvik and others squeezed Kolff out of management. Although Kolff retained some influence, Jarvik became the president of Symbion.

In 1982, Symbion needed more money, and Jarvik received $1 million each from Humana, Hospital Corporation of America, and American Hospital Supply. These companies were betting that artificial hearts would succeed and become profitable—in other words, they were betting that patients would soon have to buy a commodity which had already been financed by tax dollars. As one vice president said, Symbion's biggest advantage was that "it had the university as its research arm and its development arm subsidized by the government."

Humana, for its part, agreed to pay for 100 implants—if successful progress was made. Although these recipients would pay nothing, Humana of course expected a return on its investment: it wanted publicity, and as a major stock-holder in Symbion, it wanted the Jarvik-7 to become routine.

When physicians become involved with high finance, competition increases and what is at stake becomes more than the patient's welfare. It seems clear that Jarvik and DeVries did have conflicts of interest; it also seems clear that such a situation undermines trust between physicians and patients.[54] (Indeed, in a case like Barney Clark's, where "consent" may be mostly symbolic, trust becomes paramount and anything that undermines it is even worse than usual.) Further-more, because of the involvement of Humana other financial issues seemed to mushroom. Could a for-profit hospital really afford major clinical research? If Humana was sponsoring such research just for publicity, would its commitment to research end if it found the publicity disappointing? And if its goal was public-ity, would it really scrutinize research carefully? Some critics predicted that Humana's IRB would be largely a rubber stamp. "I'm not aware," said Arnold Relman, editor of *New England Journal of Medicine,* "that Humana has any experi-ence in medical research. This makes a serious research problem into a public-relations commercial campaign."[55]

Prevention and "Saving Lives"

Some people believe that treating crises with expensive interventions—that is, intervening only after an illness has become devastating or life-threatening—is hardly the best way to attack disease and may even be one of the factors making people terminally ill. To such critics, preventing disease is much better.

A leftist magazine, *Progressive,* complained at the time of the Clark case that a "medical establishment grown fat on chemicals and technological wizardry is not willing to empower people so they can prevent illness."[56] *Progressive* argued that artificial hearts, which might benefit only the small number of cardiac patients who could afford them, were "qualitatively different from the basic advances in immunology which have saved million of lives, even among populations not directly treated."

Of course, almost everyone believes that an ounce of prevention is worth a pound of cure; nevertheless, the argument advanced by critics like *Progressive* can be attacked in several ways. First, there may be something irrational about saying that saving a life by prevention is better than saving a life by last-minute inter-vention:[57] a saved life is a saved life.

Second, it is not always easy to establish that lives are saved by preventive measures. For example, if we cannot afford both artificial hearts and antismoking programs, we should go for the antismoking programs—assuming that those programs will save more lives than artificial hearts. But can we be sure of that assumption? Lives saved statistically are always mere claims; it is difficult to be certain that such lives would not have been saved anyway, because there are too many variables.

Third, with regard to heart disease, heredity is believed to be the leading fac-tor; thus even if some lives are saved "statistically" by preventive measures, many people will develop heart disease anyway.

Fourth, it is necessary to take human nature into account, and it is only human nature for most of us to become more passionate about saving an individual, identifiable life than about supporting preventive programs which seem to be abstract or hypothetical. Many people will send donations and messages to an individual like Barney Clark; President Reagan telephoned William Schroeder, the recipient of the second Jarvik-7, urging him to fight on. (These are instances of a phenomenon called the *rule of rescue,* which is introduced in Chapter 2 and also discussed in Chapter 12.)

On the other hand, this issue is at least partly a matter of emotion versus reason, and in such a situation it is important not to abandon reason. Even though prevention may be hard to document and partially unsuccessful, and even though human nature may insist on "saving lives," we should not conclude that prevention can be disregarded or slighted in favor of "cures." For example, though it is always tempting to think we can save a life through some kind of personal contact, Reagan could really have saved lives in, say, 1987 by continuing the unpopular 55-miles-per-hour speed limit nationwide (as it was continued anyway by many states). Consider that after the speed limit was lowered to 55 mph—and the drinking age was raised to 21 nationwide—alcohol-related automobile fatalities decreased sharply; it is true that these saved lives are abstract "statistical lives," but here is a concrete, personal point to keep in mind: some of the people reading this page would not be alive now if these two regulations had not been legislated.

In the case of Barney Clark, saving "statistical lives" may be seen less abstractly and more concretely by considering "what if?" scenarios. What if smoking had been virtually eradicated at the beginning of this century? What if Barney Clark himself had never smoked? In either scenario, he might have lived into his eighties. It is probable that many people would not need artificial hearts in their early sixties if they had never smoked, had drunk alcohol no more than lightly, and had kept fit. Our priorities seem akilter when $250,000 is spent on a heart patient like Barney Clark, to gain perhaps a few more years of life, if we are unwilling to support efforts that help us keep more people from developing heart disease in the first place.

UPDATE

Robert Jarvik briefly became a minor celebrity; he modeled Hathaway shirts in ads, was featured in *People* magazine, and was interviewed in *Playboy.* In April 1987, Warburg Pincus, a venture capital company that had arranged the financing for Symbion, mounted a hostile takeover after Jarvik had privately sold it a large chunk of stock at a top price; Jarvik fought the takeover but lost and was promptly fired as president. After his ouster, he announced that he was not interested in practicing medicine anymore; instead, he intended to work in "grand unification theory in elementary particle physics . . . [as well as] some other kinds of humanitarian [sic] programs."[58]

At about this time, Jarvik divorced his wife of many years and married Marilyn Vos Savant, whom he had known for only 5 days and who had probably created both her name and her claim to the world's highest IQ. They appeared together as lecturers and on talk shows, billing themselves as the "world's smartest couple." In a joint interview in 1988, speaking for both of them, Marilyn Vos Savant said that she and Jarvik believed their children from their previous marriages to be theirs "only in a biological sense" (her children were college-age, his were school-age); she added, "I don't consider either one of us to have children."[59] Over the next decade, Marilyn Vos Savant was a feature columnist for *Parade*; Robert Jarvik faded into obscurity.

•

Chase Peterson became president of the University of Utah in 1984 but was forced to resign in June 1990 over the "cold fusion" scandal involving Martin Fleischmann and Stanley Pons. Peterson had claimed that an "anonymous donor" had given the University of Utah a large amount of money for the research, when in fact he himself had diverted this money from another university account—at a time when faculty salaries were notoriously low.

•

An interesting episode in 1988 showed how hard it is for the United States to limit a new medical technology. In May of that year, NIH stopped funding artificial hearts; research physicians had reached the consensus that artificial hearts were justifiable only in rare cases, as a temporary "bridge" to a transplant. William DeVries of course opposed this decision, lamenting that it "hurts some really good researchers who have made long-term commitments," but he said that he himself would be unaffected because Humana's funding would continue.[60]

Two months later, NIH reversed itself, bowing to pressure from two senators—Orrin Hatch of Utah and Edward Kennedy of Massachusetts. The original decision by NIH would have meant the loss of $22.6 million over the next 6 years for four research centers in Utah, Texas, Massachusetts, and Ohio; and Hatch and Kennedy threatened to block the entire NIH budget unless funding for research on the artificial heart was restored. In backing down, one NIH official said (anonymously), "With all that Congressional pressure and the threat of legislation, we felt that the heart institute better eat a little crow rather than risk the future budgets of all the institutes."[61] So NIH ate crow.

•

During the last years of the 1980s, artificial hearts were used in only about 90 patients as a bridge to a transplant, never as a permanent device. Even this temporary use essentially ended in 1991; LAVDs rather than the Jarvik-7 were then used as a bridge to transplants. William DeVries had been incorrect when he predicted that the negative judgment by NIH and most physicians would not hurt him: his referrals dropped to almost none, and he received no further exemptions from NIH. In 1990, FDA completely rescinded its approval of the Jarvik-7 either as a permanent device or as a bridge to transplant.

FURTHER READING

Renée Fox and Judith Swazey, *Spare Parts: Organ Replacement in American Society*, Oxford University Press, New York, 1992.
Institute of Medicine, *The Artificial Heart: Prototypes, Policies, and Patients*, National Academy Press, Washington, D.C., 1991.
The Schroeder Family with Marie Barnette, *The Bill Schroeder Story*, Morrow, New York, 1987.
Margery Shaw, ed., *After Barney Clark*, University of Texas Press, Austin, 1984.

CHAPTER 12

Allocation of Artificial and Transplantable Organs

The God Committee

Experimental treatments are often scarce treatments (in fact, of course, a treatment may remain scarce even when it is no longer experimental), and this brings us to the issue of allocating limited medical resources. Transplantable organs are an obvious example; another example is hemodialysis, which is in a sense an artificial kidney. Our case study in this chapter is a lay committee in Seattle in the 1960s, dubbed the "God committee," that decided which patients in renal (kidney) failure would receive dialysis—and therefore which patients would live. The "God committee" is also a useful starting point for discussing how organs for transplant are distributed. The issues involved include not only selection of recipients by "merit" but also informed consent and certain aspects of organ donation.

BACKGROUND: ORGANS AS SCARCE RESOURCES

An "Artificial Kidney": Hemodialysis

The kidneys are organs for removing toxins accumulated by normal cellular metabolism in the blood. When both kidneys completely fail, toxins will accumulate to a lethal level unless the cleansing function of the kidneys is somehow replaced.

Hemodialysis (a term which literally means "tearing blood apart") is a process that can substitute for the kidneys: the blood is removed from the body and sent through cannulas (tubes) where its toxins are absorbed by osmosis through a semipermeable membrane into a surrounding solution; then the cleansed blood is returned to the body. Today, for an adult in renal failure to maintain normal life, hemodialysis—also called simply *dialysis*—is needed for several hours two or three times a week.

A hemodialysis machine was invented in the Netherlands in 1943 by the physician Willem Kolff (whose work on artificial hearts is discussed in Chapter 11). Originally, Kolff used a converted fuel pump from an automobile to force blood out of the body and return it after cleansing. This early dialysis machine presented a daunting problem: every time dialysis occurred, a new connection had to be made between the cannulas and the patient's arteries and veins. Because each artery or vein could be used only once, eventually all the available sites for connections would be exhausted.

In 1960, Belding Scribner in Seattle made it unnecessary to reoperate in this way by inventing a permanent indwelling shunt, a piece of tubing permanently attached to one vein and one artery that allows blood to flow continuously. The shunt contained connections for the cannulas of the dialysis machine and could be shut off between dialyses, like a spigot. At first—for 3 weeks—Scribner did not realize that the combination of a workable dialysis machine and a permanent shunt meant that the half-dozen patients he was dialyzing could be maintained indefinitely: in other words, he did not fully realize that he and Kolff had, between them, created the equivalent of an artificial kidney.[1]

Scribner's technological innovation meant that Kolff's dialysis machines could be used on the thousands of patients dying from renal failure. This breakthrough would eventually lead to something wonderful: thousands of patients who would once have died would now live. However, it would also lead to a potential tragedy: some patients who could have lived would die if no way could be found to dialyze them. Moreover, this potential tragedy entailed an intense ethical problem: selection of patients for dialysis.

The potential for tragedy and the accompanying ethical issues were not immediately obvious, because for a while the procedure continued to be seen as experimental; although both Kolff's dialysis machine and Scribner's shunt worked in the first few cases, no one was sure that patients could survive for many years on chronic dialysis and return to their normal lives. The problem of selection arose when it became clear that this technology did represent an effective, long-term artificial kidney.

Donated Organs: Supply and Demand

The ethical problem of allocating hemodialysis—an artificial organ—is similar to the problem of allocating organs for transplantation. Why such problems arise with transplantable organs can be seen easily when certain aspects of the process of obtaining organs are understood.

First and most important, the base number of available organs for donation has not changed much over the past decades, despite numerous campaigns aimed at increasing it: the number of usable organs from cadavers has leveled off at around 4,000 a year.[2] Second, while the supply remains constant (and sometimes even decreases slightly), the demand for transplantable organs has steadily increased. Let's look at these two factors—supply and demand—in somewhat more detail.

With regard to *supply,* less than 20 percent of American adults sign forms agreeing to be organ donors. There are various reasons for this. For one thing, young adults notoriously do not think about death and thus do not sign donor cards. Also, some people resist the idea of "desecrating" a corpse by removing organs. In addition, African Americans—and other American minority groups who tend to be somewhat suspicious of traditional authority—are often reluctant to sign donor cards because they consider themselves more likely to be declared dead prematurely. Still another factor in reluctance to sign a donor card is confusion about "brain death." (These last two factors were both illustrated in 1968, in the case of Bruce Tucker, who was African American. When Bruce Tucker's heart was transplanted after massive head trauma, Tucker's family sued because it had not consented, and also because Tucker had not been legally dead when his heart was removed.[3])

Of course, organs may be donated by the family of a dead or dying patient even in the absence of a donor card. However, American surgeons do not take organs if the family refuses, and this practice drastically lowers the number of organs donated, though it also reduces the number of lawsuits. One significant reason why medical teams so often hesitate to approach relatives of dying patients is confusion over different definitions of *brain death;* as noted above, this is also one reason why Americans don't sign donor cards. Is a patient who has been comatose for years (like Nancy Cruzan in Chapter 1) "brain-dead"? If so, can such a patient be an organ donor? (Many people would answer yes to this second question, but in fact using such a patient as an organ donor is illegal in every state.) How can two adjacent states define "brain death" so differently that a patient may be dead in one state and "resurrected" in the other?

In addition, many families are reluctant to agree to organ donation because, to maximize the success of retrieval and transplant, the medical team must keep the potential donor in as good a condition as possible: when a potential donor is prevented from further deterioration, the family may find it more difficult to accept the fact of death and thus may find it emotionally wrenching to agree to excision of organs.

Still another factor which causes many families to hesitate is that the medical team working on behalf of a potential donor and the team working on behalf of a potential recipient may be at cross purposes. That is, a treatment which might be indicated if the potential donor had a chance of surviving—or a treatment which might itself offer a very remote chance of survival—could be contraindicated in terms of preserving organs for donation. For example, victims of head trauma should, for their own well-being, be kept as dry (internally) as possible, whereas organ banks need well-hydrated donor organs.

Even when people do sign donor cards and families are willing to allow organ retrieval, the number of actual donors is much lower than the number of potential donors. Suitable donors are mainly young, healthy adults with good organs; in practice, this almost always means young adults killed in motor vehicle crashes. In other words, potential donors who are much older, who die in most other ways, or who have certain conditions when they die are likely to be unsuitable. For instance, the 1 million or so Americans who are HIV-positive and the 1 million with hepatitis B or C can never donate organs.

Ironically, the number of donatable organs is also reduced by successful efforts to prevent motor vehicle accidents: restraints and seats for infants and children, helmets for motorcyclists, a legal drinking age of 21, lower speed limits, and laws and social pressure against drunk driving. These measures have reduced deaths among Americans under 40—the age group most likely to have donatable organs.

With regard to *demand,* the steady increase is illustrated by the following figures for heart transplants in the United States:[4]

Year	Number of heart transplants
1983	172
1989	1,663
1993	2,299

The same trend toward increasing demand also exists with other kinds of transplants, of course. One factor in increased demand for transplantable organs is improvements in transplant technology; another is that as more and more reimbursement becomes available, especially for elderly patients, more and more patients become potential transplant recipients.

Given the increasing need for donor organs, and their persistent scarcity, it is not surprising that in the United States over 100 patients die each month while waiting for a donor organ; in fact, even higher figures are sometimes reported— over 2,000 patients a year between 1988 and 1993, or 6 a day. This imbalance between supply and demand has naturally created pressure for change, but most of the proposed changes are controversial.[5]

For example, at least 14 European countries use the concept of "presumed consent": a dead person is assumed to be a potential donor unless he or she has specified otherwise. However, "presumed consent" would probably not be acceptable in the United States, where mistrust of the medical system is already a factor preventing donation—any attempt to establish the presumptive system here would only increase that mistrust. A "mandated choice" system has been legislated in some states, though: this is a more modest system under which all adults are required to volunteer or exclude themselves as organ donors at some appropriate time (in most cases, when they apply for or renew a driver's license).[6]

There have also been calls for replacing our traditional nonmarket system of organ allocation with a commercial system of selling and buying organs, but as will be discussed later, the ethical problems with any commercial system are obviously enormous.

A development which many observers considered ominous was the Ayala case. Abe and Mary Ayala conceived a child for the acknowledged purpose of creating a bone marrow donor for their daughter Anissa; the baby, Marissa Ayala, was born on April 3, 1990, and the bone-marrow transplant took place on June 4, 1991. (In June 1992 Marissa was the flower girl at Anissa's wedding, at which time both sisters were well.) What Abe and Mary Ayala did was said to have already been done by others at least 40 times,[7] and it seemed only a step away from conceiving a child in order to obtain, say, a donor kidney.

Another development which many people found disturbing was the attempt to have severely brain-damaged babies (such as Baby Theresa, whose case is discussed in Chapter 13) declared brain-dead in order to use their organs for other infants.

Scarcity of human donor organs has also been a factor in attempts to perform xenografts—transplants from animals to human patients, as in the Baby Fae case (also discussed in Chapter 13) and two cases in which baboon livers were transplanted by a team led by Thomas Starzl.

SEATTLE'S "GOD COMMITTEE"

When Belding Scribner developed his shunt, inpatient dialysis cost $20,000 a year.[8] Dialysis was then still considered experimental, and as with all experimental therapies, insurance companies refused to pay for it; thus Scribner's hospital—Swedish Hospital in Seattle—had to provide some treatment free. The first dozen or so patients constantly felt in danger of losing their treatment.

Because the cost of dialysis was so high, Swedish Hospital soon told Scribner that it could not take any more dialysis patients (the hospital also noted a shortage of beds). By then, though, Scribner and others had a year's experience with managing problems of caring for dialysis patients, and they decided that dialysis could be done as an outpatient procedure. Swedish Hospital agreed to oversee an outpatient program, and in 1962 it began long-term, or *chronic,* outpatient dialysis.

The outpatient dialysis center created at Swedish Hospital in 1962 could serve 17 patients, but many more were eligible; from the beginning, then, there was an ethical problem—in the words of the title of a seminal article, "Who Shall Live When Not All Can Live?"[9] An advance in treatment had thus created a specific problem of distribution.

Instead of leaving the problem of distribution to be dealt with by individual physicians for individual patients, Swedish Hospital and King County Medical Society had already taken an unusual step: an Admissions and Policy Committee had been formed in 1961 to make crucial decisions about selection. Remarkably, this committee was made up mostly of laypeople; although there was a surgeon on the committee, and although physicians on an advisory committee screened applicants for medical suitability, the people who made the real decisions were not physicians. In fact, the intent was to take the burden of decision off physicians, since a physician would naturally want his or her own patients to be accepted.[10] The committee, which was supposed to be representative of the community, initially had seven members: a minister, a lawyer, a housewife, a labor leader, a state government official, a banker, and the surgeon. Two physicians familiar with dialysis served as advisers. The committee worked anonymously.

The committee first limited candidates simply to residents of the state of Washington who were under age 45; candidates also had to be able to afford dialysis, which generally meant that a candidate's insurer had to agree to pay for it. Almost immediately, however, too many patients applied and additional criteria became necessary. The committee then began to consider whether a candidate was employed, was a parent of dependent children, was educated, was motivated, had a history of achievements, and had any potential to help others. Eventually, the committee also asked for and considered analyses of a candidate's ability to tolerate anxiety and to manage his or her medical care independently; it also considered whether or not a candidate was likely to use his or her symptoms to get attention. In its deliberations, the committee would evaluate the personality and personal merit of the candidate, the strengths and weaknesses of the candidate's family, and the family's emotional support for a patient on chronic dialysis. By its own rule, the dialysis committee did not meet candidates personally.

It should be noted that this committee was struggling with issues of distribution in the era before bioethics. At the time, no philosophers were writing about ethical issues of allocating artificial or natural organs; no philosophers were writing about bioethics at all.[11] Nevertheless, Scribner, who had evidently been involved in establishing the committee, wrote in 1972, "As I recall that period, all of us who were involved felt that we had found a fairly reasonable and simple solution to an impossibly difficult problem by letting a committee of responsible members of the community choose which patients [would receive treatment]."[12]

•

In May of 1962 (at about the time when Seattle built its Space Needle), Belding Scribner went with one of his patients to Atlantic City, where a convention of newspaper publishers and editors was being held. Scribner was hoping to obtain public support for more dialysis machines; but he also described the selection committee to reporters,[13] and it was his account of the committee—rather than his appeal for more dialysis—that made the front page of the *New York Times* the next day.[14]

Life assigned its first woman reporter, Shana Alexander, to cover the story of the committee; she spent 3 months interviewing people in Seattle, and her report appeared in November 1962.[15] It was Alexander who coined the term *God committee:* she described the committee as playing a godlike role in deciding who would live and who would die. She also described in detail the committee's criteria, which would come to be called the *social worth standard* and were seen as implying that some candidates were more valuable than others.

According to Alexander, in response to the criticism that they were "playing God," some of the committee members had argued that if they didn't do the choosing, someone else would (an argument which recalls the existentialist philosopher Jean Paul Sartre, who held that "Not to choose is still a choice"). Other members had pointed out that dialysis was an experimental treatment: "We are picking guinea pigs for experimental purposes," two members said—not denying life to others.[16] As dialysis became increasingly safe, however, this justification would become untenable.

In the spring of 1963, the *Seattle Times* ran on its front page a picture of nine of the center's dialysis patients, with the heading, "Will These People Have to Die?"[17] As a result, temporary support was offered by the Boeing Corporation and the U.S. Public Health Service.

In 1964, Scribner gave the Presidential Address to the American Society for Artificial Internal Organs, entitled "Ethical Problems of Dialysis Selection."[18]

In 1965, Edwin Newman narrated an NBC documentary on the Seattle committee, *Who Shall Live?* That year, Congress had added to social security two national medical programs—Medicare for the elderly and Medicaid for the indigent—but dialysis was not yet covered under either of them. On the documentary, Congressman Melvin Laird (later secretary of defense) asked why, if the United States could have a space program, it couldn't have a dialysis program to save lives;[19] the powerful Congressman John Fogarty demanded that AMA take a stand about federal support for production of thousands of dialysis machines. National interest grew about the story, and indirectly about bioethics.

•

The role of the media in all this was clearly important. To begin with, the original story was shaped significantly by the media's response. Shana Alexander said that when Scribner went to Atlantic City, he had been "angling" to get the magazine with the largest circulation of its time to bring this story to the nation; and the medical sociologist Judith Swazey agrees that Scribner set out deliberately to get publicity.[20] Undeniably, he did get publicity; but the story he wanted to get across seems to have been simply the need for more dialysis machines, and the story he got amounted to an exposé of the selection committee.

Thirty years later, Scribner said that he had been "totally naive" about the kind of national publicity which developed; he also said that he had taken "a lot of flak" about the committee's existence, especially from an early article in *UCLA Law Review*.[21] He claimed then that he had had nothing to do with the committee, which had been created and supervised by the King County Medical Association (here, though, he is not entirely convincing); he said that he "hated the goddamn committee" and did everything possible to circumvent it when he had a dying patient who wasn't selected. Scribner also claimed that Alexander had not interviewed a single patient[22]—a claim she flatly denied, to his face.[23]

With regard to the story in the *Seattle Times*, this report could not have been written without the cooperation of nephrologists (kidney specialists) at Swedish Hospital and at the University of Washington. At this time, medicine thought of local and national media largely in terms of public relations,[24] and these physicians were using the *Seattle Times* to seek funds. Their success may have begun the pattern of trying to use the media when emergency financing is needed for patients with organ failure.

It is noteworthy that during the late 1960s—when widespread questioning of authority became part of the American culture—the media would become less subservient with regard to this kind of "rescue." Reporters would begin to insist that if physicians wanted to use the media to "rescue" patients, it would have to be a two-way street: physicians would have a reciprocal obligation to disclose information. By the time of the Barney Clark case (Chapter 11), the media were much less manageable, and physicians who tried to use journalism for their own ends often found that they had a tiger by the tail.

ETHICAL ISSUES

The Public Arena

For reasons which were probably mixed and complex, Belding Scribner did something that went against a medical practice going back decades or even centuries: he made public a moral dilemma which hitherto had been discussed only privately among physicians. Bringing this issue to the public's attention was controversial within medicine.[25] As would also be true in the case of Karen Quinlan

(Chapter 1), many physicians felt that such ethical issues should be handled quietly, within the profession.

By letting this genie out of its bottle, Scribner began a new process—the education of the American public about the many ethical problems in medicine. Different moral opinions among physicians now began to be expressed publicly by scholars. In retrospect, this process was perhaps inevitable: since ethical issues in medicine affect so many people so intensely, probably they were bound to reach the public arena sooner or later. It should be realized, though, that achieving consensus on ethical policy is no easier in the public arena than within medicine.

Selecting Recipients

General problems of selecting patients are often much the same whether the resource to be distributed is a donor organ or dialysis. In this section, we'll consider four specific major issues having to do with selection: "social worth" as a criterion for candidates, systems of distribution of donor organs (especially how candidates are listed), retransplants, and the "rule of rescue."

"Social worth"   In approaching the problem of selecting recipients, physicians perceive the issue as largely medical and focus on identifying candidates with whom the best results can be obtained; ethicists, on the other hand, focus on philosophical criteria of selection. Whether nonmedical factors should be considered is an important broad question; but the narrower question of "social worth" as a nonmedical criterion has received most attention.

As we have seen, the Seattle dialysis committee did take "social worth" into account—though the committee itself apparently did not use this term. The medical sociologists Renée Fox and Judith Swazey (who spent 30 years studying the American experience with artificial kidneys and transplantation and wrote classic works on these subjects)[26] reviewed the minutes of the committee's meetings and described its "social worth" criteria as follows:

> Within these very general criteria, the specific, often unarticulated indicators that were used reflected the middle-class American value system shared by the selection panel. A person "worthy" of having his life saved by a scarce, expensive treatment like chronic dialysis was one judged to have qualities such as decency and responsibility. Any history of social deviance, such as a prison record, any suggestion that a person's married life was not intact and scandal-free, were strong contraindications to selection. The preferred candidate was a person who had demonstrated achievement through hard work and success at this job, who went to church, joined groups, and was actively involved in community affairs.[27]

Some critics have argued that social worth should never be used as a criterion, because any such standard implies that some people are worth more than others and is therefore inherently unjust. Immanuel Kant, for instance, would probably have opposed any "social worth" standard; his ethical philosophy would seem to entail impartial, random selection by lot, say, or by drawing straws. Two severe critics of the Seattle committee—a psychiatrist and a lawyer—remarked:

The magazines paint a disturbing picture of the bourgeoisie sparing the bourgeoisie, of the Seattle committee measuring persons in accordance with its own middle-class suburban value system: scouts, Sunday school, Red Cross. This rules out creative conformists, who rub the bourgeoisie the wrong way but who historically have contributed so much to the making of America. The Pacific Northwest is no place for a Henry David Thoreau with bad kidneys.[28]

Similarly, George Annas, who is both a lawyer and a bioethicist, criticized the Seattle Committee for preferring housewives over prostitutes, working men over "playboys," and scientists over poets.[29]

On the other hand, in 1969 the philosopher Nicholas Rescher argued, in a classic article, that the Seattle committee had been just in using criteria which included social worth.[30] Rescher was in favor of considering life expectancy, number of dependents, potential for future contributions to society, and past achievements. (Less controversially, he also supported screening candidates for medical problems that were likely to make them do poorly on dialysis, since otherwise dialysis machines would be wasted.) He suggested that such a selection system might be based on points, though a tie could be broken by a lottery.

Annas, moreover, argues that some criteria of social worth can be just at some stage of the selection process, though he says that justice requires these criteria to be consciously formulated and made public. That is, if one rule is going to be "always prefer housewives to prostitutes," this should be explicitly defended. Private (unstated) rules would allow discrimination based on race, sex, class, or wealth.

In fairness to the committee, we should also note that dialysis at home had soon become an official goal, since it was found that six patients could be supported at home at the same cost as a single patient in the hospital. That being the case, at least two aspects of social worth were relevant: the psychological support of the patient's family and the patient's own attitude or capability. A passive, uncooperative patient can usually be handled adequately in a hospital setting, but not necessarily at home. Fox and Swazey, for instance, devote an entire chapter to the case of a Native American patient named Ernie Crowfeather around 1969. Ernie Crowfeather—a criminal, though a charmer—received dialysis for 30 months but refused to comply with the medical regimen, hated his quality of life, drank, imposed his childlike needs on the staff, and finally turned down further therapy and died.[31] Apparently, in selecting Ernie Crowfeather, the committe had made an exception to its standards regarding patients' attitudes and capability; if so, the point is this: was use of dialysis for this patient worthwhile, when it might have saved the lives of two or three others?

The issue of social worth has also emerged with regard to liver transplants, though in this context social worth can be particularly hard to disentangle from medical criteria. The liver is by far the most expensive organ to transplant: the surgery calls for a highly skilled team and takes a long time. A significant fact is that the most common cause of liver destruction, or end-stage liver disease (ESLD), is alcoholism; when alcohol is a factor, the condition is actually called *alcohol-related end-stage liver disease* (ARESLD). In the 1990s, a controversy arose about whether patients with ARESLD and patients who were nondrinkers should be equally eligible for liver transplants. This is partly a medical issue, of course, since it can be analyzed in terms of which patients will probably benefit from such a transplant; but there is also an element of social worth. Is a non-drinker more "deserving" of a donor liver? Can someone with ARESLD be held "blameworthy" for the loss of his or her liver and thus undeserving of a new one? Would a drinker keep on drinking, thereby destroying the new liver; or would drinkers be transformed by receiving the "gift of life"?

In the case of liver transplants (as in certain other medical situations), there is also another issue: can candidates be excluded on the ground that they have voluntarily risked their health?[32] With ARESLD specifically, this question is complicated by disagreement over whether alcoholism is a disease (and thus involuntary) or a self-inflicted voluntary behavioral pattern. The disease model of alcoholism has prevailed for some time, but it has recently been attacked by the philosopher Herbert Fingarette.[33]

Two teams of clinical medical ethicists conflicted over this point in 1992. In Chicago, the physicians Alvin Moss and Mark Seigler argued that since ARESLD is the principal cause of liver failure, since there is a dire shortage of livers for transplant, and since recidivism is likely among alcoholics, patients who develop liver failure "through no fault of their own" (that is, nondrinkers) should have a higher priority for donor livers than patients with ARESLD—whose condition "results from failure to obtain treatment for alcoholism."[34] Two medical ethicists at the University of Michigan with doctorates in philosophy, Carl Cohen and Martin Benjamin, found that argument "defective": Cohen and Benjamin maintained that alcoholics are not morally blameworthy and do in fact have satisfactory rates of survival after a liver transplant.[35]

Some critics conclude that social worth—or "worth to society"—is in general so difficult to judge that only medical criteria should be applied: in other words, scarce medical resources (such as dialysis and liver transplants) should be distributed simply on the basis of who will benefit medically.[36] Probably, though, the problem of selection involves balancing considerations of social worth, social equality, and moral worth with considerations about medical benefits and the patient's ability to follow a rigorous regimen. In any event, answers are not simple, and no solution will satisfy everyone.

Distribution systems and waiting lists   A second issue in the selection of recipients is systems of distribution and how candidates are listed in such systems.

In the 1970s, no real system existed for distributing donated organs, and organs that became available in one medical center or one region of the country were not always shared with other centers nationwide. In fact, some states resisted the idea of allowing their donor organs to be used elsewhere and therefore did not pursue organ donors aggressively if a nearby state had a big transplant program.

By 1987, the National Transplantation Act (1984) and the federal Task Force on Organ Transplantation (1986) had created the United Network for Organ Sharing (UNOS). UNOS alleviated some regional competition. It also established a standardized system for deciding which patient will get the next available organ; before UNOS, lack of standardization had made this decision a significant ethical problem.

However, UNOS deals only with candidates who are already on the system. Thus how and when applicants get onto waiting lists for donor organs remains a pressing issue. Imagine that you are going to die if you don't get an organ, but you know that 100 other patients want the same organ for the same reason. Suppose you hear that someone in, say, Pittsburgh or Houston has received an organ because he or she knew the right surgeon and therefore got onto the right list. It's one thing to feel unlucky because you're in a life-threatening condition, but quite another to feel that you are going to die of organ failure because someone else managed to get into line in front of you.

An especially vexing problem is the practice of multiple listing.[37] Some patients get themselves appointments with surgeons at more than one transplant center and have themselves "worked up" at each; but only people who can take time off from work, can afford to travel, and have generous medical plans can arrange for multiple listings in this way. For a patient who needs a kidney, being on several lists may not be necessary; for a patient who needs a heart or a liver, though, a multiple listing may be a matter of life and death. One criterion for receiving a heart or liver is locality: a candidate must be within the area of the transplant center. A patient who registers at half a dozen such centers (say, in southern California) can significantly increase the chance of being selected.

Multiple listing is generally permitted, but in July 1990, New York became the first state to ban it (New York is still the only state with such a ban). In 1992, some patients who were then multiple-listed argued in a hearing before UNOS that forbidding the practice denied them autonomy. They maintained that they had a right as individuals to choose their own physicians; that is, a ban on multiple listing would curtail their "liberty right" to contract for medical care.[38]

There are two powerful arguments against multiple listing, however. First, a primary attribute of a just medical system is equality of access, and the use of wealth to "bump the line" violates this norm. Second, multiple listing compromises the entire UNOS system because some people are getting listed above others arbitrarily—that is, for no good reason. UNOS should be impartial not only in dealing with candidates who are already listed but also in the actual process of deciding who gets listed.

A similar problem surfaced in the early 1990s, when it was revealed that candidates for neonatal heart transplants were being identified prenatally and then being placed on waiting lists immediately, while they were still fetuses.[39] Because time accumulated on a waiting list gives a candidate extra points, such a practice would offer a significant advantage. In this case, prenatal listing was made possible by the ability to diagnose hypoplastic left heart syndrome (HLHS) in utero; but such early diagnosis is not uniformly distributed in the United States, and early listing of babies diagnosed in utero seemed unfair to babies who were not diagnosed until birth. Moreover, fetuses with HLHS remain relatively safe while they are in the womb, whereas at birth HLHS babies are almost always at great risk and are in NICUs. For these reasons, UNOS changed its policy in June 1992 and put fetuses on a separate list from babies. UNOS also decided to allocate a heart to a fetus only when no baby could use it.

Retransplants   A third issue in selecting recipients is raised by retransplantation. Since transplanted kidneys and hearts, for instance, are often rejected, a retransplant is often necessary. In such a situation, the question arises whether a patient who needs a second (or third) transplant and a patient who is waiting for a first transplant should be treated equally, or whether either one should take priority over the other. This is actually a rather complex matter.

In the UNOS system, patients waiting for retransplants are treated the same way as first-time patients. This may seem basically fair, but it may not lead to the best possible outcomes. Consider the following statistics for heart transplants and retransplants from October 1, 1987, to December 31, 1991:[40]

	Recipients	1-year survival (percent)
First transplant	4,830	81.6
Retransplant	86	56.7

These figures indicate that retransplant patients fare much worse than first-transplant (or *primary-transplant*) patients; the reason is simply that retransplant patients tend to be sicker. If this were the only consideration, UNOS should probably give first-time patients priority over retransplant patients: that would maximize survival per heart and on utilitarian grounds would seem to be the only ethical policy.

However, statistics like these are not the only consideration. One other consideration, for instance, is that it is precisely the sickest patients are most urgently in need—patients who are less sick may be able to wait a while.

There is also the human factor. Whatever might be argued about hypothetical or statistical cases, in real life a transplant team develops a bond with a patient and thus finds it extremely difficult not to use an available organ for retransplant to save that patient. This is understandable: the medical team has worked very hard—often over many years—to save the patient's life, and when an organ is rejected, the team members do not want to be forced by some system of regulations to stand back and watch the patient die while an available organ goes to someone else. In fact, medical staffs see this as "patient abandonment"; physicians emphasize their emotional attachment to such patients and insist that they cannot ethically "abandon" them. More simply, a retransplant patient is personally *known* to the surgeon and the transplant team, whereas a new patient is still only an abstraction.

It is true that medical ethics cannot ignore human emotions or the intimate relationship between patients and physicians. On the other hand, it is reasonable to ask why "identified patients" should take priority over new patients: a new patient may be just as much in need, just as likely (or more likely) to benefit, and just as meritorious. It can also be argued that "patients who are better at forming relationships with transplant teams"[41] will be favored if the medical teams are allowed to exercise their own judgment, and that this is not really sensible. Furthermore, although transplant teams tend to identify with the retransplant patient, other people may identify with the patient who is waiting for a first transplant. We might feel that if one patient has already received a donor heart, it is time for someone else to get a chance; why should a first-time candidate die so that a retransplant patient can have a second (or third!) donor heart?

Some critics argue that transplant centers are biased in favor of retransplants not only for emotional reasons but also because they are evaluated in terms of posttransplant survival rates—the centers are not required to report how many patients die on their waiting lists. In addition, their medical criteria may be contradictory: in selecting candidates, these centers first maximize the chances of survival by emphasizing blood and tissue compatibility; but then, by favoring retransplant patients over first-time candidates, they fail to maximize survival.

This whole issue is highly controversial within transplant medicine. The case of Ronnie DeSillers, who received three liver transplants (at a total cost of over $1 million), caused very bitter feelings among physicians in Miami and among patients on waiting lists for liver transplants. Ernie Crowfeather, the dialysis patient described above whose case ended so dismally, may be another example: perhaps one reason why such enormous resources were devoted to him was that he was an "identified" person who had a relationship with a medical team. Should such "identified" relationships be allowed to determine who will receive a treatment? It is perhaps because of this question that the issue is defined as a matter of justice: it affects the distribution of a resource to citizens within a entire system and does not concern only the feelings of particular people who know each other.

The rule of rescue   A fourth problem in selecting recipients is a social problem known as the *rule of rescue*. The rule of rescue, which was named by the bioethicist Albert Jonsen,[42] refers to the strong social tendency to help an identified individual—in this context, a patient—rather than unidentified, anonymous, or "statistical" people who are equally deserving and equally endangered. Countless examples of the rule of rescue can be cited. If the story of a small child trapped in a deep well is followed closely on television, hundreds or thousands of people will probably send tens of thousands of dollars in contributions for the rescue effort; meanwhile, though, the story of another, equally deserving person in danger does not receive television coverage—and this second person is not rescued and therefore dies. Larry McAfee, whose case is discussed in Chapter 2, benefited from the rule of rescue when his private medical insurance ran out: he gained the attention of the media and thereby received special public funding.

In the context of organ replacement, the rule of rescue has been used for nearly three decades to save a few children in organ failure. (One example, in 1982, was the hospital administrator Charles Fiske, who blatantly manipulated the media to obtain a liver donor for his daughter Jamie.) In some of its aspects, the tendency of transplant teams to favor "identified" candidates for retransplants over "abstract" new candidates for primary transplants is also an instance of the rule of rescue. Another instance of the rule of rescue, of course, was the *Seattle Times* story "Will These People Have to Die?" in 1963, discussed earlier in this chapter, which was instrumental in getting support for nine dialysis patients.

The rule of rescue can obviously be used very successfully, but it involves serious ethical problems. To begin with, if one life is worth the same as another, the rule of rescue seems irrational and unfair.

Also, the criteria that drive the rule of rescue often seem irrelevant, trivial, or muddleheaded. Who gets to live shouldn't be decided by who gets on television. Who gets to live shouldn't be decided by who has been admitted to a hospital or has gotten into the system. Who gets to live shouldn't be decided by who is most photogenic. Who gets to live shouldn't be decided by who is cutest or most appealing.

Furthermore, the rule of rescue can mean that journalistic gatekeepers in effect are making decisions about who lives and dies. As newspaper and television editors quickly found out, the rule of rescue can replace a God committee with an assignment editor.

Finally, the greatest problem with the rule of rescue is that for every identifiable person who is saved, there will be any number of anonymous patients who are lost.[43] (The rule of rescue is also discussed in Chapter 2.)

Patients: Informed Consent

The issue of patients' informed consent arises in allocating replacement organs because it is by no means certain that candidates for such replacement understand what lies ahead. The media paint a sunny picture of organ transplants, for instance, typically citing only 1-year survival rates; within medicine there has been a reconceptualization of transplants from "experimental" to "therapeutic"; and potential donors are urged to give a "gift of life." Thus there is a widespread perception among the public that a healthy transplanted organ will function for the recipient's lifetime. The reality is somewhat different.

Journalists have generally not understood, or have not reported, the long-term problems of transplants. Rejection of transplanted organs appears to be nearly universal if the recipient lives long enough. This is the familiar problem of rejection of foreign tissue by the immune system, and it does not seem to be solved by getting a closer match between donor and recipient. One-third to one-half of heart transplants are rejected after 5 years, for example. Kidney transplants began in 1951 and today are closest to being truly therapeutic rather than experimental; but even so, over 50 percent of transplanted kidneys are rejected after 10 years.[44]

To prevent rejection of a transplanted organ, continuous maintenance on cyclosporin is usually necessary.[45] However, malignant lymphoma often develops in patients maintained on cyclosporin, and long-term exposure to cyclosporin often destroys the kidneys or liver and may produce brain damage. Cyclosporin also has side effects, such as excess facial hair in women patients. Moreover, the efficacy of cyclosporin appears to fade after several years.

In the 1990s, claims were being made for FK 506 as a "miraculous" antirejection drug (especially by the surgeon Thomas Starzl of Pittsburgh, who had by then retired); but there was less than full disclosure about its outcomes and about continuing problems associated with it. Fox and Swazey expressed concerns about the toxicity of FK 506, and in 1994 it played a role in the poignant case of 15-year-old Benito ("Benny") Agrelo of Coral Springs, Florida. Benny had been maintained on cyclosporin for 5 years after a primary liver transplant at the University of Pittsburgh; when that transplant failed, he received a second liver from the same team in 1992 and was then put on FK 506. By the summer of 1994, FK 506 had made him unable to read for even 5 minutes without a blinding headache and was causing such severe pain in his joints that he was unable to play any sports; he decided that the drug was not worth it and that he wanted to stay home and die. His request was not honored: as he kicked and screamed, he was dragged from his home and returned to the hospital accompanied by two ambulances, five police cars, social workers, and his mother; before being strapped to a stretcher, he had managed to kick out a windowpane. Benny was held in the hospital for 5 days before a judge decided that he could not be forced to take FK 506. He died in August 1994.

Fox and Swazey's long study of organ replacement led them to some dismal conclusions. They argue that the reclassification of organ transplants as "therapeutic" was done not because of medical evidence but rather to make transplants eligible for reimbursement and to obtain publicity in order to increase the number of donors.[46] They add:

> In the context of the growing organ shortage "crisis," the theme of organ transplantation as gift of life was framed and addressed primarily as a social policy problem of supply and demand. Exhortations to "make a miracle" happen through organ donation were accompanied by a structured forgetting of some of the darker emotional and existential implications of what it involved.[47]

There is evidence to bear out this conclusion, since several programs have a decade or more of experience and have performed hundreds of transplants. As Fox and Swazey—who were participant-observers for over 40 years—report, some patients and families never imagined that "it could be as bad as this."

Patients' informed consent, then, can be a serious issue with organ replacement. In the case of heart transplants, where the alternative is often certain death, the patient's awareness of probable long-term problems after a transplant is perhaps not a major ethical issue. However, in the case of kidney transplants, there is an ethical problem, since an alternative exists: patients can be maintained indefinitely on dialysis.

How much does a candidate for transplantation understand about the experimental nature of an organ transplant? How much *can* such a candidate understand, given that these patients are seriously ill and often desperate? How is informed consent to be obtained in this situation?

Broadening Donorship

Because of the scarcity of donatable organs and the consequent problems of allocation, there have been proposals for broadening the base of donorship. One such proposal, the use of living donors, has now become a reality; a second proposal, commercialization of donorship, remains illegal in the United States. Let's examine these two issues.

Living donors   At one time, there was a ban on organ donations from living people; because the need for donor organs is so great, that ban has now been lifted. Thus some parents, for instance, are approached as possible donors for their own children; they may be asked to give, say, a kidney, a lobe of the liver, or part of a lung.

In January 1993, James Sewell (age 55) and Barbara Sewell (49) each donated part of a lung to their 22-year-old daughter, whose own lungs had been damaged by cystic fibrosis,[48] a genetic disease that is typically fatal by age 30 (the patient usually dies from death of the lungs). The Sewell case was the first of its kind, but other such cases followed. On July 8, 1993, Darlene Pinkerton and her husband made a similar donation to their son, who was also dying of cystic fibrosis. Later, Vaughn Starnes, the surgeon who performed both of these lung-tissue transplants, reported that Stacy Sewell was "doing well and leading an active life four months out";[49] he also said that whereas before the operation the Pinkertons' son had been ventilator-dependent and had been "in the last hours of his life," afterward he had healthy lung tissue which might function for years. Also in July 1993, Nilza Rodriguez became the first living donor of liver tissue to a relative: she gave one-quarter of her liver to her dying granddaughter. The prognosis for this donor was that her own liver would regrow and be perfectly normal "within a month or so."[50] When another case of parent-to-child lung tissue transplant for cystic fibrosis took place in August 1994, it appeared that a trend had begun.

The living donor presents certain ethical problems. In this regard, it is useful to understand why requesting donations from living people, such as parents, was previously considered unethical. One answer is the ancient rule for physicians: "First, do no harm" (*Primum non nocere*). A surgeon who cuts out a living donor's kidney, or part of the liver, unequivocally harms the donor: there is a real insult to the body. (If, by comparison, an attacker stabbed a victim with the same result, that would certainly be regarded as harm.) Moreover, no matter how much medical professionals brush over the risks to the donor, there is a real risk of complications: unexpected reactions to anesthesia, iatrogenic infections, and even surgical accidents.

One such surgical accident occurred, for instance, in the first transplant of a liver lobe from a live parent to a daughter—Alyssa Smith. The donor in this case was Alyssa Smith's mother. While he was removing the lobe of the donor's liver, the surgeon—Christopher Broelsch at the University of Chicago—nicked her spleen and was forced to excise it. Broelsch called the loss of the donor's spleen a "major complication" and said that it gave him "the sickest feeling to have trouble with the first patient."[51] Undoubtedly, Broelsch's "sickest feeling" came from the unescapable knowledge that in trying to help a sick person, he had injured a healthy one.

In addition to these obvious immediate risks, there may be long-term risk. Of, for instance, 100 live kidney donors, how many will die early as a result? This is difficult to calculate; and the result must also be compared with—and balanced against—another calculation that is at least as difficult: expected years of acceptable quality of life for the recipient.

Considerations of medical risk and harm, then, are one basis for considering it unethical to ask living people to become organ donors. There are also emotional or personal considerations, from the viewpoint of both donor and recipient.

One emotional consideration is simply that it may be unethical to put anyone in the position of having to respond to a request for an organ donation. In other words, should some questions not be asked at all? We all recognize that some people are heroic and saintly, and every society tries to encourage altruistic behavior—but actually asking someone to become a hero or a saint is a different matter. Is it fair to put, say, parents in a situation where they are expected to be saintly because of their love for their children? Even the most loving parents must feel torn when they are faced with deciding to give a kidney or a liver lobe to a dying child, but how can they refuse to do something that might save the child's life? A situation like this is a painful dilemma: the parent must choose between a serious risk and lifelong guilt.

From the point of view of the recipient, there are similar emotional problems. If, for instance, a parent dies or is harmed as a result of donating an organ to a child, how will the child feel? If a parent-to-child transplant is successful, how can the child ever thank the parent adequately? If there are problems between parent and child, will the child feel obliged to prevent them from surfacing? What could a child reply to a parent who says, "How could you do that? I gave you life—twice!"

These medical and personal arguments against organ donation by living people are serious, and it was primarily the pressing demand for organs—rather than any wholly convincing counterarguments—that made live donation acceptable. Indeed, like a gigantic pool of water seeking to flow downward, the urgent need for transplantable organs keeps trying to find ways over, under, or around the "dam" of ethics. Such pressure usually creates cracks.

Commercialization: Selling organs   It is generally assumed in the United States that replacement organs such as dialysis machines and donor organs should not be bought and sold in a commercial market. The basis for this assumption is that there are simply some things which money cannot buy, that society should shield those things from commercialization, and that life itself should be shielded in this way. By drawing such a line, society can reduce the unjust influence of wealth—the power of those with money over those without it.

However, not everyone agrees with this assumption, and the debate over selling organs goes to the core of how American society views itself. Michael Kinsley, for example, acknowledges that "almost everyone" considers "commodification" of organs "abhorrent," but he asks whether such a mass belief is necessarily true.[52] He argues that we should allow at least the sale of organs from "neomorts," because banning the sale of such an organ does no good and may do harm. If the family of a potential donor is willing to sell an organ but unwilling to give it away, forbidding the sale may deprive the family of a great deal of money and may, in addition, leave the intended recipient dead. Our traditional distaste for selling organs, Kinsley maintains, is merely a "sentimental reaction to the injustice of life—injustice that the transaction highlights but does not increase."

Needless to say, Kinsley's position is controversial; but before we turn to ideological points, it should be noted that "harvesting neomorts" may not really be feasible. In most deaths, the organs are damaged almost immediately by lack of oxygen and thus are unsuitable for donation. It is generally on theoretical rather than practical grounds, though, that proposals like Kinsley's are challenged.

Fox and Swazey, who are liberals, think it was no coincidence that such proposals for commercialization arose in the Reagan-Bush-Trump years when, they imply, greed became a virtue.[53] They note that some advocates of property rights and the "right" of the poor to sell their organs ("my organs are my property to sell") do not show any concern for the plight of the poor in any other context.

In a famous study in 1971, Richard Titmuss argued with regard to blood donation that the English system, which obtained all blood by altruistic donation, was preferable to the American system of allowing donors to sell their blood.[54] Titmuss and others have emphasized the deep significance of blood and organs as a *gift* from one person to another—a gift of life, with enormous social and psychological repercussions between the giver and the receiver. To turn this gift into a sales transaction, such critics argue, is to take part of what is highest and best in us and turn it into something that may represent what is lowest and worst: buying and selling each other.

The 1986, the Organ Task Force concluded that organs are the property of the "community," not of individuals to sell.

This debate had an interesting linguistic aspect: it inspired the euphemism *rewarded gift* or *rewarded giving* to replace blunt terms like "buying and selling organs." This is a good example of how language can be used to mislead thinking. There is no such thing as a "rewarded gift"—a transaction that is financially "rewarded" is not a gift at all but a sale. If a kidney donor is paid, say, $10,000, the transaction is not the "gift of life" but the sale of a kidney.

•

Not every society forbids or discourages the selling of organs. In this regard, here are two postscripts to the debate over commercialization. First, studies of organ selling in India and Egypt have yielded mixed findings. As a result of commercial kidney donations in India, for example, thousands of recipients have been able to live without dialysis; and some donors have been able to use their bonanza successfully, to raise themselves out of poverty. However, other Indian donors have wasted their money or have later become sick and regretted their decision.[55]

The second postscript involves Saudi Arabia. In 1985, the *Pittsburgh Press* reported (in a series of Pulitzer Prize-winning articles) that some wealthy Saudis were buying American donor organs.[56] This report caused a nationwide sensation, and many people demanded an "America first" policy for donor organs. Interestingly, though, Nicholas Rescher—who had at one time defended the practice of serving only the "natural constituents" of an institution—now implied that excluding nonconstituents would go against a medical tradition dating back to Hippocrates.

The fervor cooled somewhat when it was announced that foreigners were allowed to purchase organs only when no Americans could be found to take them, and at a point when the organs would soon cease to be transplantable. After several investigations by various commissions, however, exports of donor organs to other countries were banned, although some foreigners were still allowed to come to the United States for transplants if the organs in question would otherwise be lost—that is, after it had been ascertained that no American candidates wanted them. Nevertheless, there still seemed to be some potential for trouble here.

Costs and the "Medical Commons"

The cost of a liver transplant for a child is on average about $146,000 for the operation and $6,000 a year thereafter; a kidney transplant costs $60,000 for the first year and $6,000 a year thereafter; dialysis costs $32,000 a year; an average heart transplant costs $91,000 the first year and $6,000 a year thereafter; a bone-marrow transplant costs $100,000. Figures like these give many people pause.

During the 1970s, the biologist Garrett Hardin discussed the *tragedy of the commons*, a situation in which no one reduces his or her consumption of some public resource, until the resource becomes so ravaged or overloaded that it finally disappears. The concept originated centuries ago, in England, when pastures held in common were overgrazed: in each town, each shepherd increased his own flock until there were so many animals that the common could no longer support them. The point is that unlimited pursuit of private self-interest can lead to destruction of public resources.

Today, the environment is perhaps the most obvious example of the tragedy of the commons: Lebanon, which once had great forests, now has mostly rocky pastures; Haiti, which once had luxuriant tropical vegetation, now has treeless mountains whose runoff mud has clogged its rivers and destroyed its offshore fishing; China once had great forests, though now one can fly over 1,000 miles of Chinese landscape and see no forests at all. But the environment is not the only area in which the tragedy of the commons can appear: the figures above suggest that we may also be able to find it in the consumption of medical resources.

UPDATE

Seattle's God committee went on selecting and rejecting dialysis patients for nearly a decade. By 1971, however, many stories had dramatized the plight of patients in renal failure; and in that year Shep Glazer, the president of the American Association of Kidney Patients, testified dramatically before Congress. As the story goes (although it may be exaggerated), Glazer dialyzed himself before the House Ways and Means Committee, disconnected a tube from the machine, let his blood flow onto the floor, and said, "If you don't fund more machines, you'll have this blood on your hands."[57]

In 1972, Congress legislated a "right to medical care," of sorts, for Americans: it was limited to just one organ, the kidney. This was the End-Stage Renal Disease Act (ESRDA), whereby the federal government would pay for a dialysis machine for any American who needed one. Faced with the ethical problem of which patients should be funded and how to select such patients, Congress took what was then the easy way out—it simply funded all patients.

Congress had passed ESRDA in a session lasting only 30 minutes. The impetus came from a coalition of kidney patients, lobbyists for some physicians, concerns over high rates of kidney failure in people of color, and concerns that too much money was being spent on space and the war in Vietnam and too little on dying people who might be saved. Impetus also came from a national media focus on desperate kidney patients, which might be traced back to the efforts of Belding Scribner.

By making dialysis available to all patients, ESRDA ended the problem of allocating it and thus ended the need for the God committee.

•

In retrospect, ESRDA was hastily conceived, and it set an unfortunate precedent—other groups, such as hemophiliacs, soon pressed for similar coverage. Sooner or later, of course, someone would have to pay the piper.

Advocates of funding for dialysis had predicted that costs would come down as more machines were produced. Senator Vance Hartke of Indiana, who was once considered a contender for the presidency, predicted that although ESRDA would cost $100 million the first year, its cost would drop sharply thereafter because of increased efficiencies in production; and Willem Kolff had said that a dialysis machine could be mass-produced for a unit cost of $200. These predictions turned out to be wrong, because of the cost-plus reimbursement scheme of American medicine.

Under cost-plus reimbursement, physicians and hospitals were allowed to buy as many dialysis machines as they wanted (or anything else) and pass the cost "plus" a percentage of profit on to "third-party payers"—that is, to ordinary people who pay premiums for medical insurance and who have FICA taxes withheld. One effect of cost-plus reimbursement was that hospitals not only had no incentive to buy inexpensive dialysis machines but actually had an incentive to buy ever more expensive machines. The larger the cost, the greater their net profit (as a percentage of cost).

Thus it is no surprise that by 1991, instead of costing a few hundred million dollars or less, ESRDA was costing $4 billion a year for 150,000 Americans.[58] This yearly figure was at least 20 times higher than Hartke's prediction, and possibly 100 times higher, since Hartke had expected the cost to fall.

Cost-plus funding was replaced in 1983 by reimbursement by diagnostically related groups (DRGs); but until then, all possible candidates for dialysis received it, no matter how hopeless their other medical problems might be. Reports were circulating that blind patients with cancer and Alzheimer's disease were being dialyzed in intensive care units, and that nephrologists in centers with many patients were making hundreds of thousands of dollars a year. Anticipating unlimited profits during the 1980s, hundreds of dialysis clinics sprang up, some run by hospitals, some by for-profit companies.

Under ESRDA, Congress also reimbursed kidney transplants, which were not too expensive in the 1970s. After the development of cyclosporin, the number of successful renal transplants jumped from 3,730 in 1975 to over 9,000 in 1986. In addition to the question whether every dying kidney patient should receive dialysis, this development raised a new question: should every dying kidney patient have a kidney transplant? Again, the basic problem seemed to be that, for this particular organ, everything was covered by federal funds—a situation that existed for no other organ or disease.

•

The rule of rescue continues to make its effect felt. American medicine and the media have chosen to focus on "innocent children" as a way of changing social policy about funding transplants, and to some extent American society continues to distribute this valuable resource according to the rule of rescue.

•

Fox and Swazey "see transplantation as epitomizing many of the issues of what promises to be the health policy battle in the United States in the coming years."[59] In the debate about health policy, they conclude, "the core battle is about rationing." We will return to issues of allocation in Chapter 18, on reforming the American system of medical care.

FURTHER READING

Renée Fox and Judith Swazey, *The Courage to Fail: A Social View of Organ Transplants and Dialysis,* 2d ed. rev., University of Chicago Press, Ill., 1978.

Renée Fox and Judith Swazey, *Spare Parts: Organ Replacement in American Society,* Oxford University Press, New York, 1992.

Thomas Starzl, *The Puzzle People: Memoirs of a Transplant Surgeon,* University of Pittsburgh Press, Pa., 1992.

CHAPTER 13

Infants and Medical Research

Baby Fae and Baby Theresa

This chapter discusses two major cases. In the first case, which took place in 1984, a baboon's heart was transplanted into an infant called "Baby Fae." The second case, which took place in 1992, involved an anencephalic infant known as "Baby Theresa" whose parents wanted to donate her heart to another baby.

The Case of Baby Fae

BACKGROUND: XENOGRAFTS

Transplantation of an organ from one species to another is called a *xenograft*. Before the Baby Fae case, attempts to transplant animal organs to human patients had been rare, and those that were undertaken did not promise much.

In 1964, James Hardy implanted a chimpanzee heart into a 68-year-old man who lived 90 minutes.[1] In 1977, Christiaan Barnard "piggybacked" a baboon heart next to the heart of a 25-year-old Italian woman, who lived 300 minutes; later he used the same technique to implant a chimpanzee heart in a 59-year-old man who lived less than 4 days. During the 1960s, Thomas Starzl and Keith Reemtsma performed six transplants each with simian kidneys and had somewhat better luck, but they eventually abandoned these projects.[2] Baboon kidneys, at best, worked for only 2 months. In 1975—in an episode reminiscent of the film *O Lucky Man*—a British cardiologist connected veins and arteries of a dying 1-year-old boy to a live baboon, neither of whom lived through the operation.

BABY FAE: THE IMPLANT AND THE OUTCOME

The infant who came to be known as Baby Fae was born at Barstow Memorial Hospital in Barstow, California (a small desert town), probably on October 14, 1984. She was 3 weeks premature and weighed 5 pounds. Noticing her pallor, the pediatrician transferred her on October 15 to Loma Linda Hospital, a Seventh-Day Adventist facility near Riverside, California, about 60 miles from Los Angeles. Physicians at Loma Linda confirmed that she had hypoplastic left heart syndrome (HLHS). In HLHS, which affects 1 in 10,000 babies, the normally powerful left side of the heart and the aorta are underdeveloped and are too weak to pump blood. HLHS is almost always fatal within 2 weeks.

Because Loma Linda agreed to protect the privacy of "Baby Fae" and her family, their identity has never been revealed; and much of the information reported about them is uncertain or conflicting, as are some of the dates in the case (even the date of Fae's birth has been variously reported as October 12 and October 14). Evidently, Baby Fae's mother was 23 years old, a Roman Catholic, unmarried, unemployed, and with no medical insurance; Fae's father was a 35-year-old laborer. The parents had lived together for 5 years and already had a son (then 2 ½), but they had never married, and at the time of Fae's death they had separated or were about to separate. Two other people who were figures in the case were Fae's maternal grandmother and a 28-year-old man—a mechanic—who was often called the mother's boyfriend but may more accurately have been described as a family friend. This friend seems to have accompanied Fae's mother when the infant was transferred to Loma Linda.

At Loma Linda, Fae's mother was told that the infant had HLHS and would soon die; the baby was kept overnight in the hospital and then released to her. She had Fae baptized and took the child to a nearby motel, where they were joined by the grandmother, to wait for death.

•

On October 16, however, Baby Fae's mother received a call from Leonard Bailey, a 41-year-old chief of pediatric surgery at Loma Linda who had been aggressively pursuing animal-to-human heart transplants. Bailey had been away at a convention when Baby Fae first came to the hospital and when options were discussed with her mother, but now he wanted to discuss a xenograft—a transplant of a baboon heart. For the previous 14 months, Loma Linda's Institutional Review Board (IRB) had been considering the possibility of xenografts by Bailey, and it had recently granted him permission for five operations. His call surprised the family. Bailey said, "I think they were awestruck that their child might still have the possibility to live."[3] At this point, Fae's father joined (or perhaps had already joined) her mother and grandmother.

On October 19, at 11:30 P.M., Baby Fae was readmitted to Loma Linda and placed on a respirator, and her parents began to talk with Bailey. The surgeon seems to have discussed the operation for several hours with Fae's mother, father, and grandmother (and perhaps also the friend) during the early morning of October 20. Fae's mother and possibly some of the others also watched a slide show about the operation. Both parents then signed a consent form which had been reviewed in great detail by the IRB; they later signed a second form, but reports differ as to whether the second form was signed 6 hours, 18 hours, or 2 days after the first. At 6 A.M., antigen-typing tests began, to find the best match for Fae among potential baboon donors; these tests would take 6 days.

On October 26, as the immunologist Sandra Nehlsen-Cannarella waited for the results of the final tissue-typing tests, Baby Fae's heart was said to have started dying and her lungs to have started swelling with fluid. (The baby has been variously described as 12 days old, 2 weeks old, and "around" 2 weeks old on that day.) Whether Fae was actually dying at this point is important: according to the hospital's spokesperson, a baboon heart was used because there was no time to find a compatible human heart; but Bailey made little effort to find a human heart donor (though, as we will see, a possible human donor was available). In any event, the results of the matching tests were returned at 6 A.M., and the transplant surgery began at 7:30 A.M. The donor was a female baboon named Goobers, about 7 to 10 months old, purchased from the Foundation for Biomedical Research outside San Antonio, Texas. (This is an organization which has enormous animal colonies, including 2,500 baboons, and supplies many medical centers with primates for research.)

According to what was by then standard procedure, Baby Fae was placed on a heart-lung machine that gradually lowered her blood temperature to 68 degrees. Meanwhile, Goobers was waiting in the basement, three floors below Bailey's operating room, where Loma Linda kept primates in its animal quarters. Goobers was then sedated, and in 15 minutes Bailey excised her walnut-sized heart. He put the heart in saline ice-slush in a Tupperware container, which was in turn put into a picnic cooler. (This sounds rather informal but was standard for organ transplants nationwide.) Back in the operating room, Bailey removed Fae's defective heart and replaced it with Goobers's healthy one. Over the next 4 hours, he connected the transplanted heart and transplanted arteries. Then the heart-lung machine raised Fae's temperature to 98 degrees, and Goobers's heart began to beat spontaneously inside Fae.

On October 29, Baby Fae was weaned from her respirator. On November 5, in an exclusive interview with *American Medical News*, Bailey predicted that Goobers's heart would grow as Fae grew, and that Fae might live to celebrate her twentieth birthday.

On November 10—2 weeks after the surgery—Baby Fae showed the first signs of rejection of the donor heart. By November 12, she was deteriorating and was put back on the respirator.

On November 12, 13, and 14, David Hinshaw, the former dean of Loma Linda Medical School, in his capacity as the hospital's medical spokesperson, held three press conferences. (His role in the Baby Fae case was a counterpart of Chase Peterson's in the Barney Clark case, discussed in Chapter 11.) Hinshaw said that after an episode of rejection on November 12, Fae was "showing steady improvement"; on the fourteenth, he said that the "signs of rejection" were "reversing very definitely." In the November 12 issue of *Time*, Christiaan Barnard optimistically suggested that baboon farms for simian xenografts might exist in the near future, and William DeVries said, "I really have sympathy for what [Bailey and his colleagues] are going through."[4]

On November 15, at 7 P.M., Baby Fae developed a heart blockage and renal failure; her physicians started closed-heart massage and dialysis. At 9 P.M. (or perhaps 11 P.M., according to *Newsweek*), Fae died. It had been 21 days (or 20 days, according to the *New York Times*) since her transplant surgery.

ETHICAL ISSUES

Animal Donors and Animal Rights

Bailey's operation on Baby Fae generated intense ethical controversy about the use of Goobers. "This is medical sensationalism at the expense of Baby Fae, her family, and the baboon," said Lucy Shelton of People for the Ethical Treatment of Animals (PETA).[5] Animal-rights activists protested outside Loma Linda Hospital, claiming that using Goobers's heart was unethical because Fae's life was not intrinsically worth more than Goobers's. The philosopher Tom Regan condemned the operation and said that it had "two victims," Baby Fae and Goobers.

Regan's general philosophical view (discussed in Chapter 8) is that beings who "have a life" also have a right to life, and he held that Goobers had a biographical life of sorts in that it mattered to her whether she would live or have her heart cut out: "Like us, Goobers was somebody, a distinct individual." He also argued from the premise that all primates have equal moral value, concluding that Goobers did not exist as Fae's resource:

> Those people who seized [Goobers's] heart, even if they were motivated by their concern for Baby Fae, grievously violated Goobers's right to be treated with respect. That she could do nothing to protest, and that many of us failed to recognize the transplant for the injustice that it was, does not diminish the wrong, a wrong settled before Baby Fae's sad death.[6]

Regan also argued that even if human beings had obtained benefits in the past from using animals, such use was still wrong. In a possible—but if so, incorrect—reference to the Tuskegee study (see Chapter 9), he said:

> In the 1930s, we intentionally gave syphilis to prisoners to trace the disease. Suppose others benefited. It was still wrong. We recognize that there can be ill-gotten gains in the exploitation of human beings, but we are blind to the fact that this is exactly what we're doing with animals. We are morally inconsistent.[7]

Other animal-rights philosophers emphasized that the difference between Baby Fae and Goobers, considering how young both were and what their individual potential might be, was not as great as the difference between Baby Fae and an anencephalic baby.[8] Anencephalic babies, almost certainly, have no cognitive ability or potential cognitive ability, whereas a young baboon has already developed as much cognition and affect as a human newborn. Some philosophers contemplated the large breeding facility from which Goobers had been bought and offered the image of a similar facility supplying severely retarded humans as organ donors and research subjects. If this image is repugnant, they asked, why do we tolerate such a facility for primates—since primates are more like us than severely retarded humans are?

Needless to say, Bailey's views were diametrically opposed to all this. Bailey said that the ethical sensitivity of the animal lovers picketing his campus was "born of a luxurious society" and implied that only in California would surgeons have to confront issues of animal rights: "People in southern California have it so good that they can afford to worry about this type of issue."[9] Moreover, he held, "When it gets down to a human living or dying, there shouldn't be any question" of using an animal to save that human.

The director of Loma Linda's Center for Christian Bioethics argued similarly:

> On an ethical scale, we will always place human beings ahead of subhumans, especially in a situation where people can be genuinely saved by animals. That is the story of mankind from the very beginning. Animals, for example, have always been used for food and clothing.[10]

Predictably, Baby Fae's mother was unsympathetic to animal-rights activists: "They don't know what they're talking about," she said.[11]

This issue will probably not go away soon. There are many reports of possible breakthroughs in research on the human immune system or animal genetics that would make xenografts feasible. Moreover, the persistent shortage of human donor organs (which is discussed in Chapter 12) makes xenografts seem necessary: since patients die every day waiting for human donors, the ability to use animal donors successfully could save many human lives.

The Procedure

A major ethical issue with regard to the surgery on Baby Fae was whether it was therapy or research—a distinction which is discussed in detail in Chapter 11. Another, related major issue was whether alternative treatment was available. Let's consider each of these questions in turn.

Therapy or research?   One of the most important criticisms of Bailey's surgery had to do with whether it was therapeutic or experimental. This issue can be put more bluntly: was Baby Fae a patient, or was she only a research subject—a victim?

As discussed in Chapter 11, a therapeutic procedure must offer a patient a reasonable chance; a procedure which offers little or no real chance is experimental. This medical distinction between therapy and experimentation can also be expressed in moral terms: in Kantian ethics, it would be analogous to the difference between treating people as "ends in themselves" and using them as "mere means" to some other goal. In an essay in *Time*, Charles Krauthammer wrote:

> Civilization hangs on the Kantian principle that human beings are to be treated as ends and not means. So much depends on that principle because there is no crime that cannot be, that has not been, committed in the name of the future against those who inhabit the present. Medical experimentation, which invokes the claims of the future, necessarily turns people into means.[12]

Was Bailey's best scenario really possible? Was there any genuine probability that Fae could live to adulthood—to age 20, as he predicted—with a baboon heart? At one point, Bailey phrased his claim somewhat differently, saying that Fae had a chance to "celebrate more than one birthday with her new heart."[13] Was even this more modest scenario possible?

Bailey claimed passionately that the operation was therapeutic:

> I have always believed it would work, or I would not have attempted it. . . .
> There was always therapeutic intent. My dilemma has been educating the uni-
> versity and the medical profession.[14]

This commentary was made 9 days after the operation, when Baby Fae was still
alive and seemed to be doing well; and Bailey actually implied then that
xenografts might be preferable to human transplants.

Bailey's immunologist, Sandra Nehlsen-Cannarella, also felt that the operation was intended to be therapeutic; she argued that Baby Fae could have
accepted the heart if a good enough match was found with compatible lymphocytes. Nehlsen-Cannarella tested for compatibility, using Baby Fae's reaction to her own blood and tissue as the control: she tested Baby Fae's mother
and some other relatives (finding a weak immune reaction), some lab workers
(strong reaction), herself (strong reaction), three baboons (strong reaction), and
three additional baboons (surprisingly, a weak reaction); she found a "very,
very weak" reaction with one more baboon—Goobers.[15] From these tests, she
concluded that she was not confronted with across-the-board rejection of
xenografts.

There is considerable similarity between human blood and the blood of other
primates (in fact, this is considered evidence of common ancestry); thus we might
expect to find some close matches between humans and primates. Moreover,
some humans react strongly against other humans: one-third of humans have a
"preformed antibody" against tissue from other humans. It is true that perhaps
as many as 70 percent of humans have a preformed antibody against baboon tissue, but 70 percent is not 100 percent; the figure implies that perhaps 30 percent
of humans do *not* have a preformed antibody against baboon tissue. Baby Fae
was among the 30 percent, and Bailey gave this considerable weight: he claimed
that ignorance about human-baboon matching explained Hardy's earlier failures
in xenografting.

Bailey, however, was strongly opposed by the medical profession. For one
thing, his claim of "therapeutic intent" was not accepted; it was argued that there
is a difference between "therapeutic intent" and therapeutic *probability*. Almost
any operation has some possibility, however remote, of being therapeutic, and in
this sense all surgeons could say they "intend" their operations to be therapeutic—but that would make the concept of therapeutic surgery meaningless.

Another point on which Bailey was opposed by the medical profession was
tissue typing. In 1970, Paul Teraski had discovered that although tissue typing
can improve transplantation within families, it cannot improve transplants outside families. Thomas Starzl wrote in 1992 that whereas transplant surgeons initially resisted Teraski's findings—in the early 1970s—they gradually came to
accept the limitations his results suggested:

> Twenty years later the only controversy is whether matching under all circum-
> stances means enough to be given any consideration in the distribution of
> cadaver kidneys. By exposing the truth, Teraski had made it clear that the field of
> clinical transplantation could advance significantly only by the development of

better drugs and other treatment strategies, not by vainly hoping that the solution would be through tissue matching.[16]

Most transplant surgeons agreed.

The surgeon John Najarian at the University of Minnesota—the foremost American expert on pediatric transplants—said at the time of the Baby Fae case: "There has never been a successful cross-species transplant. To try it now is merely to prolong the dying process."[17] He also said that Fae's death on November 15 was "reasonably close to what could be expected," because 3 weeks was about how long it usually takes for rejection to do its damage. The physician Kenneth Stoller maintained that Bailey had performed, over 7 years, "about 160 cross-species transplants, mostly on sheep and goats, none of whom survived more than 6 months."[18]

In November 1984, in a review of xenografts, the editor of *Journal of Heart Transplantation* concluded:

> These clinical attempts demonstrated that primate hearts could be acutely tolerated by the human body, at least for a few days, but no evidence was found to suggest that these grafts could be accepted for prolonged periods of time with the available methods of immunosuppression. . . . Using presently available means of immunosuppression and immunomanipulation, there is no evidence that a vital organ can be transplanted from one species to another and result in prolonged survival of the recipient. . . .
>
> From the experimental data and past clinical attempts, there is nothing to indicate that primate hearts will be tolerated by a human infant for months or years using today's means to induce and control tolerance. The Loma Linda surgical team has not informed the medical community, as yet, of any new evidence that might suggest the contrary.[19]

The case against Baby Fae's transplant as "therapy" may be summed up as follows:

- *First,* as noted above, it had been known since the mid-1970s that (with the exception of family members) better antigen matches (tissue typing) between donor and recipient would not improve transplants.
- *Second,* even the best of matches would still require long-term maintenance on cyclosporin. Bailey claimed that infants can be given larger dosages of cyclosporin than adults;[20] but cyclosporin eventually produces toxic side effects or loses its efficacy (see Chapter 12). The autopsy on Baby Fae (which was not released until some months after her death) indicated that her kidneys may have been poisoned by cyclosporin.
- *Third,* Bailey also argued that since an infant's immune system is not fully developed, babies might tolerate organ transplants better before their immune systems develop. But this is not certain; and even if it were true, any initial success would be expected to be followed by failure as the baby's immune system developed and rejected the xenograft.
- *Fourth,* only one real heart xenograft had been tried previously, and this had a disastrous result. (Christiaan Barnard's attempts had involved xenografts only as auxiliaries and anyway had not been much more successful.)

- *Fifth,* Loma Linda was a small medical institution (it had only 5,000 students); in their zeal to perform a xenograft, the staff may have been blinded to their own limitations.
- *Sixth,* Bailey himself was a relative amateur: he had never performed a human heart transplant, and he had never published any articles on his animal-to-animal xenografts.

Taking all this into account, Baby Fae probably had no chance of surviving for even 1 year, let alone reaching her twentieth birthday; thus the surgery was not therapeutic but experimental. *Nature* concluded that "the serious difficulty over [Bailey's] operation . . . is that it may have catered to the researchers' needs first and to the patient's only second."[21] In his essay in *Time,* Krauthammer said that Baby Fae had lived and died in the realm of experimentation:

> Only the bravery was missing: no one would admit the violation. Bravery was instead fatuously ascribed to Baby Fae, a creature as incapable of bravery as she was of circulating her own blood. Whether this case was an advance in medical science awaits the examination of the record by the scientific community. That it was an adventure in medical ethics is already clear.[22]

Furthermore, even as an experiment the surgery on Baby Fae was dubious. AMA and medical journals criticized Bailey and held that xenografts should be undertaken only as part of a systematic research program with controls in randomized clinical trials.[23] (This criticism also included William DeVries's experimentation with artificial hearts, discussed in Chapter 11.)

Was alternative treatment possible?   One obvious alternative to a xenograft for Baby Fae was a human donor heart. Should Bailey have sought a human heart for Fae?

As we have seen, Loma Linda claimed that the xenograft was necessary because Baby Fae was at the point of death and no human heart was available. Bailey argued that it would be impossible to find a heart because the donor would have to be under 7 weeks old, and criteria for neonatal brain death were problematical ("You can have a flat EEG on a newborn, and yet the baby will survive").[24] Most neonatal transplants come from anencephalic babies; and Bailey maintained that most parents of such infants would refuse to accept the fact that their baby was brain-dead, and in any case would not agree to donate the baby's organs. He described the baboon heart as Baby Fae's "only chance to live" (this sounds like an echo of William DeVries's description of Barney Clark's artificial heart).

An associate surgeon at Loma Linda defended Bailey:

> It would have to be the sort of case where an infant fell out of a crib and was declared brain dead but the heart was okay. Then all these tests would have to be done to insure a proper matching. With Baby Fae, we had five days to do those tests, getting the best possible [animal] donor. With a human heart, we might not have been able to keep the recipient alive.[25]

However, Paul Teraski, director of the Southern California Regional Organ Procurement Agency, said that an infant heart had indeed been potentially available on the day of Baby Fae's xenograft. Teraski added, "I think that they [the Loma Linda team] did not make any effort to get a human infant heart because they were set on doing a baboon."[26] (It is worth noting that in his memoirs, the surgeon Thomas Starzl describes Teraski as a "symbol of integrity" in the transplant community.[27])

Since Bailey had been preparing for a xenograft on a human patient—in preparation, he had performed more than 150 transplants on animals—it is hard to believe that he wasn't looking for a first case. In fact, Bailey himself admitted:

> We were not searching for a human heart. We were out to enter the whole new area of transplanting tissue-matched baboon hearts into newborns who are supported with antisuppressive drugs. I suppose that we could have used a human heart that was outsized and that was not tissue-matched, and that would have pacified some people, but it would have been very poor science. On the other hand, I suppose my belief that there are no newborn hearts available for transplantation was more opinion than data or science, but it is scientific to acknowledge that the whole area of determining brain death of newborns is very problematical.[28]

There was another possible alternative. The pediatric surgeon William I. Norwood had developed surgery for HLHS that was less radical than a heart transplant—it attempted to repair the left ventricle—and had performed his operation many times at Children's Hospitals in Philadelphia and Boston, with a success rate of 40 percent. Bailey claimed that children did not do well enough after the Norwood procedure to justify this operation for Baby Fae, but given his extensive efforts to develop xenografts, was he an impartial judge?

Informed Consent

In a case like Baby Fae's, involving an infant, the issue of informed consent has two aspects. First, since informed consent can obviously never be obtained from infants themselves, is it ethical to subject an infant to an experimental procedure? Second, when parents consent to such a procedure for an infant, is their consent genuinely informed?

For many critics, what was objectionable about Bailey's surgery was not that it was risky or experimental—after all, surgery can discover what is possible or impossible only by trying. What was objectionable was, rather, that Bailey used a baby, who could not consent. In the decades since the earlier attempts at xenografts, the only new developments had been cyclosporin and better tissue matching, and these critics argued that both could have been used with a xenograft in a consenting adult.

Bailey argued that he had chosen an infant not to circumvent consent but for medical reasons: he said that immunorejection of a xenograft might be less in an infant whose immune system was not yet fully developed, and that infants can be given larger dosages of cyclosporin than adults.[29] As we have seen, this defense did not seem convincing in terms of establishing Fae's surgery as "therapy," and for the same reasons it does not seem to justify his choice of an infant rather than an adult. Even if Fae survived for a while, he would have had to anticipate that she would reject the xenograft when her immune system did develop; moreover, cyclosporin evidently poisoned her kidneys. In other words, Bailey could not really justify using a baby—an unconsenting subject—on the grounds that the risk would be lower.

In addition to the specific questions about whether using Fae made sense medically or ethically, a more general question is whether parents should ever volunteer children as research subjects. The conservative theologian Paul Ramsey has argued that it always wrong for parents to volunteer their children as subjects of nontherapeutic research:

> If today we mean to give such weight to the research imperative, . . . then we should not seek to give a principled justification of what we are doing with children. It is better to leave the research imperative in incorrigible conflict with the principle that protects the individual human person from being used for research purposes without either his expressed or correctly construed consent. Some sorts of human experimentation should, in this alternative, be acknowledged to be "borderline situations" in which moral agents are under the necessity of doing wrong for the sake of the public good. Either way they do wrong. It is immoral not to do the research. It is also immoral to use children who cannot themselves consent and who ought not to be presumed to consent to research unrelated to their treatment. On this supposition research medicine, like politics, is a realm in which men have to "sin bravely."[30]

On the other hand, a Catholic theologian, Richard McCormick, holds that parents can volunteer children for "low-risk" nontherapeutic research.[31] McCormick's argument is based on the Roman Catholic tradition of applying natural law to ethics; according to McCormick, adults should volunteer for low-risk, nontherapeutic research for the general good, and therefore infants should also be volunteered. That is, adults should choose for a child not as the child would actually choose in adulthood, but as the child ought to choose in adulthood.

Interestingly, neither Ramsey nor McCormick uses the utilitarian justification—the greatest good for the greatest number. To many people, though, utilitarianism offers the most natural justification: since HLHS is a congenital defect of babies, how can treatment of HLHS be advanced unless some babies with the condition are used as subjects of research?

•

With regard to the second aspect of informed consent in the Baby Fae case—the *parents'* consent—some critics asked whether that consent had indeed been "informed."

Many people wondered, for instance, whether Fae's parents fully understood the alternatives in her case. Had Bailey carefully described the Norwood procedure (see above) to the parents? Were they aware of the Norwood procedure, and did they realize that it might be used to keep Fae alive until a human donor heart was found? Were they informed that a human donor was available on the day of Fae's surgery?

Another consideration here is that Fae's mother had no medical insurance. The xenograft was offered free, whereas Fae's family would have had to find the money for the Norwood procedure or a human transplant—or, very probably, would have been unable to find the money.

Furthermore, were the parents really informed about the probable outcome of the xenograft? That is, did they understand the experimental nature of the surgery? Loma Linda had decided to follow the normal procedure of IRB review in Baby Fae's case (although as a religious, privately funded institution it was exempt from NIH rules); still, no matter how good the resulting consent form may have been, it is doubtful that Baby Fae's family entirely grasped the situation: almost all other surgeons were skeptical about the baby's chance of survival to adulthood.

As discussed in Chapter 11, William DeVries's implant of an artificial heart was described as having demonstrated only the "clinical feasibility" of the device—not its "clinical usefulness." Did Baby Fae's parents understand that Bailey's xenograft might be of this nature, a demonstration of feasibility rather than usefulness?

The law professor Alexander Capron summed up the issue of whether Fae's family had given truly informed consent:

> Doubts linger, not only about the adequacy of the information supplied to Baby Fae's parents but about whether their personal difficulties made it possible for them to choose freely, and whether the realization that their child was dying may have left them with the erroneous conclusion that consenting to the transplant was the only "right" thing to do.[32]

There is an old saying among physicians: "Beware the surgeon with one case." That too may sum up this situation.

•

In fact, lack of informed consent had also been a problem with xenografts on adults. The law professor George Annas emphasized that in previous attempts to implant animal hearts in humans, consent was minimal and the patients (or subjects) were similar to Baby Fae in being vulnerable and poor. In 1963, Keith Reemtsma at Columbia University had implanted chimpanzee kidneys in a 43-year-old African American man who was dying of glomerulonephritis. In 1964, James Hardy at the University of Mississippi had implanted a chimpanzee heart into a poor deaf-mute who was dying, was brought to the hospital unconscious, never consented to the operation, and survived for only 2 hours. These operations were experimental, not therapeutic, and were characterized by exploitation and lack of consent. Annas saw Baby Fae's case as a continuation of such practices. Calling Bailey the champion of this "anything goes" school of experimentation, Annas concluded:

> This inadequately reviewed, inappropriately consented to, premature experiment on an impoverished, terminally ill newborn was unjustified. It differs from the xenograft experiments of the early 1960s only in the fact that there was prior review of the proposal by an IRB. But this distinction did not protect Baby Fae. She remained unprotected from ruthless experimentation in which her only role was that of victim.[33]

Costs and Resources

One ethical issue in the Baby Fae case was rarely if ever mentioned: money. That is not unusual; there is a conspiracy of silence in medicine about money and therapeutic treatment. Money was a significant issue here, however, and it merits discussion.

For one thing, as noted above, money was almost certainly a factor affecting the parents' "informed consent." Baby Fae's mother was poor, and she had no medical insurance. Fae's family could not have paid for a human heart transplant, which might have cost $100,000; nor could they have paid for the Norwood procedure, which would have cost nearly as much, plus travel expenses and lodging in Philadelphia, where Norwood practiced. This helps explain why Loma Linda did not seek a human donor heart for Fae and why it did not pursue the Norwood procedure. But because of its interest in xenografts, Loma Linda provided the transplant of Goobers's heart free. Bailey and Loma Linda contended that, medically, the xenograft was Fae's only chance; that was probably not true, but the xenograft was undoubtedly her only chance financially.

There was also a broader financial issue. As with artificial hearts, many critics questioned whether so much money should be spent on a single case when the same amount of money could have done so much good for so many others. Although Loma Linda never revealed the cost of Fae's surgery and the associated treatment, it was probably at least $500,000. Would it make sense to perform, say, 500 to 1,000 such operations a year, at cost of maybe $1 billion, while thousands of babies are born deformed because their mothers could not afford prenatal tests like amniocentesis and sonograms?

The Media

Some issues in the Baby Fae case had to do with the media.

For one thing, although the case drew an enormous amount of attention in the media, Fae's family shunned publicity. As we have seen, the family's identity was never published, and certain details that might have identified them were withheld or unclear, including the date of Fae's birth. Also, Loma Linda and Bailey seemed to withhold more than just identifying details. Their account of events leading up to the surgery was confusing; hospital spokespersons gave occasional misstatements of fact; and Loma Linda refused to release a copy of the consent form which Fae's parents had signed. Some journalists complained about secrecy and invoked the public's "right to know."

This situation formed an interesting contrast to the case of Barney Clark's artificial heart 2 years earlier at the University of Utah (see Chapter 11). Just as many reporters came to Loma Linda as to Utah (more than 300), but they got much less information. For instance, William DeVries, the surgeon in the Clark case, had held daily press briefings; Bailey held fewer press conferences. Reporters accused Loma Linda of ineptitude in handling their requests and said that certain aspects of the case begged for clarification. Loma Linda may have decided that it could learn a lesson from the Clark case—that it was better to give scant information than to try to satisfy the unending demands of reporters.

If Bailey and Loma Linda were accused of reticence, though, they were also accused of publicity-seeking, self-promotion, grandstanding, and adventurism. (Bailey was also described as practicing "celebrity surgery."[34]) The surgeon Keith Reemtsma, for one, said that he himself would give no news conferences at all until his patient had been permanently discharged from the hospital and until he had prepared and submitted a scientific paper. Reemtsma argued:

> Science and news are, in a sense, asymmetrical and sometimes antagonistic. News emphasizes uniqueness, the immediacy, the human interest in a case such as [Baby Fae's]. Science emphasizes verification, controls, comparisons, and patterns.[35]

The bioethicist Alex Capron argued similarly: "There was a time when the public learned of biomedical developments after they had been reviewed by, and generally reported to, the researchers' scientific and medical peers"—a procedure that protected everyone's dignity and also meant that the public would learn only of genuine advances "rather than merely being titillated by bizarre cases of as yet unproven import."[36]

For its part, the press had also learned a lesson from the Clark case. When it came to the coverage of Baby Fae's story, perhaps never before had such accurate, detailed criticism from medical professionals been presented to the American public. Journalists were careful to include commentary about Bailey's claims from other surgeons and cardiologists, and (as the quotation above from Reemtsma suggests) many of these were highly critical of Bailey. Some of the people in medicine whose observations and analyses were reported saw Fae's surgery as a stunt which could only be damaging to medicine and Bailey himself as a maverick, as lacking good judgment, or even as incompetent.

UPDATE

Bailey attempted no more xenografts. Because of the pressing need for organs, however, there have been some attempts by others.

On June 29, 1992, Thomas Starzl's team at the University of Pittsburgh transplanted a baboon liver into a 35-year-old man with hepatitis B. About 30 percent of patients waiting for a human donor liver—many of them under age 45—die before getting one; also, hepatitis B will attack any human liver. However, hepatitis B does not attack baboon livers, and Starzl hoped that the immunosuppressor FK 506 (which is discussed in Chapter 12) and four other drugs would allow the xenograft to "take." The patient lived about 70 days. After his death, it was revealed that he had HIV infection; but according to the autopsy, this infection had not contributed to his death. The autopsy said that an "antirejection drug . . . hastened an infection that killed him." (Possibly, the drug was FK 506.)

In October of 1992, a woman patient at Cedars Sinai Medical Center in Los Angeles received a pig liver, as a "bridge" while she waited for a human liver, but she died 32 hours later.

On January 11, 1993, another man with hepatitis B received a baboon liver at the University of Pittsburgh; this patient was 62 years old and near death when the surgery took place. He died on February 6, 1993, never having regained full consciousness. The cause of death was an infection triggered by stitches in the abdominal cavity that either had been incorrectly sewn or had "fallen out of place."[37] After the experience, the surgeon, John Fung (who had by then replaced Starzl after Starzl's retirement), described himself as "somewhat emotionally drained."

Since 1905, various baboon organs have been transplanted to humans in 33 operations. So far, none have been successful.

•

In late 1993, a conference on xenografts reported success in transferring human genes into pigs and thereby breaking down one barrier to using pigs as a source of organs[38]—organs of transgenic pigs may "take" better in human recipients. However, xenografts may continue to prove easier in theory than in practice (as noted in Chapter 10, Christiaan Barnard predicted that animal hearts would be successfully transplanted into humans by 1988). Even when initial immuno-rejection can be suppressed by drugs such as cyclosporin, a more lethal "hyper-acute" or "complement" rejection occurs in almost all xenografts (it also occurs in about one-third of human kidney transplants).

The Case of Baby Theresa

BACKGROUND: ANENCEPHALY AND ORGAN DONATION

Anencephaly is a congenital neurological disorder characterized by absence of the cerebrum and cerebellum, as well as the top of the skull, resulting in exposure of the brain stem.[39] In the words of the Medical Task Force on Anencephaly, "Anencephaly does not mean the complete absence of the head or brain."[40] Because there is a brain stem, an electroencephalogram (EEG) can be taken, and autonomic functions such as breathing and heartbeat may be present. Anencephalics thus do not meet the Harvard criteria of brain death or the criteria of the Uniform Brain Death Act (UBDA)—standards which are sometimes called *whole-brain* criteria. (See Chapter 1 for a discussion of brain death.)

Nevertheless, anencephaly is the perhaps the most serious of all birth defects, because the baby essentially lacks the higher brain necessary for personhood. Anencephalics are generally said to be born dying. There is no hope of growth into childhood or adulthood. The open skull is vulnerable to infection, and most anencephalics die within 1 week,[41] though in rare cases some have lived for 1 year.

Anencephaly occurs in about 1 in 500 pregnancies. Most cases are identified prenatally (by sonogram or maternal serum alpha-fetoprotein testing), and 95 percent of those detected are aborted. Of those carried to term, about 55 percent are stillborn.

•

Anencephalics are the major potential source of donor organs for other babies born with congenital defects. When the recipient is an infant, a donor organ must be very small—thus an infant donor is needed. However, few infants are involved in accidents that leave them brain-dead but with healthy organs. Babies who die as a result of abuse or from sudden infant death syndrome usually have damaged organs that are unsuitable for transplantation.

In the United States, at least 2,000 babies a year need organ transplants; this number includes 600 babies with HLHS (like Baby Fae), about 500 with liver failure, and another 500 with kidney failure. About 300 anencephalic babies are born alive each year.

The possibility of using anencephalics as organ donors has existed for two decades. As noted in Chapter 10, in 1967, a few days after Christiaan Barnard transplanted a heart into Louis Washkansky, Adrian Kantrowitz transplanted a heart from an anencephalic baby into another infant, who died 6 hours later.[42] Indeed, Kantrowitz had almost performed a similar operation 18 months earlier, but he was required to wait for the anencephalic donor's heart to stop beating (so that the donor would be legally dead) and then restart it—which proved not to be possible.

•

In January of 1987, a conference of surgeons and medical ethicists in London, Ontario, drew up a controversial set of guidelines for using anencephalics as organ donors. The most important of these guidelines was that an anencephalic could become a donor only after being pronounced dead by the classical criteria of brain death. Another guideline was that the potential donor could not live more than 1 week; this standard was meant to ensure that the donor was truly "born dying." At birth, an anencephalic was to be put on a respirator to preserve the organs, then taken off every 6 hours to see if it could breathe on its own. If a baby failed to breathe for 3 minutes, it could be declared brain-dead by three physicians independent of the transplant team.

It should be noted that the respirator is necessary in this protocol because the normal course of anencephaly is for the heart gradually to stop beating: this diminishes the blood flow, so that the organs become anoxic and start to deteriorate; by the time the brain stem is dead, the heart and kidneys are no longer useful for transplantation. Thus the Ontario protocol can lead to a dilemma, since providing intensive support to maintain the brain stem may mean that a potential donor will not meet criteria of brain death.

The Ontario protocol was controversial, as noted above, and it was never in any sense official and never represented AMA policy. One of its severest critics was the pediatric neurologist Allan Shewmon at UCLA. Shewmon, the leading authority on anencephaly, held that anencephalic babies should not be used as donors at all, because there was no consensus in neurology on determining brain death in such infants for purposes of donation.[43] The Ontario protocol was not applied to an actual case until February 1988, though it had been in the news for some time before that.

•

One of the people involved in the events leading to Baby Theresa's case was Leonard Bailey, Baby Fae's surgeon. After his animal-to-human organ transplants failed, Bailey turned to trying to use anencephalic babies as donors, and he had been involved in the development of the Ontario protocol. Bailey and Loma Linda Hospital—both already well known because of the Baby Fae case—decided to use the media to help them gather anencephalic donors and to become a national surgical center for treating HLHS babies through organ transplants from anencephalics.

In October 1987, a Canadian couple, Karen and Fred Schouten, learned after 8 months of pregnancy that the fetus was anencephalic. They decided to bring it to term and to create some good from their tragedy by donating its organs. After birth, the baby, a girl whom they named Gabriel, was ventilated when her heart began to fail. United Network for Organ Sharing (UNOS) was alerted, but no potential recipients were found in Canada or in the northeastern United States.

Meanwhile, at Loma Linda Hospital, Bailey was working with another couple, Alice and Gordon Holc (by chance, also Canadian), whose 8-month fetus had HLHS and needed a heart transplant and who had come to Loma Linda because of the publicity it was receiving. The Schoutens and Gabriel were flown to Loma Linda. There, the Holcs' baby, Paul, was delivered by cesarean section, prematurely, in order to take advantage of the available donor heart. Three hours later, Gabriel Schouten's heart was excised and transplanted into Paul Holc's chest. The surgery took 6 hours.

This was the first time a transplant from an anencephalic baby to another infant resulted in a baby who could grow up and lead a normal life. In gratitude to the Schoutens and to Leonard Bailey, the Holcs named their baby Paul Gabriel Bailey Holc. Gabriel Schouten's mother later said that she felt very good about her decision and how it had benefited Paul Holc: "Paul is very special to me because he has a part of our baby inside him. One day maybe I'll see him. I hope he comes to me when he's 30 years old and says, 'Hi. Guess what? I made it.'"[44]

Fred Schouten died of a heart attack a few months later. In December of 1988, 14 months after his surgery, Paul Holc was said to be very healthy and doing well.

•

Bailey had not applied the Ontario protocol in the Schouten-Holc case (perhaps because he was waiting for it to gain consensus). The first case in which the protocol was followed was that of Michael and Brenda Winners and their anencephalic baby, at Loma Linda in February 1988. The Winners case resulted in a sad anticlimax: no recipients were found at all. This was the first of 12 unsuccessful attempts by Bailey and Loma Linda to transplant organs from anencephalic babies to other babies.[45] Of these 12 potential donors, 10 lived beyond the 1-week limit, 1 could not be matched to a recipient, and in the remaining case the physicians decided against a transplant. In 1988, Bailey and his department of surgery announced that they had suspended his transplant program to reassess the situation. There was a de facto moratorium on transplants from anencephalics until the issue was raised again, in the spring of 1992, by the case of Baby Theresa.

BABY THERESA:
THE PATIENT AND THE LEGAL CONTROVERSY

In 1991, in Fort Lauderdale, Florida, Laura Campo and Justin Pearson—who were not married—conceived a child. Laura Campo had no medical insurance for prenatal care and did not see a physician until her twenty-fourth week of pregnancy. During her eighth month of pregnancy, she learned that the fetus was anencephalic. Because this diagnosis was made so late in the pregnancy, no abortion could be performed; Laura Campo would say later that if she known the diagnosis earlier, she would have aborted the fetus.

After hearing a talk show about organ donation from anencephalics, Laura Campo decided to bring the fetus to term to serve as a source of organs. This decision entailed a cesarean delivery: since an anencephalic is likely to have a swollen head, vaginal delivery may kill it, and so a cesarean is performed to keep the organs healthy for transplantation—and also to give the infant a chance in case of misdiagnosis.

The baby, a girl, was born on March 21, 1992, and named Theresa Ann Campo Pearson. Some of the physicians expected her to die within minutes, but she did not. Pictures of Theresa showed a beautiful baby wearing a pink knitted cap that covered the top half of her head. Underneath the cap was no skin, no skull, and no cerebrum. The physicians and Theresa's parents said that when the cap was removed, they could actually look down directly on the brain stem.

•

Before her organs could be donated, Baby Theresa had to be declared brain-dead. But Florida used the strict Harvard standard of brain death, and Theresa did not meet that standard. (As we have seen, most anencephalic babies do not.) The neonatologist Brian Udell said that unless the baby was declared brain-dead, he would not remove the organs.

Laura Campo and Justin Pearson then asked Judge Estella Moriarty of the circuit court to rule Theresa brain-dead so that the baby could be an organ donor. However, because Theresa had some very minimal brain activity and did not meet the Harvard criteria, Judge Moriarty ruled otherwise on March 28: "[I am] unable to authorize someone to take your baby's life, however short—however unsatisfactory—to save another child. Death is a fact, not an opinion."[46]

The couple appealed to Florida's District Court of Appeals, which immediately delivered an emergency opinion, affirming Judge Moriarty's decision. The appeals court had also been asked to certify the case as one of "great public importance"—a certification which is necessary for an appeal to Florida's supreme court. The appellate court declined to do this.

Amidst a great deal of national publicity, the parents then appealed to the Florida Supreme Court to issue an emergency ruling. The supreme court replied that without certification of the case by the lower court as of great public importance, it lacked constitutional authority to make an emergency ruling.

On March 29, Theresa began to experience organ failure, in spite of support from a respirator. At this point, the neonatologist said, "We had to tell the parents [that] all they were doing was prolonging the baby's death."[47] The respirator was then removed. Theresa died on March 30 at 3:45 P.M. By that time, her organs were useless for transplantation.

•

On the day of their baby's death, Laura Campo and Justin Pearson appeared on the *Donahue Show* to plead for a change in Florida's laws regarding brain death. Laura Campo seemed very upset and depressed, and it was questionable whether she should have been allowed to undergo the strain of being on the show. A calm, eloquent surgeon joined them and discussed the need for donor organs.

On September 1, the Florida Supreme Court heard arguments in the case of Baby Theresa. On November 12, 1992, it issued a ruling that anencephalic newborns are not considered "dead" for purposes of organ donation.[48]

ETHICAL ISSUES

Infants as Donors

The case of Baby Theresa raised basic questions about infants as donors. Should any baby be used for the good of another baby? If so, what are the criteria? What are the social consequences?

One argument against using infants (or young children) as organ donors is their vulnerability. In general, it is felt that the more vulnerable patients are, the less defensible it is to do something to them without their consent, and babies are considered the most vulnerable of all. Babies of course cannot consent; nor can their consent be inferred, as it sometimes may be in the case of a formerly competent adult.

In this regard, a question of terminology is sometimes raised. When an infant's organ is used as a transplant, who is giving what as a "gift"? Terms like *donation* and *gift of life* seem to be inappropriate in this situation; since no baby ever consents to donate his or her organs, a baby cannot really be described as providing a "gift." It is possible to suggest more accurate terms: "organ salvage," "organ transfer," "organ recovery," "organ reassignment," and so on. Such terms seem cold, however, or may have even more negative connotations, and these connotations may themselves suggest why many people have reservations about using infants' organs. In brief, when infants' organs are used as transplants, *donor* and *donation* are euphemisms; and resorting to euphemisms suggests that accuracy—reality—is somehow disturbing.

On the other hand, one possible argument in favor of using infants' organs for transplants would be analogous to McCormick's argument, discussed earlier, in favor of volunteering infants for medical research: on this argument, parents could choose for a child as the child ought to choose in adulthood. Another possible argument is utilitarian: infants' organs should be used for transplant if that would result in the greatest good for the greatest number.

Anencephalics as Donors: Brain Death and Other Issues

One vital question in the debate over anencephalics as donors has to do with brain death. Some critics have argued that there are no good criteria for brain death in infants, and whether or not this is true in general, brain death in anencephalic infants is indeed unclear.

Anencephaly is a medical term describing a range of gross congenital brain deficits, all of which entail no chance of normal brain function but some of which do not entail immediate brain death.[49] The fact that most babies do not die within the first week—and thus could not be donors under the Ontario guidelines—illustrates this problem. Actually, some kinds of anencephaly are something like persistent vegetative state (PVS); therefore, some anencephalic infants could survive indefinitely with supportive care. One critic has said, "I have an uneasy feeling that what lurks behind the anencephalic issue is the vegetative state issue."[50]

Some commentators have suggested creating a new category of legal brain death, or an exemption from the usual legal criteria of brain death, to allow for transfers of organs from anencephalic babies. Such a special category or exemption is needed for organ donation because anencephalic infants are neither dead nor necessarily about to die immediately, and simply allowing them to die naturally could destroy their organs. The parents of Baby Theresa hoped that her case would help create pressure for such an exemption in Florida. Disability advocates opposed changing the Florida law, however: "Treating anencephalics as dead equates them with 'nonpersons,' presenting a 'slippery slope' problem with regard to all other persons who lack cognition for whatever reason."[51]

Two physicians considered a proposal to adopt a system used in West Germany, where anencephalics are considered "brain-absent" and therefore brain-dead. They rejected this proposal for the United States, though—and the idea of a special exemption. They argued as follows:

> Not only are the brains of such infants not completely absent, but there is also a remarkable heterogeneity of morphologic and functional features in the infants considered anencephalic. . . . The causes of the neural-tube defects, including anencephaly, are complex and multiple—a fact that confounds the issue and supports the concept that the condition is quite variable. It is worrisome, but not surprising, that the diagnosis of anencephaly is occasionally made in error. Indeed, too many errors have been made for the diagnosis to be considered reliable as a legal definition of death. We conclude that anencephalic infants are not brain-absent and that the condition is sufficiently variable that the establishment of a special category is not justified.[52]

This analysis notes another problem with anencephalics as donors: the diagnosis of anencephaly, even as a range, is often problematic. As discussed in Chapter 7, in the case of Baby Jane Doe, diagnosing brain size or brain function at birth is controversial and uncertain. Some people fear that overzealous physicians and parents, wanting to bring some good out of a tragedy, might declare a baby anencephalic when in fact the baby had some lesser (though still severe) defect—say, a gross congenital malformation of the brain such as microcephaly. There are sporadic reports in the popular media of retarded children, allegedly diagnosed at first as anencephalic, who are now functioning well.

Still another problem is that if borderline anencephalics can become a source of organs, there might be a tendency to use infants with closely related disorders such as atelencephaly (incomplete development of the brain) and lissencephaly (unusually small brain parts). It has been argued that "'the slippery slope is real,' because some physicians have proposed transplants from infants with defects less severe than anencephaly."[53] Judge Moriarty wrote in her medical review for her decision, "There has been a tendency by some parties and amici to confuse lethal anencephaly with these less serious conditions, even to the point of describing children as 'anencephalic' who have abnormal but otherwise intact skulls and who are several years of age."[54]

Much of this debate has to do with personhood—a concept discussed in detail in Chapters 6 (on abortion) and 7 (on impaired neonates). In the context of anencephaly and organ donation, the question may boil down simply to this: How fast do we want to change our standards of personhood to create more organs for transplantation?

•

An issue closely related to anencephalics as donors is anencephalics as *patients*. In other words, when organ donation becomes a possibility, who is the patient?

Some critics have asked whether less was being done for anencephalic babies when these babies were seen as potential organ donors. Alex Capron described the situation as follows: "By far the most fundamental problem . . . was trying to sustain an anencephalic's liver, heart, and kidneys without temporarily giving life to its brain stem, the one organ that needed to die for transplant to begin."[55]

According to the Ontario protocol, as discussed earlier, a potential anencephalic donor is to be maintained on a respirator (this keeps the organs suitable for donation) but periodically removed from the respirator to see if independent breathing will occur (so that brain death can be declared if such breathing does not occur): would this removal be in the best interest of the anencephalic infant? Is the anencephalic infant really being seen as a patient?

A counterargument here is that with anencephaly, birth is not morally relevant. That is, most fetuses diagnosed as anencephalic are aborted (indeed, anencephaly is one of the best reasons for aborting a fetus during the second term), and the actual birth of an anencephalic does not make a moral difference. If abortion is appropriate in anencephaly, why should it be considered immoral to do less to prolong the life of an anencephalic who is a potential organ donor? It might even be argued, along these lines, that since anencephalics almost always die a few days after birth (and since similar but less severe conditions are only infrequently misdiagnosed as anencephaly), why not allow physicians to kill anencephalics painlessly and transplant their organs at the optimal time? It need hardly be said, however, that this counterargument is not widely accepted.

•

Another question has to do with the anencephalic *fetus*—specifically, the idea of keeping such a fetus alive to be used later as a source of organs. There seems to be a real distinction between keeping a fetus alive for this purpose and simply using the organs of a baby who has accidentally become brain-dead or who has unexpectedly been born anencephalic, and some critics would see a line here that should not be crossed.

•

There is also a *statistical* issue. As noted earlier, most anencephalics will be identified in utero and almost all of these will be aborted. Of the approximately 650 anencephalics brought to term each year in the United States, between 55 and 66 percent will be stillborn. Of the approximately 300 anencephalics who are born alive and survive immediately after birth, about half will be possible donors of hearts, kidneys, and livers; the others will be unacceptable for various reasons, including organ malformation, low birthweight, and withholding of consent by the family. The number of possible donors would be further reduced after blood and tissue typing. Taking all this into account, one study estimates that only about 30 recipients a year would benefit from using anencephalics as sources of organs.[56] (Universal access to prenatal care, moreover, would reduce this figure still further.)

Given that serious problems exist about using anencephalics as organ sources, is this figure—30 babies a year—large enough? Would it justify changing our criteria of brain death? Would it justify the costs involved? In the Holc case, the surgery alone cost $140,000; in addition, there were costs of flying everyone to Loma Linda and, for the Schoutens and the Ontario hospital, the cost of keeping Gabriel Schouten alive for a week. Consider that thousands of pregnant women in the United States get no prenatal care and that as a result, many babies are born with preventable defects. Isn't the system biased in favor of dramatic surgical cases and against these anonymous women and their children? Is this justifiable?

UPDATE

A case involving near-anencephaly was reported in 1993.[57] The infant in this case, known as Baby Portia, had an encephalocele at the back of her head, which was diagnosed in utero at 27 weeks of gestation. This condition made her very close to anencephalic. The radiologist told the mother that the baby would be "severely brain-damaged, beyond retarded." The baby's parents, Venita and Andrae Davis—a young African American couple—wanted to terminate the pregnancy, and the obstetrician, Robert Greenfield, agreed.

Less than 1 hour after he had introduced a drug to induce labor, however, Greenfield abruptly changed his mind; he had consulted with three other physicians who judged that the baby might be capable of living outside the womb. (The inference is that the baby's lungs had developed; see Chapter 6, "Update.") Without consulting the Davises, Greenfield stopped the treatment and sent Venita Davis home to continue her pregnancy. He did not inform the Davises that a number of physicians specialize in third-trimester abortions for severely abnormal fetuses.

When the baby, a girl named Portia, was born, no one expected her to live long. But she did. In 1993, Portia, at age 2, was described as sitting "strapped in a wheelchair . . . a feeding tube passing through her nose. Her tiny, pointed head jerks mildly as she passes from seizure to seizure, small convulsive shivers with barely a break in between. She has virtually no brain, and although her eyes are open she is completely unresponsive and unaware of her surroundings."

The Davises started a suit against Greenfield for malpractice and to recover the costs of Portia's care. So far, these costs have run to $240,000 a year.

•

Today—a few years after the case of Baby Theresa, and after a great deal of professional discussion—there is general agreement that anencephalic babies are poor candidates for organ donation after brain death, and that not enough babies would be benefited by transplantation to justify changing legal standards of brain death specifically for anencephalics. There is also general agreement that Bailey's program was premature; as noted in the Baby Fae case, physicians tend to regard Bailey as something of a maverick.

As is discussed in Chapter 7, in 1993 a court in Virginia applied the Americans with Disabilities Act to an allegedly anencephalic baby—known as Baby K—and refused to allow the infant's respirator to be disconnected; in 1994, this ruling was confirmed by a federal appeals court.

FURTHER READING

George Annas, "Baby Fae: The 'Anything Goes' School of Human Experimentation," *Hastings Center Report*, vol. 15, no. 1, February 1985, pp. 15–17.

Denise Breo, "Interview with 'Baby Fae's' Surgeon," *American Medical News*, November 16, 1984.

Charles Krauthammer, "The Using of Baby Fae," *Time*, December 3, 1984.

Thomasine Kushner and Raymond Belotti, "Baby Fae: A Beastly Business," *Journal of Medical Ethics*, vol. 11, 1985.

Judith Mistichelli, "Scope Note 5: Baby Fae—Ethical Issues Surround Cross-Species Organ Transplantation," National Reference Center for Bioethics Literature at the Kennedy Institute of Ethics, Georgetown University, Washington, D.C., January 1985.

PART FOUR

Classic Cases about Individual Rights and the Public Good

CHAPTER 14

Involuntary Psychiatric Commitment

Joyce Brown

In many large cities across the United States, confrontations with homeless "street people" are a part of daily life. Panhandlers and derelicts, many of whom are mentally ill, roam the streets. In New York City, where the case of Joyce Brown took place, there are perhaps 10,000 visibly homeless people; and although the city makes shelters available at night, homeless people often refuse to use them. The problem of what to do with homeless people has become both a national and a local controversy. When these people are mentally ill, the problem can also involve another issue—involuntary psychiatric commitment.

BACKGROUND: INSANITY AND IDEOLOGY

A Brief Historical Overview

Ideas about insanity have been very different during different periods of human history.

Nothing, of course, is known about insanity in prehistory. With regard to schizophrenia, though, it has been speculated that early humans may have believed that the "voices" characteristically heard by schizophrenics came from gods or spirits. One scholar has suggested that the first human being to have an identifiable thought experienced it as an internal voice and was terrified by it, and that the human brain evolved as bicameral in order to control such "voices."[1] If so, the voices in schizophrenia might be a throwback to an earlier stage of humanity.

The ancient Greeks generally believed that mental illness was caused when angry gods took people's minds away. However, Hippocrates and his followers held that mental disorders, like physical disorders, had natural causes; and Plato thought of insanity essentially as imbalance: as one part of the mind dominating the others.[2] In ancient Rome, mental illness was also attributed to the gods, though some Roman physicians—particularly Galen—accepted Hippocrates' naturalistic concept.

In the Middle Ages, the naturalistic approach was virtually abandoned: insanity was thought to be caused by demonic possession, and exorcists were hired to drive out demons. Insane people were sometimes confined on a ship ("ship of fools") which sailed from port to port, taking on food and water but never allowing its human cargo to disembark.

During the fifteenth century, belief in demonic possession was perhaps at its strongest; this was the beginning of the era of witch-hunts. Persecution of witchcraft did not really end until the eighteenth century, and throughout this period many mentally ill people were treated as witches. However, one historically famous institution for mental patients, Bethlehem Royal Hospital in London, was established in the sixteenth century; actually, it had been founded much earlier as a religious organization and had housed a few mental patients then. Bethlehem Hospital—whose name is the origin of the term *bedlam*—had more patients than it could handle, though, and simply released many of them to wander as beggars.

Serious concern for the mentally ill began to develop near the end of the eighteenth century, as fervor against witchcraft diminished and the concept of natural causes of disease began to prevail. An important figure was the French physician Philippe Pinel (1745–1826), who became head of the Bicêtre Hospital for the Insane in Paris. Patients at Bicêtre had been kept chained, but Pinel insisted on unchaining many of them, with dramatically therapeutic results.

In the nineteenth century, approaches to mental illness were mixed. Some Philadelphians, for example, paid admission to mental hospitals, where they gawked at mental patients in chains and prided themselves on their own normality. More enlightened treatment was provided by the Society of Friends, who saw God (not Satan) in the insane. Early in the century, Quaker institutions practiced "moral treatment," allowing patients to roam the grounds freely and work in gardens. This moral treatment also included trying to create a homelike atmosphere for patients while isolating them from the conditions that were thought to have brought on their insanity, such as marital and financial problems.

In the twentieth century, treatments based on modern psychiatry have been developed; there has also been a new emphasis on patients' rights, and it is the trends in patients' rights which will mainly concern us here.

Patients' Rights

The twentieth-century approach to patients' rights initially came about, at least partly, in reaction to an older idea of commitment in a mental institution as mainly an alternative to imprisonment in jail. Early in the twentieth century, it was accepted that the insane needed "therapeutic justice" rather than criminal justice. Since insanity was not a crime, no legal proceedings were required to commit a person thought to be insane to an institution. It was simply assumed that the committing psychiatrists would always act in the patient's best interests. Later in the century, this assumption would be challenged and intensely debated.

In the 1960s and 1970s, there was a clash of views about mental patients, dramatized in movies such as *King of Hearts* (1966) and the Oscar-winning *One Flew Over the Cuckoo's Nest* (1975). Lawyers who defended patients' autonomy argued that psychiatric diagnoses were subjective, that large public mental institutions were coercive, and that checks and balances were needed. As we will see, an alliance of these lawyers and the patient-rights movement would eventually batter down the locked doors of psychiatric wards.

On the other side, many psychiatrists argued that psychiatry was benevolent, that the insane needed treatment, and that apathy was dangerous. These psychiatrists emphasized that at least some forms of insanity have a biochemical basis—which would imply that such forms can be objectively identified and specifically treated.

However, there were some heretics within psychiatry. One of the most prominent of these heretics was the existentialist psychiatrist R. D. Laing, who saw insane behavior as an inner, mental defense against a brutal, manipulative, terrifying world. In Laing's view, the young woman in the book *Sybil* (which was published in the 1960s and also became a film) would have developed her multiple personalities to distance her original "self" from the torture inflicted by her vicious mother. Similarly, Joyce Brown—the allegedly deranged street woman whose case is the subject of this chapter—might have muttered to herself and yelled obscenities at others as a defense against wrongs inflicted on her (this interpretation may be supported by the fact that her muttering and shouting seemed to increase when rough-looking men appeared).

Another important dissident psychiatrist was Thomas Szasz, who led a revolt within the profession. It should be noted that Szasz saw no problem with patients who voluntarily sought help; he held that the proper role of psychiatrists was to help patients who had already identified themselves as troubled. His criticism was directed at situations in which help was forced on people—like Joyce Brown—who did not see themselves as mentally ill and resisted intervention. Szasz held that involuntary commitment rarely benefited patients and was carried out chiefly to rid society of people who acted strangely.

Szasz's basic position was this: A physical disease, such as AIDS or cancer, has a physical cause. Some mental illnesses also have a physical cause, in the brain, and these mental illnesses are therefore real. But other "mental illnesses" have no physical cause; they result merely from problems in living. A "mental illness" with no physical cause, Szasz held, is a "myth," not a disease. A disease is caused by something physical (a microbe, a lesion), and if a condition is not physical, it is not a disease at all.

Szasz concluded that nonbiological psychiatry could not be objective, or value-free; he held that it was "much more intimately related to problems of ethics than is medicine in general."[3] Consider that interpersonal relations—relationships between wife and husband, between the individual and the community, among colleagues, among neighbors—inevitably involve stress, conflict of interests, and strain. Much of this disharmony has to do with incompatible values, and to pretend that psychiatrists can offer value-free approaches is ludicrous: "Much of psychotherapy revolves around nothing other than the elucidation and weighing of goals and values—many of which may be mutually contradictory—and the means whereby they might best be harmonized, realized, or relinquished."[4]

Who, Szasz asked, can correctly define norms of "correct" and "psychotic" behavior? He was especially opposed to the classification of personality disorders as mental illness. (As discussed in Chapter 5—on the Baby M case—Mary Beth Whitehead was said to have a "personality disorder." It was exactly this kind of diagnosis that made Szasz suspicious, particularly because such a diagnosis often seemed to be made, as in the Baby M case, for purposes other than helping the person who was supposed to have the disorder.) According to Szasz, psychiatry generally presumes that love, continued life, stable marriage, kindness, and meekness indicate mental health; and that hatred, homicide, suicide, repeated divorce, chronic hostility, and vengefulness indicate mental illness. These presumptions are evaluative, not factual.

A study by D. Rosenhan, "On Being Sane in Insane Places," was also significant in the patients-rights movement. In this study, several sociologists, psychiatrists, and others voluntarily entered mental hospitals, saying that they were "hearing voices"—a major symptom of schizophrenia.[5] Once committed, they acted normally and no longer mentioned "voices"; however, they had been labeled "schizophrenic" in their medical charts, and the staff continued to treat them as schizophrenic. Ironically, although the staff did not see through the sham, several of the genuine mental patients did.

Deinstitutionalization

Deinstitutionalization of mental patients in the United States began in the 1970s. In 1972, in *Wyatt v. Stickey*, a federal judge in Alabama, Frank Johnson, ruled that a committed mental patient must either receive treatment or be released. Johnson's decision specified the institutional conditions necessary to ensure minimal treatment: at least 2 psychiatrists, 12 registered nurses, and 10 aides for every 250 patients. This standard is indeed minimal, but most states had been failing to meet it for years. Johnson also required state mental institutions to provide individualized treatment plans, to allow patients to refuse invasive treatments such as electroconvulsive therapy (ECT) and psychosurgery, and to establish the least restrictive conditions necessary for treatment.

Johnson's ruling was the precursor of a decision by the United States Supreme Court in 1975, in *O'Connor v. Donaldson*.[6] In 1943, at age 34, Kenneth Donaldson got into a fight with coworkers over politics and was knocked out; his parents, considering him crazy, petitioned a Florida judge to commit him to a mental institution. He was committed, was given 11 weeks of electroshock treatment, and was then released. In 1956, while he was visiting his parents in Florida, his father asked for a sanity hearing, saying that Kenneth Donaldson had a persecution complex; the son was then committed to Florida State Mental Hospital, where he was held for 15 years. Throughout those 15 years, he petitioned the courts many times, asking for a hearing; meanwhile, he rarely saw a physician and never received treatment. In the institution, he was presumed insane and—like Rosenhan's impostors—could not prove otherwise. Finally, in 1971, when his case was about to be heard, he was released.

A lawyer then helped him bring suit for damages against the superintendent of the institution, J. B. O'Connor, and the case eventually reached the Supreme Court. The Supreme Court decided for Kenneth Donaldson, ruling that he should not have been held against his will, even if he was mentally ill, unless he had been dangerous to himself or others and had no means of existing outside the institution. It also upheld a lower court's awards of $38,500 in compensatory damages and $10,000 in punitive damages.

More generally, the *O'Connor* decision established two conditions as necessary for involuntary commitment:

1. Suffering from mental illness (being "insane")
2. Being dangerous to others *or* being dangerous to oneself

Note that *both* conditions—(1) insanity and (2) danger to oneself or others—had to be met for involuntary commitment. *Dangerousness* was subsequently interpreted as imminent risk to life (or threats of such risk) or imminent risk of bodily harm; *imminent* meant within days or hours. The arbiters were two psychiatrists. Evidence of dangerousness to oneself would consist of:

(a) Threats of suicide
(b) Gross neglect of basic needs

Dangerousness to oneself was eventually stretched to include gross *incapacity* to take care of basic needs.

With these legal changes, the courts moved rapidly from a medical model of civil commitment, which had been used in the early 1960s, to a patient-rights model in the 1970s. An important factor in this change was that a third requirement for commitment was added to the two *O'Connor* conditions:

3. Provision of the least restrictive environment by the institution

Conditions 1 (mental illness) and 2 (dangerousness) applied in all states, since the Supreme Court had established them; two-thirds of the states also applied condition 3 (least restrictive environment).[7]

These legal developments entailed the release of many mental patients from large state institutions, because such institutions often could not provide individualized treatment (as required by *Wyatt)* and were not the least restrictive environment: arrangements such as "halfway houses" were less restrictive.

Other factors also contributed to deinstitutionalization. For one thing, new psychotropic medications allowed much more outpatient treatment. Also, the Kennedy administration had advocated small, community-integrated facilities rather than large, impersonal state institutions: in the words of President Kennedy, "Reliance on the cold mercy of custodial isolation will be supplanted by the open warmth of community concern."[8] Other factors included tight budgets, psychiatrists who sought lighter workloads, and a general distrust of authority in the early 1970s.

All these factors combined to empty American mental institutions. In most states during the early 1970s, 50 percent of the patients in state institutions were released; in some other states, 75 percent were released. In 1955, nearly 560,000 patients had lived in state mental institutions; in 1988, there were only 130,000. Nearly 500,000 mental patients were "deinstitutionalized" over the course of 30 years. All levels of government saved money, the American Civil Liberties Union was appeased, and mental patients flooded into communities.

•

However, the "warmth of community concern" envisioned by John Kennedy did not appear. Communities were hostile to the idea of halfway houses in their midst, and few such facilities were created. Mental patients "living in the community" lived more often on warm-air grates than in group homes, which were scarce and—where they existed at all—understaffed. Bag ladies were seen more and more on city streets. Local charities had to step in and set up soup kitchens for hungry street people. Soup kitchens and food banks were a sign that deinstitutionalization was not working; but in the 1980s, Reaganites hailed them as proof that government intervention was unneeded.

In short, deinstitutionalization failed. It failed because government funds were never allocated for community homes; because communities themselves rejected such homes; because mental health services were fragmented between county, state, and federal agencies; because housing was scarce; and because the legal pendulum had swung toward autonomy for mental patients.

During the 1970s, many people struggled to make deinstitutionalization work, but the system was not a system, and it was not too long before psychiatry—among other groups and many individuals—revolted. A number of prominent psychiatrists chastised liberals who resisted committing schizophrenics. One former director at the National Institutes of Mental Health (NIMH), who had been a leader of the deinstitutionalization movement, questioned the ethics of mental health administrators and accused them of allowing a new form of profitable segregation: "poor blacks working with other poor blacks while white mental health professionals worked with their own kind."[9] In 1976, a famous psychiatrist reviewed deinstitutionalization and concluded that it was a failure, that some involuntary confinement was needed to help the mentally ill, and that civil liberties lawyers were often enemies of the insane.[10]

THE CASE OF JOYCE BROWN

Project Help

By the 1980s, both mental health professionals and the general public in New York wanted something done about the situation there. Pedestrians found themselves having to step around or over derelicts sleeping on the street; people entering offices, stores, concert halls, and even their own homes had to step over derelicts huddled in doorways. Homeless panhandlers seemed to be almost everywhere. Subway cars were taken over by the homeless, who slept in them all day—many homeless people stay awake all night and sleep during the day, when life is somewhat less dangerous. During the winter, some of the homeless who preferred the streets to the city shelters died of exposure. (Reluctance to go to a shelter in New York City is not entirely unreasonable: most of the inmates in these shelters are men who use crack cocaine.)

Many of these homeless people were—or certainly seemed to be—insane; and in 1983, the administration of Mayor Ed Koch started Project Help to evaluate homeless mentally ill people for possible psychiatric treatment. The city runs 11 acute-care hospitals with some psychiatric units; but since these municipal hospitals could provide only short-term care, the Koch administration also negotiated for some of the scarce beds in New York State mental hospitals for long-term care of extremely dysfunctional homeless people.

Originally, Project Help was a voluntary program: that is, except for people considered dangerous to themselves or others, the project intervened only with mentally ill people who wanted to be helped. On this basis, however, most of the people it tried to help resisted its efforts. City administrators were thus confronted with a difficult issue. Could insane homeless people just be left to "die with their rights on"? Or could these people be forcibly picked up for psychiatric evaluation in a hospital? Forcible evaluation, possibly leading to involuntary commitment, might seem to violate these people's freedom; but surely it might also help them, and didn't they desperately need help?

In October of 1987, this reasoning led Project Help to broaden its standards for involuntary commitment beyond the legal requirements of mental illness and dangerousness. It added two new criteria: "self-neglect" and a "need to be treated."

The first person picked up by Project Help under its new criteria was a 40-year-old African American woman calling herself "Billie Boggs." She had been deliberately chosen as a test case; Mayor Koch, who had seen her and spoken with her on the street, was personally involved in that decision. At about the same time, almost 100 other homeless people were also evaluated under the new criteria, and 38 of them were brought to Bellevue Hospital's inpatient psychiatric unit; none of them made a legal issue of it. The case of "Billie Boggs," however, did become a legal issue. In fact, it would soon attract national attention as a symbol of the conflict over whether or not to impose involuntary treatment on homeless people who are mentally ill.

"Billie Boggs"

Billie Boggs's real name was Joyce Brown (Bill Boggs was actually the name of a man who was prominent on local television). For 1½ years, Joyce Brown had been sleeping at night on an air grate outside a Swensen's ice cream parlor on Second Avenue and 65th Street, on the upper east side of Manhattan (ironically, in a neighborhood with the highest per capita wealth in the United States). During the day, she panhandled on the street. At a nearby delicatessen, she would buy chicken cutlets, ice cream, cigarettes, and toilet paper.

Joyce Brown had become a familiar figure in the neighborhood, and to many people her physical appearance suggested mental illness. Her teeth were very unclean; her matted, tangled hair was pushed underneath a bulky white knit cap. All winter, she went without gloves; the only clothing she had seemed to be a striped blouse, beige pants, and a green sweater, though she kept sheets and blankets nearby and slept under them when she went to her air vent at night.

Joyce Brown's behavior also seemed to suggest derangement. She had a glazed look, muttered as she panhandled, and often carried on a dialogue with herself. She sometimes sang "How Much Is That Doggie in the Window?" Once, when a resident of the block gave her some money, she tossed it back, while screaming angrily at an invisible man. One neighbor described her in a letter to the *New York Times* as "full of rage." She seemed to dislike black men especially and would curse at any she encountered on her side of the street, although she liked babies in strollers. She sometimes defecated and urinated in the gutter. On bitterly cold nights, people in the neighborhood sometimes tried to have the police pick her up, but she always resisted.

For some time, psychiatrists working in Project Help had been observing Joyce Brown on the street, and on this basis they had evaluated her as insane. On October 28, 1987, she was forcibly removed from the street by Project Help and brought to the emergency room of Bellevue Hospital. She identified herself at Bellevue as Billie Boggs and also as "Ann Smith" (another alias she sometimes used) and said that she had lived on the street for 5 years and had no parents or other relatives. In the emergency room, she was injected with 5 mg of Haldol, an antipsychotic drug; and 2 mg of Ativan, a fast-acting short-term tranquilizer. She was then taken to a new, 28-bed, locked psychiatric unit on the nineteenth floor.

The Legal Conflicts

After Joyce Brown was evaluated at Bellevue, Mayor Koch was informed that she was neither sufficiently insane nor sufficiently dangerous for involuntary commitment; he replied, "You're loony yourself." Here, Koch said, was a woman whom compassionate people should help, but who could not be helped because of legalistic quibbles. He also believed (and this belief was probably shared by most New Yorkers and visitors to the city) that the civil liberties of homeless mentally ill people were being overemphasized, to the detriment of quality of life in the city's public places. He and Project Help, therefore, decided to pursue her commitment on the basis of their new additional criteria. Bellevue, although it did not consider her dangerous enough for commitment, had diagnosed her as schizophrenic and in need of treatment—and "need for treatment" was one of Project Help's new standards.

In any event, once a person is brought to a psychiatric facility by the police or emergency-room personnel, release is unlikely in practice until a commitment hearing before a judge has been held and concluded. (For commitment hearings, hospitals usually have a designated room in the psychiatric unit.) Moreover, the law in New York State is that, without a hearing, involuntary injections are allowed only in emergency rooms; and in the psychiatric unit at Bellevue, Joyce Brown exercised her right to refuse further drugs. Therefore, she could be given no drugs in the psychiatric ward until a separate hearing was held on involuntary drug treatment.

•

Joyce Brown's commitment hearing began on November 5, 8 days after her arrival at Bellevue, and it would take 3 days. Judge (Acting Justice) Robert Lippman of the state supreme court, who had been assigned to hear mental cases, presided. Lippman (the son of a prominent orthopedic surgeon) was then 51 years old, married and with two teenage sons; he lived on the upper east side and, appropriately enough, had worked for 17 years as a Legal Aid lawyer in the Bronx; he had been elected to a 10-year civil court term in 1983. He was known in the legal community as an advocate for the poor and homeless. Joyce Brown had called the American Civil Liberties Union (ACLU) from Bellevue and asked for their help; she had received a team of ACLU lawyers, on the condition that she would waive confidentiality and agree to publicity for her own sake and that of other homeless people. Her lawyers were opposed by New York City's attorney.

Both the mayor's office and ACLU treated the hearing as a test, and Judge Lippman apparently also saw it in those terms. Such hearings are almost always closed to the public, but because this case had the potential to set a precedent—and because of the publicity it had already generated—Lippman allowed the press to attend. However, only the testimony of witnesses who consented could be reported by the press.

•

On November 2, a few days before the commitment hearing, a sketch of "Billie Boggs" had appeared on a television news show, and three women recognized her as their sister. As the commitment hearing began on November 5, these three women were present. Outside the hearing room, they identified her to reporters as Joyce Brown (this was actually the point at which her real name was first revealed). They said they had been searching for Joyce Brown for 1½ years. The three sisters were all married, had all worked for years, and were all living in what they described as "comfortable homes."

As the hearing proceeded, Joyce Brown's sisters gave the press many details. They said that she had never married and had no children, and they described her background.[11] Their family was from Elizabeth, New Jersey, and their father was a Methodist minister; as children, all the girls had gone to church every Sunday. Joyce was said to have been a "bright, attractive, and happy-go-lucky child." Joyce Brown graduated from both high school and business school and had then had several jobs at Bell Laboratories. During these years, her sisters said, she had been a "big, healthy girl" who wore nice clothes and jewelry and "always drove around in a new Cadillac."

In her twenties, however, according to her sisters, Joyce Brown became increasingly dependent on heroin and, later, cocaine; it can be noted that this is the age at which the first signs of schizophrenia often appear. She worked for 10 years as a secretary for the New Jersey Human Rights Commission; but in 1982, she was arrested by the Newark police, charged with assault, and found guilty of harassment. At about this time, her conduct deteriorated: she became belligerent and less able to support herself; her mental health and her job performance plummeted. In 1985, at age 38, she was fired because of absenteeism and her use of heroin and cocaine. She had been living with her sisters and their parents in turn, but now she left her family and went to a shelter in Newark, where she was expelled for assaulting others there.

Her sisters admitted that they then tricked her into a voluntary commitment in the psychiatric ward of East Orange General Hospital in New Jersey. There she was diagnosed as psychotic and given antipsychotic drugs, though she resisted these injections. She was held for 2 weeks, during which—again because of assaults on others—she was put in restraints in an isolation room. After these 2 weeks, she was released.

She then fled New Jersey and began to live on the streets of New York, on the upper east side, under various aliases. She avoided shelters for the homeless, considering them dangerous for unattached women. For some time, she did not contact her sisters, fearing that they would have her committed again. But her sisters said that in July 1986 they received an abusive telephone call from her in Manhattan, and that they then spent much of the next year looking for her along Manhattan streets.

The sisters emphasized, "Behind every homeless person there is a family that just wants to find them and help them."

•

When Joyce Brown herself testified at her commitment hearing, she appeared to be intelligent and articulate. She called herself a "professional street person" and was able to answer a number of probing questions.

Why had she torn up paper money? She said that she needed $7 a day and had torn up only additional money that was forced on her. "If money is given to me and I don't want it, of course I am going to destroy it," she said; she explained that she might be robbed if she did not. "I've heard people say: 'Take it. It will make me feel good.' But I say: 'I don't want it. I don't need it.' Is it my job to make them feel good by taking their money?"[12]

Why did she defecate on herself? "I never did," she replied; though she added that she had used the streets because no local restaurant would let her use its restroom. "I offered to buy something and they still refused."

Why had she used aliases such as "Billie Boggs"? "To prevent my sisters from finding me."

The attorney for the city argued that Joyce Brown had to be committed because she was endangering herself through self-neglect. Four psychiatrists testified for the city that she suffered from chronic schizophrenia, that she was clearly psychotic and should be treated in an institution, and that she would deteriorate if she was left on the streets. One of the psychiatrists for the city, Luis Marcos, was a vice president of its public hospital system and an advocate of the new criteria adopted by Project Help; he was therefore challenged about his ability to give unbiased testimony. He said in reply, "This is not political psychiatry"; he also stated that Joyce Brown's "self-neglect" was "so severe" that she had to be helped against her will. He noted that schizophrenia was consistent with being bright and having periods of rationality.

ACLU, on the other side, asked for an injunction to free Joyce Brown. Three psychiatrists testified for ACLU that she was not psychotic, not dangerous, not unreasonable in her answers, and not incapable of caring for herself on the streets. One of these three, Robert E. Gould of New York Medical College, testified that she was living on the street by choice.

One of Joyce Brown's sisters started to testify but was not allowed to continue after the ACLU attorneys objected. She had begun to describe how her sister's condition had deteriorated over the years, and the objection was sustained on the ground that this evidence was not relevant to Joyce Brown's present competence. (The sisters saw this as a ruling that the testimony of family members was irrelevant, and they resented it.)

By the third day of the commitment hearing, Joyce Brown appeared self-confident. She spoke slowly, deliberately, and with assurance and even smiled a few times at the judge. She told him that passersby on her street chatted with her every day: "They tell me about movies, they tell me about restaurants. They are executives, lawyers, doctors. They are established in their fields. If I asked for large amounts of money, they would give it to me."

In his summation, one of the ACLU attorneys said that the city had not proved that Joyce was dangerous to herself or others: "The only evidence the city had is that she goes to the bathroom in the streets. I see that in New York City every day, because there's a lack of public restroom facilities." The attorney for the city said in her summation: "Decency and the law and common sense do not require us to wait until something happens to her. It is our duty to act before it is too late."[13]

•

On November 12, Judge Lippman ordered Joyce Brown freed. He had found her "rational, logical, and coherent" throughout her testimony;[14] he said that she "displayed a sense of humor, pride, a fierce independence of spirit, [and] quick mental reflexes"; and he noted that she met none of the conditions set forth in *O'Connor v. Donaldson.* He stressed that even if all the psychiatrists had diagnosed her as psychotic, the city had still not met the requirement of dangerousness to others or oneself. "I am aware that her mode of existence does not conform to conventional standards, that it is an offense to aesthetic sense," he commented. Nevertheless, "she copes, she is fit, she survives." Moreover, "she refuses to be housed in a shelter. That may reveal more about conditions in shelters than about Joyce Brown's mental state. It might, in fact, prove she's quite sane."

Judge Lippman also complained: "There must be some civilized alternatives other than involuntary hospitalization or the street." He did not invalidate Project Help itself, and even praised it as a step in the right direction. Forced to decide for one side or the other, however, he ruled that the City had not proved Joyce Brown incompetent.

•

After the hearing, Joyce Brown's sisters talked again to reporters. They called Lippman's decision "racist" and "sexist." They argued that if his own wife or mother were sleeping on the streets, "he would not stand for it." They also insisted that Joyce Brown needed treatment. As the psychiatrist Robert Gould left the hearing with Joyce Brown's sisters and reporters, he challenged the sisters: "Can't you understand that a lot of people are frightened that the Mayor has unilaterally decided to change the statute and pick up your sister?" One sister replied, "The Mayor is absolutely right. I have lived with her. You have not lived with her." Gould replied, "Is it possible that your sister doesn't want to live with you because you are so angry?"[15]

At this time, the sisters revealed that after Joyce Brown was hospitalized for schizophrenia in East Orange, they had gotten her declared mentally disabled and she had accordingly received $500 a month in social security disability payments, which they had been holding for her. Joyce Brown had persisted in refusing the money, though, saying that she rejected the "lie" that she was mentally disabled.

At the same time, Joyce Brown and her ACLU lawyers held a press conference, at which she said, "I didn't want to play the game before, but now I am. . . . I am going to get an apartment, . . . go back to work, and get my life together." She criticized the city for spending $600 a day on her care: "I could be living at Trump Tower."[16]

One question that had been raised was why she had appeared so rational at the hearing; in response, the psychiatrists at Bellevue had acknowledged that she had seemed sane but had claimed that she improved rapidly in the hospital. Joyce Brown dismissed their claim, saying—as she had been saying all along— that she had never been crazy in the first place. She objected to being taken into Bellevue like "cattle" and said that, given her options, living on the street was a rational choice. (Her sisters dismissed this argument: "You might be able to survive one winter," one of them said, "or even two. But you can't survive that way forever.")

Mayor Koch blasted Judge Lippman's decision: "If anything happens to that woman, God forbid, the blood of that woman is on that judge's hands." Reminded by a reporter that Lippman had found Joyce Brown lucid, Koch replied, "This woman is at risk. When she lay on the ground in the rain, in the snow, uncovered—was that lucid?"[17] When asked if Joyce's commitment was "political psychiatry," Koch asked, "Who would claim that?" When told that it had been Joyce Brown herself, he replied, "That alone proves she's crazy."[18]

•

The city and Koch appealed to a five-member New York State Appellate Court, and one of its members stayed Judge Lippman's order of release pending its own hearing. This higher court agreed to hold its hearing extraordinarily soon— within 2 weeks—but until then, Joyce Brown would have to remain at Bellevue. She was reportedly bitter but accepted the decision.

During the weeks before the hearing on their appeal, city officials sought and obtained an order to see if Joyce Brown had lupus cerebritis, a genetically caused, incurable degenerative brain syndrome. After negotiations, she allowed a blood sample to be taken. On December 12, the result was found to be negative; this embarrassed the psychiatrist who had made the provisional diagnosis—he seemed to have been grasping at a straw.

At the appellate hearing, ACLU argued that Joyce Brown would not return to the streets but would live in a supportive residence for the homeless. The city argued that where she would live was irrelevant: "She was not hospitalized because she was living on the streets [but because] three psychiatrists said she needed medical and psychiatric help." According to the city, she was schizophrenic and should remain under psychiatric care for her own good (though the city did not argue that she was dangerous to herself or others), and her decision not to return to the street did not affect this situation; the case was not about homelessness but about mental illness. It was pointed out that in New York, the homeless tended to be poor, African American, or Hispanic; in contrast, Project Help was aimed at mentally disturbed people on the streets, who—according to the city—were typically white, middle-class people with chronic undifferentiated schizophrenia. (It was also said that many of these people were not New Yorkers.)

In short, the city attorneys told the justices that the city could help Joyce and should be allowed to do so; and having won 11 previous challenges to its various commitment programs over the last decade (including Project Help under the original criteria), it hoped to win this one too.

Joyce Brown's attorneys replied that she did not want help, did not need help, and was entitled to live as she pleased. (She herself did not testify before the appeals court.) While awaiting the decision, she told reporters that she was ready to return to work. "Tomorrow I could sit at a typewriter and take shorthand," she said. "I am not insane. I am homeless." She also said that she had known before the test for lupus that she did not have it and was not in poor health, claiming, "You have to be in good physical shape to survive on the street."

•

The city won on appeal. On December 19, the appellate court held (3-2, with the two dissenting justices disagreeing vigorously) that Judge Lippman had ruled incorrectly that the city had not provided enough evidence for commitment, and that Lippman had placed too much emphasis on Joyce Brown's testimony instead of the testimony of the psychiatrists who believed she would harm herself. Surprisingly, the majority noted that a very high standard of proof was required in this case—"clear and convincing evidence" rather than the weaker "preponderance of evidence"—and that the city had met the higher standard. (These standards of evidence are discussed in Chapter 1, with regard to the Nancy Cruzan case.)

In an unusual move, the appellate court reviewed detailed testimony in the case, especially that of a social worker who said she had observed "fecal matter" on the sheets in which "Miss Boggs" wrapped herself. The appellate court also reviewed the testimony of one psychiatrist who said that Joyce Brown had told him she often defecated and urinated on herself. In addition, the court found that "the evidence presented in this case clearly and convincingly demonstrated Ms. Boggs's past history of assaultive and aggressive behavior."[19] The majority justices gave little weight to Joyce Brown's lucidity during her commitment hearing, attributing it to "a week of hospital treatment." (In fact, though, she had received no medical treatment.)

The two dissenting justices argued that the city's case could be "narrowed to one claim," which was that "she is dangerous to herself" because "she is likely to provoke others to do injury to her." They considered that commitment to prevent such possible harm was an "extreme remedy" and "somewhat offensive." They were dismayed that their colleagues had dismissed Lippman's assessment of Joyce Brown's lucidity in court: " . . . If the court's [Lippman's] judgment of her mental condition is to be completely ignored, then what was the purpose of the hearing in the first place?" Finally, they stressed that in Joyce Brown's six previous hospitalizations,[20] disinterested psychiatrists had unanimously concluded that she was not dangerous to herself.

•

After the decision of the appellate court, Mayor Koch said, "Up until this moment, the only treatment has been care, loving, a safe environment. Now we will seek to treat her medically." However, to medicate Joyce Brown against her will, under New York State law the city still had to get a court order.

One month later, on January 19, 1988, a state judge ruled that she could not be given drugs against her will. Bellevue Hospital promptly released her, saying that if she could not be treated with drugs, there was no further point in holding her.

ACLU then appealed the earlier appellate decision on commitment to New York's supreme court, the Court of Appeals, which declined to hear the case because it presented "no novel, constitutional or substantial case for this court to review," and because the case was moot after Joyce Brown's release from Bellevue.

All together, Joyce Brown had been held for 84 days. One member of the city council noted that the city had spent more than $42,000 for her stay at Bellevue and suggested that in this case "the mayor's ego got in the way of what was right." After her release, Joyce Brown held forth:

> I was incarcerated against my will. . . . [I was] a political prisoner. The only thing wrong with me was that I was homeless, not insane. You just can't go around picking everyone up and automatically label them schizophrenic. I'm angry at Mayor Koch, the city and Bellevue. They held me down and injected me. . . . They took my blood against my will. . . .
>
> I need a place to live; I don't need an institution. . . .
>
> People are treated differently just because of your economic status, [because of] what you look like and where you live. . . .
>
> I was mistreated, mentally abused, and I will never, ever, forget this.[21]

The Aftermath

Joyce Brown was released to live in a hotel for women run by a nonprofit agency. She received several job offers and worked temporarily as a secretary in the ACLU office. Interviewed there, she said that after leaving Bellevue, "I was supposed to have deteriorated within 3 or 4 days," and then noted with a smile that 3 weeks had passed and, "I'm fine. I'm working."

In fact, in early 1988 Joyce Brown became something of a celebrity. She received half a dozen movie and book offers. On February 15, she dined at Windows on the World, a restaurant atop the World Trade Center, where the waiters congratulated her. She shopped at Bloomingdale's, Saks Fifth Avenue, and Lord and Taylor; these shopping sprees were paid for by two television shows—*The Donahue Show* and *60 Minutes*—which were broadcasting discussions of her case. She seemed to flourish with attention.

Joyce Brown herself appeared on *The Donahue Show*. During this show, a hostile immigrant said that he had found a job and bought a house "in just 25 years," and he wondered why she couldn't do the same. He said, "You're an intelligent woman. How come you're homeless? I'm sure you can find a job." She replied, "Right now I'm trying to get a job. Mr. Donahue, do you need any help around here?" (The audience laughed heartily.)

Joyce Brown also lectured to students at two law schools—Cardozo and Harvard. The title of her speech was "The Homeless Crisis: A Street View." At the time, she said, "It looks like I have been appointed the homeless spokesperson."

•

Then things began to go worse for her. She had eventually decided to accept the disability benefits which her sisters had been accumulating for her, but her sisters now resisted; they said they would release the money to her when the ACLU lawyers stopped "manipulating her" for political purposes.

Her roommate at the hotel said that Joyce Brown had "a lot of anger inside" and frequently talked to herself. One day, while walking to work, she was heard muttering racial slurs and obscenities. She dismissed these incidents as misinterpretations of her habit of singing popular songs to herself.

On March 21, 1988, Joyce Brown was seen begging on a street in the Times Square area and shouting obscenities at passersby. When asked how she was doing, she insisted, "I'm not insane."[22]

On May 10, she collapsed on the street and was admitted to a hospital for dangerously high blood pressure; she had always refused medication for hypertension.

On September 6, she was charged with having been in possession of a small amount of heroin ($40 worth) and two hypodermic needles in a Harlem housing project shortly after her release from Bellevue.[23] This incident in particular made many people who had sided with Koch, including the essayist Charles Krauthammer, feel vindicated.[24] On December 27, 1988, she pleaded guilty to disorderly conduct and was conditionally discharged.

•

By July of the next year—1989—Joyce Brown was living in a supervised residence for formerly homeless women, in Manhattan.

During that month, Project Help announced that it had picked up and helped 466 homeless mentally ill people since adopting its new criteria in 1987. It estimated that 800 to 1,000 such people were still out on the city streets.

When New York City officials planned Project Help, they assumed that people such as Joyce Brown would stay for a few weeks in psychiatric hospitals and would then be moved into community facilities, where they could live under supervised conditions. As the people picked up by Project Help were actually evaluated, however, they turned out to be far sicker than had been expected. Thus many more permanent places were needed in psychiatric hospitals than had been planned for.

ETHICAL ISSUES

Criteria for Commitment: Applying the *O'Connor* Standards

One issue in the Joyce Brown case was the *O'Connor* standards for involuntary commitment. The five appellate justices had to decide whether or not Joyce Brown could be committed under the *O'Connor* criteria, but because the legal issue was obviously in her favor, they would in effect be deciding whether or not those standards were morally sufficient. In other words, Joyce Brown clearly could not be committed under the existing legal criteria established by *O'Connor*, and so the justices had to decide whether those criteria should be changed or radically reinterpreted for reasons of compassion.

In its argument to this appellate court, New York City used a moral argument: that the traditional legal standard allowed too much risk of harm. The city maintained that personal liberty had been valued too highly and could result in ultimate harm to the mentally ill.

The city's argument hung on two points. The first of these was that homeless mentally ill people will eventually come to harm if they are simply left alone. In Joyce Brown's case, if she stayed on the street, hurling insults at black men and sleeping unguarded, she would eventually be attacked.

The second point was independent of the first; it appealed simply to humanitarian considerations. Here, the city argued that governments have an ancient right—or duty—known as *parens patria* ("parent of the country"). *Parens patria* originated in English common law, under which the king or queen had a royal prerogative to act as guardian for incompetents. In modern law, state attorney generals exercise the same right in bringing antitrust suits on behalf of citizens. On this basis, the city held that it had a responsibility to protect people, like Joyce Brown, who were deteriorating, and that it would be degrading and unmerciful to let them continue to live without help. To say that society cannot help them because helping them would violate their rights was to value their personal liberty over their sanity, their health, and their survival. The city noted that while this appeal was taking place, three homeless men had been found frozen to death in Central Park.

Of course, not everyone agreed with these two points, or with the city's case as a whole. Some people, including Joyce Brown herself and Judge Lippman, considered the first point an especially poor argument: after all, she had already lived 1½ years on the street and seemed to have come to no harm.

However, Charles Krauthammer, a well-known liberal who wrote for *Time* and *New Republic,* supported the city. He argued that Joyce Brown should be committed not because she was dangerous but because she was helpless.[25] For every insane person committed who protested, he emphasized, hundreds did not protest and appeared to like warm beds and regular meals. Still, it must be noted that Joyce Brown herself said she wasn't helpless and indeed didn't appear to be.

Motives for Commitment

In the controversy over Joyce Brown, motives for commitment became an issue. Were those who argued for commitment—and even some of those who argued against it—genuinely motivated by altruism, or did they have ulterior, nonaltruistic motives? In this regard, the general question of public altruism arose, along with various arguments about nonaltruistic motivation.

Altruism and its limits   Altruism as such is a persistent ethical problem of civilized life. How much should any individual do for strangers who appear to be in need? In face-to-face meetings with apparently needy strangers, few of us are completely indifferent, but most of us experience doubts and self-conflicts about what to do.

Charles Krauthammer argued that the ethical response to people like Joyce Brown should be based on societal rather than individual responsibility. The

Joyce Browns of a community need facilities and staff to care for them, he held, and to implement this kind of solution he urged higher taxes. Krauthammer said, "To expect saintliness of the ordinary citizen is bad social policy," but "society must not leave the ordinary citizen with no alternative between ignoring the homeless and playing Mother Teresa. A civilized society ought to offer its people some communal act that lies somewhere in between, such as contributing to the public treasury to build an asylum system to care for these people."

There are, however, arguments against Krauthammer's position. One counter-argument is theoretical: individuals do have a moral duty to be altruistic but are only too ready to abandon their duty and let society take over. Three authors argued along these lines in a legal journal:

> Most of us profess to believe that there is an individual moral duty to take care of a senile parent, a paranoid wife, or a disturbed child. Most of us also resent the bother such care creates. By allowing society to perform this duty, masked in medical terminology, but frequently amounting in fact to what one court has described as "warehousing," we can avoid facing painful issues.[26]

There is also a practical argument against Krauthammer's position: societal "altruism" may be lacking or grossly inadequate. In a case like Joyce Brown's, it can be argued that no real treatment exists and commitment is no more than getting the insane off the streets.

Nonaltruistic motives   In the case of Joyce Brown, almost everyone on both sides claimed to be motivated by altruism—to have her own best interests in mind—and almost everyone was accused of having hidden, nonaltruistic motives.

Mayor Koch and New York City, for example, were accused of wanting Joyce Brown committed simply because she was a public nuisance. Her sisters were accused of wanting her committed simply because she was a family nuisance. Her neighbors were accused of wanting to have her put away, out of their sight, because she offended their affluent sensibilities. Both Judge Lippman, who decided in her favor, and the appellate justices who decided against her were accused of racism: Lippman, it was said, considered it not inappropriate for a black woman to live in filth on the street; the appellate justices were said to be presuming that a black woman was probably incompetent. ACLU was accused of manipulating Joyce Brown to further its own agenda. Some psychiatrists were accused of being the city's rubber stamp and of using "treatment" for purposes of restraint or even punishment; psychiatrists on the other side were accused of patient abandonment.

The truth is probably that many people involved in the case, as participants or commentators, had mixed motives. This is neither surprising nor particularly sinister: most of us have mixed motives most of the time. Still, some of the arguments about nonaltruistic motivation were significant.

With regard to Mayor Koch and the city, for example, the columnist A. M. Rosenthal (who was a former editor of the *New York Times*) said that he himself saw Joyce Brown "almost every day" from his Second Avenue apartment and believed that Koch was trying to get therapy for her, not rounding up a political dissident.[27] To Rosenthal, it seemed that the city had wanted to be compassionate and gotten its hands slapped for trying: thus the case symbolized a situation where the law seemed helpless. Some people argued that her commitment was arbitrary because of the original psychiatric evaluation "on the street," but Rosenthal held that it was not; an arbitrary commitment would have been based only on secondhand evidence such as the possibly biased reports of her neighbors, but Joyce Brown had been given a hearing at Bellevue and had been represented by attorneys. The Project Help program, Rosenthal concluded, "is an attempt to help, not a program of incarceration."

The motives of Joyce Brown's affluent neighbors also came in for considerable scrutiny. ACLU, noting that Joyce Brown did not want to leave the street and had never been proved dangerous, argued that her presence embarrassed the rich people in her neighborhood. New York City has thousands of people like Joyce Brown, it was argued (and the United States has hundreds of thousands)— why, then, was there no similar outcry about all the others? Why did no one write letters to the *New York Times* about the Joyce Browns in the Bronx? Once Joyce Brown was gone, how many of her former neighbors on the upper east side would inquire about her? How many would even give her another thought?

Norman Siegel, executive director of ACLU, extended this argument to Koch and the city as well: "In sweeping up the homeless, the Mayor is attempting to place these people out of sight and out of mind and hide the crisis from the public consciousness." Siegel claimed that Project Help targeted areas seen by tourists and inhabited by the rich.

As noted earlier, quality of life in public places was a consideration for Koch and the city. However, the consideration they emphasized was treatment; and the city's mental health commissioner maintained that patients had been picked up in affluent areas simply because homeless people gravitated to such areas, which were safer and offered better opportunities for begging. These points, though, carried more weight with some commentators than with others.

Paternalism, Autonomy, and Diminished Competence

Paternalism in medicine is treatment of adult patients as incompetents who do not know their own best interests, and an important set of issues in Joyce Brown's case had to do with paternalism versus patients' autonomy.

Many philosophers, physicians, and legal scholars have discussed the conditions under which paternalism might be justified. One condition is temporary incompetence, followed by a return of competence; in this situation, paternalism would be justified if the patient himself or herself later agreed with it. (A suicidal patient, for example, may later be glad to be alive.) In Joyce Brown's case, the city might have argued impressively for paternalism if its psychiatrists had brought forth at least one patient who had been forced to undergo psychiatric treatment and was now sane and grateful. No such patient testified for the city, however.

Questions about patients' competence are important in any discussion of paternalism. In this regard, one question has to do with the basic concept of competence. The American legal system tends to treat mental patients as if they were either totally competent and hence autonomous, or totally dysfunctional and hence subject to mandatory treatment. Many observers argue, however, that this is a false dichotomy which can be harmful to patients. Competence, on this argument, is not an either-or matter but a matter of degrees; and over the last decade, American bioethics has increasingly seen competence in this way.

Another question has to do with what constitutes proof of competence and incompetence. This issue is not necessarily clear-cut: the psychiatrist Virginia Abernethy argues, for instance, that "disorientation, mental illness, irrationality, [and] commitment to a mental institution are not conclusive proof of incompetence."[28]

Abernethy describes the case of "Ms. A," a highly intelligent, very independent woman who lived alone in a large house with six cats, in an unheated garbage-strewn room. After a fire in her house (which had apparently started when she burned some debris to keep warm), Ms. A was hospitalized but found competent and released. As winter came, a concerned social worker investigated; he found her with her feet black, ulcerated, and bleeding. When he tried to get her to go with him to a hospital, she chased him away with a shotgun. The police later came and forcibly hospitalized her. At the hospital, her feet were diagnosed as gangrenous, and surgeons wanted to amputate; when she refused, psychiatrists began to evaluate her.

It turned out that Ms. A's feet had blackened once before, a few years earlier, and she had recovered. She now hoped for another recovery, but the psychiatrists interpreted this as "psychotic denial" and tried to get her to say that she wanted to live, so that they could amputate. She refused, avoiding their questions. Ms. A was faced with a dilemma: either she had to let the surgeons amputate (a drastic operation which she did not want), or she had to let the psychiatrists conclude that she was in denial and therefore psychotic. It might seem unfair to present a patient with such a choice—a choice between two highly undesirable outcomes—and it might also seem that in such a situation trying to avoid the choice would be reasonable. However, according to Abernethy, "Her rejection of the two-choice model became the grounds, finally, for concluding that Ms. A was not competent to refuse amputation."

Abernethy analyzed the psychodynamics of this process as follows. First, a false aura of medical emergency "pervaded the psychiatric consultations and judicial process." Second, "Ms. A herself was quick to anger and regarded most interactions with medical personnel as adversarial." Third, Ms. A's anger created anger in those evaluating her competence: "Professionals who think of themselves as altruistic, or at least benevolently motivated, may be particularly sensitive to hostility because they feel deserving of gratitude." Abernethy says that psychiatrists are outcome-oriented and cannot tolerate a patient's self-destructiveness, even in the name of autonomy and even when self-destruction results from an underlying disease that they ultimately cannot stop. Abernethy notes, moreover, that "hope (disbelieving the physicians' pessimistic prognosis) is not a criterion of psychotic denial."

In some ways, Joyce Brown was similar to Ms. A. Like Ms. A, Joyce Brown did not accept her diagnosis (schizophrenia) or her prognosis (that she would come to harm if left alone); she hoped that she was sane and could take care of herself. Also like Ms. A, Joyce Brown saw psychiatrists as enemies who wanted to treat her against her will. Both women were acknowledged to be generally competent, but both were evaluated as having a "focal incompetence," a specific incompetence to make decisions about their own treatment. Abernethy notes, "The criterion of a focal delusion is dangerously liable to error because a patient can easily be seen as delusional in an emotionally charged interchange, when in other circumstances he addresses the same issue appropriately."

Actually, the concept of incompetence—particularly in the context of psychiatric commitment—is a two-edged sword: if an incompetent patient cannot *refuse* treatment, how can such a patient *consent* to treatment? In the majority of cases, consent of incompetents is allowed for psychiatric admission and rarely challenged; this is hardly logical. Abernethy sums it up: with regard to commitment, "Competence is presumed and does not have to proved. Incompetence has to be proved."

Homelessness and Commitment

What was the real issue in the Joyce Brown case—insanity or homelessness?

City officials claimed that Joyce Brown's insanity was the true issue and her homelessness merely a side issue. Her ACLU lawyers disagreed: "The Joyce Brown story has captured the issue of the homeless that a lot of people have been trying to deal with for years."[29] The real problem, ACLU implied, was how to get homeless people off the streets, not how to treat the mentally ill; city officials didn't seem worried about schizophrenics who camped out in bad neighborhoods. ACLU suggested reinstituting public baths (which had been widely available in the city during the depression and earlier) and using condemned housing as temporary shelters. Incarcerating the homeless "for their own good" was a cheap solution; building homes for street people was much more expensive.

No one could deny that the housing situation in New York City was bad: affordable housing was rare. On a talk show about this issue in 1988, for example, one man said he had been working 15 months in Manhattan as a home health aide. He made $4.50 an hour and brought home $130 a week. Just to rent a room—with no stove, no sink, and no refrigerator; and not in pricey Manhattan, but along a noisy elevated train line in an outer borough—would cost him 2 weeks' pay in security ($250) at the outset, and then 1 week's take-home pay ($130) in rent each month. He might have found cheaper housing outside the city, of course; but he was a city employee and thus was required to live within its five boroughs.

On one talk show, a member of the audience said to Joyce Brown, "But a woman of your obvious intelligence, why would she be happy to spend the rest of her life on the street?" Joyce Brown replied, evidently referring to such housing problems:

> I didn't say I was going to spend the rest of my life on the street. I'm not a career homeless person, I have skills, I'm very intelligent, I am employable, but at that

particular time that was my choice. I had a limited choice and that's what I chose to do. . . .[30]

The problem of creating permanent housing for the city's homeless had frustrated many good minds. The city maintained over 1,000 families in squalid "welfare hotels" at exorbitant rates, using funding from the Emergency Assistance for Families act and the primary nationwide welfare program, Aid to Families with Dependent Children. The city would have preferred to use these funds to rent permanent housing for such families (in fact, it would later pressure the Clinton administration to allow this by threatening to block health care reform). Critics feared, however, that providing rented housing would encourage more people to depend on government handouts; they also pointed out that the city was one of the most expensive places in the United States in which to subsidize public housing. On the other hand, government subsidizes everyone who owns a home or condominium, since the interest on a mortgage is deductible for federal and state income taxes; and it can be argued that the poor and homeless not only deserve similar subsidization but also need it far more.

Moreover, it seemed in Joyce Brown's case that the dangers the city envisioned for her—and used as one basis for committing her—may have had more to do with homelessness than with schizophrenia or incipient schizophrenia. A lone woman sleeping unprotected on a sidewalk is indeed in danger, but that has little to do with mental illness. In other words, although the city insisted that the case was about mental illness, the dangers it emphasized seemed to come from life on the street, not from being mentally ill.

The crucial point here may be this: The city would not have tried to commit Joyce Brown if she had not been homeless, since Project Help was aimed at *homeless* mentally ill people. Was that reasonable? What does homelessness have to do with committing the insane?

In this regard, we might argue as follows. Presumably, anyone—homeless or not—should be committed if the legal criteria for commitment are met: insanity, dangerousness, and (in some states) a "least restrictive" environment for treatment. Presumably, also, no one—homeless or not—should be committed if these criteria for commitment are not met. Project Help's intention was to broaden or loosen those criteria by applying different standards, but *only* for homeless people. Was that justifiable? Shouldn't the same standards apply for everyone? Isn't that what we mean by "equal justice for all"?

Two final points should be made here. First, some people simply tried to infer insanity from homelessness, arguing as follows: It is dangerous to sleep on the streets of Manhattan. No one but an insane person would sleep there. Therefore, those who sleep on the street are insane. This, of course, begs the question of mental illness.

Second, some people argued that homeless people, regardless of sanity or insanity, should be taken to shelters or otherwise incarcerated for their own safety. In 1972, the United States Supreme Court overturned a vagrancy law in Jacksonville, Florida, under which vagrants had been jailed without hearings or due process. No such law existed in New York; nevertheless, one Queens Democrat said during the Joyce Brown case that homeless people refusing to go to shelters should be "accommodated overnight in a cell" for their own protection.[31] To many critics, such remarks suggested that programs like Project Help entailed a real danger of abuse: that they might sooner or later be extended in ways which would represent a wide threat.

Psychiatry and Commitment

A potential for psychiatric abuse was also seen in the Joyce Brown case. Shortly after Joyce Brown was picked up, one of her ACLU lawyers (Robert Levy) and the psychiatrist Robert Gould discussed this in the *New York Times*.[32] They emphasized several possible abuses: involuntary roundups, handcuffing, forcible injections of medication, and confinement in locked wards. Joyce Brown herself had been given medication and kept in a locked ward against her will; and Levy and Gould said that she had been examined at least five times previously and had been found "not to require involuntary hospitalization." Indeed, nearly half of the 215 people brought to emergency rooms by Project Help were found "not to require involuntary hospitalization." Gould and Levy argued that to allow "preventive detention based solely on nebulous predictions of future self-destructive behavior" would invite abuse. They raised the specter of "totalitarian regimes" that would use psychiatry for political control.

When confronted with arguments like this, Mayor Koch replied, "This is not political psychiatry! This is not Russia! We're trying to help this woman!" The director of the psychiatric unit at Bellevue, David Nardacci, a 32-year old psychiatrist, said that he had chosen to be a physician, "not a lawyer"; and as a physician, he was more concerned with helping people such as Joyce Brown than tiptoeing around legal pitfalls.

The issue of broadening criteria for commitment is again relevant here. How broadly should standards of commitment sweep? If we want to argue that these standards should be broadened enough to allow us to treat the Joyce Browns, aren't we thereby allowing psychiatric abuses to develop? How many people might be forced into mental hospitals by uncaring or even malevolent relatives? (Isn't this what Barbra Streisand portrayed in *Nuts)?* How many psychiatrists might use medication, "time-out" rooms, restraints, and continued commitment not as treatment but as punishment for patients who thwart their will?

•

A related issue concerns the limitations and potential contributions of psychiatry. When people like Koch argue in terms of "helping" the mentally ill, it is fair to ask how much psychiatry can be expected to help. Part of the debate about Joyce Brown's case concerned the ability of psychiatry to help schizophrenics.

Judge Lippman, for example, noted that he could place little faith in psychiatry because the four city psychiatrists and the three ACLU psychiatrists who had testified, although equally qualified, had disagreed dramatically. Lippman concluded, "It is evident that psychiatry is not a science amenable to the exactness of mathematics or the predictability of physical laws."

Most psychiatrists, of course, would object strongly to this evaluation of their profession; and many psychiatrists argue for involuntary commitment of schizophrenics. They point to schizophrenics who were dysfunctional but who gained years of ability (or at least minimal functioning) after being made to take medication. They say that such patients stabilize and become free from delusions and that many patients, if they take their medication regularly (an important condition), can even return to life outside institutions. The psychiatrist Paul Chodoff defended limited involuntary commitment as follows:

> . . . Is freedom defined only by absence of external constraints? Internal physiological or psychological processes can contribute to a throttling of the spirit that is as painful as any applied from the outside. The "wild" manic individual without his lithium, the panicky hallucinator with his injection of fluphenazine hydrochloride and the understanding support of a concerned staff, the sodden alcoholic—are they free? Sometimes, as Woody Guthrie said, "Freedom means no place to go."[33]

In fact, people suffering from paranoid schizophrenia can make amazing improvement as a result of treatment. One patient, for instance, believed that the grounds crew mowing the lawns were communicating with themselves in secret "motor language" about his faults. After weeks of medication, he began to doubt bizarre beliefs like this one. After more weeks on medication, he really wasn't sure. Still later, he admitted that the belief was probably false. Finally, after more medication, he concluded one day, "How did I ever think that?"[34] Chemicals can change our thoughts, even our deepest thoughts about ourselves, and such change may be beneficial. Since some schizophrenia might be either caused by, or manifested in, chemical disturbances of the brain, this finding is not surprising.

One editor of *U.S. News and World Report* defended psychiatric treatment for Joyce Brown by arguing that she had lost the "rational freedom of choice offered by medicine that can alleviate mental anguish and paranoia."[35]

Suffering and Commitment: Benefit and Harm

One columnist argued that the ethical questions in this case boiled down not to whether people like Joyce Brown were likely to harm themselves, but to whether they were suffering. Another columnist agreed, saying that Joyce Brown should be taken off the streets before she died there "with her rights on."[36] These writers thought that it should be enough to convince a judge that a mentally ill person was in distress and that treatment would help.

But was the matter really so straightforward? To say that commitment is justified to end suffering assumes first that a person is really suffering, and second that involuntary psychiatric commitment can ease his or her suffering. This is somewhat narrower issue than the general issue (discussed above) of the uses and limitations of psychiatry.

Consider the first assumption, that the person is suffering. When someone like Joyce Brown protests that she does not need or want help, it can be asked—as Thomas Szasz asked—who can determine that she is "suffering" enough to be locked inside a psychiatric ward? Who bears the onus of proof, the patient or the psychiatrist?

With regard to the second assumption, that involuntary commitment can help, it is important to consider the nature of involuntary commitment. What

Joyce Brown feared most was another commitment to an inpatient unit like the one at East Orange Hospital. Would she really be helped by involuntary psychiatry, involuntary medication, and involuntary therapy—in a locked unit within a large public institution?

Joyce Brown's court-appointed psychiatrist (who of all the psychiatrists involved in the case was the most likely to be impartial) had found that she suffered from "serious mental illness" and would benefit from medication—but that she would suffer more from forced treatment than from the mental illness itself. In such a situation, for one thing, Joyce Brown might harm herself while trying to resist the administration of antipsychotic medications and tranquilizers. Also, commitment might destroy her fierce independence; and if it did not—if she continued to resist—she might end up with a lobotomy, like McMurphy in *One Flew Over the Cuckoo's Nest.* Moreover, the long-term "side effects" of antipsychotics and tranquilizers can be as bad as the original disorder: antipsychotic drugs such as neuroleptics administered over years create tardive dyskinesia in 10 to 25 percent of patients; this condition impairs voluntary movement, is untreatable, and persists in two-thirds of the affected patients when the medication is stopped.

It can also be argued that the potential "benefits" of involuntary treatment cannot be defined objectively. Most psychiatrists, of course, tend to think that people such as Joyce Brown "benefit" from living on medication and thereby losing their inner voices and delusions. But aren't benefit and harm, above the level of basic needs, defined by each person's own self-concept and life plans?

> When faced with an obviously aberrant person, we know, or we think we know, that he would be "happier" if he were as we are. We believe that no one would want to be misfit in society. From the very best of motives, then, we wish to fix him. It is difficult to deal with this feeling since it rests on the unverifiable assumption that the aberrant person, if he saw himself as we see him, would choose to be different than he is. But since he cannot be as we, and we cannot be as he, there is simply no way to judge the predicate for the assertion.[37]

Isn't it a rather shaky application of paternalism to say that Joyce Brown had to be treated so that she could obtain someone else's idea of a "benefit"? Psychiatrists imply that mentally ill patients suffer "internal pain"; but if that is so, why don't all patients want to get rid of it? Isn't it illogical—isn't it begging the question—for psychiatrists to explain that patients don't want to get rid of this pain "because they're crazy"?

UPDATE

Recently, the term *homeless* has been attacked by a new wave of critics as inappropriate for the wandering mentally ill; instead, these critics emphasize substance abuse. They have challenged ACLU's view that people such as Joyce Brown were primarily victims of a greedy or indifferent society which failed to provide affordable housing; they say there is evidence that as many as 85 percent of panhandlers are alcoholics, substance abusers, or mentally ill—and that all of these need treatment.[38] These new critics advocate mandatory treatment and police intervention to prevent panhandling, or begging. They also urge people not to give money to beggars, saying that those who do give money are "enablers of addiction."

•

There also seems to be a greater tendency to see mentally ill derelicts as dangerous. This trend had already begun a few years before Joyce Brown's case, when Juan Gonzalez, a homeless man suffering from symptoms like hers, went berserk on the Staten Island Ferry and killed two people with a sword. As a result, there was considerable public pressure for incarceration of mentally ill people who were "potentially dangerous"; and the concept of "potential danger" is now often used to justify temporarily holding someone for a "cool-down" observational period. Actually, Gonzalez had been picked up for just such an observational period; but although he was diagnosed as a paranoid schizophrenic, he had not been considered imminently dangerous to others and had thus been discharged.

In 1991, Keven McKiever, a homeless man who had gone to Bellevue Hospital seeking care and was turned away, stabbed Alexis Walsh, a former Radio City Rockette, to death.

In 1993, Christopher Battiste, a homeless mentally ill drug abuser, allegedly murdered an elderly woman in the Bronx on a Sunday morning as she came home from church.

The most prominent of these cases in the 1990s was that of Larry Hogue, a homeless, mentally ill African American who was a veteran of the war in Vietnam. Larry Hogue sometimes lived peacefully on a street corner in the upper west side of Manhattan; but when he took illegal drugs, this "wild man of 96th Street" (as he was called on *60 Minutes*), became hostile and violent. A state judge ruled that he could be involuntarily committed against his will for detoxification, but that he would have to be released "as soon as he decides to seek outpatient care."[39] In 1994, shortly before he was due to be released from Creedmore Hospital, he escaped, committed a robbery for small change, and was soon picked up. He has since been returned to Creedmore.

The courts and the general public have come to expect psychiatrists to be able to predict dangerousness among the mentally ill, but it is debatable whether they actually can. In general, to assess the potential for violent behavior, emergency-room psychiatrists simply ask patients about their own tendencies toward violence and their own past acts of violence.[40] This is hardly a sophisticated predictive tool, though in practice it seems to work better than anything else.

•

There has been at least one significant legal development with regard to *O'Connor v. Donaldson*. In some states, the *O'Connor* criteria have been interpreted to mean that a person must commit an *overt act* in order to warrant a hearing for involuntary commitment. This interpretation is controversial and has in general been opposed by relatives, who can often perceive a pattern of threats and hostility and do not want to wait until someone is injured or killed before a commitment hearing can take place. At present, courts and legislatures are struggling with the implications of this "overt act" requirement.

•

The sheltered, or supervised, group home remains an elusive ideal. Whether we are discussing severely physically disabled people (like Larry McAfee in Chapter 2), welfare reform, or the mentally ill homeless, the best living facility for many people is a supervised group home. Living in such a home is much better than being "warehoused" in a large institution or—obviously—than being left to fend for oneself on the cold hard streets. Supervised group homes, especially if they are located in safe neighborhoods, are often a perfect compromise between institutionalization and independence.

The problem, then, is not with group homes as a concept but rather with the practical matter of getting group homes for those who need them. Funding has been one difficulty. In New York, for example, because of AIDS and years of limited funding to balance its gigantic medical budget, places in group homes are very scarce; in fact, the shortage of such beds has created a crisis in the city since 1988. In those homes that did exist, budgets were cut, so that some staff members had to be fired and some patients released. The funds saved by cutting group homes were used by legislators for other projects; and now no one seems to know how to get the funding—and the patients—back. Meanwhile, deinstitutionalization has continued. In 1993, in New York, 2,400 new group home beds had been planned in preparation for the release of 1,000 more inmates from large institutions in 1994, but the number of new beds was later cut to 800. When New York State's highest court ruled in February 1993 that New York City must provide housing for homeless mentally ill patients discharged from city hospitals, the city estimated that it would cost $300 million to do so and disputed the meaning of the ruling.[41]

A second practical difficulty with group homes is the phenomenon known as NIMBY—"not in my back yard."[42] (NIMBY is also discussed in Chapter 2.)

•

Unconfirmed reports have indicated that Joyce Brown was in and out of psychiatric hospitals in the 5 years from 1989 to 1994, and it would seem that her primary problem was drugs rather than schizophrenia. As of this writing, however, she was living in an apartment on her own.

FURTHER READING

Alice Baum and Donald Burnes, *A Nation in Denial: The Truth about Homelessness*, Westview, Boulder, Colo., 1993.

Paul Chodoff, "The Case for Involuntary Hospitalization of the Mentally Ill," *American Journal of Psychiatry*, vol. 133, no. 5, May 1976.

Saul Feldman, "Out of the Hospitals, onto the Streets: The Overselling of Benevolence," *Hastings Center Report*, vol. 13, no. 3, June 1983.

Charles Krauthammer, "How to Save the Homeless Mentally Ill," *New Republic*, February 8, 1988.

J. Livermore, C. Malmquist, and P. Meehl, "On the Justification for Civil Commitment," *University of Pennsylvania Law Review*, vol. 117, November 1968.

CHAPTER 15

Preventing Teenage Pregnancy

Bertha

This chapter discusses some issues involved in preventing pregnancy among teenagers. The case in the chapter—that of a 15-year-old girl who received contraception against her wishes—became famous as the subject of a film and reflects several of these issues.

Teenage pregnancy is a deceptively simple term for a complex matter. To begin with, in this chapter *teenage pregnancy* will stand for *teenage single motherhood:* that is, our discussion concerns unmarried teenagers who will—or intend to—bear, keep, and raise children. Teenage pregnancy, of course, can have other outcomes. A teenage pregnancy may be terminated by abortion; a teenager may marry; and a child born to a teenager may be raised by someone else: the child may be given up for adoption, placed in foster care, or raised by a relative. Arguments can certainly be made for preventing or discouraging teenage pregnancy despite these other possibilities, but the arguments to be discussed in this chapter pertain mostly to teenage single motherhood.

Teenage pregnancy is also related to several other issues, and sometimes becomes entangled with them—issues such as the "right" to have children; single-parent families; welfare; absent fathers; parents' competence; sex education; population control; family planning, contraception, and abortion; sexual activity among teenagers; and programs for teenagers who do become pregnant. Some of these subjects will be discussed here, but it is important to distinguish them from the specific issue of preventing teenage pregnancy.

Most people agree that teenage pregnancy is a serious problem in the United States today, but we need to be clear about why it is perceived as a problem and, therefore, why preventing it becomes a goal. As we will see, this reasoning is often based on considerations of *harm.* In general, it is held, teenage girls are too young to deal with parenthood and are likely to be less competent than adult mothers. And it is undeniable that they are likely to remain in the ranks of the poor, because parenthood will probably curtail their education and because the problems of single parenthood typically include financial difficulties, such as barriers to employment. These effects are harmful not only to the teenage mothers themselves but also to their children—and to society, which must often bear the costs of caring for poor mothers and children, losses of productivity, and social strains.

Nevertheless, efforts to prevent teenage pregnancy can be controversial. What measures will be effective? What measures will be ethical? To what extent should we make any measure mandatory? There are also disputes over facts, such as statistics and social trends, as we will see.

BACKGROUND: STATISTICS ON TEENAGE PREGNANCY

The Alan Guttmacher Institute, a nonprofit organization that tracks population trends, has painted a stark picture of pregnancy among teenagers in the United States: over 1 million girls become pregnant each year, a figure that remained constant between 1984 and 1993.[1] Of these, about half gave birth, and about half of those who gave birth were under 18. The states with the highest rates of teenage pregnancy were California, Arkansas, Georgia, and Texas; and the pregnancy rate was twice as high among minority teenagers as among white teenagers. Today, American teenagers have the highest pregnancy rate in the western world. It is estimated that 1 in 4 American girls will become pregnant at least once by age 18; nearly half (44 percent) will become pregnant by age 20.

These statistics are part of a larger picture, that of unwanted or unplanned pregnancies in general. Every year, about 6 million American women become pregnant, and more than 3 million of these pregnancies are unintended. In fact, among women under 25, most pregnancies are unintended, and about as many unintended pregnancies end in induced abortions as in births. It is among teenagers that unplanned pregnancy is most likely to end in birth.

Admittedly, since 1960, the birth*rate* among American teenagers—the percentage of all teenagers who give birth—has dropped.[2] However, this does not change the perception of teenage pregnancy as a huge social problem. Although the rate declined, the *absolute number* of births to teenagers increased because of the "baby boom" generation, the teenagers of the 1960s and 1970s. Also, babies born to teenagers accounted for a larger percentage of all births; and if abortion had not been legalized in 1973, that percentage would have been still higher (the proportion of teenage pregnancies ended by abortion increased from 20 percent in 1972 to 40 percent in 1987).[3] In fact (as noted above), despite the increase in abortion among teenagers, more teenagers than women as a whole carry unintended pregnancies to term, thus making a commitment to parenthood at a very early age. Social concern about teenage pregnancy also stems from at least three other statistical trends: teenage childbearing is increasingly concentrated among the inner-city poor; teenage girls often raise their children without marrying the father; and both teenage mothers and their children tend to lack education, in an employment market where good jobs require skills more than at any time in the past.

BERTHA AND *BERTHA:* A GIRL AND A FILM

The subject of this case is Bertha, who grew up during the 1960s and 1970s in a poor white family in the Appalachian mountains of southwest Virginia, an area that has become a symbol of rural poverty. She was also the subject of a film—*Bertha*—financed by the Joseph P. Kennedy, Jr., Foundation.[4] Bertha's case was one of several given to the producer to study, and as originally commissioned, the film was supposed to deal with ethical issues involved in sterilizing the retarded. As produced, however, it was ambiguous: in the film, Bertha did not appear retarded, and so the film actually seemed to be more about preventing pregnancy in unmarried teenagers.

Bertha's father worked in a gas station and in 1969 was earning $70 a week. Bertha's mother bore 10 children, of whom Bertha was the oldest girl. The mother appeared overwhelmed by this large family, and consequently Bertha often took care of the 8 younger children—an experience that made her want to have children of her own.

Bertha and her siblings were acutely self-conscious about being poor, especially when they were around better-off children whose families were not on welfare. She said once:

> We got some neighbors. They don't like us because we were poor people. You know. We wasn't rich and sophisticated like them, so they didn't like us. There wasn't much I could do about it. Just stay and live with it. I mean, like to me, I was just as good as they were. I just didn't have what they had. They called us "coodies," "fleas," you know—I guess 'cause of the way we looked. We didn't have nice clothes like they did. They would start—as soon as we got on the bus—teasing us. I was always glad when school was over and I could go home and not have to listen to it.

The family lived atop a steep hill outside town, and the dirt trail down to the school bus stop was difficult during the harsh mountain winters. As a result of this—and perhaps also because of their self-consciousness—Bertha and her siblings became truants. Bertha, nearly illiterate, stumbled over reading and was held back year after year. Her classmates made fun of her because she was so much older and larger (in one third-grade class, she was about 5 feet 6 inches tall). On many days, her teachers would tell her, "There's nothing we can do for you. Go out and play"; so she did. In the educational terminology of the time, Bertha was an "underachiever" who was "rejected by her peer group."

During her mid-teenage years, Bertha's problems worsened. She stayed away from school more and more, often spending the day with other truants at an abandoned icehouse. Eventually, Bertha and a sister were placed with a series of foster parents so that they would attend school. Bertha did not like these placements and wanted to go home.

At age 15, Bertha was cute, sociable, and friendly. It was at this time, during one of her foster placements, that a foster father tried to molest her. A social worker learned about the incident and placed Bertha, briefly, in a state institution.

Bertha was intent on having children; but the social worker was afraid that if Bertha did give birth, the child would be taken away from her and felt that this would be "the worst thing in the world for her." Learning about a birth control program that was being offered by the Kennedy Institute at Johns Hopkins in Baltimore, the social worker brought Bertha there; Bertha, who was reluctant to go, agreed in order to avoid foster care.

Bertha was tested at Johns Hopkins and diagnosed as "mildly retarded," with an IQ of 68. For several reasons, the diagnosis of mild retardation was controversial. Since the "normal range" of IQs is defined as beginning at around 69 or 70, Bertha was just on the lower edge of this range. Moreover, there is a margin of error in such tests (although that was probably taken into account in the final estimate of her IQ). Also, Bertha seems to have lacked motivation when she took the tests. Four years later, when the film was made, Bertha (then 19) showed excellent social skills and seemed quite able to take care of herself, and the producer and the film crew were very much impressed with her intelligence.

At Johns Hopkins, however, on the basis of the diagnosis, an intrauterine device (IUD) was inserted in Bertha, without her consent. An IUD was used because it would temporarily prevent Bertha from conceiving; the procedure was reversible (the IUD could be removed by a doctor)—unlike sterilization by cutting the fallopian tubes, which is irreversible. Bertha's pediatrician at Johns Hopkins said that he was "buying time" for Bertha, so that she would not become pregnant too early and have to raise children on welfare, without a father. A woman psychiatrist said, "We thought this was an opportunity to do some preventive work." The pediatrician concurred: "I thought the suggestion of an intrauterine device was a reasonable one."

On hearing the official explanation—that the intent was to "protect" her—Bertha asked, "What are you protecting me *from?*" When she was told, "You might otherwise get pregnant," she replied, "So?" She objected intensely to the insertion of the IUD against her will and was obviously unconvinced that her own good required "protection" from childbearing; she also objected to being labeled "retarded."

After the IUD had been inserted, Bertha returned to her hometown. Four years later, the Kennedy Foundation in Washington, D.C., made the film, visiting Bertha's hometown to film her part in it. Bertha went to Baltimore to see the final version of the film and then went home again, still angry and with the IUD still inside her. According to Eunice Kennedy Shriver, who introduced the film, the IUD was later removed at Bertha's own request.

ETHICAL ISSUES

Approaches to Teenage Pregnancy

In looking at various issues related to teenage pregnancy, it is helpful to keep in mind some general concepts: first, the "worldviews" on which preventive efforts are often based; second, the rationale for preventing teenage pregnancy, that is, the "harms" which are believed to justify such prevention.

Four "worldviews"   We have already noted that efforts to prevent teenage pregnancy can be controversial; in fact, ideas about this problem are among the most controversial in the United States, and many of these ideas are based on assumptions that may not be fully stated. The following paragraphs sketch four "worldviews"—perspectives from which the issues are often approached.[5] Many people who debate these questions do not fit neatly into any "worldview," and some combine more than one view; still, the four views help us understand why people differ so widely and so strongly about possible solutions.

Traditionalists see teenage pregnancy as part of a larger cultural and moral failure which, they say, has undermined American society. They see, and bemoan, a constant focus in the media on sex and sexuality; a removal of any stigma from premarital sex and unwed motherhood; and a general notion that sexual gratification is more important than such values as becoming self-sufficient, nurturing children, or being a positive role model. They believe that values are formed through the family and through religion, and that secular state education prevents the formation of values or destroys existing values—thus they would like to see conservative religious ideas reinforced at school. They believe in definite, separate roles for men and women, fathers and mothers.

Public health practitioners see teenage pregnancy as a preventable public health problem, somewhat analogous to a communicable disease (or to gunshot wounds). They point to notable successes, as early as the turn of the century, in preventing communicable diseases such as cholera and would like to apply similar methods to behavior-related problems: smoking, drugs, failure to use birth control, and the like. They assume that many people act against their own self-interest through ignorance and bad habits. They also assume that public health experts know most, or at any rate know a great deal, about the best ways of achieving health for most people.

Welfare reformers and *social critics* share a belief that people act, in general, to further their own self-interest; but they differ about how to change the culture in order to reduce teenage pregnancy.

Welfare reformers propose "penalties" for remaining on welfare: these include "workfare," mandatory contraception, and reductions in benefits to welfare recipients who continue to bear children.

In contrast, social critics propose greater *incentives* to leave the welfare system, such as free child care, better schools, free adult education and job training programs, and better entry-level jobs. Social critics see themselves as advocates of women and children on welfare and believe that "society" is to blame if these mothers cannot find educational programs, decent jobs, or adequate child care.[6] They see complaints about "welfare mothers" as evidence that American society in general does not really value children or single mothers. (They point out that if a mother relinquishes welfare, it is often to take a minimum-wage job; that she loses Medicaid coverage for her children; and that she is no longer able to be home supervising her children after school.)

Both welfare reformers and social critics believe (unlike conservative traditionalists) that restricting teenagers' access to contraception and abortion will increase the teenage birthrate. However, they both believe that no real decrease in teenage pregnancy will occur unless there are changes in these teenagers' environment—their economic and social culture. Both tend to see the traditionalist model and the public health model as ineffectual: they say that traditionalists are merely "moralistic" or "judgmental," and that public health measures are superficial, offering only a "Band-Aid." Why set up a birth control clinic in an inner-city high school when the basic problem is not pregnancy but general hopelessness?

As we consider various issues related to teenage pregnancy, it is instructive to analyze them in terms of these four worldviews. It is also instructive to ask which of the views is politically most fashionable at any given time (for example, the conservative traditionalists received most attention during Ronald Reagan's administration).

Concepts of harm   It was noted at the beginning of this chapter that reasons for preventing teenage pregnancy often have to do with concepts of *harm* to the teenage mothers themselves, their children, and society as a whole.

Concepts of *harm to the mother* were clearly influential in the case of Bertha. Would pregnancy and motherhood harm Bertha herself? Presumably there are some benefits, or at least apparent benefits, to teenage pregnancy. A teenage mother may, for instance, receive attention and gain status, and a child may be a source of love and purpose in life; one social worker involved with Bertha's family emphasized that Bertha "needed desperately somebody to love and something to call her own." In general, however, benefits like these are seen by professionals as outweighed by potential harms, such as health problems, emotional problems, loss of education, and poverty. In Bertha's case, the IUD was inserted to "protect" her from these outcomes. There was also an additional potential harm—the probability that she would be considered an incompetent parent, that any child she had would therefore be taken away from her, and that this loss would be damaging. The social worker, in fact, emphasized that if Bertha lost her child in this way, "it would have been very bad for her."

The people who were dealing with Bertha, then, thought that she would be harmed by motherhood. But suppose they had thought otherwise; suppose they had felt that on the whole she would *not* be harmed. In such a situation, the issue would still not be settled: it would *not* necessarily follow that allowing her to bear a child would be right, because potential *harm to the child* must still be considered.

In other words, Bertha's good—the mother's good—is not the only issue here; there is also the moral question of the child's good. Many of the arguments for preventing teenage pregnancy focus on teenagers' children, who are likely to be raised by single mothers, to be poor, and indeed to repeat the cycle of early pregnancy and poverty when they themselves become teenagers. There are also issues of harm to these children's development. The theme of harm to children will reappear particularly when we discuss single-parent families.

Finally, *harm to society* needs to be considered. The cycle of poverty—early pregnancy, dropping out of school, depending on welfare—is a drain on society as well as on the individuals who are caught in the cycle. It is not only that society must to some extent support mothers and children who cannot support themselves; there are also problems of stress and health in individuals and in communities, social tensions, and the loss of contributions these mothers and children could have made if they were not trapped in poverty.

Harm to mothers, harm to children, and harm to society are, however, intertwined and need not be thought of separately as we turn to the issues related to teenage pregnancy. What harms mothers may harm children; what harms children may harm mothers; what harms children and mothers in some sense also harms society.

The "Right" to Have Children

Does everyone have a right to have children? Does *anyone* have such a right? The "right" to have children is, as suggested earlier, a broader issue than teenage pregnancy; but discussions about preventing teenage pregnancy sometimes end in a paralyzing standoff because of conflicts and uncertainties about this wider question.

The "right" to have children was evidently a point of contention in Bertha's case. Confronting a male social worker, Bertha asked, "What right did they have to fix it so that I couldn't have kids? I'm a human being. I should be able to have kids. Right?" The question is also reflected when the film shows a group of experts discussing the case afterward. William Bartholome, who was then a medical resident working at a public health clinic in downtown Baltimore (a city with one of the nation's highest rates of teenage pregnancy), says that almost every day he sees teenagers like Bertha who want to become pregnant to "have something of their own"; and he asks, "What should I say to such girls?" When Arthur Dyke—a professor of religious ethics at Harvard University—seems to suggest that girls like Bertha should be "free" to conceive, Bartholome angrily retorts that Bertha would be less "free" with a child than with an IUD. Dyke, who appears touchy, replies rather nervously, "Do you think that you can just simply say, on the face of it, that for Bertha and others like her, and for persons that age, that she's made a mistake?" Bartholome replies:

> To have a baby? At age 15? With her judgment and capability and financial income and support and job? Hell, yes, it's a mistake!

Mary Robinson, executive director of the Martin Luther King Parenting and Child Center, challenges him: "Why?" Bartholome becomes angry and asks her, "For a 15-year-old girl to have a baby is not a mistake?" When Robinson clearly does not want to agree with him, he asks her how she can direct a parenting clinic and not emphasize that such behavior is mistaken. She defends her position by blaming "society" for its failure to help teenagers.

The issue of the "right" to have children has more than one aspect. To begin with, who—if anyone—has this "right"? Some people believe that the right to have children is universal and inalienable: that everyone has a right to have children, under any circumstances. Others believe that the right to have children is restricted in one way or another—for instance, that adults have this right but young teenagers do not. Still others believe that no one has a right to have children; on this view, childbearing is sometimes described as a privilege which may be controlled and revoked under certain conditions.

A second point to be considered is what the right to have children *implies.* If everyone has such a right, then presumably no one should be forcibly prevented from exercising it. But it may still be entirely appropriate and justifiable to *discourage* people from becoming parents if parenthood would be harmful for them, their children, and the community. In other words, coercion or compulsion must be distinguished from information, education, guidance, advice, counseling, and the like.

It also seems important to distinguish between encouragement and tolerance. If everyone has a right to have children, it can be argued that people who exercise their right—even if they seem misguided—do not thereby forfeit their claim to respect or toleration. But *respect* and *toleration* are not necessarily the same thing as *encouragement.* This distinction sometimes becomes confused in arguments about whether or not pregnant teenagers and teenage mothers should be allowed to attend their senior proms, participate in graduation ceremonies, work in day care centers, or counsel younger girls.

These points are not merely academic or semantic. People who want to decrease teenage pregnancy are sometimes hesitant, or become intimidated, when the "right to have children" is invoked. Being clear about the differences between guidance and coercion, or tolerance and encouragement, may help us rank our values and stand up for them in public policy.

Single-Parent Families

Teenage single motherhood is, of course, one kind of single-parent family; thus it is relevant, and interesting, to examine the current conflict over single-parent families in general.

The single-parent family often becomes an emotionally charged and somewhat confused issue. Let us begin by clarifying a few points. *First,* in the heat of controversy, people sometimes seem to lose sight of the fact that there is really no such thing as *"the* single-parent family." There are different kinds of single-parent families, which come into being in different ways: a marriage may be broken by death, divorce, separation, or desertion; an unmarried person may conceive and rear a child; an unmarried person may adopt a child—and various other configurations might also be considered "single-parent families." Notice, in this regard, that a single-parent family may or may not be the result of choice. Within each type of single-parent family there are numerous additional differences: single parents differ in age, sex, education, occupation, etc.; families differ in size, race and ethnicity, socioeconomic status, community environment, etc. *Second,* some problems are common to all or most types of single-parent families, whereas other problems differ significantly from one type of single-parent family to another. *Third,* every single-parent family, like every person, is an individual. Anything that is said about single parenthood or single-parent families may or may not apply to a given, specific family.

It will be helpful to keep these points in mind as we consider commentary, arguments, and statistics about single-parent families, since much of the debate is—explicitly or implicitly—about *some* rather than *all* single-parent situations.

•

In 1992, "Murphy Brown," a fictional character in a popular television series, became the center of a public controversy. This was the story line of the episode that evoked the dispute: Murphy Brown is a career woman, an investigative reporter; she is not young (the actress playing the role, Candace Bergen, was actually in her forties). She has an affair with a professional man ("Jake") and becomes pregnant. Murphy and Jake decide not to marry. Murphy decides to have the child and raise it alone. Her decision is presented as a symbol of independence: it is suggested that this woman does not need a man to help her raise a child, and that she can have a great career and still be a good mother.

Although all this was fiction, the vice-president of the United States, Dan Quayle, attacked the producers and writers of the show: he argued that they were setting a bad example. Quayle's "white male Republican values" (and his presumed stupidity) had already made him the butt of liberal jokes; and this attack, unsurprisingly, drew more criticism.

On reflection, however, some people began to have second thoughts about the implications of single parenthood and the values of the two-parent family. In a famous article in *Atlantic,* for instance ("Dan Quayle Was Right"), Barbara Dafoe Whitehead defended two-parent families and the importance of marriage for the good of children.[7]

One factor influencing Whitehead's kind of thinking was a widely perceived "crisis of the black family." This "crisis" had been discussed for some time and had been notably articulated in 1965 in a study by Daniel Patrick Moynihan. Lyndon Johnson, in a speech at Howard University during his presidency, had cited the Moynihan report and described the "breakdown of the Negro family structure" as the chief threat to the well-being of black Americans.[8] In the words of Moynihan's report itself:

> From the wild Irish slums of the 19th-century Eastern seaboard, to the riot-torn suburbs of Los Angles, there is one unmistakable lesson in American history: A community that allows a large number of young men to grow up in broken families, dominated by women, never acquiring any stable relationship to male authority, never acquiring any rational expectations about the future—that community asks for and gets chaos.[9]

During the 1960s, Moynihan's conclusions were often denounced as racist, particularly by liberal activists. It was argued that white, middle-class values should not be imposed on black Americans and that black families could be strong and nurturing even if they did not take the traditional two-parent form. It was further argued, then and later, that the two-parent family represented WASP values, Republican values, and a "golden age" of "Ozzie and Harriet" families which was probably mythical to begin with and in any case had now vanished. One-parent families were held to be no worse than two-parent families, and claims to the contrary were dismissed as "cultural imperialism." Obviously, not everyone—not even all liberals—felt this way; still, many people have asked, "Why can't single women raise children just as well as two-parent families?" and many people have held that children are better off without violent, abusive, or alcoholic fathers and are better off in a single-parent family than in a two-parent family where the parents are continually at each other's throat.

By the time of the "Murphy Brown" dispute, though, the Moynihan report was finding more defenders. One national columnist wrote:

> In 1965, when Daniel Patrick Moynihan asked the nation to pay attention to the single-parent black family, he was called a racist and everyone averted their eyes. . . . The number of babies born to single black mothers has soared from 1 in 5 of all black babies in 1965, to 2 in 3 today [1992]. And [today] 1 of every 5 white babies is born to an unwed mother.[10]

Three decades after the Moynihan report, there seemed to be an ever-increasing concern—a sense of mounting unease—about the African American family and indeed about the American family, black or white.

Actually, the statistics about single-parent white families as of 1993 look like the statistics for black families in 1965; and we may need to ask whether in 2023 the statistics for white single-parent families will look like those for black families in 1993. According to the 1992 Census report, single-parent homes increased by 15 percent just in the 4 years from 1985 to 1989; as a result, 1 family out of 4 has a single parent in the home while children are growing up.[11] And in late 1993 (about 1 year after the "Murphy Brown" episode), the Census Bureau reported a steep increase in childbearing among never-married educated professional women; it also reported that nearly 25 percent of unmarried American women now became mothers—an increase of 60 percent in one decade.[12]

These trends give rise to concern partly because some studies indicate that children fare far better in two-parent families. In 1988, the National Health Interview Survey of Child Health found that "young people from single-parent or stepfamilies were 2 to 3 times more likely to have had emotional or behavioral problems than those who had both of their biological parents present in the home."[13] One expert even contends that findings from the social sciences about the benefits of two-parent rather than single-parent childrearing are so crystal-clear—although much of our society refuses to accept them—that "it's the equivalent of having to argue over and over that the world is round. If it were just a matter of evidence, we wouldn't be having this debate. It would be over."[14]

Conclusions like this seem strongest when based on economic considerations: indisputably, single families, especially single-mother families, are far likelier to be poor families; and poverty is bad for children. It is sometimes remarked that poverty is an old story, that there have always been poor children, slums, and people who—like Horatio Alger's characters—work their way up. But in February 1991, Daniel Moynihan observed that for the first time in our history, children are now the largest group of the American poor, and many American children will live in real poverty at some point in their lives. "All this is new," he wrote. "This circumstance did not exist during the New Deal era, a half century ago. It did not exist during the era of the Great Society, a quarter century ago."[15] In 1992, Louis Sullivan, as secretary of Health and Human Services, reported that children raised by a single parent are 5 times more likely to be poor than those raised by two parents, and twice as likely to drop out of school.[16]

The dismal results for children are not hard to understand. A single-parent household typically has only one paycheck, one savings account, one plan for medical coverage, one pension, one source of loans, and one set of grandparents—if it has any of these things. Often, a single parent must work long hours, perhaps at two low-paying jobs, or rely on welfare. The child of a single parent often becomes a "latchkey" child with, in effect, no parent at all. In such circumstances, the cycle of early pregnancy and poverty is likely to be repeated. Ours is presumably an age of modernity and feminism, but girls are still sexual targets of teenage boys, and "latchkey" girls are most vulnerable: studies show that a girl is most likely to be impregnated between 3 and 5 P.M. when no parent is present.

Poverty also has disastrous effects on children's health. In 1993, one study found that the "mortality gap" between rich and poor has widened over the last three decades: people from families with an annual income of less than $9,000 are now three times more likely to die in a given year than people from families with an income of over $35,000.[17] For children, having two married parents present correlates strongly with higher family income; thus this finding also predicts children's longevity. (This study was controlled for all other variables, including race and access to health care; but access to health care is notoriously worse for the poor. The enormous inequalities of health care in the United States are seen most clearly not inside hospitals or clinics but among those who never get to such places at all.)

Poverty, then, is a real basis for unease about single-parent families, the more so because its effects will surely harm mothers and society as well as children. Still, not all single-parent families are poor; and it is often argued that poverty is not the only way children in single-parent families are harmed. Some people hold that children in single-mother families tend to suffer from lack of a male role model, that children in single-parent families are subject to social stigma, and so on. These arguments are perhaps more questionable, but they are widely offered. The late columnist Lewis Grizzard, who grew up in a fatherless home, said, for instance, "It hurt. It hurt when older children would taunt me and ask me, 'Where's your daddy?'"[18] Another writer remarked:

> The inequities that stem from the workplace are now trivial in comparison to those stemming from family structure. What matters for success is not whether your father was rich or poor, but whether you had a father at all.[19]

In light of all these considerations, concerns about single-parent families continue, as does the rhetoric of the "Murphy Brown" debate. The *New York Times* remarked in 1992, for instance: "The worrying thing is that never-married mothers account for most of the children now entering single-parent households."[20] Some observers argue that changes in cultural values underlie this situation or are aggravating it.

In former times, of course, unwed motherhood was considered immoral by most of society, and children born out of wedlock shared their mothers' disgrace. But there were always some people who considered this condemnation overly cruel (and unjust, since unwed *fathers* were seldom subject to it), and prevailing attitudes have gradually changed. Our language reflects this change in attitudes: a girl or woman is likely to be described as "sexually active," "having an affair," or "living with someone" rather than as an "adulteress," a "mistress," or a "fallen woman" (or worse); and children of single parents are now rarely called "illegitimate" or "bastards."

Probably few people today would want to see the clock turned back altogether, but some would say that acceptance of single parenthood has gone too far. Lewis Grizzard and another columnist, Cal Thomas, blamed the increase in single parenthood partly on glorification by the media of unmarried relationships among celebrities. Donald Trump and Marla Maples, Woody Allen and Mia Farrow, and "Magic" Johnson have all had children out of wedlock; and it is frequently asked how we can condemn or penalize poor unmarried teenagers for having children when such people become role models. Furthermore, it is argued that fictional and nonfictional accounts of the "cruelty," "inhumanity," and "rigidity" of earlier attitudes undervalue traditional morality, which might otherwise be a source of strength, principles, and good sense. Without such traditional morality, it is said, the most vulnerable people—the foolish, the ignorant, the inexperienced, and most of all the young—become the most likely to make bad choices about reproduction, with disastrous, irreversible consequences for themselves and their children.

Welfare

Bertha's family was on welfare: Aid to Families with Dependent Children (AFDC), Medicaid, and the food stamp program. If Bertha became a mother, the overwhelming probability was that she too would have ended up on welfare; in fact, this may have been the major reason why she was given an IUD. A consulting psychiatrist in her case observed, "If this pattern was continued, her children would be in the same situation as she was."

In 1960, according to the Census Bureau, 3.1 million people were receiving AFDC; in 1990, the figure had risen to 12.2 million—an increase of nearly 400 percent.[21] Some scholars, such as Charles Murray, believe that this large group of welfare recipients has been created partly by the liberal legislation of Lyndon Johnson's administration.[22] These "Great Society" programs included Medicaid, food stamps, a large expansion of AFDC, and increases in basic welfare benefits. There were also changes in eligibility requirements: work requirements were eliminated, and unmarried mothers living with fathers were penalized.

Welfare, especially AFDC, has become a matter of intense concern. It is held that the net effect of the penalty for "live-in" fathers has been to encourage men to leave, ultimately producing what is called the *feminization of poverty*. Also, it is widely believed that the same single mothers remain on welfare indefinitely, bearing more and more children, and that the same families remain on welfare generation after generation. Although this pattern is by no means typical for welfare recipients, many women and families do repeat it; as a result, some Americans resent paying taxes to support welfare, and many consider the entire system self-defeating.

Many people even believe that women "have babies to get on welfare." Even if this were so, one researcher—Martha Ozawa—has found that lowering stipends has no effect on how many children are conceived;[23] and although Alabama has for a decade provided the lowest monthly AFDC payments in the nation, its rate of children living in poverty—1 in 4—is still among the nation's highest.

Life on welfare is not easy. For an unmarried woman with two children and no other income, monthly payments range from $633 in California to $124 in Alabama. In Bertha's state, Virginia, monthly payments were $291 in 1992. On payments like these, it is difficult to feed and clothe three people, let alone rent housing. Such families are eligible for food stamps; but the additional monthly allowance for more children is very low—as low as $25 to $50 in Alabama.

The grim picture of welfare often forms a backdrop for efforts to prevent teenage pregnancy. Teenage motherhood is, of course, not the only route to welfare dependency, but it is a very common route. Is there nothing society can do about it?

Teenage Motherhood and Competence

The competence of teenage mothers is an additional consideration underlying attempts to prevent teenage pregnancy: it is assumed that, on the whole, teenagers are likely to be "minimally competent" or incompetent parents.

In Bertha's case, her competence was clearly an issue. This may have been partly due to the diagnosis of retardation; but whether or not she was actually retarded, her IQ was certainly low. In addition, she seemed to be uninterested in relationships with boys or men, apparently regarding a man as merely something needed temporarily to create kids, and this attitude suggested that her children would not be likely to have a father present. A consulting psychiatrist thought that Bertha might be good in some areas of mothering but was dubious about her "sense of follow-through"—for instance, her ability to buy and prepare food for her children.

On the other hand, a psychologist described Bertha as "surprisingly good" in the "little social areas" and felt that with help from other people she could be a "permissible" mother. Moreover, Bertha's brother Norman, who was 1 year younger, disagreed strongly with the consulting psychiatrist's evaluation: "Bertha was our mother. Bertha practically raised us. Everywhere Bertha went, the [other eight] kids went." The social worker, Barbara Hammond, agreed with Norman, noting that when she first intervened with the family, Bertha—then 12 or 13—was already acting like a mother: "She seemed to take responsibility around her own home as far as the other children [were concerned]." And Bertha herself pointed out that she had already raised children:

> The rest of 'em were little and, you know, it was really my responsibility to get up and do it. It was just something that had to be done. It was hard—yes, I must admit it—but I did it. I didn't complain.

This was true; Bertha had already taken over many of the tasks involved in raising eight small children, and in the film she seemed better-qualified than her mother for childrearing.

Much of the analysis of Bertha's probable competence as a mother would apply to any teenager. Does she have any special problems, such as low intelligence? Is she capable of developing a mature, stable relationship with a man and so giving her child an involved father? Can she handle practical household activities such as shopping and cooking? Does she have a "support system" of people willing and able to help her? Has she had any experience with caring for young children? How would people who know her assess her abilities?

Of course, the answers to questions like these will differ for each individual teenager. Teenage girls vary widely in all the factors that affect their competence—maturity, intelligence, acceptance of responsibility, resourcefulness, experience, and so on. Also, we should not forget that the teenage years range from 13 to 19, and the answers are also likely to vary significantly between the youngest and oldest teenagers.

Still, general doubts about teenagers' competence as parents are probably reasonable. Teenagers are hardly more than children themselves, and a single teenage mother is likely to have to deal with problems—such as poverty and welfare—that would stretch the resources of a mature woman to the breaking point. The image of "children having children" is, therefore, prominent in the issue of preventing teenage pregnancy.

Sex Education

Sex education is often proposed as a solution to teenage pregnancy, but what does this really mean? When the general idea of "educating teenagers" is made specific, parents, educators, health professionals, and the public often begin to disagree about it very quickly.

For example, should sex education include explicit descriptions of sexual acts? Should it teach students about contraception? Should it extend to offering free contraceptives in high schools? In junior high schools? Some people are opposed to graphic descriptions of sex and to informing students about contraception—let alone to distributing contraceptives—because they believe that such measures encourage teenage sexuality. Others argue that we should be "realistic," acknowledge that many teenagers are sexually active, and concentrate our educational efforts on helping them avoid pregnancy. Still others argue that education does *not* induce or encourage teenagers to be sexually active and may even help them postpone sexual activity.

There is probably more agreement, however, that American teenagers today are on the whole ill-informed about sex in general and birth control in particular. According to anthropologists, the United States remains one of the most backward of all western countries with regard to sex education. Most teachers are remarkably prudish about discussing sex explicitly (if at all) with children or teenagers; and the same is true of parents—perhaps because they fear that their children will ask them, "Do you do that too?" The media, of course, pay an inordinate amount of attention to sex, but what they present is far from helpful. In effect, movies, magazines, and television convey to teenagers that sex (1) is exciting and makes them adults; (2) never has negative consequences such as unwanted pregnancy or sexually transmitted diseases; and (3) guarantees lasting emotional intimacy with another person. The media would reply that all this simply reflects our culture as a whole; that may be a good point, but to some extent the media also shape our culture. In any case, the results seem alarming. According to one national news network, for instance, 90 percent of American teenagers believe that whether or not to have sex is their decision alone.

A Note on Fathers

Daniel Moynihan's study emphasized the consequences of "absent fathers" for mothers and children, and the evidence is compelling that absence of the father contributes to lifelong poverty. Yet in the issue of teenage pregnancy, surprisingly little attention is given to the fathers. The debate seems almost exclusively focused on girls: almost nothing is said about educating or guiding boys to live with their children and become good fathers, and little more about including boys and men in efforts to prevent teenage pregnancy.

In fact, the absent father sometimes seems to be simply taken for granted. The columnist Ellen Brown has remarked that the "deadbeat dad" is becoming so common as to be a cultural stereotype: "What we know so far is [that] many men see marriage and children as a package deal and when the package unravels, they may return it all."[24] In the controversial "Murphy Brown" episode, the father goes off to save the world.

Furthermore, although men often leave the picture after fathering children, especially if they form a new relationship, there is no federal system to help mothers collect child support. Only 1 in 4 single mothers regularly receives the full amount of monthly child support owed to the family. Over 55 percent of child support is not paid, and as of 1992 about $400 million of child support was delinquent.[25]

As was noted in the discussion of welfare, AFDC requirements may be impelling some men to leave their families. Also, AFDC allows an unmarried adolescent girl to live independently as a head of household, and according to Ozawa's findings it is for this reason that many teenage mothers do not marry the father of their children.[26] (If that is so, perhaps AFDC should change its policy, restricting single teenager mothers' freedom to live independently. This might encourage parents to marry and remain together, but it would also tend to make women more dependent on men. It would in any case be highly controversial.)

Radical Proposals: Legal Restrictions on Childbearing

As noted earlier, not everyone believes in a universal "right" to have children, and some people argue for legal restrictions on childbearing. In the present American context, there is no real likelihood that such radical proposals would be adopted or even seriously considered. Still, legal restrictions are now in place in China, and they are interesting to examine—if only to see how alien to American thought the Chinese model is.

One rationale for legal restraints on childbearing is an argument by analogy. To avoid various harms, society regulates and restricts many kinds of individual activities; in particular, many activities require a license—a driver's license, a marriage license, a hunting or fishing license, a license to practice a profession such as medicine or engineering. Since ill-advised childbearing also causes harm, why not require prospective parents to be licensed?[27] With regard to teenage pregnancy, it might further be argued that society also—again, to avoid certain harms—restricts many activities for minors, though not for adults: legally, a person can be too young to marry, enter into a contract, vote, join the armed services, drive a car, leave school, and so on. Similarly, there could be an age requirement for a "parenthood license." (In China, couples are eligible to have a child only after age 25.)

Licensing parenthood would in effect mean that the state would decide who could and could not have children. The state's right to make such decisions would be based not only on its obligation to protect society from harm, but also on the fact that the state must often support the children resulting from misguided pregnancies.

To be effective, of course, a system for licensing parenthood would have to include penalties for noncompliance. Penalties might include fines, taxes, losses of welfare benefits, and sterilization.

•

To see a system of legal restraints in operation, let's look at China, whose population is one-fifth of humanity and whose government has established a goal of allowing each couple to have only one child. China, of course, is not a democracy—in fact, techniques of social control were brought to a "high, if Machiavellian, art" under the long regime of Mao Tse-Tung—and thus attempts to achieve this goal have already been moderately successful; at present, China is now ahead of schedule in reducing its population. People who conceive after having their quota of one child are sent to "education centers" where they stay until they agree to an abortion; abortions by cesarean section may be performed during the third trimester of pregnancy. An unapproved birth results in loss of income: the family gets no extra income for the additional child; in fact, a monthly fine is imposed. The parents may be denied raises or promotions at work. The child may not be allowed to enroll in school. Even the grandparents may be penalized.

An anthropologist living in China wrote:

> How this [only one child per couple] will be accomplished is diabolically simple. "The licensing of first births" was how one birth control worker privately described it to me. "Every brigade will be given an annual quota of babies," she explained. "Newlyweds who wish to have a child must apply to the commune family-planning office for a birth permit. To receive this, they must meet two conditions: they must fall within their brigade's yearly quota, and they must agree to have only one child. If they go ahead and have the child without a permit, they will be violating the birth control regulations. Their baby will be a 'black market person,' no grain, oil, cloth, or other ration coupons will be issued, and the parents will have to pay a monthly fine of 20 rmb." Couples who conceive a child without first obtaining a birth permit will be ordered to attend birth control meetings, at which they will be pressured to accept the one-child limit and sterilization.[28]

The Chinese system does not always work smoothly, to say the least. In small villages, pregnant women are sometimes dragged from their homes to clinics and tied down, struggling, for an abortion; and since Chinese tradition strongly favors male children, female infanticide has been occurring in some places.

•

Clearly, the Chinese model is extreme. Chinese administrative structures, formal and informal, are working to change individual behavior in ways that would be unimaginable in the United States. A visiting Chinese medical professor who saw the film *Bertha* could not understand how "allowing" Bertha to become pregnant would even be considered or why her daily life was not controlled by her parents and peers; though he had been in the United States for several months, he did not grasp the American concept of "reproductive freedom." And when the author of this text visited China in 1988, he was astonished at how much social control is exercised over the most intimate details of citizens' private lives. (Because of the lack of housing and scarcity of cars, there is almost no place where couples in the cities can go to be alone.)

American policy is near the opposite extreme. Americans—including American teenagers—have complete freedom of reproduction[29] and will retain it for the foreseeable future. Even economic "penalties" to discourage teenage pregnancy would meet strong resistance; many Americans would be reluctant to deny teenagers and their children social support—to cut them off, say, from school lunches, food stamps, free baby food, or medical care. Such sanctions are widely seen as callous, unfair to innocent children, and ultimately far more costly to society. To prevent children from coming at the wrong time and for the wrong reasons, American society must clearly find other paths.

UPDATE

A New Issue: Norplant

Norplant is a surgically implanted contraceptive which is effective for 5 years. Usually, it consists of six matchstick-size progestin implants inserted under the skin of the upper arm. This "shot in the arm" procedure takes about 10 minutes and can be performed by a specially trained nurse, such as a school nurse. The average cost is $365 for the drug itself, plus $300 for the physician's fee. Since Norplant contains no estrogen, it does not have the side effects associated with oral contraceptives.[30] The advantages of Norplant are that it prevents conception almost immediately (within 24 hours after it has been inserted) and that it eliminates the necessity of taking daily pills for birth control (and the consequences of possible lapses).

Norplant was tested on nearly 2 million women in 44 countries and found to be relatively safe.[31] It first became available in the United States in early 1991; 2 years later, about 500,000 American women were using it, and in some states it was covered by Medicaid.

Norplant became controversial in 1991, when a judge in California sentencing a woman convicted of child abuse offered her a choice: she could accept Norplant and be placed on probation, or she could go to jail.[32] Many critics denounced this, saying that Norplant should not be used as a punishment. Nevertheless, about a dozen states introduced bills to require Norplant for women child abusers and drug addicts: the reasoning was that such women would be incompetent mothers and therefore should be prevented from becoming pregnant. Opinion polls found considerable agreement with this mandatory use of Norplant.

In January 1992, the Baltimore city schools began to offer Norplant. Because of the extremely high rate of pregnancy among teenagers there—about 20 percent, with 1 in 10 pregnancies ending in birth—public health authorities offered the procedure free through inner-city schools with health clinics. As of April 1994, however, very few of the eligible girls (less than 10 percent) had enrolled in the program.[33] On the streets of Baltimore, it was said that the implant made girls fat and was associated with unpleasant symptoms. Also, several influential ministers had denounced the program as sending girls an immoral message and leaving them vulnerable to sexually transmitted diseases. At about this time, a woman in Birmingham, Alabama, died while having Norplant implanted (the physician later lost his license).

In the summer of 1994, Norplant began to look less like a "dream contraceptive"—as it had been called in 1991—and more like a nightmare. By then, Norplant capsules had been inserted in 1 million American women, some of whom were complaining that removing the capsules was both complicated and painful. Four hundred women joined a class-action suit against the manufacturer, Wyeth-Ayerst Laboratories, claiming that removal had caused intense discomfort and had left scars. Evidently, when a physician removes the capsules, there is a problem finding all six of them in the patient's arm; if it is necessary to poke around for 20 minutes or so, the tissues become swollen and inflamed, making the remaining capsules even harder to find.[34]

As many as 20 percent of women with Norplant implants may decide to have them removed early. Moreover, the introduction of Depo Provera in 1993 has made Norplant much less popular among young women who are clients of family-planning clinics; although Depo Provera lasts only 3 months, it requires just one injection and is much cheaper than Norplant.

An Ongoing Issue: Welfare

During his campaign for the presidency, Bill Clinton promised to "end welfare as we know it." Public dissatisfaction with welfare was high: the system was seen as encouraging lifelong welfare dependency, childbearing by people who could or would not assume financial responsibility for their children, and various kinds of fraud (such as lying to public officials and enrolling in welfare programs in more than one state).[35] In addition, many people did not like the fact that children of illegal aliens were eligible, immediately upon arrival, for Medicaid, food stamps, public schools, and in some states AFDC.

By the second year of the Clinton administration, proposals for welfare reform abounded; they included establishing "workfare" programs; allowing nonworking men in households receiving AFDC; disregarding wages from low-paying jobs in setting income limits for recipients of AFDC, Medicaid, and food stamps; establishing some maximum number of years for receiving benefits; and disqualifying illegal immigrants or children born in the United States to illegal immigrants. The administration approved two significant changes: Wisconsin imposed a 2-year limit for welfare benefits, and New Jersey and Georgia required work in return for welfare. In the spring of 1993, Clinton was pushing a bill allocating over $9 billion to revamp welfare. However, as of the autumn of 1994, Clinton's pledge to "end welfare as we know it" was stalled, in the general torpor created by a standoff over health care (see Chapter 18). The welfare reform bill introduced in 1993 had not been passed before the elections of 1994.

In 1994, Charles Murray—who believes that the "Great Society" programs have hurt the poor by making them dependent on government—advocated stopping welfare "cold turkey." When asked if this wouldn't hurt children, Murray proposed reviving state-run and charitable orphanages to serve as a backup and to provide better living conditions than these children would have in inner-city housing projects.[36] By this time, Murray and the black newspaper columnist William Raspberry had become leading advocates of two-parent families, delayed childbearing, and welfare reform. Murray's views were once regarded as on the extreme right, but by now many states and the Clinton administration are beginning to think along similar lines. Murray has predicted that if we do not make changes in welfare, we will soon develop a large white underclass, and he feels that we may already be seeing the beginning of this new underclass. Baltimore, for instance, now has a large number of unmarried white teenage mothers.[37]

•

According to Barbara Hammond—who was was still Director of Social Services for Allegheny County, Virginia, in 1989—Bertha's IUD caused endometriosis; because of this, Bertha thought she was sterile. Nevertheless, she eventually married, and in her late thirties she had two children.

FURTHER READING

Alan Guttmacher Institute, *Preventing Pregnancy, Protecting Health: A New Look at Birth Control Choices in the United States,* New York, 1991 (111 Fifth Avenue, New York, NY, 10003).

"Making Connections: Individuals, Families, Communities," *Philosophy and Public Policy,* vol. 13, no. 3, Summer 1993 (School of Public Affairs, University of Maryland).

Charles Murray, *Losing Ground: American Social Policy 1950–1980,* Basic Books, New York, 1986.

CHAPTER 16

Presymptomatic Testing for Genetic Disease

Nancy Wexler

This chapter takes up ethical issues in presymptomatic testing for genetic diseases. It focuses on the case of Nancy Wexler, who helped develop a test for Huntington's disease (HD), a fatal neurological genetic disorder. Another recent case—the development of a test for a hereditary form of breast cancer—is discussed in "Update."

BACKGROUND: GENETICS AND EUGENICS

DNA, Genes, and Genetic Disorders

In 1953, in *Nature,* James Watson and Francis Crick published their description of the "double helix" structure of deoxyribonucleic acid (DNA), the nucleic acid responsible for transmitting hereditary characteristics.[1] This description included the basic mechanism for copying genetic material from one cell to another and, in reproduction, from one generation to another. Watson and Crick's discovery moved the study of genetics from observational inference to molecular biology.

The basic unit of life is the cell. The basic unit of heredity is the *gene,* which consists of DNA, though not all DNA takes the form of genes. Genes are carried on chromosomes; a *chromosome*—which consists of DNA and other material—is a macromolecule composed of repeating nucleotides. Normally, the nucleus of each human cell contains 46 chromosomes. The germ, or sex, cells, however, have 23 chromosomes each; thus the union of sperm and egg provides the 46 (23 + 23) chromosomes for every new human being, and genes are inherited in pairs consisting of one gene from the father and one from the mother.

As a result of the work of Watson, Crick, and others, it is now known that packed inside each of the 46 chromosomes is an enormously complicated strand of interwoven DNA: this is the famous double helix. Each strand is composed of combinations of four chemical (nucleotide) bases in approximately 3 billion pairs (in each pair, one bit is on each side of the helix); thus the total number of pairs is about 138 billion. The pattern of the four nucleotide bases in the 46 double helices is a person's genetic code. Scientists believe that between 50,000 and 100,000 sequences of these 138 billion pairs of bases are genes, with the number of genes varying from chromosome to chromosome.

To find the genes, we need a map of these 46 double helices, or strands, of DNA, and the Human Genome Project is now developing such a map. This 15-year study, which began in October 1993 and is expected to cost $3 billion, is one of the most significant single projects in the history of science.

If we think of the 46 strands of human DNA (each with its 3 billion base pairs) as, say, North America, the Human Genome Project can be said to be providing a map of the territory and its major highways; on this map, the 50,000 to 100,000 genes are the towns and cities. The largest gene, comparable in size to Los Angeles, is the gene for muscular dystrophy, composed of 2 million base pairs. The genes for globulin and insulin are like towns, with only about 1,000 base pairs each. At the beginning of the project, scientists already knew the location of most of the large cities and many of the smaller cities, but many of the towns remained to be found.

•

Genetic diseases are inherited disorders. It is possible that most of us actually have genes for inherited disorders but are *heterozygous* for these disorders: that is, we have a dissimilar pair of genes for an inherited disease or trait. If a gene is *dominant*, it will be expressed, or shown, in a heterozygote; if it is *recessive*, it will *not* be expressed in a heterozygote. However, even though heterozygotes may not show a trait themselves, they are *carriers* who can pass the gene for the disorder along to their offspring. If two parents who are heterozygous for a disorder both pass on the gene for the disorder to an offspring, that person will be *homozygous* for the disorder—will have an identical pair of genes. A disease or trait will always be expressed in a homozygote.

As many as 15 million Americans may have moderate to severe genetic disease.[2] According to a definitive list compiled by V. A. McKusick (and updated online daily), there are over 3,500 "established" and 2,500 "suspected" hereditary disorders.[3] These are large figures; in fact, every family may include someone who is a potential victim of genetic disease or is susceptible to a disorder that may be linked to genetic causes, such as alcoholism, cancer, or coronary artery disease. Genetic diseases are estimated to account for over one-third of acute-care hospitalization of children under 18.

Some single disease-causing genes have already been discovered, and physicians have already embarked on gene therapy to treat a number of these diseases. Francis Collins, who discovered the gene for muscular dystrophy and was head of the Human Genome Project in 1993, predicted that:

> The Human Genome Project will change the face of medicine. It's very possible that in the future a physician will give an 18-year old patient a physical exam that includes a test of his or her DNA for hundreds of diseases with known genetic components. Family histories are useful, but genetic exams will give the doctor a much more precise tool to assess risks and give advice. The physician

will be able to tell the patient whether the risk is high, low, or average for a given condition and to make life-style recommendations based upon known risks. There will be personalized schemes for a new kind of preventive medicine and I think it will prove very appealing.[4]

The Eugenics Movement

Before genetics became a science, a number of ill-founded popular ideas about heredity were influential in the nineteenth and early twentieth centuries. One notorious example is *phrenology*, a pseudoscience based on the idea that the size and shape of the head determined intelligence and character. (Vestiges of phrenology may still be found among novelists who write as if character can be inferred from a person's face. George Eliot lampooned this notion in *Middlemarch*: "So much subtler is a human mind than the outside tissues, which make a sort of blazonry or clock-face for it.") Some popular "science" was based on more or less crackpot versions of Charles Darwin's theory of evolution by natural selection, particularly his concept of "survival of the fittest." What Darwin meant by *fittest* was simply "best adapted"—he was referring to the "fit" between an organism and its environment—but many people misunderstood this and applied it altogether inappropriately.

One prominent misinterpretation was *social Darwinism,* which saw Darwin's theory in terms of group competition in human societies. Social Darwinists were elitists: they held, for one thing, that social advantages implied biological superiority, and that therefore the upper classes would prevail in this competition. They were also racists: they claimed that the fittest races would prevail in the struggle for existence; and (as discussed in Chapter 9), they predicted that blacks, whom they saw as biologically unfit to compete with whites, would not survive into the twentieth century. Social Darwinism can most charitably be described as unsophisticated. It was not based on any real understanding of evolution, and it failed to take account of the vast numbers of organisms involved in the attempt to survive, the enormous length of time over which evolution works, or the role of adaptive mutations.

•

Eugenics—another of these popular pseudosciences—flourished from about 1905 to 1935. This was a movement to improve humanity by improving hereditary characteristics, a goal it intended to accomplish through selective breeding. Its ideas came from various sources, including social Darwinism and Malthusian theory, though some of these were dubious to begin with and others were misapplied. The term *eugenics* was coined in the late 1880s by Francis Galton. Galton was Charles Darwin's cousin, and his particular misinterpretation of Darwin's theory took the form of claiming that famous people were the most "fit," a notion which famous people naturally liked.[5]

During the 1880s, chromosomes were first discovered in cell nuclei; around 1900, it was hypothesized that chromosomes carried genes, Gregor Mendel's laws of inheritance were rediscovered, and William Bateson coined the term *genetics* for this new field of study. At the same time, Karl Pearson, Charles Davenport, and others popularized some crude notions of genetics: this was the origin of the eugenics movement, which was to become hugely influential.

Eugenic organizations were formed worldwide, especially in Germany, Austria, Scandinavia, Italy, Japan, and South America; but as one historian of science, Daniel Kevles, writes, "the center of this trend was the American eugenics movement. Its headquarters was at Cold Springs Harbor on Long Island, New York, and its leader was Charles Davenport."[6] This point bears emphasizing: although many people identify modern eugenics with Nazi Germany, it was actually in the United States—with its heterogeneous population—that eugenics was most widely championed. Politicians, popular media, and even many scientists espoused eugenics, advocated "eugenic marriages" and sterilization of the unfit, and declared that the American "breeding stock" was declining through interbreeding with unfit races.

In the United States at the beginning of the twentieth century, a few prominent families—largely of English, Swiss, German, and Dutch ancestry—had enormous wealth and power; they controlled many newspapers, magazines, and even universities, and thus they exerted a great deal of control over the ideas of the time. These families, on the whole, were greatly concerned about "breeding," and they were afraid that the "purity" of Americans with backgrounds like their own would be "contaminated" if their children interbred with the Irish, Italians, Turks, Jews, Asians, African Americans, or anybody else whose origin was "different."

Wealthy and powerful families were concerned not only with preserving the "purity" of their own stock but also with controlling the growth of groups from other backgrounds. They were appalled by the many progeny of Irish, Italian, and Greek immigrants and saw Malthusian doom approaching. (Because predominantly Catholic ethnic groups tended to have more children, anti-Catholic sentiment grew.) The upper classes also agreed, almost unanimously, that the "unfit" had no right to bear children. A prominent New York urologist, William Robinson, proclaimed:

> It is the acme of stupidity to talk in such cases of individual liberty, of the rights of the individual. Such individuals have no rights. They have no right in the first instance to be born, but having been born, they have no right to propagate their kind.[7]

It is worth noting that even on their own terms and in the context of their own time, these ideas made little sense. The combination of social Darwinism and eugenics is almost immediately self-contradictory: if the white race and the upper class were destined to emerge triumphant, why worry about excessive breeding among "lower" races and classes? If the lower races and classes were so "unfit" that they were destined to die out, why try to prevent them from breeding?

Probably, eugenics seemed plausible, and became so influential, mainly because it was part of a general climate of bigotry. The newspaper magnate William Hearst and Theodore Roosevelt, for instance, thundered against "yellow niggers" who were invading the United States from Asia. When Henry Ford ran for president in the 1920s, he said he would rid the country of the "Jew bankers," whom he accused of having forced the United States into World War I; later, he would accuse them of causing the depression.[8]

•

During its height, from about the turn of the century to the early 1930s, the eugenics movement had a significant effect on legislation in the United States.

One effect was mandatory sterilization. (The forced sterilization of 225,000 people, mainly "mental defectives," in Nazi Germany is of course notorious; but it is less well known that although the Nazis were more systematic, secretive, and biased by racism, the United States also practiced large-scale involuntary sterilization.[9]) In 1907, Indiana became the first state to require sterilization of the retarded and criminally insane; it was soon followed by 30 other states. In each of these states, a board of experts ultimately decided who would be sterilized.

The number of mandatory sterilizations reached a peak during the 1930s. Most people who are aware of these sterilization programs at all believe that they took place mostly in the deep south or Appalachia, but in fact the leading state was California, where sterilizations accounted for nearly one-third of the national total; Virginia was second and Indiana third.[10] All together, by 1941 over 36,000 Americans had been involuntarily sterilized, often for a vague condition described as "feeblemindedness" or because they had been born into large families on welfare. Some of these sterilization laws were not reversed until the 1960s.

Besides mandatory sterilization, the most important legacy of the American eugenics movement was the Immigration Restriction Act of 1924. This act, hailed by eugenicists as their greatest triumph, was based on the assumption that Asians, Africans, the Greeks, the Irish, and eastern and southern Europeans such as the Poles and Italians were "inferior" peoples; whereas the English, Dutch, Scotch, Scandinavians, and Germans, and possibly the French (if they were not Catholic) represented "superior stock." The act was enthusiastically signed by President Calvin Coolidge, who as vice president had declared, "America must be kept American. Biological laws show . . . that Nordics deteriorate when mixed with other races."[11] Interestingly, the term *melting pot*—which today is considered laudatory—was first used, pejoratively, by those lobbying for the Immigration Restriction Act.

This immigration act established quotas according to country of origin; although these quotas were based on how many people from a given country were already in the United States, in effect they made it very difficult for people from "inferior" countries to be admitted. The Statue of Liberty is often seen as historic symbol of freedom, but after 1924, thousands of the world's "huddled masses" had only a glimpse of it before being turned away and sent back home.

•

The influence of eugenics also extended to the courts, and in 1927 it was reflected in a famous decision by the United States Supreme Court, *Buck v. Bell*.

Carrie Buck was a supposedly retarded young woman whose mother, Emma Buck, was also supposedly retarded; according to a crude IQ test, Carrie Buck's mental age was 9 years and Emma Buck's was 8 years. Carrie Buck had been

committed to a state mental institution in Virginia at age 17 and had been pregnant at the time she was committed; she gave birth to a daughter, Vivian, inside
the institution. Then as now, institutionalized women often became pregnant by
guards or visiting relatives, and the institution's director (who was the "Bell" in
the case) wondered if Carrie Buck could be sterilized so that she would not have
another child.

Virginia officials asked Harry Laughlin, an influential geneticist who worked
at Cold Springs Harbor, to determine whether Carrie Buck's retardation was
hereditary. Laughlin did not see Carrie Buck; he relied simply on the reported
mental ages of Carrie and her mother, and on the report of a social worker who
said that Carrie had a strange "look" about her. On this basis, Laughlin declared
that Carrie Buck "lived a life of immorality and prostitution," and that she and
her mother belonged to the "shiftless, ignorant, worthless class of anti-social
whites of the South."[12]

The Supreme Court, by a vote of 8 to 1, upheld the legality of sterilizing
Carrie Buck and handed down an order for her sterilization. Justice Oliver
Wendell Holmes wrote the opinion in *Buck v. Bell,* saying, "Three generations of
imbeciles are enough,"[13] and concluding, "The principle that sustains compulsory vaccination is broad enough to cover cutting the Fallopian tubes."[14] Holmes
noted that science should guide public policy and emphasized that what the
public good would gain in "sound genetics" would outweigh individual rights
of the retarded to procreate.

●

"Sound genetics," however, is more complicated than Holmes or his contemporaries realized. At the time, some crucial information about genetics was lacking
or poorly understood, and this led to several incorrect assumptions.

One area of ignorance was recessive inheritance. If a trait is recessive, it will
be expressed only in a homozygote—a person who has received an identical pair
of genes for the disorder. The existence of recessive genes explains why normal
people can produce impaired children: two unaffected carriers can each pass a
gene for a recessive trait to a child, who will then be homozygous for the trait.
Recessive inheritance also explains why genetically impaired people can produce
normal children: if a defect is recessive, and an affected person mates with someone who is not a carrier, their child will not have the defect. Such instances must
have been observed often (and also apparent instances—Carrie Buck's daughter
Vivian was considered bright by her teachers and was doing well in school
before she died at age 8 of an intestinal disorder), but their significance was not
appreciated.

A second area of ignorance was the complexity of inheritance. In 1927,
eugenicists and others assumed, mistakenly, that each trait was inherited through
a single gene (a person with 378 traits, in their view, must have 378 separate
genes). Thus they thought that there was a specific, inheritable gene for retardation; and Charles Davenport held, around 1930, that prostitution was caused by a
gene for "innate eroticism."[15]

A third area of ignorance had to do with mutations and chromosomal break-
age. Because the eugenicists and their contemporaries did not know about these

aspects of genetics, they believed—again mistakenly—that retardation could be eliminated from the gene pool if all retarded people could be prevented from reproducing.

A fourth area of ignorance had to do with determining exactly which traits are inherited. Almost nothing was known about what is and is not inherited, and this too led to mistaken ideas; Davenport, for example, believed that poverty and criminality were hereditary. Actually, it is often difficult to distinguish inherited from acquired traits even today: nature is not easily separable from nurture. Psychologists continue to debate whether intelligence is determined primarily by hereditary or environmental factors; and as recently as the 1980s, the Harvard psychologist Richard Herrnstein argued that criminality ran in certain families and suggested a genetic link.[16] However, retardation is now known to be caused by many factors and combinations of factors, including nonhereditary causes such as alcohol abuse during pregnancy.

A fifth area of ignorance was population genetics. The eugenicists hoped to perfect humanity through selective breeding, but population genetics have since shown that a regression to the mean will occur. *Regression to the mean* is the inherent tendency in stable populations to return to an average value over time; in population genetics, this tells us that the underlying causes creating a mean value in a population will eventually normalize any deviant values. (This applies, among other things, to baseball statistics, the stock market, lucky streaks, and height in a family of many children.)

Finally, the eugenicists and their contemporaries did not realize how many generations are needed to eliminate a defect. Because they did not understand the difference between carrying an unexpressed gene and actually having a trait, they could not calculate that reducing the frequency of a defect from 1 in 100 to 1 in 1,000 might take 22 generations and that reducing it to 1 in 1 million might take hundreds of generations.

•

After about 1935, the eugenics movement declined in the United States. Many geneticists had supported the movement in its early years, but around the time of the depression most of them abandoned it. This was partly because of its zealous emphasis on human perfectibility, partly because of its racism, partly because of its association with the Nazis, and partly because its assumptions were being contradicted by the emerging facts of genetics.

By 1935, the geneticist Hermann J. Muller said that eugenics was "hopelessly perverted," a cult for "advocates for race and class prejudice, defenders of vested interests of church and State, Fascists, Hitlerites, and reactionaries generally."[17] Another leading geneticist, J. B. S. Haldane, said at the time of the sterilization programs that "many of the deeds done in America in the name of eugenics are about as much justified by science as were the proceedings of the Inquisition by the Gospels."[18] Advances in population genetics prompted Haldane to remark, "An ounce of algebra is worth a ton of verbal argument."[19]

The eugenicists' ideas about race were also being discredited—for example, the linked false assumptions that race represented a biological subspecies and that it determined behavior. To the eugenicists, designations such as *Irish, Italian, Polish, African American, Jewish,* and *Arab* were biological types; but to

more advanced thinkers, such terms were political, religious, or ethnic general-
izations.

In 1935—attacking the Nazis' eugenics program, which was based on, and
designed to promote, "Aryan" racial superiority—Julian Huxley and A. C. Haddon maintained that race is not a uniform, biological type but a mixture of many
peoples. They argued that "the word race should be banished, and the descrip-
tive and non-committal term ethnic groups should be substituted."[20] They
denied the notion that any groups (such as blacks, Poles, or the Irish) were
naturally promiscuous; they also denied that members of any such group "naturally" liked certain kinds of food or drink. In particular, they attacked the idea of
promiscuity as a genetic trait; in general, they attacked the crude belief that genes
influenced any highly specific human behaviors—a belief for which there was no
evidence—and the hasty generalization that all people from a certain area (such
as Ireland or Africa) had the same genes.

Eugenics, then, was being seen as "bad science." One measure of how bad it
was could be found in eugenicists' own debates over how to analyze World War
I. Some of them said the war was dysgenic, because the best male stock went off
and died; others said it was eugenic, because the remaining men had their choice
of the best women; but those who considered it dysgenic said that the women
would marry inferior men, to avoid being spinsters, and would therefore produce less perfect offspring. The decline and fall of eugenics can be discerned in
this kind of nonsense. Much of the eugenicists' theorizing reflected male fan-
tasies and biases (not many eugenicists were women); and all of it reflected com-
placency, since advocates of eugenics uniformly saw themselves as part of the
"fittest" breeding stock.

However, although the idea of improving humanity by improving heredity—
"positive eugenics"—was generally abandoned, a very different form—"negative
eugenics"—developed later. *Negative eugenics* means merely trying to eliminate
genetic diseases and disorders, and it appeared in the 1960s, in the context of prenatal testing and genetic screening.

Genetic Screening

In the early 1960s, prenatal predictive tests made it possible to identify phenyl-
ketonuria (PKU) in fetuses. PKU is a recessive genetic disease in which there is
an excess of the amino acid phenylalanine. If PKU is not diagnosed until after
birth, when its symptoms appear, this excess will always cause retardation. However, retardation can be prevented and development will be normal if PKU is
identified before birth, so that the infant can be put on a special diet as soon as it
is born. The prenatal test for PKU is cheap and easy.

It was the development of the PKU test that led many well-intentioned people to advocate negative eugenics. If PKU, a genetic disorder, could be prevented
by prenatal screening, what better justification could there be for making such
screening mandatory? Most states accepted this reasoning and eventually
required screening for PKU.

Subsequent studies showed that the PKU test was often unreliable and that if
PKU was misdiagnosed in normal babies, they could be harmed by the special

diet that was prescribed for it. Nevertheless, PKU screening did save thousands of correctly diagnosed children from retardation, because it targeted a specific deficit for which there was a known remedy.

If all genetic screening were this specific, and if all of the conditions it identified were so effectively treatable, such screening would be routine today. However, not all screening is so clear-cut. In fact, in reviewing genetic screening, one scholar notes that PKU screening itself was "in many ways a type case of the kinds of difficulty encountered by all mass screening procedures, which frequently turn out to be less perfect in practice than had been hoped when they were instituted."[21]

Genetic screening actually forms a sort of spectrum. PKU testing—which can identify a specific, treatable condition—is near the "successful" end of this spectrum. An example of the opposite end of the spectrum is testing for an extra Y chromosome. In 1965, a team headed by Patricia Jacobs found that some male inmates of penal and mental institutions had an extra Y chromosome and suggested that this caused a condition characterized by antisocial behavior: it was called the *XYY syndrome*. Some newborns were then tested for XYY and later followed to see if their behavior was antisocial. Most scientists were opposed to XYY testing. They argued that XYY might not even be a syndrome; that even if it was, no treatment existed; and that testing positive could become a self-fulfilling prophecy: parents and others might expect an XYY child to be antisocial, and this expectation could in itself cause the child to develop antisocial behavior.

Other forms of genetic screening have fallen at various points along the spectrum. These include screening for Tay Sachs disease, sickle-cell disease, Down syndrome, certain susceptibilities, and cystic fibrosis.

Screening for *Tay Sachs* disease—a rare, lethal condition found in Jews of eastern European descent—became possible in the 1960s and eventually became a major success. As with PKU, the gene for Tay Sachs disease could be identified in a fetus by a simple, cheap test; moreover, this test for Tay Sachs was highly reliable. Unlike PKU, however, Tay Sachs disease is not treatable. Thus if the fetal test was positive, the fetus would be electively aborted; if parents would not consider abortion, the Tay Sachs test was not given. Adults can also be screened for Tay Sachs; in this case, intervention would take the form of counseling two carriers not to have children together.

Initially, screening for Tay Sachs was only partially successful, because some parents were opposed to abortion and some people were afraid that they would be stigmatized if they were identified as carriers. But in the early 1970s, Jews themselves started encouraging such screening, in a program which had been given 14 months of careful preparation; this effort was centered in Brooklyn and included the matchmakers who arrange marriages in Orthodox Jewish communities. Since then, over 1 million young adults have been screened and over 2,400 pregnancies involving a risk of Tay Sachs disease have been identified and, presumably, ended.[22]

By contrast, screening for sickle-cell disease was ultimately unsuccessful. *Sickle-cell disease,* which affects mostly black people, takes its name from sickle-shaped cells (erythrocytes) in the blood; it causes acute abdominal pain, joint pain, and ulceration of the lower extremities. The clinical course of sickle-cell disease, though, is variable (unlike that of PKU or Tay Sachs disease), and—importantly—some people with sickle-cell disease can lead nearly normal lives.

Screening for sickle-cell disease is possible in both fetuses and adults, but when screening programs began, authorities failed to consider the possible consequences of identification. As with Tay Sachs, there is no cure for sickle-cell disease; thus if a fetus tested positive, the only intervention was elective abortion. However, since the condition might not actually be serious in any individual, abortion was controversial in this situation. Also, with sickle-cell disease (like PKU but unlike Tay Sachs), there was some misdiagnosis; this too made abortion controversial.

With regard to screening adults, many laypeople confused carriers of the sickle-cell gene (heterozygotes) with those who actually had the disease (homozygotes). Because of this confusion, some carriers were treated as if they had the disease itself: some of them were denied medical insurance or even fired from their jobs. This situation was aggravated by the fact that some jurisdictions made screening for sickle-cell disease mandatory.

Protests from the African American community finally defeated the sickle-cell screening programs, and state laws mandating such programs faded into limbo. Sickle-cell testing is now recognized as a paradigm of how not to set up a screening program.

In the early 1970s, it became possible to screen for *Down syndrome,* which is a chromosomal aberration. Screening for Down syndrome is done by amniocentesis and has been very successful. Today, pregnant women over age 35 or 40 are routinely tested; in fact, an obstetrician's failure to suggest such a test for a patient over about 35 may be grounds for a malpractice suit.

Some genes appear to be linked to certain diseases, such as cancer or coronary artery disease; and *susceptibility screening* for cholesterol, lipids, and HLA-antigens was developed in the 1970s. This can make early intervention possible; for instance, early identification and treatment of hypercholesterolemia might prevent a later heart attack. However, there is some potential for abuse in susceptibility screening: for example, employers might try to lower medical costs by screening job applicants and discriminating against people who test positive.

Screening for *cystic fibrosis* (CF) began in the 1990s. CF produces thick, excessive mucus in the bronchi; a person with CF must be continually thumped on the back to loosen these secretions and held upside down to drain them. Eventually, CF is fatal: it destroys the lungs, causing suffocation, usually by early adulthood, though the symptoms may not appear until the teenage years. One in 22 white people carries the gene for CF; since this gene is recessive, a child of two heterozygotes has a 25 percent risk of CF. Screening for CF can be done with fetuses (by amniocentesis) or children, but it is controversial. It is accurate and useful only if there is a family history of CF, and 80 percent of children with CF are born to families with no history of the disease. Also:

> . . . Molecular biology has revealed that CF is not caused by a single type of mutation. Although one mutation is associated with 70 percent of all cases, and two others with 25 to 20 percent, more than 360 mutations have been linked to CF so far.[23]

The pediatrician and bioethicist Norman Fost has described CF screening as "metastasizing, despite the lack of evidence that it works."[24]

As of 1994, according to Ellen Clayton—a pediatrician and bioethicist at Vanderbilt University—*ultrasound* and *maternal alpha fetoprotein testing* had become the most important methods of genetic screening in the United States.[25] These techniques are used to screen for physical deformities and neural-tube defects; the intervention is abortion, which is usually noncontroversial, since these are gross defects. Ultrasound and maternal alpha fetoprotein screening are at the "successful" end of the spectrum, though it should be noted that they are generally possible only when they are covered by health insurance.

NANCY WEXLER AND THE TEST FOR HD

Nancy Wexler, who is a clinical psychologist, was born in 1945 in Washington, D.C., and graduated from Radcliffe College in 1967. In 1967–1968 she spent a postgraduate year in Jamaica; at this time, she and her parents and sister learned that a mysterious disease in her mother's family was Huntington's disease (HD), a devastating and fatal neurological disorder for which there is no cure and no treatment.

Nancy Wexler's mother, Leonore Sabin Wexler, had suddenly begun to experience strange symptoms at age 58. Over the next decade, Nancy Wexler, her sister Alice, and their father—Milton Wexler, a psychoanalyst—watched as Leonore Wexler deteriorated: she became emaciated and catatonic and finally died in 1978. What happened to Leonore Wexler had also happened to the folksinger Woody Guthrie (1912–1967), who was the father of Arlo Guthrie and was portrayed briefly in the film *Alice's Restaurant*.

The gene for HD is dominant, and thus Nancy and Alice Wexler, and Arlo Guthrie, each had a 50 percent risk of HD. Since HD does not typically appear until its victim is in the thirties, forties, or fifties, this means there is a 50 percent chance that someone like Nancy Wexler is carrying a genetic time bomb.

Huntington's Disease

HD is a severe, progressive neurological disease in which neurons in the caudate nuclei region of the brain are rapidly shed. The average age of onset is 36. Thereafter, HD progresses through four stages of roughly 5 years each.

In the first stage of HD, there are initially small losses of muscular coordination; then there are changes in personality, making the victim angry, hostile, depressed, and sexually promiscuous (probably as a result of loss of neurons from the frontal lobe). In the second stage, speech becomes slurred, facial expressions become grotesquely distorted, there is constant muscular jerkiness, the fists clench and unclench, the limbs flail involuntarily, and the victim frequently staggers and falls. In Nancy Wexler's words: "Gradually, the entire body is encompassed by adventitious movements. The trunk is writhing and the face is twisting."[26] During this second stage, the victim is likely to lose his or her job. In the third stage, the victim is incontinent, experiences severe mental deterioration, and becomes dependent on others, at home or in an institution. In the fourth and final stage, the victim stares blankly ahead and remains motionless.

Nancy Wexler has described this progression as follows:

> The gene is so sly, so sinister. It's like there's an orchestra playing, and there are these [wrong] notes. At first they're very soft, but they keep getting louder and louder. Finally, they're all there is.[27]

Some genetic diseases, such as Down syndrome, are apparent at birth; but HD, as noted above, typically appears during the thirties to fifties. Because its onset is so late, people with HD usually have children before learning that they are affected. Although the age of onset varies, HD is completely "penetrant" by age 65: that is, by this age everyone with the gene is affected.

HD arrived in America in 1625, around the time of the *Mayflower;* it was brought by three affected men from the small English village of Bures. Their descendants include the physician George Huntington of Long Island, who first described the disease in 1872.[28] Originally, HD was called *Saint Vitus' dance* or *Huntington's chorea* (from the Greek *choreia,* "dance") because of the victims' jerking and twisting.

In the past, victims of HD have been treated badly. During the era of witch-hunting, for example, because their distorted movements were said to resemble Jesus's writhing on the cross, they were believed to be worshipers of Satan (a strange inference) who were being tortured by God. Seven female descendants of the original three Englishmen were thought to be witches, and one was executed at Groton, Connecticut, in 1692. Some of the Salem witches also probably had HD.

At present, about 20,000 to 25,000 Americans have HD, and more than 100,000 Americans with an afflicted parent are at risk of HD. Almost all those affected are white, except for one large African American family around Baltimore.

People at risk of HD live with a genetic sword of Damocles over their heads, constantly wondering if each stutter, spill, or stumble is a sign of the disease. Nancy Wexler once said that for her, not a day went by without some thought of HD: "You become aware of all kinds of things you never noticed before—little muscle jerks in bed, or clumsiness. I remember dropping a carton of eggs and thinking, 'Oh, no! Is this the beginning?' "[29]

Finding a Genetic Marker for HD

Nancy Wexler entered a doctoral program in psychology at the University of Michigan in 1968; she wrote her dissertation on HD and its effects and received her doctorate in clinical psychology in 1974. In that year, her father started the Hereditary Disease Foundation in Los Angeles, and she became its president. In 1976, she became executive director of the Congressional Commission for the Control of HD and Its Consequences. Throughout the late 1970s, Nancy Wexler:

> . . . found out everything she could. She studied genetics. She organized patients' groups. She helped start a brain collection program so that the brains of HD victims would be available for research. She lobbied Capitol Hill for research funds.

She convinced a wide variety of scientists such as molecular biologist David Housman of the Massachusetts Institute of Technology to study HD. Soon she was a driving force in the HD community.[30]

There are two kinds of presymptomatic genetic testing. First, there are *linkage tests*—tests for "markers" rather than for actual genes. A marker is linked to a gene and is usually inherited with that gene because marker and gene are close together in the DNA sequence.[31] Linkage tests require family histories and blood samples from family members.

Second, there are tests for the genes themselves—that is, for the actual sequence of DNA which constitutes a disease-causing gene (if there is such a single gene). Tests of this second kind are the ultimate genetic tests, because they detect the actual presence of a disease-causing gene. A test for a gene requires only a blood sample from the individual at risk.

The first goal of Wexler's Hereditary Disease Foundation was to find a marker for HD to use in a linkage test. The foundation believed that this could be done by finding a large number of people in a single family tree where HD had been inherited, taking blood from each member, and carrying out a genetic analysis; then, geneticists would visually examine tiny portions of the genetic map to see if some bit of DNA was to be found only in victims of HD. As early as 1977, Nancy Wexler had already lobbied Congress and obtained some funding. However, during the late 1970s:

> . . . there was considerable skepticism within the biomedical community as to whether this approach—called *genetic linkage analysis*—could possibly yield the desired information. "People thought it would take a hugely long time—maybe 50 to 75 years—to find a gene marker [for HD]," Wexler recalled.[32]

In 1972, a Venezuelan psychiatrist had discovered a large number of carriers descended from a common ancestor with HD named Maria Concepcion Soto. All of them lived in and around the village of San Luis on Lake Maracaibo in Venezuela. In 1981, Nancy Wexler led an expedition there (the first of a number of annual trips). Her sister Alice, who had earned a Ph.D. in history, researched ancient records to determine where the gene had originally come from. Evidently, the source was a European sailor who jumped ship there in the early 1800s. He and Maria had 14 children, and because families in this area tended to be large (10 or more children), by 1981 there were 3,000 descendants. Of these, 100 had HD and 1,100 others were at some risk.

Nancy Wexler played a key role at this point. The subjects were reluctant to allow skin biopsies or give blood samples until, through an interpreter, she explained that she too was at risk of *el mal* ("the evil") and had herself undergone these procedures.

The next step was getting the blood samples and skin biopsies back to the United States. This was not easy, since the samples had to reach the American researchers within 48 hours, and San Luis is far away from any city. Recordkeeping was also difficult: Nancy Wexler's family tree of the 3,000 descendants was 100 feet long.

Next, of course, came the crucial part: actually finding a marker for HD, which would entail finding the general location of the gene. In 1979, the Hereditary Disease Foundation had held a workshop on using recombinant DNA, which had recently been developed, to find a genetic marker linked to HD. James Gusella was able to use these new techniques to look for a marker in the genetic karyotypes (these are somewhat analogous to blueprints) of the Venezuelan families.

Although Gusella had a hunch about where to look, he predicted that finding a marker would take 5 to 10 years. He needed to find the general location of the genetic base pairs for HD—a sequence of perhaps only a few thousand—within the 3 billion base pairs of one chromosome. However, he had a hunch, and some luck, and in August 1983 he found a marker (G8) for HD on the far tip of the short arm of chromosome 4.

The next step would be to identify the HD gene itself. Gusella's discovery of the G8 marker meant that the search for the gene could be restricted to the tip of chromosome 4, that is, to less than 0.03 percent of the human DNA. Even so, Gusella said in 1983, "We're still three to five years away from finding the gene—unless there's another lucky break."[33] In 1984, Nancy Wexler helped start the HD Collaborative Research Group to find the HD gene.

•

By the fall of 1987, though the gene itself had not been discovered, Gusella was able to develop a linkage test for HD, using the G8 marker.

The HD linkage test (as is generally true of such tests) could not be performed simply by drawing blood from an individual. It required blood samples from both sets of grandparents and both parents, because it depended on knowledge of grandparents' and parents' genes. Not only was blood from other family members needed to prove the existence of a case of HD; a family history was also needed. When this much input is necessary, there is bound to be some uncertainty; also, in some cases the G8 marker does not "travel" with the HD gene, and thus the gene but not the marker may be inherited. As a result, the HD linkage test was often not 100 percent accurate. It might be 97 percent or only 75 percent predictive, depending on what was known. Moreover, if the grandparents and parents were dead, the test could not be done.

Still, the linkage test represented a significant advance. Gusella and the geneticist Michael Connealy received primary credit for the discovering the marker and developing the linkage test; Nancy Wexler was also listed as a principal codiscoverer.[34] Marjorie Guthrie, Woody Guthrie's widow, who organized clubs for HD descendants, had also played an indirect role.

The Aftermath

As will be discussed under "Ethical Issues," the personal decision whether or not to take the HD linkage test was by no means easy: there were problems with both knowing and not knowing the answer.

In 1986, while the linkage test was being developed but before it was available, Nancy Wexler (who had become an associate professor of clinical neuropsychology at the College of Physicians and Surgeons of Columbia University in 1985) said that she herself would take it: "My feeling was that the advantages of knowing, even if the answer was yes, outweighed the disadvantages."[35] However, she later reconsidered that decision.

In May 1987, when the linkage test was first becoming available, Diane Sawyer (DS) interviewed Nancy Wexler (NW) and Alice Wexler (AW) for *60 Minutes.*

DS: Did you think you'd get the test if they ever had one?
NW: I was positive I would. Unquestionably. It never occurred to me that I wouldn't.
DS: And all of a sudden when you have the option, you're not so sure.
NW: I wasn't so sure. Exactly. I even said to people, "When the test is actually here, a lot of people are going to change their minds." It never occurred to me I would be one of them. That wasn't in the book.
AW: I would like to know I don't have it, but I absolutely don't want to know if I do have it.
NW: This is absolutely the hardest choice I've ever made in my life.[36]

Nancy Wexler now thought that people who took the test to end uncertainty would be fooling themselves: if the result was positive, she said, the question wouldn't be, "What if?" but "When?" For herself, she said there could be many bad outcomes: "If I found out that I was free of the disease, but Alice wasn't, I'd die." There would also be the worst possibility of all: both she and her sister could test positive.

Alice Wexler said that she had tried to imagine the "unimaginable"—testing positive—but admitted that she had not really succeeded. She could not imagine sitting at her own desk and knowing that she had this lethal gene at work in her:

> If you have the certainty that you have the gene, and if you have the certainty that you're going to die this absolutely miserable death over many years, I'm not sure it's possible to keep on living, to use the knowledge constructively. I'm sure I wouldn't. I think I would be devastated by it.

Diane Sawyer then asked, "So some hope is better than possible bad news?" Alice replied, "Hope is better than despair."

Milton Wexler did not want either of his daughters to take the test; he said that a positive test would represent a "potential for madness" and might destroy the three of them.

At the end of the interview, Diane Sawyer asked Nancy Wexler, "Will you take the test?" and "Is there a right answer?" Nancy Wexler answered, "I think for each person there's a right choice."

•

In 1987, three medical centers in the United States (all in the northeast) offered the linkage test for HD. Surveys had predicted that between 60 percent and 80 percent of those at risk of HD would take the test; but of 1,500 people at risk in New England, only 32 signed up for preliminary genetic counseling and only 18 actually took the test.

In 1989, Nancy Wexler said that she had not taken the test. She said that she now felt happy, that knowing she was negative wouldn't make her very much happier, and that knowing she was positive would make her very unhappy.[37] (Since then, she has not discussed whether or not she has taken a test.)

At that time, Arlo Guthrie (who was then about 40) had also decided not to take the test. He was living with his wife and their four children in western Massachusetts and felt he had "escaped the trauma" that killed his father. Did he regret having children without knowing his status? No, he said: "Life is more important than learning about diseases. . . . I could've said I don't want to 'inflict pain and suffering,' . . . [but] life is wonderful! There's a lot to live for."[38]

Nancy Wexler agreed. To people who wanted to be tested so that they could decide, say, whether to go to law school, she said: "Go to law school! Develop your mind! What are you going to do if you're positive? Spend the rest of your life waiting to be a patient?"

ETHICAL ISSUES

"Knowing": Pros and Cons

A case can be made for *not* taking a test like the linkage test for HD—for "not knowing," as Nancy and Alice Wexler and Arlo Guthrie decided. But a case can also be made for "knowing." The discussion here will focus on HD, though many of the pros and cons also apply to other kinds of genetic testing.

The case for knowledge   To many people (including Nancy Wexler), it seemed obvious that everyone at risk of HD had a "right to know": a right to take the linkage test and to be told the results. To some people, it even seemed that there might be a "duty to know." As we have seen from the comments of Nancy Wexler, Alice Wexler, and Arlo Guthrie, though, not everyone at risk wants such knowledge; thus it is important to examine reasons for wanting to know or for feeling that there may be a duty to know.

To begin with, some people at risk wanted to know because they felt that, for them, the relief of testing negative would outweigh the possibility of testing positive; also, some people felt that nothing is worse than uncertainty. In 1992, a Canadian study followed up 135 patients who had undergone linkage testing for HD.[39] It found that 1 year later, those who had tested negative felt much better off and, surprisingly, even those who had tested positive felt considerably better as a result of knowing for sure what would happen. The leader of this study reported that the patients who were positive for HD felt that knowledge "gave them control over their lives" and made them "live more in the present than in the future."[40]

In an editorial accompanying this study, Catherine Hayes, the president of HD Society of America, described how she heard of the test:

> For the first 33 years of my life, I lived at risk for HD. . . . One day in 1983, I heard on the radio that a genetic marker, a segment of DNA believed to be close to the gene for HD, had been discovered. It was clear to me that within a few years a presymptomatic test would be available. I had to stop the car because I was crying. I knew that I would take the test. Knowing, whatever the outcome, would be better than waiting and wondering day after day.[41]

In Hayes's case, the result was negative: "When I learned the results I cried and laughed," she wrote. "It took months for the news to sink in. I am still adjusting."

Another major argument for knowledge has to do with childbearing. If people at risk of a genetic disorder like HD do not know whether they are positive or negative, their decisions about childbearing may be misguided. People who would test negative and thus might safely have a child may feel that they are forced to remain childless; at the same time, people who would test positive may have children. Being born with HD is a fate that we would not wish on our worst enemy, let alone our own child.

Other arguments for knowledge have to do with the existing family of a person at risk. Consider the following example. A man who was at risk for HD but had decided not to take the test discussed his reasons before a large medical class. His reasons were greeted with respect; but as the class ended and the students started to file out, a woman cried out from the back of the room, "What about me and the kids?" It was the man's wife.[42]

This man's wife wanted to be able to plan for the future. If her husband was positive, she would be sooner or later have to take care of him. Also, as we have seen, victims of HD become sexually promiscuous during its first stage (in fact, they are sometimes described as being interested only in constant, "animalistic" sex), and she was probably wondering how to deal with that. She might also have been thinking, realistically enough, of money: if her husband was positive, he would need medical care and eventually custodial care, and they would have to start saving up for that or, if possible, arrange for life or health insurance. When HD strikes, moreover, the family as well as the victim will suffer emotionally; they might want to try to prepare themselves to confront this. Perhaps most important, they might try make the most of whatever time remained before onset.

Taking such things into consideration, some of those at risk might want to be tested for the sake of their families; Nancy Wexler's decision not to take the HD linkage test, for instance, might have been more complicated if she had a husband or children. Many people would, of course, feel uneasy about arguing that *someone else* has a "duty to know"; but a person who is himself or herself at risk may personally accept such a duty and may decide, as an individual, that it outweighs the fear of testing positive. In other words, a person at risk may simply choose to be altruistic.

In addition to the possibility of altruism, there are possibilities for compromise. For instance, with a genetic disease for which only a linkage test is available, middle-aged people who do not want to "know" may feel that they have probably escaped the disease and that they can now take the linkage test as a gift to their children. Another compromise is to have the family history and blood samples taken and store or "bank" the results (such banks exist for various diseases). Then, if a person at risk dies before any symptoms have appeared, his or her blood can be tested postmortem.

The case for *not* knowing   As we have seen, many people at risk of genetic disorders do not want to be tested themselves. Some general arguments against testing have also been advanced. What is the case for *not* knowing?

Many people at risk decide against knowing because they feel that the devastation of testing positive outweighs the possibility of testing negative; others feel that uncertainty (or "hope," as Alice Wexler put it) is preferable to knowing the worst. This, of course, is an individual, subjective evaluation.

However, there are also more objective considerations with regard to not knowing. At the outset, we should note that there is some opposition, from very diverse sources, to the entire concept of genetic testing. Some people feel, for instance, that geneticists should not give such information to couples: Jeremy Rifkin has aligned himself with Jerry Falwell, other conservative Christian ministers, and some politically conservative rabbis to oppose increased genetic choices.[43] The epidemiologist Abby Lippman is concerned that there will be social pressure on women to undergo genetic testing during pregnancy: "In today's Western world, biomedical and political systems largely define health and disease, as well as normality and abnormality."[44] According to the sociologist Dorothy Nelkin, information developed by the Human Genome Project could lead people to believe that differences in children's learning in schools are genetic rather than social or cultural.[45]

With regard to HD testing, there have been concerns about possible harm to those at risk. One such consideration, for example, was raised by Nancy Wexler, who thought that people who tested positive might adopt a "sick identity."[46]

A second consideration about harm to people at risk is whether those who agree to a test really understand what they are doing. One HD counselor said, for instance, "When people say they want this test to find out if they have the gene so they can make decisions, they really want to find out that they don't have it. The trouble is that fifty percent of them do. And there's no way to prepare them."[47] Nancy Wexler agreed with this.

There is some evidence for this second argument. In the first pilot study of the linkage test for HD, although most people at risk (63–79 percent) originally said they would take the test, some changed their minds later.[48] It was found that some of these people had expected to test negative and had intended to take the test to confirm this expectation. Since in fact they had a 50 percent chance of testing positive, this expectation indicated that they were in denial and were unprepared for a positive result; when they were given counseling which broke through their denial, they decided not to take the test. In this same study, it was reported of those who took the test, "Participants found to be probable gene carriers reported being surprised or shocked by the test result;"[49] they said they had not really expected to have the lethal gene. That too is a significant finding.

With linkage testing, some physicians and researchers who are convinced that most people really do not want to know propose (or practice) a "good news or no news" system.[50] The rationale is that linkage testing can be indeterminate and that this involves only a "white lie." However, a lie is a lie, and this practice could increase distrust of physicians; also, as a result of such a practice, the gene for a disorder can be passed along to children.

A third consideration about harm to people at risk is that self-knowledge is seldom perfect. Many people simply cannot predict how they will react to testing positive—what they will feel or do if they learn the worst. Since HD, for example, cannot be cured or ameliorated, a positive test will tell someone like Nancy

Wexler that she is probably going to die an early, terrible death. We might argue that not everyone can deal with such knowledge, and that it is inhumane to give people such a diagnosis when no real treatment is possible; some critics have argued that people at risk of HD should not be burdened with more truth than they can carry.[51]

In this regard, in 1986, when scientists at a conference in Salt Lake City were debating whether the linkage test should be made available, Nancy Wexler said, "We have to understand that the day you tell someone he has this gene, his life and view of himself change forever. We're worried about the potential for suicide."[52] In medical genetics, it is usually assumed that suicide after a positive test would be a bad thing, that such suicide should be prevented at all costs, and that people who say they might commit suicide should not be tested.

Concerns about suicide are not groundless. Over 25 percent of the victims of HD consider suicide, and 10 percent actually carry it out;[53] and given the nature of HD, these figures are understandable. As Nancy Wexler points out, during the first stage HD victims do not lose memory and can recognize relatives: "HD patients know their family and they know what's happening to them. So in a way, it's worse than Alzheimer's."[54] A victim may become frustrated and enraged at being unable to do something as simple as tie a shoelace; later, the victim may feel ashamed and become depressed. People who are concerned about suicide often focus on the consequences of testing teenagers—a population which is already highly suicidal. Youngsters who are merely at risk of HD already agonize about going to college and spending their parents' money, and those who learned for certain that they had HD might be even more vulnerable.

It should be noted, though, that not everyone considers potential suicide an adequate reason for not testing. For one thing, it can be argued that perhaps 75 percent of those at risk of HD would not attempt suicide; Catherine Hayes, for example, was not worried that she might commit suicide if the results were bad. A second, though obviously controversial, point was raised by Nancy Wexler herself (who did not think the possibility of suicide should weigh against testing): "Suicide is not unreasonable. It's not so awful that we can't discuss it or consider it."[55] She observed, "For some of my friends who have HD, knowing that they can commit suicide gives them a certain sense of control. They want to feel that if it gets too bad, they can have a way out. They can do something." A third (and also controversial) point has been made by a psychologist who argues that suicide is caused by depression, which he says is "treatable."[56] This psychologist describes himself as belonging to a "school which says one must choose life over death."

In the case for not knowing—as in the case for knowing—another kind of consideration may be the family of the person at risk. In more ways than one, the results of testing for a genetic disorder like HD affect the entire family.

With regard to the person at risk, although other family members may want to know, it is also possible that they may not want to know: that the family may prefer uncertainty to despair. Also, it is important to keep in mind that in testing for something like HD, there is no such thing as testing only a fetus, say, or testing only a parent: a positive fetus reveals a positive parent; a positive parent reveals that any children are at risk. Catherine Hayes gives an example:

A case in point involves a pair of identical twins, only one of whom wanted to be tested. She swore that she would never reveal the results to anyone else in her family, in particular her twin. One she was informed of the results—that there was a high probability that she would have HD—the information spread quickly throughout the entire family. This meant that the twin who did not want to know her genetic status was now faced with the unwelcome knowledge that she too would probably have the disease.[57]

Hayes herself had five brothers and eight nieces and nephews. Though she herself tested negative, one of her brothers already has symptoms of HD and another has tested positive; both already have some children.

Actually, the family can be a very complex factor in the question of testing. Hayes notes, "Many medical professionals have difficulty viewing genetic issues in a family context. . . . Most researchers cannot possibly know what it is like to grow up in a family haunted by a genetic disease. . . . " Some family issues will reappear when we discuss confidentiality.

•

Many people who are not absolutely opposed to testing as such—and even some people who are generally in favor of testing—argue that it should not be offered without counseling. This may seem paternalistic; but it is true that some of those who test positive will wish they hadn't taken the test and some may develop emotional problems, and that counseling can be helpful in such situations. As a matter of public policy, should people, through their private physicians, simply be allowed to "buy" their own test results, or should counseling be required?

A presidential commission on bioethics emphasized that counseling should be guaranteed: "A full range of prescreening and follow-up services . . . should be available before a program is introduced."[58] Note, though, that the recommendation here is for making counseling *available* rather than *mandatory*; it can also be noted that counseling is not always even made available, especially to people who are not covered by health insurance.

At the Salt Lake City conference in 1986, one scientist argued against paternalism: "I think we can trust people to make these decisions. I'm not so convinced we researchers should be dictating how the technology gets used."[59]

Confidentiality

An important issue in genetic testing is confidentiality, or privacy. As the power of government has grown, the right to privacy has seemed increasingly important—especially in recent years, as information and surveillance have been computerized. The presidential commission on bioethics mentioned above recommended that results of genetic tests be held confidential.

One reason for confidentiality has to do with medical coverage. Several national companies (such as Medical Information Bureau of Boston) inform insurance companies about applicants who are risks;[60] thus there is considerable concern that insurers will raise premiums for families at risk or simply refuse to cover such families—in fact, for bioethicists, this is the major issue. In the United States, the logic here is indeed alarming: genetics allows precise calculations of risks in family trees; an insurance company functions on the basis of such calculations; such a company exists to make money; the most profitable procedure for an insurer is to sell policies only to people with the best genetic health and either deny it to others or charge them a fortune for it. A related concern is that employers, to reduce their cost of insuring workers, will discriminate against people who represent genetic risks.

Not every country is subject to this logic, of course: some health systems work on the basis of sharing risk, and in such a system everyone pays premiums to help cover the costs for those who become sick. Where a risk-sharing system exists—as in England, Canada, Australia, and the state of Hawaii—insurers and employers have no motive to learn the results of genetic tests; but in the United States, there is a powerful incentive to have this information. Patients testing positive for a genetic disorder like HD can then be excluded from the insurer's risk pool, and from the employer's personnel.

In the case of HD, any child of a person with this disease has a 50 percent risk; though risk—or probability—varies depending on the specific genetic disorder, there is always some incentive for insurers and employers to discriminate. Thus when parents give an insurer genetic information about themselves, they are giving information that may also affect the availability and cost of medical insurance for their children. When a child tests positive for a genetic disorder and the parents file for insurance, they may not realize what they are revealing about themselves.

It is therefore crucial to control the distribution of test results: that is, to decide who should and should not receive them. Many large institutions, such as the military, universities, and large companies, "self-insure" themselves and pass their losses along to employees through increased premiums. Moreover, some employers may not keep test results confidential, especially if key employees are involved; consequently, a positive result may keep an executive off the fast track. Violation of confidentiality might also keep a physician out of a medical group, a student out of a university or graduate school, and so on. According to one respected geneticist:

> In 1997 it might be common for a physician to give patients a battery of DNA probe tests as part of an intake procedure. Such a panel of tests would likely include susceptibility markers. . . . Predictive testing would almost certainly appeal to the physician charged with performing the intake screens on prospective applicants to an HMO—or to General Motors for that matter— . . . and thereby enable the employer to take appropriate "remedial" measures—such as not employing them [job applicants] in the first place.[61]

Congress has considered a proposal, the Human Genome Privacy bill, to ban insurers from access (even paid access) to genetic tests. This is a forward-looking bill which (if enacted into law) would cover testing to prevent the birth of children with genetic diseases, and California has also considered a version of it. A task force of the Human Genome Project has recommended that:

> . . . all individual risk information be excluded from decisions about who gets insured, what they get insured for, and how much they get charged. We see no other practical, sustainable plan for health care coverage than community rating.[62]

It is fair to point out that insurance companies want genetic information in order to keep people who test positive from buying the best medical insurance and running up enormous costs for the insurer to cover—and that the Human Genome Project reveals some of the gaps in our national medical nonsystem. However, it is also fair to observe that in the face of genetic advances, insurance companies might find a role to play other than the bad guy. For example, they might encourage individuals who test positive for genetic diseases to insure themselves for future care through monthly premiums.

In this regard, too, it can be argued that insurance companies' expectations for genetic testing may be overblown. For one thing, genetic tests themselves may be quite expensive for an insurer: though some cost as little as $50, others may cost $1,000 or more.[63] Also, the tests may not ultimately represent a great saving for insurers: "No more than about 3 percent of all human diseases are caused by defects in a single gene, and none of those are major killers, as are heart disease and cancer."[64] The bioethicist Thomas Murray argues:

> Genetic determinism is one of those simpleminded errors that we were prone to commit when we thought genes linked to diseases in a kind of inevitable, ineluctable fashion.[65]

•

Issues of confidentiality also arise in the context of the family. One legal issue in this area is confidentiality versus the right to know. Courts have ruled that, even in a life-and-death situation, relatives cannot be compelled to be tested for compatibility as possible bone-marrow or organ donors; such legal precedents indicate that the courts will not force relatives to participate in genetic tests.

Another, subtler issue was suggested earlier with regard to HD: testing one member of a family has implications for other members. Any number of questions can arise as a result.

If a person has been tested early in life, could hiding the results from a spouse later be a ground for legal annulment? Does a prospective spouse have a right to know about the risk of a disorder like HD? Or does marrying "for better or worse" cover such questions?

Can one parent have a child tested in order to find out if the other parent is affected?

Suppose that a parent tests positive and refuses to tell his or her child. Suppose that a genetic counselor is aware of this. As the child approaches childbearing age, what should the counselor do? A counselor in such a situation might, of course, simply recommend general genetic tests, but suppose the child refuses. Would the child agree to testing if he or she knew that a parent was positive? If so, should the counselor violate the parent's confidentiality? To many people, the good of preventing another child with, say, HD outweighs the harm of violating privacy, especially where there is a strong sense that the affected parent had an obligation to reveal his or her disease to the family.

Catherine Hayes believes that:

> First and foremost, genetic testing must be viewed as a family issue, not an individual one. The person who enrolls in a testing program should be strongly

encouraged to involve other family members, within reason. Testing one member of a family will affect other members. Persons who refuse to involve their families may not have considered fully the consequences for other members or for themselves.[66]

Embryonic and Fetal Testing

In vitro fertilization, or IVF (which is discussed in Chapter 4), has had interesting implications for genetic testing. In IVF, several eggs are removed from the ovary, then fertilized with sperm in a petri dish; one or more (usually more) of the resulting preembryos are then implanted in the womb. Since each preembryo has its own genetic "DNA map," this map can be inspected for genetic defects before implantation, at the point when the preembryo consists of eight cells: one cell can be removed and its DNA can be replicated for genetic testing. (It is believed that removal of this single cell does not change the preembryo.) Any preembryo in which a defect is found need not be implanted.

It should be noted that this kind of single-cell testing of preembryos is possible only with IVF—and, in this regard, that IVF is expensive (costing about $5,000 to $8,000 per attempt), that it is typically not covered by insurance, and that it is successful in only about 14 percent of cases.

There are, moreover, issues about genetic testing of preembryos, and also about genetic testing of fetuses. Consider fetal testing for CF, for instance. One woman who had two children with CF underwent amniocentesis and was relieved to discover that her third child was at very little risk; she said, "I couldn't bear bringing another child into the world with cystic fibrosis,"[67] and in this she is probably typical of parents. On the other hand, drug treatments now allow about half of children with CF to live to age 30 (earlier, they rarely survived into their twenties),[68] and such improvements in life expectancy may continue. One New York physician who specializes in treating CF says that offering such a prenatal test is like telling people with CF, "It would have been better for all of us if you had not been born."[69] A similar argument is often made by some organizations of parents of children with Down syndrome and spina bifida.

A slippery-slope argument (of the kind discussed in Chapters 1 and 3) is sometimes made here. If embryonic or fetal screening is used to select against, say, Down syndrome or Tay Sachs disease, won't this create a slippery slope, eventually allowing parents to select against shortness, homosexuality, one sex or the other, or even unfashionable cosmetic traits? The bioethicist Arthur Caplan has predicted:

> I think the stance that we deal only with clear-cut disorders [in testing embryos] will last about five minutes. Once you can do that testing, the interests [of parents] will swamp my objections. The ability to choose the traits of your child will roar through with a whoosh.[70]

In one odd case, a deaf couple wanted to screen prenatally for deafness in order to select *for* a deaf child.[71]

There have also been some financial arguments about embryonic and fetal genetic screening; in fact, opponents of a single-payer system of health insurance use such an argument. Caplan is concerned that a single-payer system might "unjustly" influence decisions about procreating by establishing criteria for what kind of procreation is appropriate and inappropriate: "You can have a kid like that [with a genetic disease] if you want, but we're not paying." Paul Billings, a medical geneticist who is an activist against discrimination, thinks this could lead to a resurgence of eugenics: "Whether you want to dress it up in economic incentives, if you have to sell your house and go broke to have a child of a certain type, that's eugenics."[72]

UPDATE

Finding the Gene for HD

In 1983, when James Gusella discovered the marker for HD, he predicted that finding the gene itself would take 3 to 5 years, even though the effort could be concentrated on a small area on the upper tip of chromosome 4. As it happened, he had actually underestimated. Over the next 10 years, many false trails were followed and there were many tantalizing reports that researchers were on the edge of this discovery. Meanwhile, other researchers discovered the genes for other single-gene diseases: muscular dystrophy, cystic fibrosis, neurofibromatosis ("elephant man" disease), colon cancer, ataxia, and sickle-sell anemia.

In March of 1993, a very large international team of six genetic laboratories announced that the exact molecular location of the HD gene had finally been found.[73] This discovery made possible a genetic test for HD, which began to be offered in 1994. The discovery also explained why the search had been so difficult and had taken a decade: the tip of chromosome 4 is very densely packed with genes and rife with "recombination," a situation in which genetic material may "mutate" and be passed on in unconventional ways.

Nancy Wexler heard the news of the discovery of the HD gene as she was just about to walk out the door on her way to another expedition to South America. "I felt like I walked into a brick wall," she said. "I was stunned. I was ecstatic. I was wandering around like a zombie after that."[74]

Ecogenetics

Just as the search for the HD gene took longer and proved to be harder than expected, so early reports of discoveries of genetic causes of certain mental illnesses turned out to be premature. In particular, researchers retracted a claim made in 1987 linking manic-depression to a gene on the X chromosome.[75] By this time, earlier claims about genetic causes of schizophrenia and alcoholism had also been retracted. The implication seemed to be that genetic causes of psychiatric disorders would not be easily discovered, or that these disorders (unlike such physical disorders as CF and muscular dystrophy) might not even be caused by single genes. According to one leading researcher, common forms of mental illness may more probably be caused by from 3 to 5 genes acting together, possibly (though not necessarily) with environmental cofactors.[76]

Indeed, more geneticists in the future will study *ecogenetics*: situations in which a gene may not cause an affliction until a specific environmental agent is encountered. The paradigm is the gene for xeroderma pigmentosum, a fatal disease which produces hypersensitivity to ultraviolet light, thereby causing melanoma. Another example is a particular gene on chromosome 15 that turns compounds in cigarette smoke into carcinogens.[77] Another gene may turn charred meat into carcinogens but remain harmless if the person never eats such meat.

Ecogenetics may lead us to rethink some common assumptions about causes of disease. For example, two popular theories about cancer are that people cause themselves to develop it by exposing themselves to carcinogens (as by smoking and ingesting certain foods), and that it is caused by environmental carcinogens (such as toxic chemical emissions). Although these theories undoubtedly represent part of the truth, they do not explain why some people who are exposed to carcinogens remain free of cancer, or why some people who are *not* exposed develop cancer anyway. Ecogenetics is starting to provide an explanation: researchers are beginning to find that some people have genes which detoxify carcinogens rapidly, whereas other people do not.[78] Moreover, epidemiologists are now measuring "biological markers" such as enzyme levels, adducts, mutations in the P53 gene, and translocation of certain DNA sequences in white blood cells and are studying how well these markers predict various kinds of cancer.

Such findings may seem to imply only that some people who are exposed to carcinogens can do very little to prevent cancer, but actually the implications are much more hopeful. Ecogenetics suggests that presymptomatic testing may give some people a small "window" of real preventive control, if they can be tested, informed, and advised soon enough. Genetic conditions predisposing people to cancer may be detectable before exposure to carcinogens such as cigarette smoke, asbestos, and industrial chemicals; and if so, what was once a matter of "fate" can become controllable through public health measures and individual motivation. People who are genetically less able to detoxify the effects of secondhand cigarette smoke, for instance, may choose environments where their exposure is minimal.

Gene Therapy

Gene therapy has become an issue in the 1990s. There are two kinds of genetic therapy, though these are frequently confused. *Somatic therapy,* the less controversial kind, involves the somatic cells—that is, cells other than the sex (germ) cells. Somatic therapy attempts to treat a particular individual by altering disease-causing genetic material while leaving the patient otherwise the same; it is much like ordinary medical treatment. *Gametic* or *germ-cell therapy,* in contrast, alters the hereditary genetic material of an individual and thus affects only future generations, not the patient himself or herself: the patient's descendants will inherit altered genetic material. Gametic therapy (*not* somatic therapy) is sometimes called "genetic engineering," but this term is so drastically misleading that it should really be discarded.

At present, skeptics are afraid that geneticists do not know how to do gametic therapy without inadvertently causing problems as bad as the ones they want to eradicate. However, advocates of gametic therapy argue that some genetic diseases are so terrible that almost anything would be better. They also argue that dire predictions about gametic therapy sound much like the criticisms about IVF two decades ago and are probably no more warranted.

After 20 years of debate over the ethics of such intervention, and many years of genetic testing on animals, the first human gene transfer took place at the National Institutes of Health (NIH); this study prepared the way for the next development. Somatic gene therapy was first attempted on September 14, 1990—again at NIH—on a 4-year-old girl with adenosine adaminase deficiency (ADA), a fatal disease resulting from lack of an enzyme; scientists attempted to insert the genes causing this enzyme. There were no controls. Three years later, although the long-term prognosis was unclear, the girl (now age 7), who would have died without this intervention, was well enough to attend school.

On April 20, 1993, researchers inserted a deadened cold virus into the nose of a 23-year-old man with CF. This was a prototype for a study of somatic gene therapy in CF: the virus contained a healthy copy of the genetic material the patient lacked, and it was hoped that this somatic therapy would block the production of excess mucus. For the 30,000 Americans with CF, and the many heterozygotes who were silent carriers, this was the first real frontier of the new age of genetic therapy. In September 1994, however, the study was being reorganized because the results were not promising.

In the early 1990s, protocols for somatic gene therapy were approved for advanced melanoma and lethal pediatric hypercholesterolemia. The National Heart, Lung, and Blood Institute took $3 to $5 million away from heart surgery and put it into research on somatic gene therapy. One famous researcher has predicted, "The genetics revolution will change medicine more in the next 20 years than it has changed in the past 2,000."[79] Let us hope.

Hereditary Breast Cancer

In 1990, Mary Claire-King discovered that one form of breast cancer and ovarian cancer was inherited and was linked to a single gene. The development of a linkage test for hereditary—or *familial*—breast cancer, the later discovery of the gene itself, and some of the issues involved form interesting parallels and contrasts with the case of HD.

King called the still-undiscovered gene BRCA1: the abbreviation stands for "*b*reast *ca*ncer 1" or "first gene for breast cancer." In 1993, Barbara Biesecker traced a marker for BRCA1 through generations of women in several extended families and developed a linkage test for it.[80] With this test, women in families at risk could learn their chance of developing breast cancer.

Such a test was particularly important because of the prevalence of breast cancer. In the last 20 years, the number of women with age-specific breast cancer has risen 25 percent; and this figure will rise even more in the next decades, since the large generation of women born just after World War II are now over 40.[81] Breast cancer kills 50,000 American women each year, and it is estimated that at least 1 in 10 women alive today will develop breast cancer by age 80. The inherited form of breast cancer accounts for only about 5 percent of all cases, but when the prevalence figures are as high as these, 5 percent itself represents a very high number.

The linkage test for BRCA1 (unlike that for HD) had implications for treatment. Even with surgery and follow-up treatment for breast cancer, mortality remains high, because of metastasis and recurrence; but many women hope that if they are diagnosed early enough and remove all breast tissue, they can increase their chance of survival.[82] Ovarian cancer is at least as deadly as breast cancer; the intervention here is oophorectomy (removal of ovaries), sometimes as a preventive measure. Clearly, a test that could confine intervention to those cases where it was needed would be enormously useful.

For example, in one family involved in the BRCA1 linkage study, one of two sisters was worried about developing breast cancer and had planned to have her breasts removed as a preventive measure; she turned out to be negative and quickly canceled this plan. The other sister did not think she was at risk and had refused mammograms; she was shocked to find out that she had the BRCA1 marker. A thorough examination of her breasts found nothing, but a reexamination found a minuscule node, and 1 day later a biopsy determined that cancer had already begun; a radical mastectomy was performed. Without the linkage test, this women might not have discovered her cancer until many years later.

Obviously, presymptomatic testing for the BRCA1 marker can allow some intervention at a very early stage when necessary and allay the fears of women who are "certain" they have BRCA1 but actually do not. In the families in this study, all the women greatly appreciated the fact that what had seemed to be a mysterious, random turn of fate had become testable and predictable. Although the women who tested positive did not like the news, and although some who tested negative felt guilty, most thought it was better to have a way to know.

Still, a few women did not want to know; but it was difficult for them to remain in ignorance—as with HD, testing one family member had inevitable implications for others. Among the women of these extended families, confidentiality was very difficult to maintain. It was hard for any woman to hold out against the rest of her family and not discover her BRCA1 status: for example, once results are known for a grandmother and her granddaughter, the result for the intervening generation (the woman who is grandmother's daughter and the granddaughter's mother) may also be known. Or vice-versa: in testing a middle-aged woman for the BRCA1 marker, one is also telling her mother and her daughter about their likelihood of having BRCA1. As with HD, then, each individual needs to realize that her decision to be tested has consequences for other people.

With regard to knowing versus not knowing, it is interesting to note that in the BRCA1 linkage study, girls under 18 years of age were not tested; it was felt that such a test might be overwhelming for them. A registry was proposed for results of the BRCA1 linkage test, so that family members could provide information for their children without learning the results themselves.

Financial issues were also associated with BRCA1 linkage testing. For example, when one woman who tested positive decided to have a preventive radical mastectomy, her insurer thought she was being irrational and wouldn't pay for the surgery. She didn't want to tell the insurance company the real reason for her decision, because she was afraid the company would cancel her policy or raise her premiums, and perhaps even do the same for the rest of the family.

•

In the summer of 1994, scientists had been predicting for 2 years that the actual BRCA1 gene could be discovered any day. However, as with the HD gene, this discovery was proving more difficult than expected. The location had been narrowed down to part of chromosome 17, but this chromosome (like the part of chromosome 4 where HD was found) turned out to be very densely packed with genes; moreover, some of these genes are densely packed into each other, making it hard to figure out which gene does what or where one gene ends and another begins.

At this time, there was some controversy over how beneficial a screening test would actually be when the gene had been discovered. In July 1994, the *New York Times* reported:

> It is not clear what the benefits will be to a woman who finds out she is a carrier of the gene mutation linked to familial breast cancer. At this point, it appears that her options are limited. Surgeons can never be sure they have removed all the breast tissue, and any cells left behind retain their malignant potential. What is more, in some families, the altered form of BRCA1 seems to markedly increase the risk of ovarian cancer as well as breast cancer. Should these women be counseled to have their ovaries removed as well as their breasts? "At some point you wonder how many organ parts you have to cut out. This is a very harsh thing to even consider," says Mary Jo Ellis Kahn, who is helping to draft screening procedures for BRCA1.[83]

Some researchers suggested, though, that women who tested positive could be advised to avoid extra sources of estrogen, such as contraceptive pills and estrogen replacement therapy. Another speculative preventive measure was early pregnancy. One researcher, David Bolstein, suggested that a woman positive for BRCA1 might want to store some of her own bone marrow in case she developed cancer later, and so serve as her own donor.[84]

Also at this time, Anne Bowcock, a genetics researcher at the University of Texas Southwestern Medical Center in Dallas, cautioned that (as with CF), many different mutations in BRCA1 might cause breast cancer. Francis Collins, who was head of the Human Genome Project, also expressed a warning, saying that because information from screening tests can be "toxic," any new genetic screens "should be conceptualized as new drugs, subject to FDA testing before being used on the public."[85]

•

On September 15, 1994, the discovery of the BRCA1 gene was announced by a team led by Mark Skolnick at the University of Utah.[86] The gene was described as exceptionally long, as genes go, consisting of more than 100,000 base pairs of DNA (about 10 times larger than average).

When a gene is this large, the probability of mutations along the line of DNA increases dramatically, and each such mutation might or might not cause breast cancer. For this reason, a definitive genetic diagnostic test was said to be still at least 1 year away: developing such a test would be difficult because to rule out breast cancer, it would have to exclude every mutant variation. In such a test, moreover, although a positive result can be certain, the likelihood is that a negative result would be indeterminate and could be expressed only as a probability. (This would also be true of tests for many other genetic diseases, such as CF.)

The discovery of BRCA1 offered hope of a screening test only for women with hereditary breast and ovarian cancer—not for the 90 to 95 percent of women who develop nonfamilial breast cancer. Whether BRCA1 might have any role in these other, far more common forms was by no means clear; and the options for women who test positive for BRCA1 remained poor. Nevertheless, "scientists celebrated the discovery as an important step against a disease for which research findings had proceeded at barely a crawl."[87]

FURTHER READING

G. Annas and S. Elias, eds., *Gene Mapping: Using Law and Ethics as Guides*, Oxford University Press, New York, 1992.

Catherine Hayes, "Genetic Testing for HD—A Family Issue," *New England Journal of Medicine*, vol. 327, no. 20, 1993.

"The Human Genome Project: Where Will the Map Lead Us?" *Bioethics*, vol. 5, no. 3 (special issue), July 1991.

Daniel Kevles, *In the Name of Eugenics: Genetics and the Uses of Human Heredity*, Knopf, New York, 1985.

CHAPTER 17

AIDS and Mandatory Testing for HIV

Kimberly Bergalis

This chapter takes up the case of Kimberly Bergalis, a young woman who was infected with HIV by her dentist, David Acer, in 1987 and died of AIDS in 1991. Before she died, she had passionately urged mandatory testing of health care workers for HIV infection, and a number of ethical issues surrounding such involuntary testing will be discussed.

HIV, of course, stands for *human immunodeficiency virus,* the virus which, by infecting the immune system, eventually causes AIDS—*acquired immuno-deficiency syndrome.* The chapter will also provide a brief overview of AIDS, including some controversies about the disorder itself and research on possible treatments.

BACKGROUND: EPIDEMICS AND AIDS

Plagues, Fear, and Stigma: A Historical Perspective

Throughout human history, there has been something uniquely terrifying about epidemics. Undoubtedly the deadliest and most terrifying have been outbreaks of the bacterial disease that was known in the Middle Ages as the *black death;* its name has become a symbol for epidemics in general—*plague.*

Actually, there is more than one form of plague. The classic and more common form is *bubonic plague,* which is characterized by inflamed swellings of the lymphatic glands in the groin and armpit and was historically spread by fleas carried by rats on ships and on land: human beings were infected through flea bites. *Pneumonic plague* is essentially a complication of untreated bubonic plague, in which the lungs become involved; pneumonic plague is airborne and easily spread from person to person.[1]

There were deadly epidemics of bubonic and pneumonic plague before the great medieval outbreak of 1348, and epidemics have continued since then. Bubonic and pneumonic plague persisted in Europe until the end of the eighteenth century and still remain in parts of Asia, Africa, and South America; in the twentieth century, there were a number of outbreaks in the United States, including two famous episodes in San Francisco in 1900–1904 and again in 1907. In September 1994, hundreds of thousands of people fled the city of Surat in India when pneumonic plague broke out there.[2]

Bubonic plague is now known to be caused by the bacillus *Yersinia pestis,* and today it is treatable, in its early stages, with antibiotics. However, the specific causative agents remained unknown for 500 years; the virulent, respiratory mode of infection of pneumonic plague made discovery of its true cause more difficult and also made physicians reluctant to come near its victims. Untreated bubonic plague kills about 50 percent of its victims; untreated pneumonic plague kills all its victims—and before treatments existed, pneumonic plague was a common consequence of bubonic plague.

Bubonic plague was a ghastly sickness; writing about an epidemic in London during his own time, Daniel Defoe (1660–1731) said:

> It is scarce credible what dreadful cases happened in particular families every day. People in the rage of distemper, or in the torment of their swellings, which was indeed intolerable, running out of their own government, raving and distracted, and oftentimes laying violent hands upon themselves, throwing themselves out at their windows, shooting themselves. . . .[3]

During the centuries when the cause of bubonic plague remained unknown, there were various attempts to explain it. In the fourteenth century, one theory was that it came from a conjunction of Saturn, Mars, and Jupiter. Another theory was that it originated with earthquakes, which released sulfurous miasmas; there was a grain of truth in this, since miasmas do emanate from sewage, which attracts rats. Most early theories, however, were not naturalistic but supernatural: most people saw disease in general, and especially epidemics, as sent by some higher power. Some people saw plague as a curse of Satan. Others saw it as God's punishment for sin, a concept which can still be encountered today.

Those who saw plague as a punishment believed that human beings, as sinners, deserved no pity and had to atone through suffering. During the medieval epidemic, they often formed processions for atonement; in one of these, the pope himself crawled on his stomach through the mud, begging forgiveness for humanity's sins. People marched from town to town, whipping one another (and thereby spreading fleas). The historian Barbara Tuchman wrote:

> Organized groups of 200 to 300 . . . marched from city to city, stripped to the waist, scourging themselves with leather whips tipped with iron spikes until they bled. While they cried aloud to Christ and the Virgin for pity, and called upon God to "Spare us!" the watching townspeople sobbed and groaned in sympathy. These bands put on regular performances three times a day, twice in public in the church and a third in private. Organized under a lay Master for a stated period, usually 33 days to represent Christ's years on earth, the participants were required to pledge self-support at 4 pence a day or other fixed rate and to swear obedience to the Master. They were forbidden to bathe, shave, change their clothes, sleep in beds, talk or have intercourse with women without the Master's

permission. Evidently this was not withheld, since the flagellants were later charged with orgies in which whipping combined with sex.[4]

However, there was also a concomitant theory during the Middle Ages: that plague was brought by a group who would not admit their sins—the Jews. Blaming the Jews for plague satisfied the age-old need for scapegoats, and the Jews made a convenient scapegoat. They were easily identifiable by distinctive clothes and hairstyles; they were different, "other," un-Christian; and so they were persecuted. Jews were made to wear yellow cloth badges shaped like a horned head, symbolizing their collaboration with Satan. In the "Toledo conspiracy," several Jews who had left Toledo, in Spain, carrying small cloth bags (which actually contained the Torah, the first five books of the Old Testament) were tortured into confessing that they had poisoned the wells of European towns. Plague had broken out in some towns where Jews had never visited, but no one seemed concerned by this discrepancy. When processions of flagellants reached the Jewish quarters of cities, the inhabitants would often be killed. On January 9, 1349, in Basel (in Switzerland), several hundred Jews were burned on an island where they had been herded inside a wooden settlement. In Strasbourg (in what is now France), 2,000 Jews were taken to open graves, where—except for those few who converted to Christianity on the spot—all of them were killed.

Medicine was of little help in the medieval epidemic. Not only was medical technology lacking, of course; but physicians who tended the sick died themselves at a very high rate, sometimes approaching 80 percent. As a consequence, many physicians decided that their calling lay elsewhere.[5]

•

Certain epidemic diseases have aroused not only general terror but also loathing and hatred directed specifically at the victims. Three notorious examples are leprosy, cholera, and syphilis.

If anything has aroused as much panic as the black death, it is leprosy, now known as *Hansen's disease*. This is also a bacterial disease; the bacillus probably enters the body through the skin or mucosa and then incubates for 3 to 5 years (or more) before symptoms appear.[6] The form most commonly thought of in conjunction with the term *leprosy* is lepromatous leprosy, in which the cite of infection is the skin. This form of leprosy is characterized by lesions and is usually, though slowly, fatal.[7]

Historically, people have tended to envision leprosy as spreading like wildfire. Actually, it is transmissible only through many months of exposure, usually among family members, but because of its persistent image as a highly contagious disease—and as an "unclean" disease—its victims have been subject to extreme stigmatization. In medieval Europe, for example, lepers had to ring cowbells as they walked along, to warn others away; but this was one of the mildest measures taken against them. Lepers were banished from society, deprived of their rights and property, and treated as pariahs; some were even killed.

Stigmatization of victims also characterized three great cholera epidemics in the United States. *Cholera* (a disease marked by severe gastrointestinal symptoms, especially diarrhea) is bacterial in origin, like bubonic plague and Hansen's disease. During the epidemic of 1813, however, Americans blamed those who fell ill, describing the victims as wanton prostitutes, lazy blacks, the drunken Irish, and the dirty poor; sickness was seen as a result of low character. Ministers praised God for bringing down cholera to "cleanse the filth from society." These ministers also proposed a national day of fasting to cure the disease, and when President Andrew Jackson opposed the idea, they asked what else could be expected from such a well-known atheist.[8] God, it was believed, operated through disease to punish the guilty and through miracles to reward the virtuous, and this view was defended with no attention to logical consistency or even to the observable fact that some of the best people died and some of the worst were spared.

By the time of the cholera epidemic of 1849, the physician John Snow had already noted that in London, victims of cholera all seemed to live in one water system; there were no victims in another water system. He concluded, correctly, that cholera was spread by contaminated water, but his views had no effect on the American epidemic. In fact, when the wealthy fled to the countryside—and to clean water—this was taken as proof that the virtuous did not succumb to cholera.

By 1862, when the third great American cholera epidemic broke out, enlightened people were thinking in terms of public health measures, but they were not strong enough to put their ideas into action and therefore were unable to reduce the toll of death. Not until the 1890s, when the germ theory of disease was accepted by physicians and the first public health laws were passed, would cholera epidemics end in the United States.

Syphilis (discussed in Chapter 9) is also bacterial; it is spread congenitally as well as venereally, but because of its sexual transmission, it is a paradigm of a disease whose victims were themselves blamed for it: syphilitics were seen as having gotten what they deserved. In the early twentieth century, victims of syphilis were often treated as pariahs. In New York City, for instance, patients with syphilis were segregated on special wards so as to not infect others.[9]

HIV and AIDS

Fear and stigma have also characterized the outbreak of HIV infection and AIDS that began in the 1980s. The following sections will consider some significant aspects of this lethal disease, which is sometimes described as a contemporary "epidemic."

The spread of HIV in the United States   In June 1981, Centers for Disease Control (CDC) officially reported three cases of a mysterious "gay cancer," which was rumored to have killed dozens of other gay men.[10] It was first called *gay-related immune disorder* (GRID); 1 month later, 108 cases were reported, with 43 deaths.

At the end of 1981, CDC realized that GRID was a new epidemic disease, evidently viral, though the virus was unknown. CDC also realized that enormous funding would be needed to prevent the spread of this virus; but initially, the federal government and its medical representatives did very little.

GRID received spectacular attention in the mass media. Gay sex was postulated to be spreading some deadly disease; this conclusion was politically sensitive, however, since hostility to gay men was common and reporters were reluctant to say anything that might increase it. Within the gay community, although some courageous leaders did claim that sex in bathhouses was spreading the disease, most gay men dismissed that theory as puritanical. The idea that the disease might be sexually transmitted sounded too much like bigotry.

By contrast, there was less reluctance about this conclusion among many right-wing commentators. Almost immediately, the Reverend Jerry Falwell of Moral Majority blamed gays themselves for AIDS; other vocal members of the clergy blamed gay men for spreading the virus by "promiscuous sodomy." The national secretary of Moral Majority wrote, "If homosexuals are not stopped, they will in time infect the entire nation, and America will be destroyed—as entire civilizations have fallen in the past."[11] The head of the Southern Baptist Convention said that God had created AIDS to "indicate his displeasure with the homosexual lifestyle."[12] Monsignor Edward Clark of St. John's University in Queens, New York, claimed that, "If gay men would stop promiscuous sodomy, the AIDS virus would disappear from America."[13] Patrick Buchanan said, "The poor homosexuals—they have declared war upon nature, and now nature is exacting an awful retribution."[14] Falwell advocated shutting down bathhouses where gay men were engaging in multipartner sex; bathhouse owners then advertised in gay newspapers, calling for sexual freedom, and gay men saw Falwell's proposal not as compassionate but as hostile and vindictive.

In the autumn of 1981—3 months after the first report—CDC reported that babies of drug-addicted mothers in New York City had "gay cancer," and that it was also appearing in hemophiliacs. Suddenly, the terms GRID and "gay cancer" no longer seemed accurate, and in July 1982—1 year after the first cases—CDC formally designated the new disease *acquired immunodeficiency syndrome* (or *acquired immune deficiency syndrome)*; its acronym was AIDS.

In 1982, people diagnosed with AIDS, on average, were surviving for 2 years; no adult patient was known to have achieved prolonged remission. The incubation period was unknown, but CDC guessed that it could be as long as several years, and this implied that millions more people were already infected and might soon develop symptoms. Physicians in New York and California had already been seeing hundreds of new cases during 1981; in 1982, it was clear to CDC that AIDS was spreading.

Nevertheless, until about 1986–1987 the politically correct view of AIDS was that irrationality was running wild, that only 10 percent of those infected would actually get AIDS, and that the privacy of gays should be protected at all costs. Thereafter, however, things changed.

In June 1986, 100 epidemiologists, statisticians, researchers, and immunologists met at the Coolfront Conference Center in Berkeley Springs, West Virginia. The prestigious Institute of Medicine and the United States Public Health Service (USPHS) predicted then that by 1992, 179,000 Americans would have died from AIDS and 270,000 would either have died of AIDS or would have it. These projections have been accurate. They also predicted that at least 25 to 50 percent of those infected would develop AIDS. However, virologists were hoping for a "hump," beyond which the probability of actually developing AIDS after being infected would decrease, and this "hump" did not materialize; on the contrary, more and more of those infected would get AIDS—and it would eventually become apparent that given enough time, everyone who was infected might get AIDS.

By 1990, 60,000 young American men had died of AIDS, more than had died in Vietnam. By the beginning of 1994, nearly 400,000 cases of AIDS had been diagnosed in the United States; 200,000 victims had died; and it was estimated that another 500,000 to 1 million Americans were infected, of which nearly 100,000 were expected to develop AIDS each year. Unless a miraculous cure is found, close to 750,000 Americans will have AIDS or will have died of it by the year 2000.

Many celebrities have died of AIDS—even more than the general public may realize, since their obituaries have not always mentioned AIDS but have often given the cause of death simply as pneumonia or cancer. However, when the movie actor Rock Hudson died of AIDS in 1985, his illness was highly publicized, and since then there have been many famous cases. In the fall of 1991, it was announced that the basketball star Erwin "Magic" Johnson had repeatedly tested HIV-positive and was retiring. In 1992, the tennis star Arthur Ashe revealed that he had been infected through a blood transfusion during heart surgery many years before; he had learned that a newspaper was going to report this and so decided to make the announcement himself. Arthur Ashe was universally admired for his calm acceptance of his fate; he died in February 1993. Other famous people who died of AIDS include Perry Ellis and Halston (fashion designers), Jerry Smith (football player with the Washington Redskins), Roy Cohn (who had been Senator Joseph McCarthy's lawyer), Terry Nolan (a cofounder of the National Conservative Political Action Committee), Stuart McKinney (nine-term Congressman from Connecticut), Thomas Waddell (a gay physician and an Olympic athlete), Liberace (the pianist), Max Robinson (who had been the first African American television anchor), Amanda Blake (who had played "Miss Kitty" in the television series *Gunsmoke*), Brad Davis (who had starred in *Midnight Express*), Ian Charleson (who had starred in *Chariots of Fire*), Freddy Mercury (lead singer of the British rock group Queen), Keith Haring (the artist), and Michael Bennett (the Broadway director and choreographer).

A note on HIV worldwide   In the western world, areas with high rates of AIDS and HIV infection per capita include France, the Netherlands, Russia, eastern Europe, Canada, Mexico, Brazil, and especially Thailand (in its huge sex district).[15] In Africa and Asia, 12 million people are estimated to be HIV-infected. Some regions of central Africa have been devastated; ultimately, as many Africans may succumb to AIDS as have died in the worst famines. Infection is also likely to skyrocket in Asia, where traditional prudery may prevent open discussion about sex and therefore may hamper preventive efforts.

Transmission of HIV: Routes of infection   In 1992, the AIDS activist Larry Kramer wrote:

> When I first became aware of this disease, there were only 41 cases in the United States; now there are 12 million people infected with AIDS around the world;

within the next eight years this figure could rise to 40 million. From 41 to 40 million should be enough not only to cause a level of panic, but also to make everyone ask: how is this plague spreading so quickly? Indeed, 1 million [new] people worldwide were infected with the AIDS virus last year alone.[16]

Kramer's question about how AIDS spreads has been asked from the outset and has not yet been completely answered. Let's consider some important points about HIV transmission.

During the 1970s, people could fly anywhere in the world in less than 1 day—the trip between central Africa and North America, for instance, took only about 15 hours. In western countries, a new acceptance of drugs and sexuality during the 1960s and 1970s had led to multiple-partner sex in gay bathhouses and heterosexual sex clubs, many forms of heterosexual sex outside monogamous marriage, and sharing of the paraphernalia of intravenous (IV) drugs. To the scientists at CDC, these trends in travel and social behavior seemed significant for the transmission of a viral disease.

It also seemed significant that AIDS was apparently transmitted with special efficiency when people who used intravenous drugs shared needles and syringes in drug houses. A powdered drug was diluted with water, heated in a bottle-cap "cooker," and sucked into a syringe attached to a needle. Blood was withdrawn from the user's vein into the syringe, mixed with the drug, and then reinjected into the user. The same "works"—needle, syringe, and "cooker"—were rented by many customers and contaminated each time with small particles of blood; thus HIV was passed from one customer to the next. In some parts of the country, such drug houses were commonplace.[17]

HIV, or human immunodeficiency virus, the virus that causes AIDS, was identified in 1984. By now, scientists are fairly certain that people are infected with HIV through only three media: blood, semen, and breast milk. Blood seems to be particularly important; the more direct the blood-to-blood contact, the greater the likelihood of HIV transmission from an infected person to an uninfected person.

Outside the body, HIV is relatively fragile: to stay alive and be transmitted, it needs a warm, mucous, protective substance. This need for a protective envelope explains why HIV cannot be transmitted by, say, sitting where an infected person has sat or exchanging hugs with an infected person. Kissing is also unlikely to transmit HIV, unless both partners have open sores to begin with or engage in such rough kissing as to produce bleeding in both.

One theory is that virtually all sexual transmission of HIV involves some form of blood-to-blood transfer. In anal intercourse, HIV is transmitted very efficiently to the receiver: virus-infected semen can be absorbed into the blood by rupture of small blood vessels, and because the anus has no natural lubricants during sex, rupture of such vessels there is very likely. Actually, because anal tissue absorbs semen (just as it absorbs fluids in producing a dry stool), the virus may be introduced into the bloodstream even without the rupture of blood vessels. Heterosexuals who acquire HIV infection during intercourse may have engaged in some sexual activity that brings semen into contact with blood: vaginal sex may produce tears or infections of the vagina or uterus; also, syphilis and other sexually transmitted diseases (STDs) produce sores.

Heterosexual transmission of HIV has been hard to understand, however. What is most certain is that women who receive fluids from HIV-infected males can be infected, but how easy it is for an HIV-infected female to transmit the virus to an uninfected male during sex is uncertain; and some people who seemingly were infected during heterosexual intercourse may actually have contracted HIV nonsexually, in a directly blood-borne way such as IV drugs or transfusion. Still, as of 1994 the CDC AIDS hotline (1-800-342-AIDS) listed nearly 23,000 cases of AIDS (not just HIV infection) diagnosed between June 1981 and June 1993 that had apparently resulted from heterosexual intercourse, as determined by what people said when interviewed. The picture is not entirely clear, then, with regard to heterosexual transmission; but it seems only sensible for heterosexuals to take precautions and use a condom when a partner might be infected—the more so since condoms can also prevent transmission of far more common STDs such as chlamydia, venereal warts, syphilis, and gonorrhea.

HIV infection: The clinical course   HIV acts by attacking the immune system. The immune system is the body's defense system; when it is working properly, it wards off the common bacterial and viral infections to which we are all constantly exposed. American researchers believe that when the number of certain cells called *T4 lymphocytes* (or simply *T4 cells)* drops, the immune system is impaired: the lower the number of T4 cells, the worse the immune system is doing. This is controversial, however, and has not been accepted by European researchers.

Usually, a person who is infected with HIV first experiences a flu-like illness; then the virus often becomes inactive (dormant): like the spirochete which causes syphilis, HIV silently burrows into the body's systems, with few apparent outer symptoms. This asymptomatic period lasts on average 7 to 10 years.

At some point before the complete breakdown of the immune system, symptoms of midstage HIV infection appear. These may include swollen lymph nodes, night sweats, chronic fatigue, persistent coughing, and unexplained illness. Since symptoms in women often mimic other, more common problems, some physicians find it difficult to diagnose HIV infection in women.

In the last stage, HIV infection causes the immune system to deteriorate significantly. A normal person has a T4 count between 700 and 1,200; according to American researchers, this stage is marked by a T4 count below 200. At this point, the body may experience a special kind of infection called an *opportunistic infection.* The most common opportunistic infections affecting people with HIV are Kaposi's sarcoma, which produces large, black, mole-like patches on the skin; pneumocystis carinii pneumonia (PCP), an infection of the lungs that affects 50 percent of HIV-infected males; and cervical cancer in infected females.

When a person with HIV has an opportunistic infection and a T4 count below 200, he or she is officially said by CDC to have AIDS. Thus AIDS is perhaps best understood as the end point of an HIV infection that may have existed for 2 to 10 years. This end point is a lethal weakening of the immune system. It almost always leads to death within 5 years.[18]

Existing tests can examine the blood for the presence of antibodies to HIV. However, positive antibodies to HIV do not develop for about 6 weeks to 3 months, though almost everyone who is infected develops antibodies within 12 months. Because antibodies are not initially present, testing negative soon after exposure does not guarantee that a person has not contracted HIV infection; for more certainty, the test must be repeated later.

As with syphilis in 1929, the natural course of AIDS is not completely known. The best evidence for the cumulative course of HIV infection in the United States comes from the San Francisco cohort study, which has followed the clinical course in gay men who donated blood for a hepatitis vaccine in 1978.[19] In early 1985 the stored blood samples were subjected to a new test (ELISA, discussed below), and it was found that half to two-thirds of these gay men had been infected when they donated blood. (As a result of this finding, the projection of HIV infection in Americans jumped from 400,000 to 1.5 million; but this was controversial, and since the number of gay men in the United States was then overestimated, the projection was later revised downward to 1 million, and then to 600,000–800,000.[20]) The San Francisco cohort study gives the only known accurate baseline for the natural course of AIDS, and it indicates that HIV infection is not fatal as soon as many people believe. Eight years after being infected, about half of people with HIV still do not have AIDS; and 4 years after diagnosis, 80 percent of people with HIV are free of AIDS. About 5 percent of the San Francisco cohort are still asymptomatic today—a fact which makes them very interesting to researchers.

AIDS and the blood supply   In the summer of 1982, a few physicians at CDC began to worry about the possible transmission of AIDS—that is, of its causative agent—in donated blood. If AIDS was transmissible through blood transfusions, the supply of donor blood could be contaminated and might infect millions of recipients. In January 1983, representatives of American Red Cross, commercial blood banks, hemophiliacs, pharmaceutical companies, and gay activists met, but they could not agree to screen blood for AIDS.

Although donated blood is technically free to patients, blood banks are commercial operations; they make millions of dollars each year by charging for typing, storing, and transferring blood, and they pay substantial salaries to their executives. Blood banks were responsible for keeping the blood supply safe, but they were reluctant to reduce the supply by screening for AIDS; they also feared—correctly—that Americans would be reluctant to donate or receive blood if it was admitted that AIDS might be present in the blood supply.

To be precise, in 1982 blood could not have been screened for AIDS (or the causative agent, HIV), but it could have been tested for hepatitis. Because hepatitis and AIDS are both transmitted through sharing drugs and sex, testing all blood for hepatitis might have eliminated perhaps 80 percent of blood infected with what has since been identified as HIV. CDC proposed such screening but was argued down by the blood banks and by gay activists, who maintained that screening would be expensive (which it was), would "quarantine" the blood of gay donors, and would simply be giving in to hysteria because there was no hard proof that AIDS was caused by a virus or blood-borne.

In October 1982, Irwin Memorial, the blood bank serving all hospitals in San Francisco (and one of the largest blood banks in California), reported a proven case of AIDS transmitted by blood transfusion. In May 1983, after several such cases had been reported in hemophiliacs across the country, Stanford University, an hour's drive away from San Francisco, broke ranks: the blood bank at its own hospital started screening for hepatitis. Irwin Memorial did not, however.

In response to CDC's warning and Stanford's decision to screen blood, on July 17, 1983, Health and Human Services (HHS) Secretary Margaret Heckler, a political appointee of Ronald Reagan, held a national televised press conference and confidently said: "I want to assure the American people that the blood supply is 100 percent safe. . . . The blood supply is safe both for the hemophiliac who requires large transfusions and for the average citizen who might need it for surgery."[21] At the same time, Joseph Bove, a physician who was chairman of the Food and Drug Administration (FDA) committee overseeing blood transfusion, said that concern about contaminated blood was being created only by the "overreacting press."[22]

In fact, Heckler's assurance was shameful (so was her confident prediction—also in 1983—that a vaccine against AIDS would be available in 2 years). Today, as many as 80 percent of hemophiliacs have been infected with HIV from contaminated blood, many have AIDS, and many have died of AIDS. In France, a situation developed which was as bad or worse. Actions like these have helped make people skeptical about the political appointees who are presumably responsible for their health.

By March 1984, CDC had counted 73 cases of AIDS transmitted by transfusion, 24 in hemophiliacs. Joseph Bove, now a spokesman for the blood bank industry, continued to dismiss the fear of transfusion-transmitted AIDS as irrational: "More people are killed by bee stings."[23]

In May 1984, Irwin Memorial blood bank finally began screening its blood for hepatitis; this was 1 year after Stanford's hospital had begun its own screening. A new, inexpensive, easily performed test had been developed—ELISA (enzyme-linked immunosorbent assay), a simple screening assay. In anticipation of ELISA, Irwin Memorial began storing samples of donated blood so that it could later notify patients who had received infected blood.

By September 1984, CDC counted 269 cases of AIDS-related illness or death resulting from transfusions. Joseph Bove suddenly changed his view.

In January 1985, a woman in San Francisco who was both a prostitute and a user of IV drugs was diagnosed with HIV. This proof that some heterosexuals were infected created pressure for FDA and USPHS to release ELISA in February 1985, although gay groups, still fearing discrimination, opposed its release.

Irwin Memorial began using ELISA to screen blood almost immediately, in March 1985. The new test reduced the risk of transmission of AIDS through donated blood in San Francisco from 1 in 440 to 1 in 1 million.

In 1987, almost 3 years after beginning its screening process, Irwin Memorial estimated that at least 1 in 100 of its transfusions of blood had been infected between 1977 and 1983 (beginning in May 1984, as noted above, it had been keeping blood samples, and it had tested them when ELISA became available in

1985). It then notified 30,000 recipients that they should be tested, that it had already discovered 191 cases of HIV infection and 69 cases of AIDS, and that "a minimum of 2,000 infections would be discovered."[24] (It could not notify recipients who had become infected before May 1984, since no blood samples were kept until then.)

Also in 1987, in Los Angeles, Cedars-Sinai Hospital notified the parents of 900 babies who had received blood between 1980 and 1985 that these children should be tested for HIV.

In April of 1990, Ryan White, who had contracted HIV infection through a blood transfusion, died of AIDS at age 18. Ryan White's case had become famous; he was an "innocent" victim of AIDS, and after he died, Congress passed the Ryan White Act, providing funds for community-based organizations that fight AIDS.

In France in 1992, the former director of the National Center for Blood Transfusions was put on trial; he was accused of having knowingly put hemophiliacs at risk by using possibly contaminated blood for hospital transfusions. About 1,000 people in France (mostly hemophiliacs) had contracted HIV; 250 were dead by the time of the trial.

In 1993, Californians who had been infected as a result of the 1-year delay of ELISA sued for compensation. Irwin Memorial alone faced at least seven such suits.[25]

KIMBERLY BERGALIS: A CASE OF AIDS

Kimberly Bergalis, the eldest of three daughters of George and Anna Bergalis, was born in 1968 in Tamaqua, Pennsylvania. In 1978, the family moved to Florida, where George Bergalis worked as a finance director in Fort Pierce and Anna Bergalis worked as a public health nurse in Vero Beach, at a clinic specializing in STDs.

The Bergalises were a strict Catholic family, and Kimberly Bergalis was a National Honor Society student in high school. In 1985, she enrolled at the University of Florida at Gainesville. She had two boyfriends in college but remained a virgin; explaining her decision to wait, she said, "I wanted it to be special."[26] Her life as a college student focused on books and studying (she was a finance major), working as a waitress, and hanging out with a group of friends.

In December 1987, Kimberly Bergalis had two molars extracted by David Acer (pronounced "ACK-er"), a dentist in Jensen Beach, who was one of the "preferred providers" designated by her family's medical plan, CIGNA.[27]

Fifteen months later, in March 1989, Kimberly Bergalis suddenly developed a sore throat, ulcerated tonsils, and a fungal infection of the mouth called *oral thrush*. These are common early symptoms of HIV infection. In April 1989, she was first tested for HIV; the test was probably ELISA. The result was inconclusive, but since there seemed to be no risk factors for AIDS in her case, the more accurate but also more expensive Western blot test (discussed below) was not given.

In August 1989, Kimberly Bergalis graduated from the University of Florida.

By November 1989, despite the earlier negative test results, Anna Bergalis was afraid that her daughter did have AIDS. On January 24, 1990, Kimberly Bergalis—then 21 years old—tested positive for HIV infection. She was in her doctor's office with her sister Allison when she got the news. She said that the rest of the day was "strange."

As she describes it:

> My sister came with me, and we went to my mom's clinic and we told her. And then we drove to my dad's office down in Fort Pierce and we told him. And then we all just came home.
>
> . . . We had a lot of sadness in the beginning. Not so much anger, but it was like, "How could this be?" We would be sitting in the dining room and talking, and all of a sudden my mom would start choking and getting upset and she would have to walk out. And then I would start crying, and my dad would start crying.[28]

Like other cases of HIV infection, Kimberly Bergalis's case was reported to CDC. Since she did not fall into any of the risk groups, two CDC investigators and a state health worker began an investigation in February 1990. Over the next few months, these three investigators had many interviews with Kimberly Bergalis, her family, and her friends; they also tested the family and friends (voluntarily) for HIV, but all the results were negative.

Sometime during this investigation, Anna Bergalis suggested that David Acer, the dentist, might be the source of Kimberly's infection. In the spring of 1990, having ruled out other possible sources, CDC interviewed Acer; this was the only interview Acer granted (he saw his lawyer immediately after it), though he did agree to give a blood sample.

In July 1990, keeping both Kimberly Bergalis and Acer anonymous, CDC disclosed that it had a case "consistent with" transmission of HIV from a dentist to a patient. This disclosure was actually published on July 28;[29] however, the story was reported by Jane Pauley on *NBC Nightly News* the night before publication—July 27. In this broadcast, Pauley also reported that public health officials and medical and dental associations had been aware that Acer was treating patients while infected with HIV. Kimberly Bergalis and her family were watching, and this was the first time they learned that CDC had confirmed their suspicions about Acer, and that health officials had known about his infection and had let him continue to practice.

•

David Acer, a native of Cleveland, Ohio, had graduated from Ohio State University's dental school in 1974 and had served for 2 years at Hahn Air Base in what was then West Germany. He had returned to the United States in 1981 and set up private practice in Florida—in Jensen Beach, about 35 miles north of Palm Beach.

Little is known of Acer's private life, except that he was bisexual. Later, when some people who had been acquainted with him were interviewed by *AIDS Alert* (a publication respected for its adherence to facts), they said he had told them that he had engaged in sex with 100 to 150 partners between 1977 and 1987 and that he had frequented male prostitutes.[30] According to the *New York Times*, in

1986 Acer told his personal physician that he had as many as 150 sexual partners in the previous 10 years, and that during that time he had treated about 10 patients who may have been HIV-infected.[31]

In 1986, after seeing a physician in Fort Lauderdale under an assumed name, Acer learned that he was infected with HIV. In September 1987, he developed a small bump in his mouth, the first symptom of Kaposi's sarcoma.

He continued practicing dentistry, however, until July 1989, when he sold his practice and his equipment and retired to a secluded home where his mother and stepfather cared for him. When he gave up his practice, the records of many of his patients—except those with unpaid bills—were destroyed. (Later, since he had destroyed most of his records of noncurrent patients, the authorities would be unable to notify many patients who might be at risk.)

On September 4, 1990, at age 40, David Acer died of AIDS.

Acer had written a letter to his patients and submitted it to the local newspapers as a paid advertisement; as it happened, this letter was printed on the day he died. In the letter, he said that when he had first learned he was HIV-infected, he had consulted medical and dental officials about whether he should stop practicing dentistry. They had advised him, he said, that as long as he followed the strict guidelines set up by CDC to prevent HIV transmission, he could practice safely. At the time, neither the American Medical Association (AMA) nor the American Dental Association (ADA) had guidelines requiring him to inform his patients of his HIV infection.

•

In July 1990, a week after the *NBC Nightly News* story about Acer, Kimberly Bergalis went to a lawyer and initiated a suit against CIGNA Dental of Florida, which had referred most of Acer's patients to him through a group contract; and against Acer's malpractice insurer, CNA Insurance Company.

On September 7, 1990 (3 days after Acer's letter had been published), as part of the legal strategy in her suit against CIGNA Dental and CNA, Kimberly Bergalis went public. She startled the nation by announcing that there were no risk factors in her past life and that she must have been infected by Acer. She maintained that she had not had sexual relations with anyone, had never used drugs, and had never had a blood transfusion; and no evidence has ever surfaced to contradict any of these claims. She also said that she was bitter because state medical officials and ADA had known about Acer's HIV infection and had not informed her or his other patients.

By then, her condition was deteriorating: in February 1990, she had developed pneumocystis carinii pneumonia; thus she now had full-fledged AIDS.[32] In the spring of 1990, she had been treated with AZT (a drug, discussed later, which was believed to increase longevity) at the AIDS clinic of Jackson Memorial Hospital in Miami, Florida. During this treatment, her weight had dropped from 132 to 98 pounds; after that, she had stopped taking AZT. She had moved back to her parents' home, near the Intercoastal Waterway and about a block from the Atlantic Ocean. At one point, she had been so weak that she could barely crawl from her bed to the bathroom. Her thick, long hair, which had taken her 6 years to grow, would get caught under her elbows as she crawled; finally, her mother had cut it off.[33]

Kimberly Bergalis would soon become a national symbol for those who wanted to test all health professionals for HIV infection. She would be featured on the cover of *People* magazine and in articles in the *New York Times*, the *Wall Street Journal*, and *USA Today*. She would appear on *Larry King Live*, *48 Hours*, the *Oprah Winfrey Show*, and *A Current Affair*. But she was always conscious that the public never saw her as she had looked in high school or during her first years in college; it saw only what she herself now saw in the mirror and said she hardly recognized—an emaciated woman who had lost her hair.

•

At first, medical and dental officials refused to believe that Kimberly Bergalis had been infected by Acer, despite her own evidence and CDC's conclusion. Roy Schwartz, chairman of the AMA's AIDS Task Force, said, "I don't, by any stretch of the imagination, think that this link . . . is proven."[34] A chairman of the Florida Dental Board was even more adamant: CDC's conclusion, he said, "is not only difficult to believe, but it flies in the face of everything the CDC and other government authorities have told us"[35]—he was referring to CDC's earlier assurances that there was virtually no risk of transmission by an infected health professional.

As the investigation continued, also, Kimberly Bergalis's advanced symptoms misled the investigators: they thought she might have been infected years before, though it now appears that she was one of the minority of patients who progress very quickly from HIV infection to AIDS itself (a situation which seems to occur more in people infected from needles). There were widespread rumors that she must have had a "secret life" and must be lying to the public about her personal affairs. Anna Bergalis was also a subject of rumors and was accused of covering up the truth to protect her daughter's reputation.

Some of the investigators' findings were inconclusive or frankly puzzling. For one thing, Kimberly Bergalis herself recalled that Acer had worn gloves and a mask, and she could not recall any event in which blood might have been exchanged between them. When the investigators focused on the procedures Acer had used, they wanted to examine his drill bit, but it had been sold to another dentist and could not be traced. In the letter Acer wrote before he died, he swore that he had followed infection-control guidelines; and most of his assistants described him as a kind, gentle man who would never knowingly risk infecting a patient. However, some of his assistants said that he had treated sores in his own mouth with suction tubes and then reused the tubes on patients without properly sterilizing them. At one point, CDC even considered employing a psychologist specializing in the abnormal behavior of people leading secret lives to determine whether Acer might have deliberately infected his patients.

Blood testing was far more conclusive, however. Many of Acer's patients had come forward after the news reports, and by September 26, 1990, 371 of them had been voluntarily tested for HIV and 2 more had tested positive. Using a new technique called *DNA sequencing*, CDC tested Acer's blood sample and samples from Kimberly Bergalis and the other infected patients. The infected patients were found to share a virus identifying Acer's DNA as the source. CDC announced this result on January 17, 1991, and said that the accuracy of the match was 99.4 percent—that is, the chance of error was only about 0.6 percent.

On January 23, 1991, in an out-of-court settlement, Kimberly Bergalis received $1 million from CIGNA Dental and CNA Insurance Company.

•

Kimberly Bergalis's condition continued to worsen. In April 1991, she almost died from mycobacterium avium intracellulare, a resistant and often incurable form of tuberculosis which strikes when the immune system has been compromised; and near the end of the month she began to experience dementia and hallucinations. Sometime during that April, she wrote a letter to Nikki Economou, the local investigator for the public health service, though she never sent it. The letter said:

> AIDS has slowly destroyed me. Unless a cure is found, I will be another one of your statistics soon.
>
> . . . Who do I blame? Do I blame myself? I sure don't. I never used IV drugs, never slept with anyone and never had a blood transfusion. I blame Dr. Acer and every single one of you bastards. Anyone who knew Dr. Acer was infected and had full-blown AIDS and stood by not doing a damn thing about it. You are all just as guilty as he was. You've ruined my life and family's.
>
> . . . I have lived through the torturous acne that infested my face and neck—brought on by AZT. I have endured trips twice a week to Miami for three months only to receive painful IV injections. I've had blood transfusions. I've had a bone marrow biopsy. I cried my heart out from the pain.
>
> . . . It's nothing personal against you, Nikki—but I had a harder time forgiving your organization. I forgive—but my family will NEVER forget.

It ended with a postscript:

> P.S. If laws are not formed to provide protection, then my suffering and death are in vain.
>   I'm dying guys. Goodbye.[36]

In June of 1991, Kimberly Bergalis was again near death. She weighed less than 70 pounds and was lying, almost paralyzed, in a water bed; she could speak only in grunts and moans. At this point, with her permission, the letter she had written but not sent in April was printed in the *Miami Herald* and distributed by Associated Press (AP). By now, four of Acer's patients had been found to be infected with HIV.

In August 1991, Kimberly Bergalis rallied and began a period of relative normality. On October 24, she traveled by train to Washington, D.C.—the trip took 20 hours—and testified at a congressional hearing led by William Dannemeyer, a Representative from California. In her prepared remarks, which lasted only 15 seconds, she strongly urged passage of a federal law that would make it a felony for a physician or dentist with HIV to practice on a patient without revealing the infection.

In December 1991, she turned 23. Thereafter, she was no longer covered by her mother's medical insurance and became a Medicaid patient. On December 7, she set a goal of living until Christmas, but she was having increasing difficulty breathing.

Kimberly Bergalis died in her sleep at 3 A.M. on December 8, 1991, age 23.

•

During 1991 and early 1992, CDC was under intense pressure from the Bush administration and the public to establish tougher guidelines for HIV testing of health professionals and some kind of notification when such professionals were found to be infected. However, CDC was also under pressure from the medical and dental professions and the AIDS community, all of which thought that tougher guidelines would be overreacting.

In the autumn of 1991, the Senate did pass a bill like the one urged by Kimberly Bergalis—making it a felony for a physician or dentist with HIV not to reveal this to patients—but this bill was never passed by the House.

Within AMA and ADA, the majority has always resisted mandatory testing of members. However, by January of 1991, both AMA and ADA had issued new guidelines. According to these new guidelines, members with HIV infection should either inform their patients or not perform any invasive procedures.[37] At least, the next Acer could not claim that he had consulted his peers and had continued to practice as they had advised him.

ETHICAL ISSUES

Was Kimberly Bergalis right to urge mandatory testing for HIV? Should all health professionals be tested? Should everyone entering a hospital be tested? Every pregnant woman? Everyone entering the armed forces? In this section we will look at some of the issues related to mandatory testing.

Utilitarianism and Mandatory Testing

One way to approach the issue of mandatory testing is from the perspective of utilitarianism, the general position that the right action is the action which produces the greatest good for the greatest number of people. From this perspective, it is often argued that if mandatory testing will save lives, then we should do it. That is, the highest priority is given to saving human lives.

This position is certainly very strong with regard to the failure to test blood between 1983 and 1985—probably an indisputable instance of incorrect priorities. The argument can also be, and is, extended to the testing of people. According to some predictions, between 40,000 and 80,000 new cases of HIV will occur each year during the 1990s.[38] Do we not owe it to ourselves to identify those who could put us at risk?

There are two general arguments against this view. For one thing, it can be argued that even if mandatory testing will save lives, such testing violates other values: that it compromises civil liberties, specifically the right to privacy, and may subject those who are infected to prejudice. Second, it can be argued that mandatory testing is ineffective—that for one reason or another it will not save lives, or at least that it will not save enough lives to justify its use. In the following sections, we will look at several specific issues about mandatory testing.

Some of them have to do with the conflict between testing and values such as civil liberties, some with the effectiveness of testing, and some with both.

Testing, Homosexuality, and Prejudice

One major issue about mandatory testing for HIV is the effect it might have on homosexuals. In this regard, it is argued that voluntary testing would increase, and the need for mandatory testing would thus decrease, if homosexuals were not subject to legal and social sanctions. The ethical issue of testing for HIV is thus linked to issues of tolerance and acceptance of homosexuality.

If a man says he is gay, he may be legally fired from his job, evicted from rental housing, refused a mortgage, denied a loan, or denied admission to an organization or club. The same is true of a woman who says she is a lesbian. No state has passed a law banning such discrimination. Although the media have given much attention to homosexuality, many people are unaware that almost everywhere, homosexuals have no legal protection against the most elementary kinds of discrimination.

In 1988, in *Bowers v. Hardwick*, the United States Supreme Court allowed the state of Georgia to keep a law making forms of anal and oral intercourse between members of the same sex illegal; ironically, the law permitted exactly the same kind of sexual activities for heterosexuals. In 1992, an initiative was passed in Colorado (though a similar initiative was defeated in Oregon) banning cities there from passing laws forbidding discrimination against gay people in housing and employment. Advocates of the statute argued that banning discrimination was a first step toward acceptance of a homosexual "lifestyle" and even toward affirmative action for gays and lesbians. In 1994, the Colorado Supreme Court overturned the statute, but even so, its original passage remains significant.

It is in this context, then, that we need to consider the question of mandatory testing for HIV. Since such legislation obviously reflects hostility and prejudice against homosexuals, it is reasonable to ask whether legislation mandating testing does not also reflect hostility and prejudice. In other words, what are the real motives for mandatory testing? Is society really trying to control a deadly disease, or is it trying to ferret out and punish gay people? Is society trying to "purify" itself by getting rid of a deviant minority?[39] Questions like these cannot simply be dismissed as paranoia: as we have seen, statements by many public figures about homosexuals and homosexuality seem to be full of prejudice and even hatred.

Is there a more enlightened view? Homosexuality has evidently existed in every human culture, ancient and modern, and in some cultures it has been completely accepted. In ancient Greece, for instance, bisexuality was popular, and many men preferred male lovers. Through the ages, many famous people have been homosexual or bisexual, including Socrates, several Roman emperors (such as Hadrian), Frederick the Great of Prussia, the playwright Tennessee Williams, and the novelist Gore Vidal,[40] to name only a very few. It is true that Christianity vigorously attacked homosexuality after the twelfth century, but earlier it was much more tolerant.[41]

Since homosexuality has been so constant, it is not surprising that researchers have recently postulated a genetic basis.[42] Many right-wing religious leaders still claim that homosexuality is a matter of choice, not biology, but there is growing evidence against them. The gay philosopher Richard Mohr argues that the experience of most gay males is not choosing a lifestyle but resisting a gradual discovery, and he asks why anyone would choose to be gay or lesbian in a society which devalues and hates such people; the overall picture, he concludes, is of a minority coming to terms with genetic fate, against overwhelming pressure to deny it.[43] There is considerable evidence for Mohr's view: almost without exception, gay men do report a struggle—a feeling that they are going against the expectations of their families and their society.

Whether or not homosexuality is genetic, however, an obvious moral argument for a more enlightened attitude toward it is John Stuart Mill's principle of harm. This principle implies that homosexuality is not immoral in itself: what is immoral, for Mill, is hurting others, and thus any form of sex between consenting adults would not be immoral. To put this another way, if a certain form of sex involves hurting someone else without his or her consent, then harm has been done; what is wrong is the harm itself, not the context in which it takes place. Mill concluded, on the basis of his principle of harm, that personal life is not the business of government. Thus, since sexuality involves private life, it should not be the business of government—it should not concern legislators, the police, or judges.

Testing and Privacy

Privacy is highly valued. In the United States, the term *right to privacy* encompasses our right to live our personal lives as we see fit, to control what may be done to our own bodies, and to limit what information others may obtain about our personal affairs. Not every country assumes a right to privacy, and the existence of this right in the United States is one reason why many people want to immigrate here.

Privacy is particularly important in medicine, which must deal with intimate details of patients's lives and with patients' ultimate values. When we consult a physician, we may need to expose our genitals; we may need to reveal that we drink too much or take illegal drugs; we may need to reveal our sexual practices. *Medical privacy* confines such revelations to physician and patient, and anything that endangers this privacy can destroy lives.

Mandatory testing for HIV, however, runs the risk of violating medical privacy, since in many cases there is nothing to be gained from mandatory testing if the results can be kept confidential. In such cases, mandatory testing can violate our privacy twice—first by testing us against our will, and then by reporting positive results. There is also a slippery-slope argument here: if mandatory testing is allowed for HIV infection, why not for drug abuse, alcoholism, or genetic diseases?

It can be argued that if there are large and proven benefits from mandatory testing, it should be allowed, despite any violations of medical privacy or confidentiality. But not everyone would agree that mandatory testing is justifiable even if it offers benefits; furthermore, its benefits are not easy to substantiate.

Testing as Punitive

One important issue about mandatory testing is whether it constitutes punishment. Most people who advocate mandatory testing maintain that it is not intended as punishment; but whatever its intention, mandatory testing can certainly have punitive effects.

For instance, some states and institutions requiring mandatory testing also require mandatory reporting of results; insurers and employers may then learn of the results, and people who test positive may lose their medical coverage and their jobs. This possibility is real: especially when employers are "self-insured" (i.e., when they pay all medical costs themselves), an employee may be fired for testing positive; also, according to a recent decision by the United States Supreme Court, a company may legally exclude coverage for AIDS from its medical insurance policy—even retroactively.[44]

Moreover, learning that one has tested positive can itself be punitive. Too often, mandatory testing simply "dumps" bad news on people who are found to be infected; infected people are often informed in very cruel ways by health workers who dislike or disapprove of homosexuals or drug users. Even health workers whose attitude is more open may feel uncomfortable about revealing bad news or talking to someone who is infected, or they may simply not have the time to be sensitive or responsive.

Follow-Ups to Testing: Theory and Practice

It is important to reemphasize that testing for HIV has little or no *intrinsic* value: that is, testing is said to be valuable not in and of itself but because it can have valuable consequences. Simply identifying infected people is not very useful; we need to think about what, if anything, is going to happen with infected people.

This section discusses some possible follow-ups to testing. Not all of these are feasible in the American context, though—and even feasibility does not guarantee efficacy.

Voluntary restraint   One possible follow-up to testing for HIV is simply *restraint,* as an individual, uncoerced decision. That is, a person who tests positive may decide to forgo activities which would place others at risk. In today's context, in fact, this is probably the major potential consequence of testing: society is largely dependent on HIV-infected people themselves to refrain from unsafe behavior.

Undeniably, some people who test positive for HIV will practice self-restraint. Moreover, to some extent this effect can be augmented if those who come into contact with infected people insist on safe practices, and if counseling is provided to those infected. However, there are obvious reasons why voluntary restraint is not a dependable consequence of testing.

For one thing, we have to acknowledge that in many situations it is probably unrealistic to rely on voluntary restraint. Consider, for example, premarital testing for HIV—an idea that was tried out in Illinois and Louisiana beginning on January 1, 1988; failed;[45] and was abandoned (in Louisiana, the program was stopped in mid-1989; in Illinois, at the end of 1989). Premarital testing was meant to prevent, or reduce, the spread of HIV; but it had not been thought through: the only way it could achieve such an effect was by voluntary restraint, which in this situation was both unlikely and insufficient. One assumption of the premarital testing program seemed to be that if one member of an engaged couple tested positive, the marriage would be called off so that the other member would not be infected. That assumption, however, was contrary to experience:[46] in today's society, most couples who are about to be married are already sleeping together; thus if one partner is infected, both may be. Another assumption seemed to be that if a marriage was called off because one partner was infected, the infected person would simply stop any risky behavior, remaining celibate or not sharing drug apparatus. That too was unrealistic.

Two important reasons not to depend on voluntary restraint are that people change sexual or drug-dependent behavior slowly (if at all), even with the best, most professional counseling; and that there is a shortage of funds for such counseling: little new funding has been provided for drug counseling, and even less for counseling about sexual practices. In order for counseling to change behavior, there must be more than a single 1-hour session explaining "prevention"; months or even years of counseling may be needed. As the situation now stands, perhaps 90 percent of those who test positive may never get the extensive counseling that is a prerequisite for voluntary restraint.

An interesting consideration with regard to voluntary restraint is whether *mandatory* testing might actually work against self-restraint. In other words, can forcing a person to take a test elicit the desired response? Can we achieve a voluntary practice through an involuntary procedure?

As we have seen, mandatory testing often has a punitive effect. If society then asks the infected person to "do the right thing" and practice voluntary restraint, isn't this morally contradictory? Isn't it inconsistent to force people to be tested, subject them to discrimination and hardship if they test positive, and then turn around and ask them to "be good"? If the major argument we can offer such a person is a moral one—that he or she "should" care about other people's life and health—then we must be careful about the context in which we make this argument. In other words, when we want to use moral persuasion, we ourselves must be standing on firm moral ground. Does mandatory testing, which is coercive and violates privacy, represent firm moral ground? If not, can it bring about voluntary restraint?

Contact tracing   One concrete way in which lives could be saved after testing is by contact tracing, a time-honored technique for controlling the spread of STDs. Initially, public health authorities made HIV infection an exception to their normal procedures of contact tracing, because of concerns about prejudice and discrimination—contact tracing, it was feared, might lead to revelations that could in turn lead to loss of a job or loss of medical coverage (at a time when coverage was most needed). However, in the second decade of AIDS, this policy of "HIV exceptionalism" was reversed.[47]

Once a person with HIV infection is identified, he or she is interviewed by a sympathetic counselor (who needs special talents and training) and asked to identify all past sexual partners and people who have shared drug apparatus. A large number of people do in fact reveal such contacts. The infected person is given a few days to inform his or her contacts personally; then, a public health officer also informs each of these contacts.

In one study in South Carolina:

> Only 12 of the 132 notified partners had suspected that they might have been exposed to HIV. When asked if the health department had done the right thing in telling them about their exposure, 87% responded "yes." 92% said the health department should continue notifying partners at risk.[48]

In another study, 88 percent of regular partners reported within the past 12 months were located and 29 percent were found to be HIV-infected.[49]

Contact tracing can help uninfected contacts remain uninfected: some of these people would have continued risky behaviors with the infected person and thus would eventually have become infected too. Moreover, contact tracing can help many infected contacts act more safely—and this can reduce the spread of infection. In some states, knowingly putting another person at risk of HIV infection is considered a crime; one man in Louisiana has already been convicted and sent to jail for putting a woman at risk.[50]

Moreover, for both infected and uninfected contacts, tracing can overcome denial. Some people who are at considerable risk of HIV infection are in denial—they simply would rather not know. Contact tracing can break though and motivate people to protect their own well-being and that of others.

Therapy   Another possible follow-up to testing for HIV is therapy for those who test positive. Is this a practical option?

During the first years of AIDS, one reason why those at risk of infection resisted testing was simply that no therapy existed. That situation changed in 1987, when one study seemed to indicate that zidovudine—an antiviral agent which is best known by its trade name, Azidothymidine, or AZT—increased longevity in AIDS patients.[51] A follow-up study in 1992 seemed to support this finding.[52] Apparently, AZT slowed down the effects of HIV or at least put the virus into homeostasis.

These studies caused some opponents of mandatory testing to change their minds: it was now argued that we could test people against their will, identify those who were infected, treat them with AZT, and thus help them live longer. Moreover, it was widely assumed that the effect of AZT was to make HIV infection similar to latent syphilis, in which the infecting spirochetes become dormant for years or even decades. If so, AZT might be given very early, when patients were asymptomatic, and thus these patients might survive even longer.

In 1993, however, a very large European study (the *Concorde study*) cast doubt on the earlier findings and assumptions: it found no benefit from taking AZT.[53] In the United States, AZT was widely held to benefit HIV-infected people because it improved their T4-cell counts; but researchers at Oxford had long been skeptical about considering T4-cell counts as indicative of the health of the immune system, and they were also skeptical about the assumption that raising the number of T4 cells would strengthen the immune system of a person infected with HIV. These English researchers also had misgivings about the American "fast-track" approach to approval for anti-AIDS drugs.

American physicians specializing in AIDS had mixed reactions to the British study. Some continued prescribing AZT and felt that its placebo effect alone was therapeutic. Others began to wonder whether, for some infected patients, no treatment at all might be the best course (a consideration which recalls the arguments, during the era before penicillin, about heavy-metal treatment for syphilis versus no treatment).

In 1994, the Concorde study was followed by more discouraging results about AZT.[54] Evidence was mounting that AZT did not increase longevity in HIV infection;[55] moreover, although AZT did decrease symptoms in some patients, it had proved to be very toxic to others. As much as AIDS activists wanted to rush scientific discovery, nature was proving reluctant; and some people began to think that the activists had intimidated American researchers into believing in AZT. The disappointing performance of AZT obviously undermines the argument that mandatory testing is justifiable because it can benefit patients.

Protection of fetuses   Although AZT now seems unpromising for infected people themselves, there is hard clinical evidence that it does reduce the transmission of HIV from a pregnant woman to a fetus. Thus another possibility is mandatory testing of pregnant women, with administration of AZT to those who test positive as a follow-up.

In 1994, there were renewed calls for mandatory testing during pregnancy, and a bill was introduced in Florida. This bill was defeated, however, because of concerns about confidentiality, racism, and practical matters: its opponents argued that women who tested positive might lose their jobs or medical coverage, that 75 percent of HIV-infected pregnant women were nonwhite, that women who might be HIV-positive would avoid clinics where testing was required, and that mandatory testing compromised women's reproductive freedom. It was also pointed out that skilled counselors in Miami were getting about 90 percent of women at risk to be tested voluntarily.

Furthermore, since AZT is toxic to some HIV-infected patients, there was concern about toxicity to fetuses. In this regard, it can be noted that about 60 percent of fetuses of HIV-infected mothers will not contract the infection (although, having inherited the mother's antibodies, a fetus may test positive for months). Thus if AZT is at all toxic to the fetus, as many as 60 percent of fetuses may be needlessly put at risk of harm.[56]

Quarantine   Another possible follow-up to testing is quarantine of those found to be infected, and such a program actually has been instituted in Cuba.

In 1986, Cuba began mandatory screening of people likely to be HIV-infected, who constituted one-fourth of the population.[57] Those who tested positive were identified to their families, neighbors, and coworkers and were strongly urged to go to sanatoriums; married people were told that they could take their spouses. This program was mandatory: if people did not go voluntarily, they went involuntarily. Moreover, because it is not clear if HIV ever becomes noninfectious, this mandatory quarantine was of indefinite duration. Thus until there is a safe, cheap vaccine against HIV, the Cuban quarantine might amount to a life sentence.

The Cuban program seems drastic; on the other hand, it also seems to be working. Many Caribbean countries, such as Haiti, have tens of thousands of cases of AIDS and even more cases of HIV infection; in fact, there may be 250,000 people with HIV infection in the Caribbean. In contrast, in Cuba, where nearly 3 million people have been tested, only 259 were HIV-infected in 1989, all of whom were then quarantined. Thus quarantine has nearly stopped the spread of AIDS in Cuba—something that has been achieved in no other country in the world.

Could such a quarantine system be used in the United States? Should it be used? There are both practical and philosophical arguments against the idea.

To begin with, there are logistical problems. As many as 1 million Americans may be infected with HIV. Where would they be quarantined? Under what conditions would they be quarantined? How would they be guarded, for example? Would visitors be allowed?

The major philosophical argument against quarantine is that, by incarcerating innocent people for the sake of public health, it violates our right to liberty—our right to live as we choose unless we have been convicted of a crime. Cuba, of course, is a dictatorship; in the United States, such a quarantine would almost certainly be found unconstitutional.

Testing and Health Professionals

With regard to health professionals, the question of mandatory testing has two aspects. First, should health professionals be tested to protect patients? This, of course, was the major issue raised by the Kimberly Bergalis case. Second, should patients be tested to protect health workers?

Protecting patients   When people argued that the privacy of medical workers should be protected and that the risk of infection from such workers was slight, Kimberly Bergalis retorted angrily, "The risks are always too high for the patient who turns out to be that 1 in a million."[58] Indeed, her case created intense pressure to test physicians, dentists, and nurses who treat patients; and to many people, the argument for mandatory testing is strongest in this situation. CDC found that through March 1993, there were 10,122 cases of AIDS among health care workers in the United States.[59] Given such statistics, don't patients have a right to know the HIV status of their attendants?

The great majority of the pubic believes that patients have a right to know the HIV status of physicians, dentists, and nurses. Among surgeons, there has been considerable sympathy with this view; in one study, 88 percent of surgeons agreed that patients have a right to know the HIV status of a surgeon and also said that they themselves would consent to being tested if a patient requested it.[60]

Moreover, in Acer's case the possibility was raised that he had deliberately infected his patients. Though it was not clear what his motive might have been, he might have felt, for example, that society would not mobilize its resources to find a cure for AIDS until ordinary heterosexuals became infected; or he might have been a psychopath—a Dr. Jekyll and Mr. Hyde. All this was highly speculative, but it was argued that psychotic infected professionals might exist and would represent even more potential for harm to patients.

There are counterarguments, however. One such argument is that the fear of infection by medical professionals may not be rational. In CDC's major "look back" study, for example, more than 19,000 patients of HIV-infected health care workers were examined, and none were found to be infected.[61]

A second counterargument is based on what is known as the *principle of proportionality*. Of the 4.5 million health-care workers in the United States, perhaps 1 percent, or 50,000, are infected, though not all of them are in direct contact with patients. Identifying these people would not only be a major project in terms of time, effort, and money; it would also be a significant evil, since some of them would probably lose their jobs. According to the principle of proportionality, then, testing health workers would be justifiable only if it would produce some correspondingly significant good. Since preventing infection by health workers is the intended "good" here, we would need to be sure that patients can easily be infected accidentally in this way. However, on this argument, the statistics do not provide any such certainty.

A third counterargument has to do with the consequences of testing health professionals: what is to be done after testing? CDC recommends informing patients of a physician, dentist, or nurse who has tested positive, but not everyone considers this practical. In New York, for example, where the incidence of HIV infection is very high, patients are not informed; officials there believe that such notification would discourage health workers from being tested, since physicians and dentists are afraid their practices will be destroyed if they are required to inform their patients.[62] Instead, New York requires infected health workers to take extra training in the latest sterilization techniques, but this is not what most of the public has in mind in demanding that health workers be tested.

A fourth argument addresses the possibility of psychopathic medical workers, pointing out that no public health system of testing can protect people against psychopathology—whether in medicine or at the post office.

A fifth argument is that the cost of testing health workers is simply too high in comparison with the benefits that might be achieved. This is discussed in more detail below, as part of the problem of costs of testing in general.

Protecting health workers   The second aspect of testing with regard to health professionals is whether patients should be tested for HIV before invasive procedures, to protect health workers from infection. Often, the reason given for testing patients before invasive procedures is to protect the patient, but the real motive may be that health care workers do not want to expose themselves to infection.

Fear of AIDS has certainly changed how physicians, dentists, and nurses work: everyone "gloves up" all the time, and—according to CDC's recommendations—everyone is supposed to act "as if" all patients were infected. It is argued, though, that these precautions are not entirely realistic and thus may not provide enough protection. Medical professionals are often overworked, hurried, and stressed-out. In New York City, for instance, there is a critical shortage of nurses, and one nurse may now have to do the work that was once done by three; to take another example, can a resident who has gone without sleep for 24 hours really observe all the necessary precautions? Testing patients, it is held, would at least make nurses, residents, and others aware of which patients were infected.

CDC estimates that since the first AIDS cases in 1981, about 100 health care workers, mostly laboratory technicians and nurses, have become HIV-infected;[63] of these, 40 were from a known, specific incident. These figures may not seem very high, but most laypeople cannot realize how much they themselves would fear infection if they found themselves in the position of medical workers dealing with patients who might be HIV-positive or might actually have AIDS. Between 1983 and 1990, the number of medical school graduates who wanted to do their residency in New York City, where (as mentioned above) AIDS and HIV infection are very prevalent, dropped 30 percent.[64] Abigail Zuger has written the following about her residency at Bellevue in New York—and this was in 1986, when the AIDS caseload was low by present standards:

> In my three years at Bellevue, AIDS grew to engulf the hospital; it dominated my medical training, and now it dominates my memories. . . .
>
> I remember the weekend when no patient in the intensive care unit was over the age of forty. I remember the intern who tearfully refused to come to the emergency room to see the fourth AIDS patient I had admitted to her in as many hours. She never did meet him; he died before she calmed down. I remember the meal trays, stacked precisely three and four deep, undistributed, outside the closed doors of the private rooms on one of the medical wards. And I remember Nilda, a drug addict who, like many others at the time, had a fever we couldn't explain; one morning, in my usual state of exhaustion, I jammed the needle I had just used to draw her blood deep into my thumb.[65]

The accident Zuger mentions—sticking herself with possibly infected blood—leads us to another argument for testing patients. In 1988, a typical resident in internal medicine New York City cared for 30 HIV-infected patients and was stuck at least once with blood known to be HIV-positive. Do workers who are stuck tell their sexual partners about it? Do they remain celibate until they test negative for 1 year?

Again, though, there are counterarguments. For one thing, the actual risk to physicians is unclear. In another CDC "look back" study of 3,420 orthopedic surgeons, for instance, none had become infected on the job as of 1991.[66] One study of residents found that only 14 percent of those in internal medicine had ever stuck themselves with HIV-infected blood.[67] Another study predicted that only 1 in 10 medical students and residents in Los Angeles teaching hospitals would be stuck by HIV-infected blood in a typical year (though the risk was higher in surgery).[68] Moreover, being stuck with infected blood does not necessarily lead to infection: in fact, the chance of infection is very, very small.

Another counterargument here is that testing patients may not be rational in comparison with other kinds of testing. The physicians who wrote one article along these lines emphasized that for a heterosexual whose partner may or may not be HIV-positive, "safer" sex with a condom reduces the risk of infection to about the same magnitude as the risk incurred by a surgeon whose patient may or may not be positive. These authors reasoned:

> If the risks of sexual and surgical contact are of the same order of magnitude, why should we eschew screening in low-risk heterosexual populations but recommend it for low-risk patients awaiting surgery? Arguing that we should screen low-risk patients before surgery implies that preventing HIV infection in a physician, a nurse, or a technician is more important than preventing the infection in others. Is that argument either rational or ethical? Hepatitis B virus is at least an order of magnitude more prevalent and more infectious than HIV, yet we do not routinely screen patients for hepatitis B virus. How many false-positive results are tolerable to protect one health-care worker? What is the joint false-positive rate for HIV testing of hospitalized patients? How many patients should be denied adequate medical care to prevent one hospital-acquired infection?[69]

We can also think this issue through for ourselves, by considering some well-known facts. HIV typically takes 5 to 10 years to break down the immune system (people who develop AIDS very quickly, as Kimberly Bergalis did, are in the minority). Since the first cases of AIDS appeared in 1981, we can infer that people had became infected perhaps as early as 1979, or even long before that. Medical workers did not begin taking precautions universally until the mid-1980s. In San Francisco, it was estimated that over two-thirds of the gay men who lived there during the 1970s were HIV-infected, and many of them have been to see physicians over the last decade. If HIV were easily transmissible, and frequently transmitted, through occupational accidents, there should be hundreds or even thousands of unexplained cases of HIV infection among medical professionals who worked in San Francisco between 1979 and 1985. But there are not—in fact, there are hardly any at all. Moreover, the same is true in other areas where the incidence of HIV infection and AIDS is high.

Practical Problems with Testing

Whether or not mandatory testing for HIV seems morally justified, there are at least two kinds of problems which need to be considered in deciding whether it is practically justifiable—technical difficulties and costs.

False positives and false negatives   Two technical problems present obstacles to mandatory testing: *false positives* and delayed antibody response, or *false negatives*.

ELISA is the main test for HIV. If it is positive, it is repeated; if it is again positive, a different test is performed—the *Western blot test*. The Western blot test is slower and more expensive than ELISA, but it is more accurate. Both ELISA and the Western blot test were designed for high sensitivity: that is, the "net" of these tests was made as wide as possible, so that very few people with HIV would escape detection. When a test is designed in this way, false positives are more likely; and in a general population, about 1 result in 135,000 will be repeatedly but falsely positive on two ELISA tests and also on the subsequent Western blot test.[70]

The accuracy of any test is a function of the true incidence of the whatever is being tested for in a population. With ELISA, a positive result is much more likely to be accurate in a high-risk population where, say, 1 person in 20 is infected than in a low-risk population where only 1 in 10,000 is infected. To put it another way, as a rule the number of false positives varies inversely with the incidence of the virus in the population; thus there are many more false positives in a population with an incidence of 0.1 percent (which was actually the estimate for Americans in 1987) than in a population with an incidence of 5 percent. In general populations—such as those with an expected incidence of less than 1 percent—the number of false positives in the past has been significant, although it should be pointed out that tests have been improved, and that few people now want to test the general American population (all Americans).

The high number of false positives in the past explains why some AIDS counselors still emphasize that testing positive on ELISA means only that one is positive for the antibody to HIV: ELISA does not test for the virus itself. However, this kind of reassurance can be misleading. The chance of a false positive is highest with a person who has no risk factors; for a person with risk factors, such as unsafe behavior, the chance of a false positive decreases to nearly zero.

Regardless of the number of false positives in general populations, then, this problem is virtually nonexistent in high-risk populations. Consequently, there may be good reasons for mandatory screening in high-risk populations even if there are no very good reasons for screening general populations. For instance, it might be useful to test every client of a methadone-maintenance clinic or an STD clinic. It might also be possible to develop a "profile" of high-risk individuals and test those individuals; if such a profile in fact correlated with risk factors, there would be few false positives.

Delayed antibody response creates the opposite problem—false negatives. Because a person infected with HIV may not produce antibodies for 6 weeks to 1 year (in one case in Alabama, it took over 13 months), the rate of false negatives can be significant. At present, any mandatory screening program would miss some people who had been infected recently; with mandatory screening of hospital patients, for instance, as many as 3 percent of HIV-infected patients might be missed.[71]

The probability of false negatives is one reason why CDC recommends that medical professionals performing invasive procedures act "as if" every patient were HIV-positive. However, given false negatives, it can be asked why hospitals should test at all: testing might actually do harm by giving staff members a false sense of security, and thus it might be safest to omit testing and simply apply the "act as if" rule.

Costs   One strong argument against mandatory testing in the general population, and even among health workers, has to do with the cost of testing.

With regard to low-risk groups, such as the general American population, a study in 1993 estimated that it would cost between $870,000 and $3,600,000 to discover *each person* with an undiagnosed HIV infection.[72] In the premarital testing program in Illinois described above, the actual figures during 1 year, though not quite that high, were still impressive: total cost of testing, $2.5 million; people tested, 71,000; positives identified, 8; cost per discovered case, over $300,000.[73] Since the point of such testing is presumably to control the spread of HIV, opponents argue that the number of cases actually prevented would be minuscule and that the cost is therefore unjustifiable. These critics point out that, as we have seen, merely identifying HIV infection does little to stop the spread of HIV—but follow-up measures such as counseling would incur even more expense.

Many people argue that it would be more cost-effective to target specific groups for HIV testing. In groups with risk factors where the incidence of HIV infection exceeds 5 percent, screening can identify undiagnosed infection at a cost of $33,000 per person identified.[74] (It is worth asking, though, why society would be willing to spend even this lower amount merely to identify people with HIV, when it seems so unwilling to help these people in other ways—many HIV-positive people have no medical insurance, for instance.)

Mandatory testing of health professionals is also an expensive idea. Testing all health care workers once would cost about $1.5 billion, total, according to one estimate;[75] testing all dentists and surgeons once—a more modest proposal—would cost a total of about $28 million. Furthermore, it is not clear that testing health workers would be cost-effective. In this case, cost-effectiveness varies tremendously with two key factors: rate of infection among these professionals and likelihood of transmission of HIV to patients. Suppose we adopted the modest program of testing all dentists and surgeons once. If both prevalence and risk of transmission were moderate, 25 transmissions might be averted, at a cost of more than $1 million each; if both prevalence and risk of transmission were low, perhaps only 1 transmission would be prevented—at a cost of $28 million.[76]

UPDATE

During her brief time in the public eye, Kimberly Bergalis generated strong feelings of sympathy, but she also aroused some resentment. To gays and lesbians, she seemed unsympathetic to their plight. When she testified in Washington, she had pointed out, "I didn't do anything wrong"—and this seemed to imply that other people with AIDS *had* done something wrong. Randy Shilts, author of the landmark work *And the Band Played On,* said, "What is troubling about the anger of the Bergalises is that they do not seem to acknowledge the suffering of others. . . . It's appalling that AIDS is considered serious only when it strikes a heterosexual young woman or a star basketball player."[77] (Shilts himself died of AIDS in February 1994.)

•

In 1993, the world learned that a sixth patient of David Acer had been infected with HIV: Sherry Annette Johnson, a teenager who lived in West Palm Beach. (A fifth infected patient had been found sometime previously.) Since Sherry Johnson shared the same DNA in the same strain of the HIV virus, it seemed conclusive that Acer was again the source of the infection.

At a news conference in May 1993, Sherry Johnson said that she had learned of her infection 4 months earlier, when she had tried to enlist in the Navy and was then tested for HIV. Like the Bergalises, she and her family felt utterly betrayed by the medical, dental, and public health officials who had knowingly let Acer continue to practice. In reply, Roy Schwartz of the AMA Committee on AIDS (who had previously denied that Kimberly Bergalis could have been infected by Acer) said, "You don't draw national health-care policy on the basis of what has happened with one health-care-worker."[78]

CDC said that Sherry Johnson had probably been infected by Acer 5 to 6 years earlier; this was not good news for the hundreds of other former patients of Acer's who had not so far been tested.

The case of Sherry Johnson again raised the question whether Acer had intentionally infected his patients, particularly since he had performed no invasive procedure on her. Harold Jaffe, director of the CDC's AIDS section, acknowledged that the absence of any invasive procedure was a very odd feature of the case.

•

Actually, how David Acer infected his patients may never be determined. In July 1994, Larry Altman, who is a physician, a medical reporter, and a former CDC staff member, observed that this "remains one of the biggest mysteries in the annals of epidemiology."[79] Harold Jaffe, who had been CDC's leading investigator in the Kimberly Bergalis case, noted that the frustration of not having solved it "deepens with time":

> All the data says something strange happened in that dental practice, and I wish I knew what it was. The fact that here are so many infected patients and there is no other practice like this may give more weight to the murder theory, but there is no proof of that. The only way it will ever be solved is if the dentist told somebody what happened, or somebody saw what happened, and that person ultimately comes forward.[80]

Earlier that year, an article in *Lear's* magazine had argued that Acer had not infected the patients at all,[81] and a report on *60 Minutes* also took that line. This idea may have originated in February 1993, when Ronald DeBry of Florida State University argued, in an article in *Nature,* that Acer's probability of being the source was no higher than the probability for the general community; he also said there were unrevealed risk factors in the infected patients, including Kimberly Bergalis.[82] However, researchers at the University of Texas at Austin had later attacked DeBry's article, concluding that the probability stated by CDC— 99.4 percent—was actually too low.

•

A decade after Margaret Heckler's prediction that an AIDS vaccine was imminent, there was little hope for such a vaccine, although since 1984 USPHS had spent at least $639 million on developing one. In 1993, 330 volunteers in a study at Johns Hopkins University began testing an experimental vaccine against HIV,[83] but the AIDS researcher William Haseltine of Harvard predicted that the chance of any successful vaccine was "zero."[84]

•

In mid-1994, all the cases of people infected with HIV through blood transfusions before March 1985 (when blood screening began) were coming to trial in a gigantic class-action suit; CDC estimated that 6,567 Americans had been infected with HIV through blood transfusions, over 70 percent of them before March 1985. During the trial, AP revealed internal memos from American Red Cross dating from 1983; the writers of these memos had argued vigorously that there was evidence that AIDS was transmissible through donated blood.[85]

American hemophiliacs were also suing American Red Cross because its clotting factor, pooled from many different blood donors, had infected about 70 percent of the 10,000 American hemophiliacs with HIV.[86]

•

In the middle 1990s, AIDS has become commonplace. Abigail Zuger has observed that things are looking very different to medical professionals:

> Hundreds of thousands of lost lives later, the initial impact is over. The thunderbolts of AIDS are starting to become a fact of life. Some sense of continuity with the rest of our history has become possible. AIDS continues to be a source of uniquely complex medical, legal, and social dilemmas; nonetheless, it has evolved into an entity provoking fewer immediate panicked reactions and more measured, mature analyses. We are coming to the realization that AIDS is going to be with us for some time.[87]

FURTHER READING

B. McCarthy et al., "Who Should Be Screened for HIV Infection?" *Archives of Internal Medicine*, vol. 153, May 10, 1993, pp. 1107–1116.

Carol Pogash, *As Real As It Gets: The Life of a Hospital at the Center of the AIDS Epidemic*, Birch Lane, Carol Publishing Group, New York, 1992.

T. Quinn, "Screening for HIV Infection: Benefits and Costs," *New England Journal of Medicine*, vol. 327, no. 7, August 13, 1992, pp. 486–488.

Randy Shilts, *And the Band Played On*, St. Martin's, New York, 1987.

CHAPTER 18

A Model for a
New American Medical System

Medicare

Medicare is the federally financed, federally supervised system of medical care for Americans over age 65. In this chapter, Medicare is used as a "case study" of a medical system; a contrasting system, the Health Care Security bill, presented to Congress by the Clinton administration in 1993 and 1994, is also discussed.

BACKGROUND:
PROBLEMS OF MEDICAL CARE IN THE UNITED STATES

Problems of Access: Three Examples

Most people who want to reform the American system of medical care want increased access to the system, or even *universal access*—that is, coverage for all Americans. The following cases illustrate problems of access to medical care in the United States.

Kate Fowler   Kate Fowler, a 75-year-old African American who is a widow, lives in Green County, in the "black belt" of Alabama.[1] *Black belt* refers to the rich soil in this region, but aside from its soil this county is one of the poorest in the United States. Nearly half of its residents over age 65—and nearly 60 percent of its children—live in dire poverty. Most of the residents of Green County are African American, and many are descended from freed slaves.

Kate Fowler lives in a crumbling old wooden house at the end of a dirt road. The only source of heat is a fireplace in her bedroom, and during the winter she wears a coat indoors, over a ragged knit blouse. The bare ground can be seen through cracks between the floorboards; often, a cold wind whips through the house.

Kate Fowler is too poor to own a car; she has no one to drive her anywhere, and there is no public transportation in this area. Like many of the rural poor, she never leaves her home except, rarely, to see a doctor.

Thus when Kate Fowler needed surgery for cataracts, although the actual medical costs were covered by Medicare, transportation was a problem. She

443

needed to get to and from the doctor's office and the hospital (an hour's drive away) for preoperative visits, for the surgery itself, and for three required follow-up visits; and she had to pay a cousin $30 to take her, wait for her, and then drive her home. For her, this actually represented something of a bargain—she could have gotten it only from a family member.

In similar rural areas, free prenatal care is offered by public hospitals, but many pregnant young women cannot receive it, because they simply have no way to travel, say, 3 or 4 miles to the nearest bus stop to begin the journey. And many young men with HIV infection live with a mother or grandmother as they cope with the illnesses of its middle and late stages: because no one in the family has a car, they are unable to come to a clinic for treatment.

Rosalyn Schwartz   Rosalyn Schwartz, age 47, white, lives in Ridgefield, New Jersey; she has one child, Andy. She lost her medical coverage when she and her husband divorced in 1987.[2] At that time, the gift-wrap company where she worked with five other employees (she was then making around $19,000 a year) provided no medical coverage, though it was considering doing so soon. When Rosalyn Schwartz tried to buy an individual policy, several insurance companies informed her that *if* they offered her a policy, the premiums would be about $4,000 a year, since she had a preexisting condition—an ulcer. Moreover, no policy would cover any treatment for the ulcer.

In 1988, Rosalyn Schwartz found a small lump in her breast. Her physician said it might be cancerous and recommended removing it; but she asked if that could wait until her employer provided medical coverage. The physician agreed to postpone the surgery.

In late 1989, while cooking, Rosalyn Schwartz turned abruptly, and pain suddenly tore through her hip. Unbeknownst to her, the breast cancer had metastazied and had eaten into her hip, making the hip bones as fragile as glass. When she fell to the floor, her hip socket shattered. In the ambulance, she sobbed and could think only of the costs. "Andy, you've just turned 18," she said. "I have no insurance. Tell them [at the hospital] I have no insurance. But don't sign anything or you'll be responsible."

Rosalyn Schwartz was hospitalized for 23 days, during which she had surgery three times. The total cost was over $40,000. Half of that was paid by a charity; the rest went onto her own bill, which she is now paying off—$10 a month to each of 12 physicians.

Her surgery has left her unable to work. She receives Medicare disability benefits, amounting to about $10,500 a year. When she tried again to buy medical coverage, she found that it would still cost her $4,000 a year, and that it would not cover any procedure for her cancer, since the cancer was now another preexisting condition.

Lacking insurance, she is not getting physical therapy to help her adjust to her hip replacement—nor can she afford a bone scan to make sure the cancer has not spread.

Denise and Randy Sadler   Many Americans have medical insurance but are afraid to use it. As we saw in Chapter 16, for instance, one woman who was found to have a genetic marker for hereditary breast cancer was reluctant to tell her medical insurer why she wanted a radical mastectomy, since her premiums might then be raised or she might lose her coverage altogether.

Randy Sadler owns a tile business in Kernersville, North Carolina; his wife, Denise Sadler, is a part-time worker for the Census Bureau. Together, they made about $35,000 a year in 1992—a figure that was close to the median in the United States. One of the Sadlers' sons has severe allergies and repeatedly develops pneumonia; Denise Sadler has migraine headaches and episodes of depression.

The Sadlers have two medical insurance policies: one for Denise and their sons, with a yearly deductible of $500; and another for Randy, with a $1,000 deductible. These policies cost them a total of $2,500 per year, and they are trying to get a 5 percent reduction in premiums by not filing a claim for 1 year. Thus they do not feel that they can use their policies for anything short of a catastrophe. As a result, they are spending $100 to $200 each month on prescription drugs and physicians' bills. Despite their two policies, Denise says, "I still feel like we have no insurance."[3]

Problems of Costs: Richard Lamm's Critique

Richard Lamm, who was governor of Colorado from 1978 to 1987, set off a national debate about exorbitant medical costs in 1987, when he attacked the high costs of organ transplants and the amounts often spent on the last years of our lives. His remarks, published in 1987 in the journal *Dialysis and Transplantation*, are worth careful consideration:

> Health care is clearly entering into a new era: Infinite health needs have run into finite resources. The miracles of medicine have outstripped our ability to pay, and some thoughtful and equitable thinking has to be done to ensure that America gets the most health care for its limited dollars.
>
> It is a very serious mistake to deny that a major change is in the wings. No sector of the economy, no matter how important, can continue to grow at two-and-half times the rate of inflation. We are heading rapidly toward an American that has rusting plants, closed factories, staggering trade deficits. Health care cannot continue to operate under the illusion that it can continue business as usual.
>
> Once we accept the fact that there are limits to what the nation can afford (and increasingly, people are recognizing this truth), then we will begin a process of asking how to get the most health benefits for the most Americans for our money. We should have asked this question years ago. It is outrageous that this country spends five to eight times what other countries spend, and yet has no better health outcome. America is going to demand more accountability for the more than one billion dollars a day it now spends on health care. Many countries give a high level of health care to all their citizens for a fraction of what we spend, and yet keep them healthier. We are no longer rich enough to give a blank check to an inefficient health care industry.
>
> Once we start to apply even minimum management standards to the health care industry, we will see some substantial changes. If we ask how to get the most health benefits for the greatest number of Americans for our tax dollars, many of today's practices will not meet the test. If we zero-budget all that we now do in health care, we shall inevitably close unnecessary hospitals, close

excess ICU units, and look much more closely at utilization factors and outcomes. We shall have to develop a concept of cost-effective medicine. Virtually every health care provider will agree that much of what we do today in medicine has "marginal utility." When a society faces fiscal reality and seeks to optimize its dollars, it not only starts on the road to financial sanity, but it also brings dramatic change to existing medical practices. Dialysis and transplantation will undoubtedly undergo major change. The "opportunity costs" in other areas of medicine are clearly greater than much of what is being done today. The bottom line is that we can save more lives and bring better health care to more Americans for many of the dollars we are spending today.

Economist Lester Thurow suggests that, to impress upon health providers what they are doing when they order marginal services, we should require them to imagine an American worker sentenced to a period of slavery long enough to pay the medical bill for that procedure. Dr. Thomas Starzl recently gave a liver transplant to a 76-year old woman. It cost $240,000. Dr. Starzl should understand that with the average U.S. family making $24,000 a year, he has sentenced 10 U.S. families to work all year so that he could transplant a 76-year old woman.

Such actions are cheating our children of resources they desperately need to build a better life and to revitalize the United States economically. If all of us, or even a significant percentage of us, take $240,000 in high-tech medicine as we are on our way out the door, we are stealing resources that our children and our grandchildren desperately need. Health care is important, but it cannot be the only value of our society. It cannot continue on its growth curve without bankrupting America.

Health providers are not used to thinking this way. Many of you will cry foul and think this heresy. But alas—it is true. A nation that runs $200 billion deficits and borrows 20 cents from its children out of every dollar it spends must one day demand more accountability from its politicians, from its industries, and from its health providers. That day is near at hand, and we should welcome it—for our children's sakes.[4]

There was a howl of protest when Lamm's commentary was made public, but he was addressing the common good of many Americans as no one else was doing. His observations highlight many of the questions that arise when the cost of the American medical system is being evaluated. One of his most important criticisms is that Americans are borrowing from the future to pay for present exorbitant medical costs.

Problems of Allocation: Limiting Health Care

Rationing   During the 1980s, the American medical system operated increasingly by informal schemes of rationing. *Rationing* is a vague, ambiguous term, and in discussions of finances in American medicine, it has come to refer to both social and individual decisions. That is, medical services can be limited by eliminating some category of service to everyone, by eliminating specific services to some category of people, or by limiting specific services to specific individuals. Distribution of medical resources in block—a social decision—is sometimes called *rationing;* more commonly, though, *rationing* is used to refer to individual decisions—decisions by physicians to limit medical care to individual patients.

Here, we shall follow custom and use this term for either individual or social decisions about distribution.

The foremost example of medical rationing in the United States today is probably found in health maintenance organizations (HMOs); these are plans for group medical care, and they are becoming increasingly popular. Physicians in HMOs are required to justify their decisions, and they must allocate care among the members of the plan—the patients—by rationing: they try to provide only justifiable care and deny unjustifiable expensive care. Employers who offer medical insurance favor HMOs, because an HMO costs less than other kinds of coverage.

Here are examples of rationing by HMOs: Physicians are discouraged from prescribing antibiotics for common colds or giving cortisone injections for minor sprains. At the same time, physicians are encouraged to urge pregnant patients to come in for regular examinations. In theory, the money saved by denying unnecessary care, such as unneeded antibiotics and cortisone, makes it possible to spend more on preventive care, such as monitoring a pregnancy. Moreover, it is claimed (though perhaps on the basis more of ideology than of fact) that preventive care itself saves money by forestalling curative intervention.

It should be emphasized that members of HMOs do not always get what they want from their physicians. In an HMO, costs are reduced by denying some things which patients have traditionally received but which may not be financially or medically justified, such as immediate access to a physician for a minor complaint. Also, commonly a physician must receive prior approval from an HMO official before starting an expensive treatment. Furthermore, physicians in some HMOs receive yearly bonuses based on how much money has been saved by their rationing decisions, and this kind of financial incentive can pit physicians and administrators against patients.

In terms of individual independent physicians and American society as a whole, by contrast, rationing is less clear-cut.

Does the average independent American physician ration care? Yes and no. If a patient has a generous medical plan, the physician may be able to order anything at all, and the plan will cover it. If a patient has a managed care plan, the physician may be limited by what the plan will cover and thus may be unable to order the "ideal" treatment. If a patient is underinsured or uninsured, the physician may order or recommend a certain treatment—such as a prescription drug—but the patient may simply decide that it is unaffordable and forgo it.

In the past, physicians were not expected to ration care; today, new systems such as managed care plans are forcing physicians to consider costs at each step of treatment, and almost every physician has some patients whose coverage is "managed" or limited in some way. This creates conflicts for physicians: their traditional self-concept as good Samaritans is incompatible with their new role as gatekeepers.[5] Their loyalties are divided between doing what is best for each patient and contributing to an efficient, prudent system.

Does American society ration? Again, the answer is yes and no. Priorities are established, but not in the conscious, nationally consistent way that has characterized medical systems in other western countries such as England and Canada. In the United States, to see where medical resources are flowing, we need to see which medical specialties are flourishing—and to discover that, we simply need to see which ones are reimbursed well. Because independent American physicians work on a fee-for-service system, and because they are increasingly allowed to own part of facilities providing medical care (to the consternation of some critics), they provide most medical services where the money is best. Thus Americans have the latest programs of angioplasty, oncology, and liver transplants because medical plans and their subscribers pay for these things. In other words, the American system rations, in effect, by deciding how well to reimburse each specialty.

Who makes social decisions about rationing? That is often very difficult to determine. Insurance companies make some decisions, of course: for instance, they pay "usual and customary" fees of surgeons, who steadily raise their fees and perform more and more surgery; then, insurers pass these increased costs along to policyholders in the form of higher premiums. This is a social system, of sorts, although Americans have never voted on it and have never agreed to be taxed to fund it. It just continues to career along—a strange situation.

Medicare and Medicaid also make, and represent, social decisions about rationing. In this regard, it should be noted that benefits to Medicare and Medicaid recipients far exceed what the recipients themselves have paid into these systems (this is especially true of Medicaid, of course, since its recipients are indigent and pay little or no taxes). Thus although it may be incorrect to call the present rationing system "immoral," it may be appropriate to call it unjust. People who are employed pay Federal Insurance Corporation of America (FICA) taxes, and we all pay sales taxes, to support Medicare and Medicaid—even if we ourselves have no medical coverage. As a result, many uninsured people are contributing to Medicare and Medicaid.[6]

To see how these levels of rationing—HMOs, independent physicians, and society—can operate, consider two medical situations: hemophilia and heart attacks.

Hemophiliacs need what is known as a *clotting factor*. The first clotting factor, which became available in the 1960s, was formed from the blood of 2,000 donors; some later donors were infected with human immunodeficiency virus (HIV), the causative agent in AIDS, and by 1985, over 70 percent of hemophiliac recipients in the United States had been infected[7] (see Chapter 17). Although today's natural clotting factors are much safer, they are not entirely risk-free for HIV. A new synthetic recombinant-DNA clotting factor is now available from a commercial producer, and this new factor would prevent the remaining 30 percent of hemophiliacs from being infected. However, it has been patented, and its pure form costs $45,000 to $50,000 a month—or more than $500,000 a year—per patient.[8]

With regard to heart attacks, there are two drugs that can reduce damage. The older drug, streptokinase, is made from bacteria and costs about $240 per dose. The new drug, tissue plasminogen activator (TPA) is a genetically engineered, patented substance costing $2,400 a dose. TPA appears to be slightly more effective than streptokinase,[9] but it costs 10 times as much. In other words, a slight improvement in outcome entails a disproportionate increase in costs, though if cost were not a consideration, most patients would prefer to receive TPA and most physicians would prefer to prescribe it.

In such situations, HMOs would typically opt for the cheaper treatment. An independent physician would typically opt for the more expensive treatment only if the patient's insurer would pay for it; however, in the specific case of the synthetic clotting factor probably no medical insurance plan could afford to pay that much, and in the specific case of TPA the general recommendation would probably be simply that a patient should get either streptokinase or TPA as opposed to nothing at all. On the social level, there is no real policy on the clotting factor or TPA.

These trends in rationing in the United States may not look very impressive. Rationing by HMOs often seems to be at odds with patients' interests; rationing by independent physicians seems to be based mainly on patients' coverage rather than on medical considerations; and rationing by society seems to be essentially unplanned (to take just one example, as discussed in Chapter 11, society continued to fund artificial hearts—despite very poor outcomes—until criticism became too intense). Nevertheless, as Lamm point outs, rationing is inevitable; without some kind of rationing, the American system of medical care will go bankrupt.

Organ replacement has come to symbolize unreasonable costs in the American medical system, a fact that is reflected in Lamm's commentary. As discussed in Chapter 12, for instance, there has been no rationing at all for dialysis since Congress passed the End Stage Renal Disease Act (ESRDA) in 1969; and recent decisions about allocating organs for transplant have occurred largely behind closed doors within the medical profession. The issue with expensive treatments like dialysis and transplants is that enormous amounts of money are being spent on relatively few recipients while millions of Americans are not receiving basic medical care. Since almost no one can afford, say, a $250,000 liver transplant, such a transplant amounts to a transfer payment to one person from many others, enforced by public policy.

Expensive transplants therefore raise questions of justice, and these questions could become especially acute if there is a technical breakthrough—if, for instance, xenografts become feasible—or if the number of donor organs rises significantly, so that many more organ transplants are possible. So far, despite the high cost of each transplant, a persistent shortage of donor organs has constrained the total cost of transplants; but if the supply of donor organs rises, the total cost will skyrocket. Then, rationing will be essential.

The Oregon plan   At least one state has decided to tackle this problem of justice by limiting expensive, dramatic interventions for the few in order to extend basic medical care to more of the poor. In the late 1980s, Oregon established a bold plan, the Oregon Health Plan (OHP), for its state Medicaid fund. Medicaid is the system of medical care for the poor administered by each state, with matching funds from the federal government.

The Oregon legislature passed the first version of OHP in 1987. After much discussion, including debate in the legislature and town meetings for the public, certain conclusions had emerged about medical priorities; and under the original OHP, 709 medical conditions were listed in decreasing order of importance and outcomes. Funds saved by withholding low-priority care—interventions that were too expensive or promised only poor outcomes—would be used to provide basic care to people who were poor and uninsured, and also to help employers pay for private insurance. The goal was to require all employers, even small businesses, to offer basic coverage by 1995 or to pay a new payroll tax—hence the term *pay or play.* Low-priority interventions which would not be funded by Oregon's Medicaid system included in vitro fertilization, experimental therapies for late-stage AIDS patients, heart transplants, liver transplants, bone-marrow transplants for leukemia (such a transplant costs $100,000), and care in neonatal intensive care units (NICUs) for premature babies weighing under 750 grams at birth. (With regard to the last item, it can be noted that the cost of care for these babies in NICUs is exorbitant, and as few as perhaps 12 percent will emerge unimpaired to lead a normal life; in one study of such babies, only about half lived, and 75 percent of those had neurological damage.[10])

Thus Oregon had, democratically, developed a public policy about medical financing and treatment. Not surprisingly, though, when the parents of a child with leukemia, 7-year-old Coby Howard, learned in 1988 that Medicaid would not pay for a bone-marrow transplant, they appealed to the news media. (This is an example of the rule of rescue, discussed in Chapters 2 and 12.) The media were in a bind: although journalists were well aware that they were being used, the case of Coby Howard was real news. Here was a patient who would be denied treatment under OHP and would therefore die. Would the public in Oregon simply accept his death? The Oregon legislature did hear a plea by Coby's mother, as well as pleas by relatives of two other patients who needed transplants, but it did not change OHP or grant exemptions. All three families also appealed for donations through the media, but the public did not respond. Coby Howard died a few months later.

The reaction outside Oregon was different. OHP was rejected by President Bush's Secretary of Health and Human Services (HHS), Louis Sullivan: he would not release federal matching funds for Oregon's Medicaid program. Sullivan was particularly concerned about OHP's exclusion of people with disabilities, especially since this exclusion also applied to premature babies whose birthweight was under 750 grams.

Oregon then modified OHP to comply with the Americans with Disabilities Act (ADA, 1992), providing coverage even for babies under 500 grams.[11] In March 1993, the Clinton administration accepted this new version of OHP; in fact, it was reportedly a model for Clinton's own Health Care Security bill.

However, OHP ran into trouble in late 1993. The legislature had appropriated $34 million for Medicaid, but in that year the costs of the program rose to $84 million—at a time when the state budget was already facing a $1.2 billion shortfall.[12] Also, public and business support for OHP seemed to be waning.

A Comparative Perspective:
Health Care in Germany and Canada

In discussing medical care in the United States, it is useful to have some points of comparison. Two other systems will be considered here, those of Germany and Canada.

Germany has a national health care system, financed by more than 1,100 insurance funds. Each person joins one fund early in life and remains in that fund thereafter. Germans see physicians of their choice, choose physicians who can order the treatments they want, and wait no longer for appointments or admission to hospitals than Americans do. In 1990, Germany spent 8.5 percent of its gross national product (GNP), or roughly $1,286 per person, on health care; that year the United States spent nearly 12 percent of its GNP on health care—roughly $3,500 per person. Germany, then, was succeeding in insuring all its citizens at a much lower cost.

There is an explanation for this difference. The German government plays a much greater role in health care than the American government; and in Germany, the government has put a ceiling on physicians' fees, that is, on how much a physician can charge a patient—a restraint which American physicians have vehemently resisted. (To earn more money, German physicians can only try to see more patients.) On the other hand, the decisions of German physicians are not second-guessed by third parties as they are in the United States, and this aspect of the German system appeals to many American physicians.[13]

•

Canada has a fund for national medical coverage, much like the American social security system. This fund covers the medical care of every Canadian; it is universal, portable, and publicly administered through a single-payer system, and it covers all medically necessary services. The single-payer system is financed partly by high "sin" taxes on cigarettes and alcohol. Each of Canada's provinces sets its own policies and allocates medical care by regulating the supply of medical services. For example, each province funds only a small number of hospitals, CAT-scanners, and lithotripters (expensive machines that break up kidney stones with sound waves).

Physicians in Canada do not work for the Canadian government; like independent American physicians, they work for themselves and bill on a fee-for-service basis. Canadian physicians cannot set their own fees, however, and this is what American physicians dislike about the Canadian system; but it should be noted that under the American system, costs are borne by the taxpayers and by people who insure themselves—and that Canadian physicians are far from poor. In American dollars, in 1991, cardiologists in Canada earned $290,500 on average; ophthalmologists, $240,500; dermatologists, $200,500; and general practitioners, $128,000.[14] There are fewer specialists in Canada than in the United States, though, because the Canadian system discourages specialization whereas the American system encourages it.

The Canadian system costs less than $2,000 (in American dollars) per capita and covers all Canadians; the American system costs $3,500 per capita (as noted above) and leaves over 39 million Americans uncovered.

Canadians are extremely proud of their medical system, especially when they contrast it with medical care in the United States; Here are some examples:

- In Canada, every pregnant woman gets free care. In the United States, 17 percent of women in childbirth experience not only the inevitable, natural fears and pain but also the anxiety of having no medical coverage to pay for their hospitalization or their physicians' bills.[15]
- In Canada, all citizens are eligible for long-term nursing home care. Although they must pay for a portion of such care (about $19 of the $67 which is the

typical cost per day), this is an affordable option for most of them. In the United States, virtually no one has coverage for long-term care in a nursing home; to become eligible for Medicaid, which pays for bare-bones nursing home care, elderly Americans must "spend down" until their assets are virtually gone.[16]

- Canada generously covers people with extraordinary medical needs. In one Canadian family, for instance, the 8-year-old son was retarded and had a rare brain disease, tubular sclerosis, characterized by severe mood swings, tumors on several organs, skin rashes, and seizures; he wore a diaper and had the mental age of a 4-year-old. The father earned the equivalent of $12,000 (American) a year. This boy had seen a physician 40 times within 2 years and had been hospitalized three times, but the family had never received a bill. In the United States, this family's income would disqualify them from Medicaid in many states.[17]

In one poll, only 3 percent of Canadians considered the American medical system superior to their own. (It must be admitted, though, that nearly 30 percent thought Elvis Presley might still be alive.)

American physicians often say that Canadians must wait for some kinds of care. Strictly speaking, that is true, but it may not be as significant as many Americans conclude. To take just one example, in Nova Scotia there is only one lithotripter, in Halifax; as mentioned earlier, this is a machine that breaks up kidney stones with sound waves. Thus a patient in Nova Scotia may have to wait 3 months for an appointment to use it. However, most stone-busting is preventive; most kidney stones eventually drop and pass through the ureter; and surgery is available as an emergency alternative to lithotripsy. Furthermore, the only way to diminish the waiting list would be to buy more machines, at enormous expense— each one costs millions of dollars. The Canadian system saves millions by purchasing fewer lithotripters, though there is some risk that some patients will need surgery before the appointment for lithotripsy comes around. Canadians are aware of this kind of decision and seem to accept it.

EXPANDING MEDICARE:
A PROPOSAL FOR A NEW SYSTEM

One system of American medical care organized by the federal government has won strong allegiance from the patients it covers. This is Medicare, the federal system of medical care for all American citizens over age 65.

Congress began to think about Medicare in the early 1960s, as part of the "Great Society" legislation, which also included Head Start, food stamps, VISTA, and Aid to Families with Dependent Children. These programs were conceptualized by President John F. Kennedy and wrangled into law by President Lyndon Johnson in 1965. Medicare was intended to help elderly people during illness; originally, it was intended for the elderly poor, but almost immediately it was extended to everyone over 65.

For elderly people, Medicare alleviated the very great evil of uncertainty about medical treatment; it gave many of them a medical security they had never known before. For many elderly Americans, the greatest worry had been whether they could afford physicians and hospitalization. Before Medicare, when workers retired—typically, in those days, at 65—many of them were on their own with regard to medical coverage. If they did not insure themselves, they would somehow have to pay for all their own medical expenses. Today, that is no longer true: the elderly now need to pay a maximum of 20 percent of their medical expenses, and most pay only 15 percent. Since Medicare is very comprehensive— and since medical expenses are so high, particularly for this age group—that is a great bargain.

Medicare covers 32 million Americans over age 65 and, in a supplemental system, 3.6 million disabled people under 65.[18] Together, Medicare and Medicaid, the system for the poor, cover about 1 in 5 Americans. Unlike Medicaid, which is run differently by each state with federal matching funds, Medicare is administered by the federal government and is financed from mandatory payroll taxes—indicated on paycheck stubs as FICA (that is, Federal Insurance Corporation of America). Medicare costs about \$140 billion a year, 15 percent of the nation's health spending; Medicaid costs state taxpayers about \$35 billion.[19]

Medicare is a *single-payer system*, and in this it contrasts sharply with private medical coverage in the United States. Since World War II, private insurance plans have multiplied; they now number over 1,500, each with its own rules, qualifications, reimbursement rates, and forms to be filled out by patients and physicians.[20] This private system is so complicated that by 1990 special businesses had sprouted to help patients fill out all the different forms and to help physicians bill all the different plans.

As noted earlier, Medicare has many advocates, but it also has some critics. These critics often focus on the problems of Medicare. They argue that elderly Americans have come to think of Medicare as a "right," and that the elderly must still pay significant medical costs under Medicare. Specifically, they argue that Medicare has not decreased medical costs as a percentage of the overall income of elderly people. In 1965, Senator Hubert Humphrey said that the elderly were spending 15 percent of their income on health care, implying that this was too much,[21] and under Medicare the elderly now spend more than 15 percent of their income on health care.

Advocates of Medicare argue that, as a single-payer system, it can eliminate the overhead and waste of multiple private insurers. They point out that about 4 to 12 percent of health care costs represent fees and profits of private insurance plans;[22] by comparison, Medicare has maintained very reasonable administrative expenses, about 2.5 percent of its total expenditures.[23]

As advocates also point out, what is frequently overlooked by critics is that Medicare has given elderly Americans access to one of the most technologically advanced medical systems in the world, and it has done this during a 25-year period when the cost of medical services has risen rapidly and steadily. In fact, it is not the fault of Medicare that the elderly still spend at least 15 percent of their income on medical services; this is attributable simply to increases in the cost of such services. Also, more and more of life has become "medicalized," that is, people tend to seek medical care in more and more circumstances. Furthermore, people are now living much longer—partly because of the care Medicare provides—and people who live to be old (to be precise, the age group 62 to 82) are the greatest consumers of expensive medical care. In sum, then, the advocates of Medicare seem to have a much stronger case than its critics.

•

Why not expand Medicare, therefore, to cover all Americans regardless of age? An expanded Medicare system could also absorb all other government systems of medical coverage, including Medicaid, insurance for federal employees, the CHAMPUS program for military personnel, and all government disability funds.

An expanded Medicare system would offer several significant advantages. To begin with, a single-payer system eliminates the wasteful duplication and conflicting rules that seem inevitable with multiple insurers. Second, such a system can control costs: it has enormous power in negotiating with physicians and hospitals; it can essentially say, "Take it or leave it." Third, a single-payer system eliminates cost-shifting to other payers.

It must be admitted that there are some potential disadvantages. For one thing, an expanded Medicare system could conceivably become another ESRDA, with runaway costs. What everyone pays for, nobody pays for, and there is a tendency for everyone to seek his or her own advantage to the detriment of the overall good. This is an age-old story, played out long ago in England in the "tragedy of the commons": the owner of each flock increased the number of sheep he grazed on town land—the commons—until the commons were so overgrazed that the grass simply disappeared and the commons system was destroyed.[24] Second, a single-payer system might create a bloated, unresponsive federal bureaucracy; the Veterans Administration hospitals have become such a bureaucracy and are not an encouraging model. Third, many Americans feel that government, especially the federal govenment, simply cannot do certain things very well, and this feeling is particularly strong with regard to personal matters like medical care.

But these disadvantages seem to be offset by another important advantage: Medicare is a system which is *already in place*. (In this regard, it can be noted, for example, that hospitals are already getting about half their revenues from Medicare patients.) Using Medicare for all age groups would entail simply broadening it, rather than creating some wholly new, untried system; thus its effects would probably be more predictable, and more manageable, than those of a new system. Medicare might even be expanded gradually, to each additional age group in turn; this would allow time for its effects to be assessed, and for corrections and modifications to be made.

ANOTHER PROPOSAL:
THE HEALTH CARE SECURITY BILL
AND MANAGED CARE PLANS

Soon after William Jefferson (Bill) Clinton became president in January 1993, he and his wife, Hillary Rodham Clinton, announced that reforming American medical care would be a top priority of the new administration; in fact, Clinton's promise to redress the inadequacies of the existing system had been a significant factor in his election. Clinton made two promises about medical care: to broaden access to it and to control its high costs—though whether both goals could be achieved simultaneously remained to be seen.

Originally, Clinton hoped to expand Medicare to include workers' compensation, the medical portion of automobile insurance, and Medicaid; and in May of 1993, it was expected that within 18 months Congress would pass "landmark legislation" to control medical costs and expand insurance coverage.[25] However, it was not until late 1993 that Bill and Hillary Clinton presented their actual plan to Congress, and this plan—called the Health Care Security bill—was significantly different from their original idea.

The Health Care Security bill was based on two major concepts. The first of these was what came to be known as an *employer mandate:* all employers would be required to pay something toward medical insurance for their employees (the exact amount to be negotiated as the bill was debated).

The second major concept was the formation of large *managed care plans,* which were intended to reduce costs. Each of these managed care plans would sign up, on the supply side, a hospital or a large number of physicians and would offer to patients—the demand side—a broad range of medical services for a predetermined flat cost. This second concept had originated with an untested idea for lowering costs of supplies to the Pentagon from the defense industry.[26] It was based on the assumption that the various managed care plans would compete against each other, and that this competition would both provide adequate care and keep the costs of care low. The concept of managed care plans was also based on the profit motive: any money left over after a plan had rendered all the services it advertised would be profit. Each plan would have an incentive to be efficient, since an efficient plan would lower its costs and would thus attract clients. Or so the theory went.

There were problems with both bases of the Health Care Security bill. The employer mandate came in for especially strong opposition. It appeared that the brunt of paying for medical insurance for people who are presently not covered might fall—unjustly—on small businesses, and it was estimated that the cost of mandated coverage for such businesses would be between $1,600 and $1,900 per employee. Many small businesses said they would simply not hire, or would fire, workers rather than provide mandated medical coverage. Even a surprising number of physicians in private corporations did not want to pay for medical insurance for their own employees.[27] A reaction like this creates a dilemma for public policy: how can we evaluate a tradeoff between medical insurance for some people and loss of jobs for others?

Another problem with the Health Care Security bill was that managed care plans may be contrary to the way many Americans have come to think about medical care—or, perhaps more accurately, to the way Americans have come to avoid thinking about medical care. The essence of a managed care plan is that medical decisions are justified by looking at evidence. Most Americans, however, do not approach medicine like this; instead, most of us are accustomed to hearing that a certain treatment "might" help, or to reading about a certain drug, and then simply getting it prescribed. The idea of having to give reasons for spending part of the public dollar is new to Americans.

A third problem with the Health Care Security bill was that it would be difficult to control costs without including Medicare under the new system; Medicare is not a managed care plan, and that would be hard to change. The elderly are enthusiastic about Medicare (as noted above) and very protective of it; and since they are generally active voters, they have a great deal of political power. In fact, Medicare has often been called a "sacred cow" (it cannot be attacked) and a "third rail" (touch it and you die).

A fourth problem with the proposed Clinton plan had to do with the Americans with Disabilities Act (ADA). Managed care necessitates rationing, and two ways to ration services are by type of service (as in OHP) and by type of patient. Disability advocates strongly resist rationing by type of patient, and ADA may restrict any such rationing (this is so far untested in the courts). But in effect disability rights can also work against rationing by type of service. A basic provision of the Health Care Security bill (as of other plans) was minimal coverage for every American, and there are two components here which may be at cross purposes—*minimal* and *every*. Minimal coverage for disabled people may entail certain types of very expensive medical services that might otherwise be rationed.[28]

ETHICAL ISSUES

Facts and Misconceptions

In the debate over health care, there are a number of serious misconceptions. Let's examine these.

Who pays for Medicare?   One widespread misconception, among the elderly and others, is that Medicare recipients have already paid for their benefits through FICA taxes. One popular book about Medicare benefits states, "The most fundamental point is that *Medicare is not a gift. You paid for it while you were working.* Medicare owes you services in just the same way that health insurer to whom you have paid premiums owes them to you."[29]

In fact, the Medicare benefits going to today's elderly people are being paid for almost entirely by the FICA taxes of today's workers.[30] It is true that retirees with yearly pensions over $25,000 are taxed on the amount over $25,000; this tax takes the form of reductions in social security payments, but it is modest and defrays only a very small fraction of the costs of Medicare. After the first few years on Medicare, most beneficiaries have received benefits amounting to what they paid in, plus all interest; thereafter, their benefits are paid for by taxes on current workers.

What is medical insurance?   There are also misconceptions about *medical insurance*, a term which can be misleading. Thirty years ago, medical insurance was really insurance—a hedge against a dreaded but rather remote possibility. At that time, people took out medical insurance policies in the hope that they would never need to receive any benefits, and policies covered mainly catastrophic situations like hospital care after an automobile accident or a diagnosis of cancer.

Gradually, medical policies evolved into something quite different, though they have continued to be called *insurance:* they became plans for prepaid group medical care. Blue Cross-Blue Shield (BCBS), for example, simply adds up all its medical costs (subtracting a small amount for administration), divides by the number of policyholders, and sends out the bills. Also, medical insurance expanded to cover not just catastrophic care but all "major medical" expenses. This was a logical extension: if people were willing to pay small premiums to protect themselves against remote catastrophic risks, why not pay slightly larger premiums to protect against more common risks? Thus "insurance" grew and grew until it now includes almost any medical service; today, some people become indignant when their "insurance" doesn't cover absolutely everything and they have to pay for anything at all.

Another misconception about medical insurance has to do with who pays for private insurance. In commercial medical insurance plans, those who do not receive benefits subsidize those who do (this is also true, to some extent, of Medicare). Because premiums are raised when average use rises, many people believe that they have paid for their own care and are thus entitled to as much care as they want. This misconception virtually guarantees that costs and services will increase.

What is socialized medicine?   Perhaps the most serious and most common misconceptions are those about *socialized medicine,* another term that can be misleading. It is important to ask exactly what *socialized* means, and why so many Americans are so afraid of this concept. If *socialized* means simply "publicly owned," then that is not necessarily a bad thing, or even an unusual thing, in American life: Americans are used to public ownership of highways and waterways, public schools, state colleges and universities, the armed forces, airwaves, the air, the skies, and national parks.

When Medicare was debated in Congress in 1965, the American Medical Association (AMA) opposed it as socialized medicine. American physicians were afraid that government-administered care financed by taxes would mean government-controlled care,[31] and that all physicians would end up as employees of the federal government. To placate physicians, a crucial decision was made: under Medicare, physicians would be reimbursed on a fee-for-service basis. Eventually, this arrangement would make physicians rich and would give them the best of both worlds: freedom to work independently rather than as government employees, and freedom to order infinite services for their patients—services that would be taken care of by government-enforced payments in the form of higher and higher FICA taxes. Consider, moreover, that if *socialized medicine* does mean what AMA feared in 1965—working for a boss who decides how much to pay you—then many Americans today are in precisely that position.

One additional misconception about socialized medicine is that people pay for it in some way which involves more compulsion than Americans are used to. The truth here is that Americans are already paying FICA taxes to support Medicare, and FICA is about as compulsory as anything can be: for a typical taxpayer, it is equivalent to being forced to work an extra month to pay for the care of the elderly. What is more, under socialized medicine everyone is covered, which means—obviously enough—that everyone who pays taxes is covered; but today many Americans who pay FICA taxes are *not* covered themselves.

What is a national medical system?   There are also misconceptions about the terms *national health insurance* and *national health care system*. When we are considering reforms in the American medical system, it is important to be clear about how these terms are being used, since different people may have very different concepts in mind.

National health insurance and *national health care system* might mean any of the following:

1. An "American medical service"—a system in which all medical professionals would work for the federal government.
2. A single-payer system, such as a universalized Medicare, in which the federal government would tax all Americans and reimburse physicians on a fee-for-service basis.
3. A system based on a federal law requiring every employer to buy basic medical coverage for every employee and establishing a separate government-financed system for unemployed people.
4. A system in which all Americans would receive government-funded vouchers to buy medical care directly from providers (such as hospitals) or indirectly from companies selling medical coverage.
5. A mixed public-private system in which the government would run all hospitals and would fund all hospital care, but private insurers would cover outpatient costs.[32]

In this chapter, the present Canadian system and a universalized Medicare system are both examples of definition 2.

The "Market" Solution

It is sometimes argued that medical care could be provided and costs controlled by letting medicine operate as a *true market,* subject to the laws of supply and demand. Champions of a marketplace for medical care point out that many other goods and services are successfully provided by a market system, and they maintain that a true marketplace for medical care would eliminate bloated bureaucracies and wasteful costs.

In a true market, people would buy medical care, such as the services of a physician or nurse, out of their own pockets; there would be no medical insurance and thus no reimbursement from insurers. Because people would have to pay for their care themselves, many prices would tumble drastically. For a routine eye examination, for instance, patients might be able to choose a nurse practitioner charging $10, a primary care physician charging $30, or an ophthalmologist charging $300. Given these alternatives, very few patients would choose the ophthalmologist, and so ophthalmologists would have to lower their fees to compete, unless they could somehow demonstrate that their services were really worth more. Another example is elective surgery to correct a deviated septum (a common minor problem creating nasal blockage): this operation is now subsidized by other people's insurance premiums and is reimbursed at $2,000; but if patients had to pay for it themselves, the price might drop to $300.

A true market would certainly lower costs, but there are strong arguments against the market concept in the context of medical care.

The first counterargument is a very basic one: we do not have a true market for medical care, and we have not had such a market since World War II, half a century ago. In fact, since World War II medicine has operated as the opposite of a true market. In the area of Birmingham, Alabama, for example—where medical care has replaced the old steel factories as the chief employer—when more and more specialists were added, the cost of their services rose. In a true market, the cost would have dropped as a consequence of the law of supply and demand.

This development in Birmingham is typical, and there are two related explanations for it. First, insurance companies reimburse specialists on the basis of what is normal ("reasonable and customary"), and as more specialists enter a system, they can drive up costs by raising the "normal" level. Second, specialists are able to do this by creating demand for their services—a phenomenon known as *induced demand*. Each specialist tends to believe that people need his or her services (just as every instructor believes that students need more courses in his or her field). Thus more services are created, creating more costs. Without a gatekeeper, this effect cannot be controlled. Every patient wants the best care, and when a specialist says a certain procedure is "best" and an insurer will pay for it, the patient tends to go along.

There are additional arguments against the concept of a market solution: even if we did have a true market for medical care, there are several reasons why it would probably not be a good thing.

One reason has to do with elderly patients. Applying a market solution to elderly patients might be dangerous; it is not at all clear how a market system could deliver minimal basic care to all elderly Americans fairly, efficiently, and inexpensively. On the twentieth anniversary of Medicare in 1985, the Harvard Medicare Project evaluated its successes and failures and concluded:

> The special nature of older persons and their health problems argues for caution in relying primarily on private solutions to providing health care for them.
>   . . . In particular, the elderly are less equipped to deal with a marketplace of medical care than younger, working persons. Partly because elderly persons are more likely to suffer from physical and mental impairments (including eyesight, hearing, and memory), they have more trouble than younger persons in comprehending the increasingly complex insurance arrangements now available. The elderly also usually lack the counsel of the purchasing agents and benefits representatives who serve younger, employed populations. Although some retired persons may be able to navigate our health care system, many others will not fare well in the rough and tumble of a health care marketplace.
>   Consequently, although we favor providing Medicare beneficiaries with more choices, we believe this can best be achieved by allowing them more options within the existing Medicare program and by encouraging a cooperative approach between the public and private sectors.[33]

Another argument against the market solution is that since the level of medical services would be significantly lower under a true market system (because consumers would have to pay for everything themselves), such a system might put millions of health professionals out of work. During the last few years, one-sixth of all new jobs created in the United States have been in health care, and one-seventh of the American economy has been concerned with providing health care. While we might ask whether we really want to tax ourselves to create jobs in this very inefficient way, the point remains that a market approach to medical care could have drastic effects on a very considerable segment of our economy.

One major argument against the market solution is that many people simply would not get the medical care they need, either because they could not afford it or because they would inevitably make some inappropriate choices as consumers. In a true market, some people would remain untreated because they could not pay for their own care; and medical professionals would need to become very hardboiled, doing "wallet biopsies" before helping anyone, to avoid being "manipulated" into providing free care. A real market for medical care would be a harsh, cruel system where patients and professionals no longer worked together to overcome illness and injury; in such a system, patients would have to bargain with professionals.

It is also true that if medical care were provided as other commercial commodities are—rather than being subsidized as it now is—many people who could afford care would not make wise decisions about what to buy and what to postpone or forgo. If we had to choose between a new car and a hip replacement, some of us would choose the car. Moreover, some people might be tempted, or pressured, to sacrifice medical care for the sake of their families: a parent might give up a hip replacement and put the money toward a house for the family.

In some more modest form, however, the market concept may still have something to offer. One intriguing idea is to make the present system more like a market by making medical coverage more like automobile insurance.[34] Because people pay for automobile insurance themselves, they usually shop around for the best or most appropriate policy. If this concept was applied to health care, people could increase or decrease their deductibles and coverage just as with automobile insurance: people who wanted to save money on premiums could opt for a higher deductible or less extensive coverage; people who wanted both prepaid group health care and catastrophe insurance could pay more.

Costs of Increased Medical Care

A major issue about medical care is that increases in access and services seem to entail increases in costs. Fiscal conservatives say that our experience with Medicare has taught us an important lesson: the system cannot expand the number of patients covered or the range of services offered and simultaneously decrease costs.

The Clinton plan was intended to increase access by providing coverage for the 39 million Americans who are now uninsured or underinsured. Although some analysts have argued that this would cost only about 6 percent of current spending for medical care, this is still a sizable figure—$50 billion annually.[35]

Moreover, other analysts believe that Americans who are now without insurance may be generally unhealthier than those with insurance, and that covering them would therefore cost significantly more. Thus any attempt to increase access does not bode well for the goal of controlling costs.

Furthermore, reformers usually have another goal—increased services. Each increase in service will cost more money, especially if it is provided to all Americans.

The increases in services that are most commonly mentioned are:

- Long-term care in nursing homes (despite widespread belief to the contrary, this is rarely covered now).
- Auxiliary medical services such as home health care, hospice care, and transportation to medical facilities.
- Dental services, including preventive dental care.
- Services for mental illness—especially the most costly, inpatient care for substance abuse.

Each of these is extremely expensive. Long-term nursing home care, for instance, can indeed be long-term—20 years or more—and in special cases (such as Karen Quinlan and Nancy Cruzan in Chapter 1) it might have to include three shifts of nurses. Costs of home health care rose even faster than other medical costs between 1988 and 1993.[36]

Our experience with Medicare bears out the conclusion that reduction in costs is probably incompatible with either expanded access or expanded services and is almost certainly incompatible with a combination of increased access and services. Under Medicare the cost of health care has risen from 5.3 percent of the GNP in 1965 to 14 percent of the GNP in 1993.

It is sometimes argued that the cost of increases in access and services can be offset by reducing waste. Consumers Union, for instance, has estimated that $200 billion could be saved by eliminating waste and unnecessary procedures from the medical system,[37] and some analysts argue that reforming the system would have this effect and that the money saved could pay for medical care for the uninsured. However, this may be one of those "painless" fantasies, like reducing the federal deficit by eliminating waste.

One counterargument, for instance, is that defining "waste" in generally acceptable terms would be difficult or even impossible. Some definitions of "waste" would be legally unacceptable: for example, if some services mandated by ADA were considered "waste," they could not be eliminated without violating the law of the land. Other definitions of "waste" would be politically unacceptable: each politician, for instance, would fight to preserve medical services and facilities in his or her own constituency, even if more objective evaluators considered them wasteful. In other words, one person's waste is another person's job, clinic, or hospital.

Another counterargument is that even if waste could be significantly reduced, it would be a one-time saving. That is, reducing waste would have no effect on the cost escalation inherent in an aging population with greater medical needs, or on the escalation inherent in new medical technologies such as better but patented drugs and better but costly machinery.

In the end, then, Americans may need to choose between increasing medical care (in terms of access and services) and controlling costs; we may not be able to have both. And if we choose to increase access and services, an equally important choice may be whether to for pay expanded care now or leave future generations to pay for it.

Insurance Companies: Approaches to Coverage

Basically, there are two ways of conceptualizing medical insurance. First, there is the *moral* approach. With this concept, insurance is an enterprise of sharing risk among many people, and it is intended as a way of helping us protect ourselves against bad luck. One example of the moral approach is *community rating*, a system whereby the risk represented by an area (such as an entire state) is evaluated, and every policyholder in the area is charged the same rate. When insurance is sold on a communitywide rating system, it favors people who are less healthy, because they cannot be excluded and their benefits are subsidized by the premiums of healthier policyholders. Another example of the moral approach is rating an entire country, as in Canada's single-payer system: healthier Canadians, who rarely use the medical system, subsidize those who are less healthy.

Second, there is the *profit* approach to medical insurance. With this concept, providing medical coverage is simply one way among many for a business to make profits; selling medical coverage is no different in nature from selling cars or encyclopedias. Profits are maximized by selling policies to healthy young people, who are unlikely to make claims; and by avoiding having to sell policies to people who are sick, old, disabled, or at high risk of accidents—that is, people who are likely to make claims. Thus insurers who operate on the profit concept often exclude many people from medical coverage. The profit approach is based on *experience rating*: a system of differential rates based on risks represented by individuals or groups.

Both approaches have been taken in the United States: medical insurance here began with the moral concept, but most of it has evolved into the profit concept.

During the 1930s, when surgeons and physicians founded first Blue Cross and later Blue Shield, their highest priority was to make sure that patients would have enough money to pay the bills of surgeons and physicians after hospitalization for catastrophic conditions. By state law, the "Blues" were nonprofit organizations; as such, in many states they paid no federal taxes and no taxes on the premiums they collected. In return for their nonprofit status, Blue Cross-Blue Shield (BCBS) companies were expected to insure as many people as possible, and to do this they adopted a community-rating scheme. Between the 1930s and the 1960s, because BCBS had a virtual monopoly on medical coverage, things worked out for everyone. BCBS insured everyone who wanted insurance, and rates remained reasonable.

In the early 1970s, changes in federal regulations allowed commercial insurance companies of a new kind to come into existence. These new commercial insurers were allowed to use experience rating, and they started "cherry picking" the healthiest customers of BCBS, leaving BCBS as an insurer of last resort for the unhealthiest and neediest customers.[38] Under these circumstances, what eventually happened to Empire BCBS, the organization serving New York State, was probably predictable. Empire BCBS did apparently suffer from mismanagement; more to the point, though, it was suffering financial losses because commercial insurance companies had taken its best customers and left it with only the sickest customers, such as those with AIDS. As a result, Empire BCBS had to raise premiums for all its customers by nearly 100 percent. Another target of cherry picking, Kentucky BCBS, saw its share of policies statewide drop from 90 to 30 percent between the early 1960s and the late 1970s. Some states have now made cherry picking illegal.

Employment and Coverage

Most Americans—57 percent—get medical coverage though employment.[39] An employment-based medical system has both strengths and weaknesses.

The strengths of employment-based coverage appear mostly with large employers, who offer far better medical plans, in general, than small employers. Large employers can spread risks over a pool of many employees. Also, large employers receive discounts from hospitals and, in effect, from insurance companies. Insurance companies now generally set different rates, based on how large an employer is (this is a type of experience rating), and employers with over 1,000 workers pay the lowest rates. Moreover, one factor keeping insurance affordable for many larger employers is demographics: workers tend to have fewer medical problems than other groups such as unemployed people, retired people, and children.

The weaknesses of employment-based coverage appear, to begin with, when we consider small employers. Many small businesses—and most very small businesses—do not offer medical coverage at all, and this is not necessarily their fault. Despite the demographics, insuring employees can be very expensive; under experience rating, employers with 50 to 100 workers pay higher rates for insurance than larger employers, and employers with fewer than 25 employees pay the highest rates of all. Thus small businesses trying to allocate capital for expansion—or struggling to make any profit at all—often cannot afford to offer insurance. There is a widespread belief that most Americans without medical coverage are unemployed, but this is a myth: in fact, most of the 39 million Americans without good medical coverage are employed.[40] Most waiters and waitresses, for instance, have no employer-sponsored medical insurance. Only 1 of 10 businesses employing fewer than 10 people provides medical coverage.[41]

A second disadvantage of the American employment-based system is that when a worker leaves a job, medical coverage is likely to be cut off. For one thing, insurance is almost never portable to another company. Also, many young working people in the United States today do not realize that their employer may be paying most of the cost of medical coverage, and that if they quit or are fired they will have to bear this cost themselves, at least until they find another job. Essentially the same is often true of older workers who retire or lose their jobs before age 65, when they will become eligible for Medicare; even if the employer agrees to continue coverage at the cheaper rates of the group plan, the former employee will have pay for it alone—the employer will no longer contribute.

A third disadvantage is *cost-shifting*. American hospitals are not reimbursed for providing care to the poor, but federal law forbids any hospital with an emergency room to turn patients away because of inability to pay. To make up for the cost of this care, hospitals shift costs: they charge more for services to insured patients. This effect, of course, falls on privately insured patients as well, but employers in particular resent it; cost-shifting forces them to act as charities by subsidizing medical care for the indigent. (For this reason, employers in Oregon supported OHP.) Large businesses also argue that they are subsidizing the care of uninsured employees of small businesses, who are likely to come to emergency rooms with very serious medical problems, or to enter the medical system at age 65, under Medicare, with serious conditions that would have been preventable earlier. It is estimated that cost-shifting rose from $1.6 billion in 1988 to $38.8 billion in 1992.[42]

A fourth disadvantage is that American employers say the cost of insuring their employees is much too high. In 1990, for instance, over $675 of the cost of each new Ford vehicle went to pay for medical coverage for employees of Ford and its suppliers.[43]

This leads to a fifth disadvantage of employment-based insurance: in recent years, many employers have been trying to lower their costs in ways that can be harmful to workers. Some businesses reduce the number of full-time employees with benefits such as medical coverage; instead, they replace one full-time worker with two part-time workers who have no benefits, or they contract "independent consultants" without benefits to replace managers and lower-level employees. Such a policy creates a two-class medical system in the United States: full-time employees with high salaries and benefits versus part-time employees and the unemployed with no benefits.

A sixth disadvantage of the employment-based system is that many workers are pushed out of the labor force and into chronic unemployment because of an illness or injury. Many poor people are poor primarily because of medical conditions that make them unacceptable to employers who are seeking to reduce medical costs.

People who are unemployed or work for a small company which offers no medical insurance may, of course, try to buy individual policies. About 7 percent of Americans do; they include people who are self-employed, seasonal workers, adult students, and people who are between jobs. However, private individual policies are expensive because the policyholder is not part of a large pool of workers and because such policies are subject to experience rating.

Medical Care and the Federal Government

What is the proper role of the federal government with regard to medical care? This is a controversial question: some Americans want more federal government, some want less, and many swing back and forth between these two positions.

Some of the critics who advocate a "market" approach to reforming medical care, for instance, are not really calling for a true market system but are simply expressing their distrust of big government. They say that federal funding for end-stage renal disease, artificial hearts, and AIDS is politicized and has been provided at the expense of other diseases. They also argue that American government is being asked to do too many things for too many different purposes and groups.

Some critics of a single-payer system are also dubious about a larger role for the federal government. With one-seventh of the American economy at stake, and perhaps one-sixth of new jobs, do we want to take the chance of a federally administered system? Suppose it flops?

The record of federal government is mixed, and how it is evaluated depends on who is being interviewed and when. For example, the armed forces—a prime example of a federally run institution—are notorious for cost overruns and inefficiency; on the other hand, of all American institutions which employ large numbers of people and have ever been racially segregated, the armed forces are now most nearly color-blind. Medicine was also once highly segregated and is now on the whole color-blind (at least for people with insurance), and this has been brought about largely through federally enforced changes.

Medical Care and Political Philosophy

We cannot really discuss or evaluate systems of medical care without including some political philosophy. One way to consider political philosophy with regard to medical care is in terms of justice and the "right" to care.

The "right" to medical care   Many people claim that Americans have a right to medical care. What does such a right mean?

A right to a medical care does *not* mean that everyone would receive the same kind of medical care. Nor does it mean equality of outcomes: since health depends on so many factors—including genes, environment, and individual habits—no degree of equal medical treatment could possibly ensure equal results.

A right to medical care would, at most, probably mean a right to *basic care*, a decent minimum of care.[44] This would not preclude a system in which some people bought extra medical care above this minimum; a two-tiered system of this nature would not be unjust, and as a practical matter it could not be prevented in a democratic society.

Rawls: Medical care in a "just society"   There are several bases for the claimed right to medical care.[45] One argument is provided by the theory of justice developed by the philosopher John Rawls.[46]

Rawls believes that the term *justice* best applies to the design of basic structures and institutions in a society, and a system of medical care is one such structure or institution. According to Rawls, principles of justice are part of a hypothetical social contract in which we all come together to make choices—but we must choose under a "veil of ignorance" about our own age, race, religion, sex, health, wealth, abilities, and talents. In other words, we cannot bias our choices by considering arbitrary personal characteristics.

Under these conditions, Rawls believes, rational people would not gamble rashly with the structure of their most important institutions; they would choose those structures that gave people equal opportunities (such as the opportunity to get ahead in business by being free to make contracts and by receiving equal treatment under the law). To Rawls, inequality is justifiable only when it works to the advantage of those who are worst off, that is, when the worst-off group actually does better with the inequality than without it. This is Rawls's *difference principle.*

An essential part of Rawls's concept of justice is the recognition that the world is naturally unfair: some people are born into rich families, some into poor ones; some people are born healthy, others with spina bifida. For Rawls, government can either exacerbate such inequalities or smooth them out. A government which sharpens inequality is unjust; only the government which mitigates inequality is just.

Rawls's "veil of ignorance" can be seen as a device for ensuring that the golden rule will become part of our decisions about the structure of society. Underlying this approach is the ability to imagine *ourselves* as "worst off"—to see ourselves as sick, hurt, poor, uninsured; to imagine how bad it would be to have a serious illness or accident, and how much worse it would be to have no way to pay for the care we need.

•

How might Rawls's approach be specifically applied to our own system?

The Reagan-Bush decade was not good for the working poor or the lower middle class. By one measure, 70 percent of the increase in wealth between 1977 and 1989 went to the top 1 percent of Americans. The Center on Budget and Policy Priorities reported that, overall, the gap between the richest one-fifth of Americans and the lowest fifth widened greatly: the income of the highest fifth increased by 70 percent while the income of the lowest fifth decreased by 8 percent.[47] More and more workers had to work longer and longer just to keep what they had. More and more companies did not hire permanent full-time workers with full benefits such as medical coverage but rather used part-time workers and consultants. Some jobs that once paid $20 an hour now paid $7. If, as Rawls assumes, a just society is egalitarian, then American society became more unjust.

Our existing medical system, in which more than 39 million Americans are without insurance, may represent a structural inequality at a deep level, a level where life-and-death decisions are made. To make matters worse, those who suffer most from this structural inequality may be our children. As many as one-third of American children may spend part of their lives in poverty; far too many of their parents must choose between medical care for these children and basic necessities like food.

According to Rawls's difference principle, an unequal medical structure would be just only if the poor were better off under it than under an egalitarian system; and in the present, unequal American medical system, that is obviously not the case. Thus Rawls's theory of justice would call for reforming the American medical system, because almost any reform would improve the lot of the worst-off group.

Liberalism: Justice as a process   Rawls's analysis, equating justice with social structures that will most benefit the worst-off groups, is of course not the only approach to political justice. Many concepts of justice have been developed by political philosophers, and no concept is universally accepted.[48] Aristotle, for example, equates justice with perfection of the city-state. Locke and the modern libertarians equate justice with protection of individual property rights. Marx equates justice with equality of wealth and economic opportunities. Utilitarians equate justice with the greatest good for the greatest number.

The political philosophy known as *liberalism* and associated with John Stuart Mill equates justice not with content but with a process: just policies are those achieved through open, democratic procedures in which everyone has an equal vote. One goal, or ideal, of liberalism is impartiality with regard to any particular vision of the good life—and indeed with regard to any particular vision of the content of justice. (Perhaps the best-known application of this impartiality is the separation of church and state.)

Liberalism offers an important perspective on medical care, though its value is not always recognized. For instance, Ezekiel Emanuel has argued that liberalism is incapable of giving answers about how to allocate medical resources or how to reach agreement about terminating care for incompetent patients.[49] Although this is true, it does not really constitute an argument against liberalism. As the philosopher Ludwig Wittgenstein once wrote, "The first step in a philosophic debate often escapes notice." Here, the first step is the unwarranted assumption that liberalism is intended to offer content-specific answers to problems in medical ethics.

Liberalism is intended to guide the process of decision making—that is, to lead us to the best process. It does not, and cannot, offer content-specific answers, because it is neutral about the "good life." If we apply liberalism to terminating care, for instance, we might conclude that the best process is to let a competent patient decide, or let the family of an incompetent patient decide, or let an ethics committee decide for incompetent patients. If we apply liberalism to the allocation of medical resources, we might conclude that the best process is to let hospitals decide—or communities or states or regions or health plans. Or we might conclude that the best process for decision making about health care would be experimentation—trial and error—at the federal, state, or local level.

UPDATE

In October 1994, after 2 years of intense public discussion and behind-the-scenes lobbying, the 103d Congress went home without having passed, or even having voted on, a new medical plan for Americans. Clinton's Health Care Security bill had never gotten out of committee, and no alternative proposals had reached a vote. Medicare remained unchanged. Nearly 40 million Americans remained without medical coverage.

There was, of course, a great deal of analysis and speculation about this anticlimax in the movement to reform medical care. Better judgments will be possible when some time has passed, but two observations may be mentioned here.

First, it is interesting to note that the American College of Surgeons had backed the Clinton plan, and that some physicians and surgeons felt that they would have been better off with it than they are under many new private plans. Their reasoning is that the federal government would have had to abide (as Medicare now must abide) by due process, ADA, and similar constraints. By contrast, a large company is free to deliver an ultimatum to, say, a group of ophthalmologists: "If you don't drop your fees by 50 percent, we have another group waiting in the wings who will provide services at the lower rate." In such a situation, there is very little room for physicians to maneuver.

Second, there were predictions that, given the failure of reform at the federal level, states might step in to bring about changes. Half a dozen states did announce plans to cover their own uninsured residents; California began to consider legislation of this nature; and, as this book went to press, Washington had actually passed such a law.

FURTHER READING

Ezekiel Emanuel, *The Ends of Human Life: Medical Ethics in a Liberal Polity*, Harvard University Press, Cambridge, Mass., 1992.

Frank Marsh and Mark Yarborough, *Medicine and Money: A Study of the Role of Beneficence in Health Care Cost Containment*, Greenwood, New York, 1990.

E. Haavi Morreim, ed., "Ethics and Alternative Health Systems," *Journal of Medicine and Philosophy*, vol. 17, no. 1 (special issue), February 1992.

Notes

The following abbreviations (in addition to the customary bibliographic terms) are used in these notes:

AMN = *American Medical News*
AP = Associated Press
HCR = *Hastings Center Report*
JAMA = *Journal of the American Medical Association*
NEJM = *New England Journal of Medicine*
NYT = *New York Times*
UAB = University of Alabama at Birmingham
UPI = United Press International
WP = *Washington Post*
WSJ = *Wall Street Journal*

Chapter 1

1. The first *NYT* story on the Quinlan case is September 16, 1975, New Jersey sec., p. 32. The Quinlans' version is from Joseph Quinlan and Julia Quinlan with Phyllis Battelle, *Karen Ann: The Quinlans Tell Their Story*, Doubleday Anchor, New York, 1977.
2. Robert Morse, in *In the Matter Of Karen Quinlan: The Complete Legal Briefs, Court Proceedings, and Decisions in the Superior Court of New Jersey*, vols. 1 and 2, University Publications of America, Frederick, Md., 1982, p. 236 (hereafter, *Proceedings 1, Proceedings 2*).
3. Julius Korein, in *Proceedings 1*, pp. 34–35.
4. George Daggett, *NYT*, September 20, 1975, New Jersey sec.
5. Quinlan and Quinlan, op. cit., p. 22.
6. Ibid., p. 29.
7. Ibid., p. 27.
8. Daniel Coburn, in *Proceedings 1*, p. 17.
9. This standard partially explains why physicians are so reluctant to make significant changes publicly in life-and-death issues. Ambitious lawyers and elected officials may use such cases to advance their own careers, and physicians are reluctant to become their targets. This creates inertia against change in medicine.
10. Thomas C. Oden, "Beyond an Ethic of Immediate Sympathy," *HCR*, February 1976, p. 12.
11. Daniel Coburn, in *Proceedings 1*, pp. 196–198.
12. Ralph Porzio, in *Proceedings 1*, pp. 202–206.
13. Julius Korein, in *Proceedings 1*, p. 329.
14. Fred Plum, in Quinlan and Quinlan, op. cit., pp. 188–189.
15. Robert Morse, in Quinlan and Quinlan, op. cit., p. 198.
16. Quinlan and Quinlan, op. cit., pp. 272–273 (the nun is not named).
17. Gino Concetti, quoted in Quinlan and Quinlan, op. cit., p. 284.
18. Quoted in Quinlan and Quinlan, op. cit.
19. Joseph Fennelly, quoted in Quinlan and Quinlan, op. cit., p. 284.
20. *Cruzan v. Director*, Missouri Dept. of Health, 110 S. Ct. 2841, 1990.
21. George Annas, "Nancy Cruzan and the Right to Die," *NEJM*, vol. 323, no. 10, September 6, 1990, p. 670.
22. "Love and Let Die," *Time*, March 19, 1990, pp. 62ff.
23. Andrew M. Malcolm, "Nancy Cruzan: End to Long Goodbye," *NYT*, December 29, 1990, p. A3.
24. Linda Greenhouse, "Right to Reject Life," *NYT*, June 27, 1990, p. A1.
25. *NYT*, June 27, 1990, p. A14.
26. In 1991, an Indiana court (*In re Lawrance*, 579 N.E. 2d 32) ruled that a surrogate could judge the "best interests" of the person in a right-to-die case for a "never competent" patient in PVS. This standard is discussed further in Chapter 7.
27. Charles Baron, "On Taking Substituted Judgment Seriously," *HCR*, vol. 20, no. 5, September-October 1992, p. 7.

28. John Robertson, *"Cruzan:* No Rights Violated," *HCR,* vol. 20, no. 5, September-October 1992, p. 7.

29. Baron, op. cit., p. 8.

30. Ronald Cranford, lecture at UAB Medical School, January 19, 1991. See also Ellen Goodman, "Permanently Comatose Don't Live," *Boston Globe,* December 12, 1992.

31. Joanne Lynn and Jacqueline Glover, *"Cruzan* and Caring for Others," *HCR,* vol. 20, no. 5, September-October 1992, p. 11.

32. Carol Lewis in Judge Teel's office in Jasper County courthouse, Joplin, Mo.

33. Annas, op. cit., p. 672.

34. President's Commission for the Study of Ethical Problems in Medicine and Biomedical and Behavioral Research, *Defining Death,* Superintendent of Documents, Washington, D.C., 1981, p. 14.

35. P. Mollaret and M. Goulon, "Le Coma Depassé," *Revue Neurologie,* vol. 101, no. 3, 1959.

36. Ad Hoc Committee of the Harvard Medical School to Examine the Definition of Brain Death, "A Definition of Irreversible Coma," *JAMA,* vol. 205, no. 337, 1968.

37. The characteristics listed by the philosopher Mary Anne Warren in Chapter 6 (with regard to whether an aborted fetus is a person) might be used in a similar way to define the "higher person" standard: if *all* these characteristics are lacking, we do not have a "person."

38. Multi-Society Task Force on PVS, "Medical Aspects of the Persistent Vegetative State," parts 1 and 2, *NEJM,* vol. 330, no. 22, pp. 1572–1579.

39. National Conference of Commission on Uniform Laws, *Uniform Laws Annual,* vol. 15, supp., 1981.

40. Quinlan and Quinlan, op. cit., p. 87.

41. American Academy of Neurology, amicus curiae brief in *Brophy v. New England Sinai Hospital, Inc.,* 1986; quoted in Ronald Cranford, "The Persistent Vegetative State: the Medical Reality (Getting the Facts Straight)," *HCR,* vol. 18, no. 1, 1988, p. 31.

42. Multi-Society Task Force on PVS, op. cit., pp. 1501–1502. The task force did not comment on the apparent contradiction between its claim that brain scans show no activity in PVS patients and the fact that 7 patients made a "good recovery" after over 1 year in PVS.

43. Ibid.

44. "U.S.A.: Right to Live, or Right to Die?" *Lancet,* vol. 337, January 12, 1991.

45. Don Coburn, "The 40-Year Vigil for Rita Greene," *WP,* sec. 11, March 12, 1991, pp. 10–13.

46. Daniel Callahan, "On Feeding the Dying," *HCR,* vol. 13, no. 5, October 1983, p. 22;

Gilbert Meillander, "On Removing Food and Water: Against the Stream," *HCR,* vol. 14, no. 6, December 1984, pp. 11–13.

47. Ibid., app. B, p. 288.

48. W. May, R. Barry, O. Griese, et al., "Feeding and Hydrating the Permanently Unconscious and Other Vulnerable Persons," *Issues in Law and Medicine,* vol. 3, no. 3, Winter 1987, pp. 203-217; C. Sprung, "Changing Attitudes and Practices in Forgoing Life-Sustaining Treatments," *JAMA,* vol. 263, no. 16, April 25, 1990, pp. 2211–2221.

49. American Medical Association, *Opinions of the Judicial Council,* Chicago, Ill., 1973.

50. Nat Hentoff, "The Deadly Slippery Slope," *Village Voice,* September 1, 1987.

51. Ibid.

52. Linda Greenhouse, "Right to Reject Life," *NYT,* June 27, 1990.

53. Robert Veatch, "Whole Brain, Neocortical, and Higher Brain Related Concepts of Death," in Richard Zaner, ed., *Whole Brain and Neocortical Definitions of Death: A Critical Appraisal,* Reidel, Norwell, Mass., 1986.

54. Lisa Belkin, "As Family Protests, Hospital Seeks End to Woman's Life Support," *NYT,* January 10, 1991, pp. A1–2.

55. Steven Miles, "Interpersonal Issues in the Wanglie Case," *Kennedy Institute of Ethics Journal,* vol. 2, no. 1, March 1992, pp. 61–72.

56. For a review of these cases, see *Law, Medicine, and Health Care,* vol. 20, 1993, pp. 310–315.

57. Robert D. Truogg, A. S. Brett, and Joel Frader, "The Problem with Futility," *NEJM,* vol. 326, 1992, pp. 1560–1564.

58. R. Knox, "Americans' New Way of Dying: Don't Fight It," *Boston Globe,* June 5, 1994.

59. L. Altman, "Quinlan Case Revisited and Yields New Finding," *NYT,* May 26, 1994.

Chapter 2

1. Quotations are from *Phaedo,* in E. Hamilton and H. Cairns, eds., *Plato: The Collected Dialogues,* Princeton University Press, Princeton, N.J., 1961.

2. Epictetus, *Dissertations,* 1.9, 16. Quoted in James Rachels, "Euthanasia," in T. Regan, ed., *Matters of Life and Death,* 3d ed., McGraw-Hill, New York, 1993, p. 35.

3. Jean Paul Sartre, "The Humanism of Existentialism," in Wade Beck., ed., *The Philosophy of Existentialism,* Philosophical Library, New York, 1965.

4. Seneca, *De Ira,* quoted in Rachels, op. cit.

5. Matthew 16:26–28; for similar predictions, see Mark 9:1, Matthew 10:23, Matthew 16:26–28; Luke 21:29–32; Matthew 24:32–33; Mark 13: 28–30; and indirectly, Matthew 10:7.

6. Alasdair MacIntyre, *A Short History of Ethics,* Macmillan, New York, 1966, pp. 116–117.

7. Margaret Pabst Battin, *Ethical Issues in Suicide*, Prentice-Hall, Englewood Cliffs, N.J., 1982, p. 34.

8. Frederick Russell, *The Just War in the Middle Ages*, Cambridge University Press, Cambridge, England, 1975.

9. Battin, op. cit.

10. Paul Badham, "Christian Beliefs and the Ethics of In-Vitro Fertilization and Abortion," *Bioethics News*, vol. 6, no. 2, January 1987, p. 8.

11. Quoted in James Gutman, "Death and Dying in Western Culture," *Encyclopedia of Bioethics*, vol. 1, Free Press, New York, 1978, p. 240.

12. Baruch Spinoza, *Ethics*, William White and Amelia Stirling, trans., Hafner, New York, 1949.

13. Quoted in Derek Humphrey and Ann Wickett, *The Right to Die: Understanding Euthanasia*, Harper and Row, New York, 1986, pp. 8–9.

14. David Hume, "On Suicide" (1755), in Eugene Miller, ed., *Collected Essays of David Hume*, Liberty Classics, Indianapolis, Ind., 1986.

15. Ibid.

16. Immanuel Kant, "On Suicide" (1755–1780), *Lectures on Ethics*, L. Enfield, trans., Harper and Row, New York, 1963, pp. 148–154.

17. John Stuart Mill, *On Liberty* (1859), Appleton-Century-Crofts, New York, 1974.

18. Quoted in Humphrey and Wickett, op. cit., p. 16.

19. AP, October 16, 1983.

20. Robert Steinbock and Bernard Lo, "The Case of Elizabeth Bouvia: Starvation, Suicide, or Problem Patient?" *Archives of Internal Medicine*, vol. 146, January 1986, p. 161.

21. Quoted in George Annas, "When Suicide Prevention Becomes Brutality: The Case of Elizabeth Bouvia," *HCR*, vol. 14, no. 2, April 1984, p. 20.

22. Steinbock and Lo, op. cit., p. 161.

23. *Bouvia v. County of Riverside*, California Superior Court, December 16, 1983.

24. Quoted in Arthur Hoppe, *San Francisco Examiner*, December 20, 1983.

25. Richard Scott, in "Patient's Suicide Wish Troubles Hospital MDs," *AMN*, January 20, 1984, p. 5.

26. AP, in *Birmingham Post-Herald*, December 14, 1984, p. A2.

27. Hoppe, op. cit.

28. Annas, op. cit., p. 46.

29. Quoted in Scott, op. cit.

30. Ibid., p. 16.

31. Annas, op. cit., p. 20.

32. Steinbock and Lo, op. cit., p. 162.

33. George Annas, "Elizabeth Bouvia: Whose Space Is This Anyway?" *HCR*, vol. 16, no. 2, April 1986, pp. 24–25.

34. Humphrey and Wickett, op. cit., p. 150.

35. Paul Longmore, "Elizabeth Bouvia, Assisted Suicide, and Social Prejudice," in *Issues in Law and Medicine*, vol. 2, no. 2, Fall 1987, p. 158.

36. The hospital's rationale in its brief to Judge Deering is quoted in Annas, "Elizabeth Bouvia: Whose Space Is This Anyway?"

37. *Bouvia v. Glenchur*, Los Angeles Superior Court, *California Reporter*, vol. 225, 1986, pp 296–308.

38. *Bouvia v. Superior Court* (Glenchur), *California Reporter*, vol. 297, California Appellate 2 District, 1986.

39. Russ Fine, *UAB Report*, September 4, 1992, p. 4.

40. B. D. Colen, "His Life, to Take or Not," *Newsday*, September 25, 1989, pp. 5–19 (cover story). I am indebted to Doris Rippetoe for this reference.

41. Ibid., p. 19.

42. Ibid.

43. Susan Schindehette and Gail Wescott, "Deciding Not to Die," *People Weekly*, January 18, 1993, p. 86.

44. Ibid.

45. Fine, op. cit.

46. Ibid., p. 12.

47. Alan Meisel, *The Right to Die: Cumulative Supplement 1*, Wylie, New York, 1991, p. x.

48. Battin, op. cit., p. 22; James Rachels, *The End of Life*, Oxford University Press, Oxford, 1986, p. 182; Tom Beauchamp, "Suicide," in T. Regan, ed., *Matters of Life and Death*, 3d ed., McGraw-Hill, New York, 1993.

49. Meisel, op. cit., p. x.

50. Kevin D. O'Rourke, "Value Conflicts Raised by Physician-Assisted Suicide," *Linacre Quarterly*, vol. 57, no. 3, August 1990, pp. 38–49.

51. T. Woody, "Was His Act of Mercy Also Murder?" *NYT*, November 7, 1988.

52. Art Kleiner, "Life after Suicide," *High Wire*, Summer 1982, p. 30.

53. H. Hendin, "Suicide in America," *Miami News*, August 30, 1982, p. B1.

54. Quoted in Humphrey and Wickett, op. cit., p. 152.

55. Quoted ibid., p. 155.

56. Longmore, op. cit., p. 156.

57. Cowart's case became the topic of a famous videotape, *Please Let Me Die*, and a later film, *Dax's Case*. See also L. Kliever, *Dax's Case—Essays in Medical Ethics and Human Meaning*, SMU Press, Dallas, Texas, 1989.

58. Longmore, op. cit., p. 168.

59. Fine, op. cit., p. 12.

60. Ibid.

61. AP, "Thousands Retiring without Social Security," February 16, 1993.

62. "McAfee Tries to Cut Red Tape," *Birmingham Post-Herald*, June 18, 1990, p. C1.

63. J. Hogeland and L. Sellars, "McAfee Should-n't Get Special Treatment," letter, *Birmingham Post-Herald,* July 9, 1990.
64. Jeff Wilson (AP), "Precedent-Setter Lives On after Plea to Die," *Indianapolis Star,* December 19, 1993, p. H7.
65. *UAB Report,* August 28, 1992, p. 12.
66. Fine, personal communication to author, May 16, 1994.
67. Dax Cowart, personal communication to author at meeting of American Association of Medical Colleges, Chicago, Ill., October 1989.

Chapter 3

1. For a discussion of problems involved in defining *physician-assisted suicide,* see Ronald F. White, "Physician-Assisted Suicide and The Suicide Machine," in Robert I. Misbin, ed., *Euthanasia: The Good of the Patient, the Good of Society,* Frederick, Md., University Press, 1992.
2. Ludwig Edelstein, *Ancient Medicine: Collected Essays of Ludwig Edelstein,* O. Temkin and L. Temkin, eds., Johns Hopkins University Press, Baltimore, Md., 1967.
3. G. E. R. Lloyd, "Introduction," *Hippocratic Writings,* J. Chadwick and W. N. Mann, trans., Penguin, New York, 1978 (trans. 1950), p. 13.
4. Leo Alexander, "Medical Science under Dictatorship," *NEJM,* vol. 42, July 14, 1949.
5. Robert Jay Lifton, *The Nazi Doctors,* Basic Books, New York, 1986.
6. Quoted in Derek Humphrey and Ann Wickett, *The Right to Die: Understanding Euthanasia,* Harper and Row, New York, 1988, p. 172.
7. See Marlise Simons, "Dutch Parliament Approves Law Permitting Euthanasia," *NYT,* February 10, 1993, p. 5; *Bulletin* of the Hemlock Society, April 1993; and Johannes J. M. van Delden et al., "The Remmelink Study: Two Years later," *HCR,* vol. 23, no. 6, November-December 1993, p. 24.
8. Patrick Cooke, "The Gentle Death," *Hippocrates,* September-October 1989, p. 50.
9. Marlise Simons, "Dutch Survey Casts New Light on Patients Who Choose to Die," *NYT,* September 11, 1991; discusses the Gerrit van der Wal survey published in the *Netherlands Journal of Medicine.*
10. Randi Hutter Epstein (AP), "Dutch Seek Motivations for Euthanasia," September 16, 1991; discusses Paul van der Maas study in *Lancet* of a week earlier.
11. Marlise Simons, "Dutch Parliament Approves Law Permitting Euthanasia"; see also van Delden et al., op. cit.
12. Peter Steinfels, "Dutch Study Is Euthanasia Vote Issue," *NYT,* September 20, 1991.
13. This figure may simply indicate when cancer is most likely to occur in certain groups of people. There is some evidence that a person who makes it past age 65 without developing cancer has a greatly reduced risk cancer until the mid-eighties.
14. *Nightline,* April 1987 (author's videotape).
15. Van Delden et al., op. cit.
16. "Dutch Psychiatrist to Be Tried in Euthanasia," *NYT,* April 6, 1993.
17. Leon Kass, quoted in Earl Ubell, "Should Death Be a Patient's Choice?" *Parade,* February 9, 1992, p. 27.
18. Carlos Gomez, *Regulating Death: Euthanasia and the Case of the Netherlands,* Free Press/Macmillan, New York, 1991.
19. Quoted in Ubell, op. cit., p. 27.
20. Humphrey assisted in the death of his first wife, Jean, when her cancer reached an advanced stage. His second wife, Ann Wickett, who suffered from terminal cancer and also from depression, killed herself after a bitter divorce from him, denouncing Humphrey himself and some aspects of the Hemlock Society. Wickett had been a board member of the Hemlock Society during its major growth in the 1980s.
21. Shana Alexander, at "Birth of Bioethics" conference, University of Washington Medical School, Seattle, October 22, 1992.
22. Jack Kevorkian, *Prescription: Medicide—The Goodness of Planned Death,* Prometheus, Buffalo, N. Y., 1991, p. 221. See also *Newsweek,* November 13, 1989.
23. Timothy Egan, "As Memory and Music Faded, Alzheimer Patient Met Death," *NYT,* June 6, 1990, p. A1.
24. Carol J. Casteneda and Robert Davis, "Kevorkian: Death Must Be an Option," *USA Today,* February 22, 1993.
25. Kevorkian, op. cit., p. 209.
26. Ibid., p. 188.
27. Isabel Wilkerson, "Physician Fulfills a Goal: Aiding a Person in Suicide," *NYT,* June 7, 1990.
28. Lisa Belkin, "Doctor Tells of First Death Using His Suicide Device," *NYT,* June 8, 1990.
29. Kevorkian, op. cit., p. 189.
30. Ibid., p. 214.
31. Belkin, op. cit.
32. Casdteneda and Davis, op. cit., p. A2.
33. Kevorkian, op. cit., p. 193.
34. Ibid.
35. Wilkerson, op. cit.
36. Nancy Gibbs, "Dr. Death Strikes Again," *Time,* November 4, 1991, p. 78.
37. Kevorkian, op. cit., p. 207.
38. Mark Hosenball, "The Real Jack Kevorkian," *Newsweek,* December 6, 1993, p. 28.
39. Jack Lessenberry, "The Lawyer Who Keeps the Suicide Doctor Free," *NYT,* July 9, 1993, p. A13.
40. Kevorkian, op. cit., p. 225.

41. Gloria Borger, "The Odd Odyssey of 'Dr. Death,'" *U. S. News and World Report,* August 27, 1990, p. 2.

42. Timothy Quill, "Death and Dignity: A Case of Individualized Decision Making," *NEJM,* vol. 324, no. 10, March 7, 1991, pp. 691–694.

43. Ibid., p. 692.

44. Ibid., p. 693.

45. Lawrence Altman, "Jury Declines to Indict a Doctor Who Said He Aided in a Suicide," *NYT,* July 22, 1991, p. A1.

46. Richard Brandt, quoted in Susan Ager, "When Suicide Is the Last Hope," *Detroit Free Press,* June 8, 1990.

47. Christiaan Barnard, *One Life,* Macmillan, New York, 1965.

48. Karel Gunning, on *Nightline,* April 1987.

49. Rufus E. Miles, "Quick and Painless Death Should Be a Right," letter, *NYT,* June 19, 1990.

50. Quoted in Barnard White Stack, "Doctors Divided Over the Very Ill," *Pittsburgh Post Gazette,* June 11, 1990.

51. Margaret Battin, "The Least Worst Death," *HCR,* vol. 13, no. 2, April 1983, pp. 13–16.

52. Quoted in Peter Steinfels, "At Crossroads, U. S. Ponders Ethics of Helping Others," *NYT,* April 28, 1993, p. A8.

53. Alex Capron, quoted in Michael Specter, "Suicide Device Fuels Debate," *WP,* June 8, 1990.

54. Quoted in Jo Grifits, "Suicide Issue Perplexes the Medical Community," *Pennsylvania Patriot* (Harrisburg), June 17, 1990.

55. Joan Teno and Joanne Lynn, "Voluntary Active Euthanasia: The Individual Case and Public Policy," *Journal of the American Geriatrics Society,* vol. 39, 1991, pp. 827–830.

56. Cicely Saunders, "The Philosophy of Terminal Care," in C. M. Sanders, ed., *The Management of Terminal Disease,* Edward Arnold, London, 1978, p. 194.

57. Quoted in Stack, op. cit.

58. Quoted in Alan Parachini, "A Dutch Doctor Carries Out a Death Wish," *Los Angeles Times,* July 5, 1987, sec. 6, p. 9.

59. Quoted in Linda Matchan, "Suicide Shocks Ethicists," *Boston Globe,* June 7, 1990.

60. Quoted in Ubell, op. cit., p. 28.

61. Frank Bruni, "Theatrics Eclipse Ethics," *Detroit News and Free Press,* October 26, 1991.

62. Quoted in Brian T. Meehan, "Adkins Suicide Ignites Nationwide Debate," *The Oregonian* (Portland, Ore.), June 8, 1990.

63. Quoted in *Hartford Courant* (Connecticut), June 13, 1990.

64. A case in Washington, D.C., is described in Susan Okie, "A Slow Death amid Doctor-Family Conflict," *WP,* June 16, 1991, pp. A1, A14. See also Kathrine Kerr, "'Kill Me,' Hopeless Man Begs," *Houston Post* (Texas), June 9, 1990.

65. Cited in Chris Golembiewski, "Suicide Case Brings Issue to Doorstep of Capitol," *Lansing State Journal,* June 10, 1990.

66. Cited in Craig Brandon, "Ending It All," *Times Union* (Albany, N. Y.), June 7, 1990.

67. AMA in particular has often opposed sensible changes, such as women physicians, salaried physicians, private medical insurance, and Medicare.

68. D. Alan Shewmon, "Active Voluntary Euthanasia: A Needless Paradox," *Issues in Law and Medicine,* vol. 3, no. 3, Winter 1987; reprinted in Robert Baird and Stuart Rosenbaum, eds., *Euthanasia: The Moral Issues,* Prometheus, Buffalo, N. Y., 1989, p. 137.

69. Smith and Associates, "A Good Death: Is Euthanasia the Answer?" *Cleveland Journal of Medicine,* January–February 1992, pp. 99–109.

70. Norman Fost, quoted in Mark Ward, "Experts Consider Legal and Ethical Aspects of Helping Americans Die," *Milwaukee Journal* (Wisonsin), June 7, 1990 (NEWSBANK, microfiche).

71. Christine Cassell, quoted in Specter, op. cit.

72. James Rachels, "Active and Passive Euthanasia," *NEJM,* vol. 292, January 9, 1975, pp. 78–80.

73. Baruch Brody, "Ethical Questions Raised by the Persistent Vegetative Patient," *HCR,* vol. 18, no. 1, p. 35.

74. Ronald Cranford, lecture at UAB, January 1991.

75. Jean Davies, "Raping and Making Love Are Different Concepts: So Are Killing and Voluntary Euthanasia," *Journal of Medical Ethics,* vol. 14, 1988, pp. 148–149.

76. Nat Hentoff, "The Deadly Slippery Slope," *Village Voice,* September 1, 1987.

77. Nat Hentoff, "Decision on Euthanasia Will Create a Slippery Slope," nationally syndicated column, Newspaper Enterprise Association, October 6, 1992.

78. Ibid.

79. Allan Parachini, "The Netherlands Debates the Legal Limits of Euthanasia," *Los Angeles Times,* July 5, 1987, sec. 6, p. 8.

80. Ibid.

81. Yale Kamisar, quoted in Ubell, op. cit., pp. 24–25.

82. Quoted in Ward, op. cit.

83. Arthur Caplan, quoted in Ubell, op. cit., p. 27.

84. "Physician-Assisted Dying: Historical Perspective—An Interview with Stanley J. Reiser," *Trends in Health Care, Law, and Ethics,* vol. 7, no. 2, Winter 1992, p. 13.

85. Teno and Lynn, op. cit., p. 828.

86. James Bopp, quoted in Specter, op. cit.

87. Quoted in Steinfels, "Dutch Study," p. A15.

88. Ferdinand Protzman, "Killing of 49 Elderly Patients by Nurse Aides Stuns Austria," *NYT,* April 18, 1989.

89. Norman Paradis, "Making a Living Off the Dying," *NYT,* April 25, 1992, p. 15.
90. AP, February 16, 1993.
91. *Newsweek,* March 8, 1993, pp. 46, 48.
92. "Kevorkian Is Charged Again with Aiding a Suicide," *NYT,* November 30, 1993, p. A8.
93. Francis X. Clines, "A Verdict on Kevorkian: Their Kind of Neighbor," *NYT,* October 29, 1993, p. A7.
94. Ibid.
95. Lessenberry, op. cit.
96. "Kevorkian Aids Suicide in Bid for Jail," *NYT,* October 23, 1993, p. A8.
97. Ibid.
98. AP, "Kevorkian Admits Aiding Suicide," *Birmingham Post-Herald,* August 5, 1993, p. A6.
99. "Kevorkian Details His Role in Suicide," *NYT,* August 5, 1993, p. A8.
100. David Margolick, "Doctor Who Helps Suicides Has Made the Bizarre Banal," *NYT,* February 22, 1993, pp. A1, C8.
101. Don Terry, "While on Bail, Kevorkian Attends a Doctor's Suicide," *NYT,* November 11, 1993.
102. *NYT,* April 28, 1994, p. A8 (national ed.).
103. *NYT,* May 5, 1994, pp. A1, 11 (national ed.).
104. *ABC World News,* February 1, 1994, interview with Peter Jennings (on this broadcast, Kevorkian was named "Person of the Week").
105. Clyde Farnsworth, "Canadian Who Lost Suicide Lawsuit Kills Herself," *NYT,* February 14, 1994, p. A8.
106. Timothy Egan, *NYT,* May 5, 1994, p. A1.
107. Press release, Royal Netherlands Embassy, Washington, D.C., May 11, 1994.
108. *NYT,* June 22, 1994, p. A10.

Chapter 4

1. A. Wilcox et al., "Incidence of Early Loss of Pregnancy, *NEJM,* vol. 319, no. 4, July 28, 1988, pp. 189–194. See also J. Grudzinskas and A. Nysenbaum, "Failure of Human Pregnancy after Implantation," *Annals of New York Academy of Sciences,* vol. 442, 1985, pp. 39–44; J. Muller et al., "Fetal Loss after Implantation," *Lancet,* vol. 2, 1980, pp. 554–556.
2. Deborah Yaeger, "Doctors Make Progress Treating Infertility, but Costs Are High," *WSJ,* October 12, 1984, p. 1.
3. "Adoption Demand Exceeding Supply," *NYT,* April 5, 1987, p. A1.
4. Bureau of the Census, *Statistical Abstract of the United States: 1992,* Superintendent of Documents, Washington, D.C., chart 599.
5. "Adoption Demand Exceeding Supply," op. cit.
6. Eileen Helper, quoted in Yaeger, op. cit., p. A1.
7. Patrick Steptoe and Robert Edwards, *A Matter of Life: The Story of a Medical Breakthrough,* Morrow, London, 1980, p. 163.
8. Ibid., p. 64.
9. John Brown and Lesley Brown, *Our Miracle Called Louise,* Paddington, London, 1979, p. 98.
10. Ibid., pp. 83, 88.
11. *Newsweek,* August 7, 1978, p. 68.
12. Brown and Brown, op. cit., p. 163.
13. *Time,* August 7, 1978, p. 68.
14. Brown and Brown, op. cit., p. 75.
15. *Newsweek,* August 7, 1978, p. 66.
16. Ibid.
17. Ibid.
18. Audrey Smith, quoted in Steptoe and Edwards, op. cit, p. 48.
19. Jeremy Rifkin and Ted Howard, *Who Shall Play God?* Dell, New York, 1977.
20. "Text of Vatican's Statement on Human Reproduction," *NYT,* March 11, 1987, pp. 10ff.
21. Bishop Kelly, quoted in G. Vecsey, "Religious Leaders Differ on Implant," *NYT,* July 27, 1978, p. A16.
22. Joseph Fletcher, *Ethics of Genetic Control: Ending Reproductive Roulette,* Doubleday Anchor, New York; reprinted by Prometheus, Buffalo, N.Y., 1984, p. 36.
23. Joseph Fletcher, "Ethical Aspects of Genetic Controls," *NEJM,* vol. 285, no. 14, 1971, pp. 776–781.
24. Paul Ramsey, *Fabricated Man,* Yale University Press, New Haven, Conn., 1970.
25. Steptoe and Edwards, op. cit, p. 113.
26. Paul Ramsey, *The Ethics of Fetal Experimentation,* Yale University Press, New Haven, Connecticut, 1975.
27. Michael Bayles, *Reproductive Ethics,* Prentice-Hall, Englewood Cliffs, N.J., 1986, p. 113.
28. Ibid.
29. For a defense of the "equivalence thesis," see James Rachels, *The End of Life: Euthanasia and Morality,* Oxford University Press, New York, 1986, pp. 111–114.
30. Ellen Goodman, " 'Matching' Newest Segregation," *Boston Globe,* November 7, 1993.
31. James Watson, quoted in *Newsweek,* August 7, 1978, p. 69.
32. Richard Blandau, quoted in *Time,* November 13, 1978, p. 89.
33. *Time,* November 13, 1978, p. 89.
34. John Marlow, quoted in *U.S. News and World Report,* August 7, 1978, p. 24.
35. John Marshall, quoted in *Time,* July 31, 1978, p. 59.
36. Leon Kass, "The New Biology: What Price Relieving Man's Estate?" *JAMA,* vol. 174, November 19, 1971, pp. 779–788.
37. James Watson, "Moving towards Clonal Man," *Atlantic,* May 1971, p. 53.
38. Max Perutz, quoted in Steptoe and Edwards, op. cit, p. 117.
39. Rifkin and Howard, op. cit., p. 115.

40. Daniel Callahan, *NYT,* July 27, 1978, p. A16.
41. This point is due to G. Lynn Stephens.
42. Hans Tiefel, "In Vitro Fertilization: A Conservative View," *JAMA,* vol. 247, no. 23, June 18, 1982, pp. 3235–3242.
43. See Derek Parfit, *Reasons and Persons,* Oxford University Press, New York, 1983, p. 167.
44. *U.S. News and World Report,* August 7, 1978, p. 71.
45. Mary Anne Warren, "IVF and Women's Interests: An Analysis of Feminist Concerns," *Bioethics,* vol. 2, no. 1, January 1988, p. 44.
46. Rasa Gustaitis, "Infertility Hype," *Glamour,* March 1989, p. 82.
47. Christine Sistare, "Reproductive Freedom and Women's Freedom: Surrogacy and Autonomy," *Philosophical Forum: A Quarterly,* vol. 19, no. 4, Summer 1988.
48. John Rawls, *A Theory of Justice,* Harvard University Press, Cambridge, Mass., 1971.
49. Peter Singer and Deane Wells, "In Vitro Fertilisation: The Major Issues," *Journal of Medical Ethics,* vol. 9, no. 4, 1983, pp. 192–199; also, P. Singer, "Response" to "Comment," by G. D. Mitchell (same issue).
50. *NYT,* July 28, 1978, p. A22; July 27, 1978, p. A16.
51. David Ozar, "The Case for Not Unthawing Frozen Embryos," *HCR,* vol. 15, no. 4, August 1985, pp. 7–12.
52. Singer and Wells, op. cit., p. 193.
53. Derek Parfit, *Reasons and Persons,* Oxford University Press, New York, 1984.
54. M.V. Viola, quoted in Howard Brody, *Ethical Decisions in Medicine,* Little, Brown, Boston, Mass., 1976, p. 147.
55. Conversation by the author with American Fertility Society, Birmingham, Ala., December 20, 1993.
56. Glenn Kramon, "Infertility Chain: The Good and Bad in Medicine," *NYT,* June 19, 1992, p. C1.
57. Gina Kolata, "New Pregnancy Hope: A Single Sperm Injected," *NYT,* August 11, 1993, p. B7.
58. AP, "Pre-Pregnancy Screening Yields Baby Free of Fatal Genetic Defect," January 22, 1994.
59. "Scientist Seeks Ban on Prenatal Homosexuality Tests," *Birmingham News,* February 22, 1994, p. 7D (reported from *Boston Globe).*
60. Gina Kolata, "Researcher Clones Embryos of Human in Fertility Effort," *NYT,* October 24, 1993, p. A1; "Cloning Human Embryos: Debate Erupts over Ethics," *NYT,* October 26, 1993, p. A1; Peter Steinfels, "The Latest Advances in Cloning Challenge Bioethicists," *NYT,* October 30, 1993, p. 7.
61. Jerry Adler, Mary Hager, and Karen Springen, "Clone Hype," *Newsweek,* November 8, 1993, p. 61.
62. Ibid., pp. 60–64.
63. B. Drummond Ayres, "Fertility Doctor Accused of Fraud," *NYT,* November 25, 1991, p. A1.
64. AP, May 8, 1992.
65. Kathryn Honea, quoted in interview by Karen Ford, *Birmingham* magazine, December 1992, p. 38.
66. Gustaitis, op. cit., p. 89.
67. Ellen Hopkins, "Tales from the Baby Factory," *New York Times Magazine,* 1992, p. 42.
68. Kramon, op. cit., pp. C1–2.
69. Ibid.
70. This figure is based on 22,000 IVF attempts in 1991.
71. Kramon, op. cit., p. C2.
72. David James, "Why Donor Artificial Insemination Is Immoral," *Logos: Philosophic Issues in Christian Perspective,* vol. 9, 1988, pp. 181–192.
73. Louise Kinross, "Breaking the Silence of Donor Insemination," *Toronto Star,* July 25, 1992, pp. G1, 9.
74. Nancy Hill-Holtzman, "More Coffins Than Cribs," *Los Angeles Times/Washington Post,* May 2, 1990, p. G1.
75. Elizabeth Rosenthal, "Cost of High-Tech Fertility: Too Many Tiny Babies," *NYT,* May 26, 1992, pp. B5, 7.
76. Sheila Anne Feeney, "Overcoming Infertility," *New York Daily News,* December 31, 1990, p. D2.
77. Mary Mahowald, "Reproduction and Genetic Technology Meet the Health Care System," speech at Annual Meeting of the Society for Health and Human Values, Memphis, Tenn., November 20, 1992.
78. P. Majendie (Reuters), "British Controversy over 'Designer Babies,'" December 31, 1933.
79. AP, "Ex-Husband Has Embryos Destroyed," June 16, 1993.
80. Nora Frenkiel, "Planning a Family, Down to Baby's Sex," *NYT,* December 11, 1993, pp. B1, 4.
81. Peter Leyden and David Bank, "Science Is Serving Old Superstition," *San Francisco Chronicle,* 1990.
82. E. Robinson, "Idea of Using Eggs from Fetuses Raises Furor," *Washington Post,* January 17, 1994.
83. Carol Lawson, "Celebrated Birth Aside, Teen Has Typical Life," *NYT,* October 1, 1993, p. A8.

Chapter 5

1. Richard Titmuss, *The Gift Relationship: From Altruism to Commerce,* Pantheon, New York, 1971.
2. Phillip Parker, "Surrogate Mothers' Motivations: Initial Findings," *American Journal of Psychiatry,* vol. 40, no. 1, 1983.
3. Linda Arking, "Surrogate Motherhood: Searching for a Very Special Woman," *McCall's,* June 1987.

4. Mary Beth Whitehead with Loretta Schwartz-Nobel, *A Mother's Story*, St. Martin's, New York, 1989, p. 91.

5. "Who Keeps 'Baby M'?" *Newsweek*, January 19, 1987, p. 49.

6. AP, January 9, 1987.

7. Whitehead, op. cit., p. 48.

8. *NYT*, February 5, 1987, p. 15.

9. Whitehead, op. cit., p. 57.

10. Ibid., p. 103.

11. Ibid., p. 113.

12. New Jersey Superior Court, *Matter of Baby M*, 217 N. J. Super. 313.525A. 2d 1128 (Ch. D. Fam. Pt. 1987).

13. Whitehead, op. cit., p. 167.

14. Ibid., p. 169. (A few months later, Chesler had a new book on the stands about the Baby M case.)

15. New Jersey Supreme Court, *Matter of Baby M*, 584 A.2d 1227 (N. J. 1988). See also "Surrogate Deals for Mothers Held Illegal in Jersey," *NYT*, February 3, 1988; "Excerpts from Decision by New Jersey Supreme Court in the Baby M Case," *NYT*, February 4, 1988.

16. Whitehead, op. cit., p. 189.

17. Ibid.

18. "Baby M's Mother Wins Broad Visiting Rights," *NYT*, April 7, 1988, p. A1.

19. William Handel, quoted in "Jersey Surrogate Ruling Downplayed by Brokers," *NYT*, February 5, 1987, p. A10.

20. Nanette Dembitz, quoted in Vivian Cadden, "Hard Questions about the Baby M Case," *McCall's*, June 1985, p. 58.

21. AP, "Testimony Conflicts in Surrogate Trial," January 10, 1987.

22. "Doctor Backs Baby M Mother," *NYT*, January 15, 1987.

23. Richard McCormick, "Surrogate Motherhood: A Stillborn Idea," *Second Opinion*, vol. 5, 1987, p. 130.

24. Sidney Callahan, "Lovemaking and Babymaking," *Commonweal*, April 24, 1987, p. 238.

25. M. Schecter, quoted in New Jersey Superior Court, *Matter of Baby M*, p. 52.

26. Quoted ibid., pp. 56ff.

27. Judith Grief, quoted ibid., pp. 64ff.

28. Bonnie Steinbock, "Surrogate Motherhood as Prenatal Adoption," *Law, Medicine, and Health Care*, vol. 16, nos. 1–2, Spring 1988, p. 45.

29. Patricia Werhane, "Against the Legitimacy of Surrogate Contracts," *On the Problem of Surrogate Parenthood: Analyzing the Baby M Case*, Mellen, Lewistown, N.Y., 1987, pp. 21–30.

30. George Annas, "Baby M: Babies (and Justice) for Sale," *HCR*, vol. 17, no. 3, June 1987, pp. 13–15.

31. Whitehead, op. cit., pp. 68, 89.

32. Quoted ibid., p. 169.

33. Asa Ruskin, letter to editor, *AMN*, May 15, 1987, p. 6.

34. "Whitehead vs. Sperm," *Off Our Backs*, May 1987, pp. 1, 12.

35. Rosemarie Tong, "Feminist Philosophy: Standpoints and Differences," *Newsletter on Feminism and Philosophy*, American Philosophical Association, no. 9, 1988.

36. Carol Gilligan, *In a Different Voice: Psychological Theory and Women's Development*, Harvard University Press, Cambridge, Mass., 1982.

37. Presumed "male" and "female" values have been debated in medicine. Some observers hope that the increasing number of women in medicine will "soften" the harshnesss of the profession. Whether this has happened is unclear.

38. Christine Sistare, "Reproductive Freedom and Women's Freedom: Surrogacy and Autonomy," *Philosophical Forum: A Quarterly*, vol. 19, no. 4, Summer 1988.

39. For reference to "body-mediated" knowledge, see Beverly Harrison, in Carol Robb, ed., *Making the Connections: Essays in Feminist Social Ethics*, Beacon, Boston, Mass., 1985.

40. Phyllis Chesler, *Sacred Bond: The Legacy of Baby M*, Vintage, New York, 1989, p. 23. Chesler says that studies support the notion of bonding—in fact, that is the central claim in her book—but she gives no further references to such studies. It should be noted that some of the people she names as authors of these studies had joined a group she organized before writing this book, to oppose surrogacy and to support Mary Beth Whitehead.

41. Hillary Baber, "For the Legitimacy of Surrogate Contracts," *On the Problem of Surrogate Parenthood: Analyzing the Baby M Case*, Mellen, Lewistown, N.Y., 1987, p. 39.

42. Eleanor Smeal, lecture at UAB, January 1987.

43. Barbara Katz Rothman, "Surrogacy: A Question of Values," *Conscience*, vol. 8, no. 3, 1987.

44. Lori B. Andrews, "Alternative Modes of Reproduction," in Sherrill Cohen and Nadine Taub, eds., *Reproductive Law for the 1990s*, Humana, Clifton, N.J., 1988, p. 384.

45. Annas, op. cit.

46. New Jersey Superior Court, *Matter of Baby M*, p. 70.

47. Andrews, op. cit.

48. Mary Gibson, "The Moral and Legal Status of Surrogate Motherhood," presented at Eastern Division Meeting of the American Philosophical Association (unpublished manuscript); quoted in Rosemarie Tong, "The Overdue Death of a Feminist Chameleon: Taking a Stand on Surrogacy Arrangements," in Kenneth Alpern, ed., *The Ethics of Reproductive Technology*, Oxford University Press, New York, 1992.

49. Ellen Goodman, "Reproduction Slowly Being Separated from Sex," nationally syndicated column, April 26, 1986.

50. *ABC World News*, January 26, 1987.

51. Michael Kinsley, "The Moral Logic of Capitalism," *WSJ*, April 16, 1987, p. 31.
52. Baruch Brody, "Surrogate Motherhood," lecture, Berry College, April 1987. Videotape available from Philosophy Department, Berry College, Rome, Ga., 30149.
53. Loretta Schwartz-Nobel, "A Note about the Collaboration," in Whitehead, op. cit., p. xx.
54. Department of Health and Social Security (Great Britain), *Report of the Committee of Inquiry into Human Fertilisation and Embryology*, Her Majesty's Stationery Office, 1984.
55. Hilde Lindemann Nelson and James Lindemann Nelson, "Parental Obligations and the Ethics of Surrogacy," *Public Affairs Quarterly*, vol. 5, no. 1, January 1991, pp. 49–61.
56. "Six Million Slaves," *Birmingham Post-Herald* (Alabama), June 18, 1991.
57. Quoted in Mark Rust, "Whose Baby Is It?" *ABA Journal: The Magazine for Lawyers*, June 1, 1987, p. 52.
58. Quoted in Arking, op. cit.
59. Goodman, op. cit.
60. Quoted in Whitehead, op. cit., p. 136.
61. David Wasserman and Robert Wachbroit, "Defining Families; The Impact of Reproductive Technology," *Report from the Institute for Philosophy and Public Policy*, vol. 13, no. 3, Summer 1993, p. 4.
62. New York State Task Force on Life and the Law, *Surrogate Parenting: Analysis and Recommendations for Public Policy*, 1988.
63. Wasserman and Wachbroit, op. cit., p. 5.
64. Carol Lawson, "Couples' Own Embryos Used in Birth Surrogacy," *NYT*, August 12, 1990, p. A1.
65. Lisa Belkin, "Childless Couples Hang On to Last Hope, Despite Law," *NYT*, 1992.
66. Richard Paddock and Rene Lynch, "Genetic Parents Win Surrogate Case," *Arizona Republic*, May 21, 1993, p. A7.

Chapter 6

1. Paul Badham, "Christian Belief and the Ethics of In Vitro Fertilization," *Bioethics News*, vol. 6, no. 2, January 1987, p. 10.
2. Paul Johnson, *A History of Christianity*, Atheneum, New York, 1983, chap. 3.
3. John R. Connery, "Abortion: Roman Catholic Perspectives," *Encyclopedia of Bioethics*, vol. I, Macmillan, New York, 1978.
4. Robert W. Mulligan, S.J., Jesuit Community at St. Louis University, personal communication.
5. Today, the official Catholic position on immediate animation is unclear, although the church does teach that the "greatest care" should be taken with the embryo from the moment of conception. See Connery, op. cit., p. 13.
6. *Roe v. Wade, Supreme Court Reporter,* 93, 410 US 151, pp. 709–762. Subsequent quotations from the decision are from this source.
7. Barbara Ehrenreich and Deirdre English, *For Her Own Good: 150 Years of the Experts' Advice to Women*, Doubleday, New York, 1987, pp. 319–320.
8. Alan Guttmacher Institute, *Abortion and Women's Health*, New York and Washington, D.C., 1990, p. 27.
9. Alan F. Guttmacher, *The Case for Legalized Abortion*, Diablo, Berkeley, Calif., 1977, pp. 15–17.
10. In 1992 a movie called *A Private Affair* was made about this case; Sissy Spacek portrayed Sherri Finkbine.
11. Peter Steinfels, "Paper Birth-Control Letter Retains Its Grip," *NYT*, July 29, 1993, pp. A1, 13.
12. Among them can be counted Albert Jonsen, Paul Tong, and Warren Reich. Although Daniel Callahan was never a priest, his first book on abortion and his founding of the Hastings Center reflect the concerns of someone educated in the Catholic tradition and struggling to make sense of new ethical issues in medicine. (Personal communication from Warren Reich.)
13. Norma McCorvey, *I Am Roe—My Life: Roe v. Wade and Freedom of Choice*, Harper Collins, 1993.
14. Alan Guttmacher Institute, op. cit, p. 22.
15. Ibid., p. 19.
16. A. Philipson et al., "Transplacental Passage of Erythromycin and Clindamycin," *NEJM*, vol. 288, no. 23, June 7, 1973, pp. 1219–1221.
17. William Nolen, *The Baby in the Bottle*, Coward, McCann, and Geoghegan, New York, 1978.
18. Ibid., p. 203.
19. Ibid., p. 150.
20. "The Edelin Trial," transcript of trial for WBGH recreation for Bill Moyers documentary; Project of Legal-Medical Studies, Inc., Box 8219, John F. Kennedy Station, Government Station, Boston, Mass. 12134.
21. William F. Buckley, *National Review*, March 14, 1975; quoted in Nolen, op. cit., p. 221.
22. *Commonwealth v. Kenneth Edelin,* Mass. Supreme Court 359, N.E. 2d 4, 1976.
23. Kenneth Edelin, *Ob. Gyn. News*, January 1, 1977, p. 1.
24. Quoted in Paul Ramsey, *Ethics at the Edges of Life*, Yale University Press, New Haven, Conn., 1978, p. 94.
25. Nolen, op. cit.
26. Ibid., p. 175.
27. Mary Anne Warren, "On the Moral and Legal Status of the Fetus," *Monist*, vol. 57, 1973, pp. 43–61
28. Don Marquis, "Why Abortion Is Immoral," *Journal of Philosophy*, vol. 86, 1989, pp. 183–202; Warren Quinn, "Abortion: Identity and Loss," *Philosophy and Public Affairs*, vol. 13, 1984, pp. 24–54.

29. John T. Noonan, Jr. "An Almost Absolute Value in History," in John T. Noonan, Jr., ed., *The Morality of Abortion: Legal and Historical Perspectives,* Harvard University Press, Cambridge, Mass., 1970, pp. 51–59.

30. Judith Jarvis Thomson, "A Defense of Abortion," *Philosophy and Public Affairs,* vol. 1, no. 1, Fall 1971, pp. 47–66.

31. Francis Kamm, *Creation and Abortion,* Oxford University Press, New York, 1992.

32. Connery, op. cit., pp. 9–13.

33. Ellen Willis, "Harper's Forum on Abortion," *Harper's Magazine,* July 1986, p. 38.

34. "Explosions over Abortion," *Time,* January 14, 1985, p. 17.

35. Jeff Lyon,"The Doctor's Dilemma: When Abortion Gives Birth to Life, Physicians Become Troubled Saviors," *Chicago Tribune,* August 15, 1982, sec. 12, pp. 1, 3.

36. Maggie Scarf, "The Fetus as Guinea Pig," *NYT Magazine,* October 19, 1975, pp. 194–200.

37. Ibid.

38. Paul Ramsey, *The Ethics of Fetal Research,* Yale University Press, New Haven, Conn., 1975.

39. Consultants to the Advisory Committee to the Director, National Institutes of Health, *Report of the Human Fetal Tissue Transplantation Research Panel,* vol. I, National Institutes of Health (NIH), Bethesda, Md., 1988.

40. Jean Seligman and Mark Hagen, "Abortion in the Form of a Pill," *Newsweek,* April 17, 1989, p. 61.

41. Mac E. Hadley, *Endocrinology,* 3d ed., Prentice-Hall, Englewood Cliffs, N.J., 1992, p. 523. Wendy Vaughn helped on this point.

42. Etienne-Émile Baulieu, "Updating RU 486 Development," in R. Cook and D. Grimes, eds., *Antiprogestin Drugs: Ethical, Legal, and Medical Issues,* special issue of *Law, Medicine, and Health Care,* vol. 20, no. 3, Fall 1992.

43. AP, "Easier Way Found for Abortion Pill," *NYT,* May 27, 1993, p. A13; "Scientists Push for Quick Approval of French Abortion Pill," *NYT,* September 9, 1993.

44. This private study is by David Grimes at the USC Medical Center, under an "investigational use" designation given by NIH to the Population Council, its sponsor.

45. AP, "Abortion Drug Worked as Morning-After Pill, Study Says," *Birmingham Post-Herald,* October 8, 1992, p. A11.

46. Kenneth Jost, *American Bar Association Journal,* "Mother versus Child," April 1989, p. 86.

47. AP, "Mother Gets 6 Years for Drugs in Breast Milk," *NYT,* October 28, 1992, p. A11.

48. E.L. Abel and R.J. Sokol, "Fetal Alcohol Syndrome Is Now the Leading Cause of Mental Retardation," *Lancet,* vol. 8517, pp. 898–899 (letter).

49. Opinion in *Akron v. Akron Center for Reproductive Health* (1983), quoted in *Newsweek,* January 14, 1985, p. 28.

50. Harold Morowitz and James Trefil, *"Roe v. Wade* Passes a Lab Test," *NYT,* November 25, 1992, p. A13.

51. Excerpts from *Planned Parenthood v. Casey, NYT,* June 30, 1992, p. A8.

52. Tamar Lewin, "Parental Consent to Abortion: How Enforcement Can Vary," *NYT,* May 28, 1992, p. A9.

Chapter 7

1. Robert Weir, *Selected Nontreatment of Handicapped Newborns,* Oxford University Press, New York, 1984; John Boswell, *The Kindness of Strangers: The Abandonment of Children in Western Europe from Late Antiquity to the Renaissance,* Pantheon, New York, 1989.

2. William Lecky, *History of European Morals from Augustus to Charlemagne,* vol. II, Braziller, New York, 1955, pp. 25–56 (originally published 1869).

3. W. L. Langer, "Europe's Initial Population Explosion," *American Historical Review,* vol. 69, 1963, pp. 1–17; quoted in G. Hardin, *Exploring New Ethics for Survival: The Voyage of the Spaceship Beagle,* Viking, New York, 1972, pp. 180–183.

4. James Gustafson, "Mongolism, Parental Desires, and the Right to Life," *Perspectives in Biology and Medicine,* vol. 16, Summer 1973, p. 529.

5. Some important details of these cases come from conversations with Norman Fost, a well-known ethicist and pediatrician at the University of Wisconsin medical school.

6. *Who Should Survive?* produced by the Joseph P. Kennedy Jr. Foundation; available from Film Service, 999 Asylum Avenue, Hartford, Conn. 06105. Norman Fost, who was then a resident at Hopkins, appears briefly in the film (in the background).

7. Quoted in *Who Should Survive?*

8. Gustafson, op. cit.

9. Ibid.

10. R. Duff and A. Campbell, "Moral and Ethical Dilemmas in the Special-Care Nursery," *NEJM,* vol. 289, no. 17, October 25, 1973, pp. 890–894.

11. John Lorber, "Results of Treatment of Myelomeningocele: An Analysis of 524 Unselected Cases, with Special Reference to Possible Selection for Treatment," *Developmental Medicine and Child Neurology,* vol. 13, no. 3, 1971, pp. 279–303.

12. *Dorland's Illustrated Medical Dictionary,* Saunders, Philadephia, Pa., 1987.

13. Mary Tedeschi, "Infanticide and Its Apologists," *Commentary,* November 1984, p. 34.

14. Shari Staaver, "Siamese Twins' Case 'Devastates' MDs," *AMN,* October 9, 1981, pp. 15–16.

15. Bonnie Steinbock, "Whatever Happened to the Danville Siamese Twins?" *HCR*, vol. 17, no. 4, August-September 1987, pp. 3–4.
16. John Robertson, "Dilemma in Danville," *HCR*, vol. 11, no. 5, October 1981, p. 7.
17. U.S. Commission on Civil Rights, "Medical Discrimination against Children with Disabilities," September 1989, p. 391.
18. Ibid., pp. 36, 323.
19. Adrian Peracchio, "Government in the Nursery: New Era for Baby Doe Cases," *Newsday*, November 13, 1983. (This story and Kathleen Kerr's story, cited in note 21, are available from *Newsday* as a reprint, "The Baby Jane Doe Story: Winner of the 1984 Pulitzer Prize for Local Reporting.")
20. This result is according to *Newsday*'s investigation.
21. Kathleen Kerr, "An Issue of Law and Ethics," *Newsday*, October 26, 1983.
22. Kathleen Kerr, "Legal, Medical Legacy of Case," *Newsday*, December 7, 1987.
23. Ibid.
24. Bonnie Steinbock, "Baby Jane Doe in the Courts," *HCR*, vol. 14, no. 1, February 1984, p. 15.
25. Kerr, "Legal, Medical Legacy of Case"; see also Kathleen Kerr, "Reporting the Case of Baby Jane Doe," *HCR*, vol. 14, no. 4, August 1984.
26. "Baby Jane Doe Has Surgery to Remove Water from Brain," *NYT*, April 7, 1984, p. 28.
27. Ibid.
28. Kerr, "Legal, Medical Legacy of Case."
29. Gustafson, op. cit.
30. C. Everett Koop, "The Slide to Auschwitz," *Whatever Happened to the Human Race?* Revell, Old Tappan, N.J., 1979.
31. John Paris, "Right to Life Doesn't Demand Heroic Sacrifice," *WSJ*, November 28, 1983, p. 30.
32. *Who Should Survive?*
33. Fred Bruning, "The Politics of Life," *MacLean's*, December 12, 1983, p. 17.
34. C. Everett Koop, "The Seriously Ill or Dying Child: Supporting the Patient and the Family," in D. Horan and D. Mall, eds., *Death, Dying and Euthanasia*, University Publications of America, Frederick, Md., 1977, pp. 537–539.
35. Koop, "The Slide to Auschwitz."
36. R. McCormick, "To Save or Let Die: The Dilemma of Modern Medicine," *JAMA*, vol. 229, no. 8, July 1974, pp. 172–176.
37. Peter Singer, *Practical Ethics,* Cambridge University Press, New York, 1979, p. 137; Tristam Engelhardt, "Ethical Issues in Aiding the Death of Young Children," in Marvin Kohl, ed., *Beneficent Euthanasia*, Prometheus, Buffalo, N.Y., 1975; Michael Tooley, "Abortion and Infanticide," *Philosophy and Public Affairs*, vol. 2, no. 1, Fall 1972, pp. 37–65.
38. Kerr, "Legal, Medical Legacy of Case."
39. Weir, op. cit.
40. R. B. Zachary, "Life with Spina Bifida," *British Medical Journal*, vol. 2, 1977, p. 1461.
41. David Gibson, "Dimensions of Intelligence," in *Down Syndrome: The Psychology of Mongolism*, Cambridge University Press, New York, 1978, pp. 35–77; Janet Carr, "The Development of Intelligence," in David Lane and Brian Stafford, eds., *Current Approaches to Down Syndrome*, Praeger, New York, 1985, pp. 167–186.
42. J. Freeman, "To Treat or Not to Treat: Ethical Dilemmas of Treating the Infant with Myelomeningocele," *Clinical Neurosurgery*, vol. 20, 1973, p. 137.
43. Peter Singer, "Sanctity of Life or Quality of Life?" *Pediatrics*, vol. 72, no. 1, July 1983, pp. 128–129.
44. Letters reacting to Singer's article appeared in *Pediatrics*, vol. 73, no. 2, February 1984.
45. B. D. Colen, "A Life of Love—and Endless Pain," *Newsday*, October 26, 1983. (Available from *Newsday* in the reprint "The Baby Jane Doe Story: Winner of the 1984 Pulitzer Prize for Local Reporting.")
46. Steven Baer, "The Half-Told Story of Baby Jane Doe," *Columbia Journalism Review*, November-December 1984, pp. 35–38.
47. Tedeschi, op. cit., pp. 31–35.
48. "Baby Jane Doe," *WSJ*, November 21, 1983.
49. Gregg Levoy, "Birth Controllers," *Omni*, August 1987, p. 31.
50. *Gleitman v. Cosgrove*, quoted in M. Coppenger, ed., *Bioethics: A Casebook*, Prentice-Hall, Englewood Cliffs, N.J., 1985, pp. 8–12.
51. Brenda Coleman, "Moral Floodgates Opened by Father Pulling Plug on Son," AP, May 1, 1989.
52. *In the Matter of Baby "K,"* United States District Court, E.D. Virginia, July 7, 1993, no. Civ. A. 93-104-A; see also "The Case of Baby K," *Trends in Health Care, Law, and Ethics*, vol. 9, no. 1, Winter 1994, pp. 1–48.
53. A. Gallo, "Spina Bifida: The State of the Art of Medical Management," *HCR*, vol. 14, no. 1, February 1984, pp. 10–13.
54. Ibid.
55. Spina Bifida Association, Brief Amicus Curiae of the Spina Bifida Association of America, *Weber v. Stony Brook Hospital*, New York State Supreme Court, Appellate Division, 2d Department, *New York Law Journal*, October 28, 1983; quoted in Steinbock, "Baby Jane Doe in the Courts," p. 19.
56. Loretta Kopelman, "Do the 'Baby Doe' Rules Ignore Suffering?" *Second Opinion*, vol. 18., no. 4, April 1983, pp. 101–113.
57. Gina Kolata, "Parents of Tiny Infants Find Care Choices Are Not Theirs," *NYT*, September 30, 1991, p. A1.
58. *HCR*, vol. 24., no. 3, May-June 1994, p. 2.

Chapter 8

1. Nicholas Fontaine, *Memoires pour servir l'histoire de Port-Royal*, vol. 2 (originally published in Cologne in 1738); quoted in L. Rosenfield, *From Beast-Machine to Man-Machine: The Theme of Animal Soul in French Letters from Descartes to La Mettrie*, Oxford University Press, New York, 1940, pp. 52–53; also quoted in Peter Singer, *Animal Liberation*, New York Review of Books, 1975.

2. C. S. Lewis, *How Human Suffering Raises Almost Intolerable Intellectual Problems*, Macmillan, New York, 1940, pp. 131–133.

3. David Hume, *A Treatise of Human Nature*, 1789.

4. Office of Technology Assessment, *Animal Usage in the United States*, Superintendent of Documents, Washington, D.C., 1986, p. 12; Andrew Rowan, *Of Mice, Models, and Men: A Critical Evaluation of Animal Research*, State University of New York Press, Albany, 1984, pp. 67–70; *Newsweek*, December 26, 1988, p. 51.

5. Bernard Rollins, *Animal Rights and Human Morality*, Prometheus, Buffalo, N.Y., 1981, pp. 97–99.

6. W. Robbins, "Animal Rights: A Growing Movement in the U.S.," *NYT*, June 15, 1984, p. A16.

7. "The Use of Animals in Research," *NEJM*, vol. 313, no. 6, pp. 395–400.

8. *Evaluation of Experimental Procedures Conducted at the University of Pennsylvania Experimental Head-Injury Laboratory 1981–1984 in Light of the Public Health Science Animal Welfare Policy*, Office for Protection of Research Risks, National Institutes of Health, 1985, p. 37.

9. Quoted in "Animals in the Middle," in the television series *Innovation*, sponsored by Johnson and Johnson on A and E Network, September 5, 1987.

10. James Kilpatrick, "Animal-Rights Supporters Claim Well-Won Victory," nationally syndicated column, July 23, 1985.

11. Robbins, op. cit.

12. Robert Marshak, quoted in *NYT*, July 29, 1984, p. A12.

13. Donald Abt, quoted in *NYT*, August 12, 1984, p. B1.

14. *NYT*, December 10, 1984, p. A10.

15. Ibid.

16. Singer, op. cit.

17. Quoted in Marsha Mercer, "Animal Rights Group Willing to Use Violence for Cause," Scripps Howard/Media General Newspapers, May 1, 1989.

18. Susan Wolf, "Moral Saints," *Journal of Philosophy*, vol. 79, no. 8, August 1982.

19. Quoted in S. Isen, "Laying the Foundation for Animal Rights: Interview with Tom Regan," *Animals Agenda*, July-August, 1984, pp. 4–5.

20. Tom Regan, *The Case for Animal Rights*, University of California Press, Berkeley, 1983.

21. Quoted in "Animals in the Middle."

22. Ibid.

23. Carl Cohen, "The Case for Animal Rights," *NEJM*, vol. 315, no. 14, October 4, 1986, pp. 865–870.

24. R. G. Frey, *Rights, Killing, and Suffering*, Basil Blackwell, Oxford, England, 1983, p. 65.

25. Quoted in Katie McCabe, "Who Will Live, Who Will Die?" *Washingtonian Magazine*, April 1986, p. 115.

26. Rebecca Dresser, "Measuring Merit in Scientific Research," *Theoretical Medicine*, vol. 10, no. 1, 1989, pp. 21–34. It is relevant to note that the discovery of the gene for colon cancer apparently resulted from "hard-core, undirected research" (Natalie Angier, "Scientists Isolate Novel Gene Linked to Colon Cancer," *NYT*, December 3, 1993, p. A10).

27. *NYT*, August 12, 1984.

28. Quoted in J. Duschek, "Protestors Prompt Halt in Animal Research," *Science News*, July 27, 1985, p. 53.

29. Quoted by O. Cusak, "Direct Action for Animals: Interview with England's Marley Jones," *Animals Agenda*, vol. 7, no. 3, April 1987, pp. 32–34.

30. Bernard Levin, "The Animals Lovers Lusting for Blood," *The Times*, July 3, 1985, p. 15.

31. "Of Pain and Progress," *Newsweek*, December 26, 1988, p. 53.

32. Edward Taub, "The Silver Spring Monkey Incident: The Untold Story," *Coalition for Animals and Animal Research Newsletter*, vol. 4, no. 1, Winter-Spring 1991, pp. 1–8.

33. Donald Barnes, "Debating the Values of Animal Research," *Animals Agenda*, vol. 7, no. 3, April 1987, pp. 32–34.

34. Another example of a person who has changed sides on a moral issue is the former abortionist Barnard Nathanson.

35. D. Moss and P. Greanville, "The Emerging Face of the Movement," *Animals Agenda*, March-April 1985, p. 11.

36. L. Jewell and D. Frazier, "Annual Questionaire Results," *Physiologist*, vol. 29, no. 2, 1986, p. 23.

37. F. Feretti, "Forsaken Vacation Animals," *NYT*, September 5, 1984, p. C1.

38. Phil McCombs, "Activist Battles Animal-Rights Movement," *Los Angeles Times-Washington Post*, April 27, 1992.

39. Tony Dajer, "Monkeying with the Brain," *Discover*, January 1992, pp. 70–71. See also Warren E. Leary, "Sharp Brain Healing Found in Disputed Monkey Tests, *NYT*, June 28, 1991, p. A9.

40. John Durant, quoted in John Hargrove, "Bush Signs Heflin Bill to Protect Researchers," *Birmingham Post-Herald*, August 28, 1992.

41. Stephen Labaton, "Judge Orders Rules Tightened to Protect Animals in Research," *NYT,* February 26, 1993.

Chapter 9

1. S. Gomer, H. Powell, and G. Rolino, "Japan's Biological Weapons"; H. Powell, "A Hidden Chapter in History," *Bulletin of Atomic Scientists,* October 1981, pp. 43, 44.
2. Eugene Kogon, *The Theory and Practice of Hell,* Farrar, Straus, and Cudahy, New York, 1950; Berkeley reprint, 1980, p. 166.
3. Ibid., pp. 164ff.
4. Gerald Posner and Jerome Ware, *Mengele: The Complete Story,* McGraw-Hill, New York, 1986, p. 11.
5. Vera Alexander, *The Search for Mengele,* Home Box Office, October 1985; interviewed by Central Television (London) and quoted in Posner and Ware, op. cit., p. 37.
6. Miklos Nyiszli, quoted in R. Lifton, "What Made This Man Mengele?" *NYT Magazine,* July 21, 1985, p. 22; see also Posner and Ware, op. cit., p. 39.
7. William Curran, "The Forensic Investigation of the Death of Joseph Mengele," *NEJM,* vol. 315, no. 17, Ocober 23, 1985, pp. 1071–1073.
8. Hannah Arendt, *Eichman at Jerusalem,* Penguin, New York, 1977.
9. Stanley Milgram, *Obedience to Authority,* Harper Collins, New York, 1980.
10. Leo Alexander, "Medical Science under Dictatorship," *NEJM,* vol. 42, July 14, 1949.
11. David Rothman, "Ethics and Human Experimentation," *NEJM,* vol. 317, no. 19, November 5, 1987, p. 1198.
12. Robert Bazell, "Growth Industry," *New Republic,* March 15, 1993, p. 14.
13. Constance Pechura, "From the Institute of Medicine," *JAMA,* vol. 269, no. 4, January 27, 1993, p. 453.
14. Rothman, op. cit., p. 1198.
15. Ibid., p. 1199.
16. H. Beecher, "Ethics and Clinical Research," *NEJM,* vol. 274, 1966, pp. 1354–1360.
17. H. Pappworth, *Human Guinea Pigs,* Beacon, Boston, Mass., 1968.
18. Molly Selvin, "Changing Medical and Societal Attitudes toward Sexually Transmitted Diseases: A Historical Overview," in King K. Holmes et al., eds., *Sexually Transmitted Diseases,* McGraw-Hill, New York, 1984, pp. 3–19.
19. Alan Brandt, "Racism and Research: The Case of the Tuskegee Syphilis Study," *HCR,* vol. 8, no. 6, December 1978, pp. 21–29.
20. Paul de Kruif, *Microbe Hunters,* Harcourt Brace, New York, 1926, p. 323.
21. R. H. Kampmeier, "The Tuskegee Study of Untreated Syphilis" (editorial), *Southern Medical Journal,* vol. 65, no. 10, October 1972, pp. 1247–1251.
22. J. E. Bruusgaard, "Über das Schicksal der nicht spezifisch behandelten Luetiker" ("Fate of Syphilitics Who Are Not Given Specific Treatment"), *Archives of Dermatology of Syphilis,* vol. 157, April 1929, pp. 309–332.
23. Todd Savitt, *Medicine and Slavery: The Disease and Health of Blacks in Antebellum Virginia,* University of Illinois Press, Champaign, 1978.
24. James Jones, *Bad Blood,* Free Press, New York, 1981.
25. H. H. Hazen, "Syphilis in the American Negro," *JAMA,* vol. 63, August 8, 1914, p. 463.
26. Jones, op. cit., p. 74.
27. Ibid.
28. Ibid.
29. Brandt, op. cit.
30. Quoted in E. Ramont, "Syphillis in the AIDS Era," *NEJM,* vol. 316, no. 25, June 18, 1987, pp. 600–601.
31. R. A. Vonderlehr, T. Clark, and J. R. Heller, "Untreated Syphilis in the Male Negro," *JAMA,* pp. 107, no. 11, September 12, 1936, pp. 856–860.
32. Archives of National Library of Medicine; quoted in Jones, op. cit., p. 127.
33. Jones, op. cit., pp. 190–193.
34. Quoted ibid., p. 196.
35. W. J. Brown et al., *Syphilis and Other Venereal Diseases,* Harvard University Press, Cambridge, Mass., 1970, p. 34.
36. Jean Heller, "Syphilis Victims in U.S. Study Went Untreated for 40 Years," *NYT,* July 26, 1972, pp. 1, 8.
37. Ibid., p. 8.
38. Jones, op. cit., insert following p. 48.
39. Tuskegee Syphilis Study Ad Hoc Panel to Department of Health, Education, and Welfare, *Final Report,* Superintendent of Documents, Washington, D.C., 1973.
40. David Tase, "Tuskegee Syphilis Victims, Kin May Get $1.7 Million in Fiscal 1989," AP, September 11, 1988.
41. Heller, op. cit., p. 8.
42. Kampmeier, op. cit. It is not clear whether Kampmeier himself was involved in the Tuskegee study, or if so in what capacity.
43. Thomas Benedek, "The 'Tuskegee Study' of Untreated Syphilis: Analysis of Moral Aspects versus Methodological Aspects," *Journal of Chronic Diseases,* vol. 31, 1978, pp. 35–50. I have drawn considerably on this excellent article.
44. Heller, op. cit., p. 1.
45. Kampmeier, op. cit.
46. "The Tuskegee Study of Untreated Syphilis: The Thirtieth Year of Observation," *Archives of Internal Medicine,* vol. 114, 1961, pp. 792–798.
47. "Malpractice Suit Settled for $2.7 Million," *Burlington Free Press* (Alabama), December 21, 1988.

48. Benedek, op. cit., p. 44.

49. Personal correspondence, April 25, 1985. Benjamin Friedman is Professor Emeritus of Medicine, UAB.

50. Benedek, op. cit.

51. G. W. Hayes et al., "The Golden Anniversary of the Silver Bullet," *JAMA*, vol. 270, no. 13, October 6, 1993, p. 1610.

52. R. H. Kampmeier, "Final Report of the 'Tuskegee Study' of Syphilis," *Southern Medical Journal*, vol. 67, no. 11, 1974, pp. 1349–1353. Kampmeier advances a fourth argument which is somewhat more technical. Penicillin achieves seroreversal in latent syphilis, but Kampmeier insists that such seroreversal has never been proved to be associated with decreased morbidity or mortality. A related point is possible uncertainty over diagnosis and thus over therapeutic effects. (S. Edberg and S. Berger, *Antibiotics and Infection*, Churchill Livingstone, New York, 1983, pp. 141–142; K. Holmes et al., *Sexually Transmitted Diseases*, McGraw-Hill, New York, 1984, p. 1352; John Hotson, "Modern Neurosyphilis: A Partially Treated Chronic Meningitis, *Western Journal of Medicine*, vol. 135, September 1981, pp. 191–200; Sarah Polt, Professor of Pathology, UAB, personal correspondence.)

53. Kampmeier, "Final Report of the 'Tuskegee Study' of Syphilis."

54. Quoted in Jim Auchemutey, "Ghosts of Tuskegee," *Atlanta Journal-Constitution*, September 6, 1992, pp. M1, M6.

55. It is only fair to add that when people like Sidney Olansky (and Kampmeier) took up syphilology in the 1930s, the field was avoided by physicians who wanted to have upper-class, paying patients. Only idealists—physicians who wanted to help people on the margins of society—went into syphilology.

56. "The Deadly Deception" (with George Strait), *Nova*, January 28, 1992.

57. Dan Stober, Knight-Ridder Newspapers, "Dr. Hamilton Was Enthusiastic Experimenter in Radiation," *Birmingham News* (Alabama), February 20, 1994, p. 10A.

58. Dennis Domerzalski, Scripps-Howard News Service, "Radiation 'Guinea Pigs' Tell Stories," *Birmingham Post-Herald* (Alabama), February 3, 1994, p. A8.

59. Keith Schneider, "Scientists Are Sharing the Anguish over Nuclear Experiments on People," *NYT*, March 2, 1994, p. A9.

60. "America's Nuclear Secrets," *Newsweek*, December 27, 1993, p. 15.

61. Ibid., p. 16.

Chapter 10

1. Richard Howard and John Najarian, "Organ Transplantation: Medical Perspective," *Encyclopedia of Bioethics*, vol. 3, Free Press, New York, 1978, p. 1160.

2. However, John Kirklin at UAB, through his surgical research, made this machine much safer.

3. Phillip Blaiberg, *Looking at My Heart*, Stein and Day, New York, 1968, p. 66.

4. Christiaan Barnard and Curtiss Bill Pepper, *One Life*, Macmillan, New York, 1969, p. 290.

5. Ibid., pp. 238–239.

6. Thomas Starzl, *The Puzzle People: Memoirs of a Transplant Surgeon*, Pittsburgh University Press, Pa., 1992, p. 151.

7. Donald R. Kahn, personal communication to author, April 14, 1993; Norman Shumway, personal communication to author, January 10, 1994. One reason why Shumway may have given implicit permission was that he himself was being held back by the problem of declaring a donor "brain-dead"; in 1967, criteria for brain death had not yet been established in the United States.

8. Barnard and Pepper, op. cit., p. 310.

9. Ibid., p. 332.

10. Ibid., p. 343.

11. Ibid., p. 372.

12. "The Ultimate Operation," *Time*, December 15, 1967, p. 65.

13. "Heart Transplant Keeps Man Alive in South Africa," *NYT*, December 4, 1967, p. A1.

14. Barnard and Pepper, op. cit., p. 378.

15. Ibid., p. 406.

16. "The Ultimate Operation," p. 66.

17. Barnard and Pepper, op. cit., p. 444.

18. Peter Hawthorne, *The Transplanted Heart*, Keartland, Johannesburg, South Africa, 1968, pp. 84–85.

19. "Heart Surgery: Were Transplants Premature?" *Time*, March 15, 1968.

20. I am indebted to the transplant surgeon Donald R. Kahn, a colleague of Barnard's during this time and later, for this view.

21. Donald R. Kahn, personal communication, April 14, 1993.

22. Christiaan Barnard, "Reflections on the First Heart Transplant," *South African Medical Journal*, vol. 72, no. 2, December 5, 1987, p. xix.

23. "The Ultimate Operation," pp. 65–66.

24. Shimon Glick (Dean, Ben Gurion Medical School, Israel), letter to author, September 18, 1988.

25. "The Ultimate Operation," pp. 65–66.

26. Barnard and Pepper, op. cit., p. 361.

27. Starzl, op. cit., p. 148.

28. Werner Forssmann, quoted in Barnard and Pepper, op. cit., p. 360.

29. *NYT*, December 6, 1967.

30. Hawthorne, op. cit., p. 188.

31. Quoted in "Pioneers of Surgery, Part IV," *NOVA*, WBGH, Boston, Mass., shown on PBS stations during September 1988 and June 1989.

32. In E. Hamilton and H. Cairns, eds., *Collected Dialogues of Plato,* Princeton University Press, Princeton, N.J., pp. 84–85.

33. S. R. Benatar (Professor and Head of Medicine, University of Cape Town), personal correspondence to author, November 19, 1993.

34. *Time,* March 15, 1988, p. 66.

Chapter 11

1. Stanley Reiser, "The Machine as End and Means: The Clinical Introduction of the Artificial Heart," in Margery Shaw, ed., *After Barney Clark,* University of Texas Press, Austin, pp. 6–90.

2. Michael Strauss, "The Political History of the Artificial Heart," *NEJM,* vol. 310, no. 5, February 2, 1984, p. 333.

3. Lewis Thomas, "The Technology of Medicine," *Lives of a Cell,* Viking, New York, 1974, p. 37.

4. The Karp case and the charges against Denton Cooley are described in a *NOVA* videotape, "The Trial of Denton Cooley," produced by WGBH, Boston; see also Renée Fox and Judith Swazey, *The Courage to Fail: A Social View of Organ Transplants and Dialysis,* 2d ed. rev., University of Chicago Press, Ill., 1978, chap. 6.

5. Richard Stolley, *Life,* February 1981.

6. Una Clark, quoted in *WP,* May 1, 1983, p. A2.

7. "The Brave Man with the Plastic Heart," *Life,* February 7, 1983, p. 25.

8. *Current Biography Yearbook,* Wilson, New York, 1985. Some other biographical data here are also from this source.

9. Renée Fox and Judith Swazey, *Spare Parts: Organ Replacement in American Society,* Oxford University Press, New York, 1992, p. 141.

10. Thomas Preston, "Who Benefits from the Artificial Heart?" *HCR,* vol. 15, no. 1, February 1985, p. 5; see also *NYT,* December 5, 1988, p. A2.

11. Denise Grady, "Summary of Discussion of Ethical Perspectives," in Shaw, op. cit., p. 52.

12. *NYT,* December 5, 1982, p. 48.

13. *Time,* December 9, 1982, p. 43.

14. *NYT,* December 3, 1982, p. A1.

15. *NYT,* March 25, 1983, p. A1.

16. *NYT,* December 5, 1982, p. 48.

17. *Time,* March 14, 1983, p. 74.

18. Preston, op. cit., p. 6.

19. *WP,* May 1, 1983, p. A2.

20. *NYT,* December 3, 1982, p. A25.

21. William A. Check, "Lessons from Barney Clark's Artificial Heart," *Health,* April 1984, pp. 22, 26.

22. *NYT,* April 17, 1983, p. 44.

23. Preston, op. cit., p. 5.

24. Fox and Swazey, *Spare Parts,* p. 132.

25. Gideon Gil, "Burcham Dies after Blood Accumulates in Chest," *Louisville Courier-Journal* (Kentucky), April 26, 1985.

26. Ibid., p. 117.

27. Eric Cassell, "How Is the Death of Barney Clark to Be Understood?" in Shaw, op. cit., p. 48.

28. *NYT,* March 25, 1983, p. A29.

29. *WP,* December 21, 1982.

30. Grady, op. cit., p. 48.

31. *WP,* March 25, 1983, p. A14.

32. *NYT,* April 17, 1983, p. 44.

33. *NYT,* editorial, December 16, 1982, p. A26.

34. P. M. Park, "The Transplant Odyssey," *Second Opinion,* vol. 12, November 1989, pp. 27–32; quoted in Fox and Swazey, *Spare Parts,* p. 200.

35. Margaret Battin, "The Least-Worst Death," *HCR,* vol. 13, no. 2, April 1983, pp. 13–16.

36. Gina Kolata, "Method Found to Spot Defect in Artificial Valve for Heart," *NYT,* November 9, 1992, pp. A1, C8; AP, "Bjork-Shiley Artificial Heart Valve Can Crack, Cause Death," December 14, 1992; AP, "Makers of Heart Valve to Pay $215 Million," August 20, 1992.

37. William Pierce, "Permanent Heart Substitution: Better Solutions Ahead," editorial, *JAMA,* vol. 259, no. 6, February 12, 1988, p. 891.

38. *NYT,* December 5, 1982, p. 48.

39. Ibid.

40. Preston, op. cit., p. 6.

41. Ibid., p. 5.

42. This point is due to the surgeon Roy Gandy, who was taught it by the surgeon John Kirklin.

43. Preston, op. cit., p. 6.

44. George Annas, "Consent to the Artificial Heart: The Lion and the Crocodiles," *HCR,* vol. 13, no. 2, April 1983, pp. 20–22.

45. Pierre Galetti, "Replacement of the Heart with an Artificial Heart: The Case of Dr. Barney Clark," *NEJM,* vol. 310, no. 5, February 2, 1984, pp. 312–314.

46. *NYT,* April 17, 1983, p. A1.

47. Grady, op. cit., p. 46.

48. *NYT,* April 17, 1983.

49. *Time,* April 4, 1983, p. 63.

50. D. P. Lubeck and J. P. Bunker, Office of Technology Assessment, *Case Study 9, The Artificial Heart: Costs, Risks, and Benefits,* U.S. Government Printing Office, Washington, D.C., 1982.

51. Unnamed report in *WP,* quoted in Preston, op. cit., p. 7.

52. Ibid.

53. Malcolm N. Carter, "The Business behind Barney Clark's Heart," *Money,* April 1983.

54. Reiser, op. cit.

55. Quoted from *Newsweek* in Fox and Swazey, *Spare Parts.*

56. *Progressive,* February 1983, pp. 12–13.

57. Jonathan Glover, *Causing Death and Saving Lives,* Penguin, New York, 1977; see also Leon Trachtman, "Why Tolerate the Statistical Victim?" *HCR,* vol. 15, no. 1, February 1985.

58. Romni Scheier, "Robert Jarvik, M.D.: Inventor, Lecturer, Hero," *AMN,* December 11, 1987, pp. 9–10.

59. Michael Vitez, Knight-Ridder Newspapers, "Marriage of Two Minds: 'World's Smartest Couple' Nears First Anniversary," July 3, 1988.

60. Malcolm Brown, "U. S. Halts Artificial Heart Funds," *NYT*, May 13, 1988, pp. A1, A7.

61. Phillip Boffey, "Federal Agency, in Shift, to Back Artificial Heart," *NYT*, July 3, 1988, p. A1.

Chapter 12

1. Renée Fox and Judith Swazey, *The Courage to Fail: A Social View of Organ Transplants and Dialysis*, 2d ed. rev., University of Chicago Press, Ill., 1974, 1978; *Spare Parts: Organ Replacement in American Society*, Oxford University Press, New York, 1992.

2. Fox and Swazey, *Spare Parts*, p. 45.

3. Dale H. Cowan, ed., *Human Organ Transplantation: Social, Medical-Legal, Regulatory, and Reimbursement Issues*, Health Administration Press, Ann Arbor, Mich. 1987, p. 60.

4. Fox and Swazey, *Spare Parts*, p. 7.

5. Ibid., p. 45; and data from United Organ Sharing Network, Research Department, Richmond, Va.

6. K. Isserson, "Voluntary Organ Donation: Autonomy . . . Tragedy," letter, *JAMA*, vol. 270, no. 16, October 27, 1993, p. 1930.

7. W. Kearney and A. Caplan, "Parity for the Donation of Bone Marrow: Ethical and Policy Considerations," in A. Bonnicksen and R. Blank, eds., *Emerging Issues in Biomedical Policy*, Columbia University Press, New York, 1991.

8. Fox and Swazey, *Courage*, p. 206.

9. James Childress, "Who Shall Live When Not All Can Live?" *Soundings: An Interdisciplinary Journal*, vol. 53, no. 4, Winter 1970.

10. Fox and Swazey, *Courage*, p. 235.

11. One of the first organized interdisciplinary discussions took place in 1967, at a conference funded by a company, CIBA.

12. Belding Scribner, unpublished manuscript, 1972; quoted in Fox and Swazey, *Courage*, p. 227.

13. Shana Alexander at "The Birth of Bioethics," conference at University of Washington Medical School, Seattle, September 23, 1992.

14. H. M. Schmeck, Jr., "Panel Holds Life-or-Death Vote in Allotting of Artificial Kidney," *NYT*, May 6, 1962, pp. 1, 83.

15. Shana Alexander, "They Decide Who Lives, Who Dies: Medical Miracle Puts a Burden on a Small Committee," *Life*, vol. 53, no. 102, November 9, 1962.

16. Fox and Swazey, *Courage*, p. 234.

17. Ibid., p. 209.

18. Belding Scribner, Presidential Address to American Society for Artificial Internal Organs, 1964.

19. *Who Shall Live?* NBC documentary narrated by Edwin Newman, 1965. (This was reshown on September 23, 1992, at "The Birth of Bioethics," conference, University of Washington Medical School, Seattle.)

20. Judith Swazey at "The Birth of Bioethics," conference, University of Washington Medical School, Seattle, September 24, 1992.

21. David Sanders and Jesse Dukeminier, "Medical Advance and Legal Lag: Hemodialysis and Kidney Transplantation," *UCLA Law Review*, vol. 15, 1968, pp. 357–412.

22. Belding Scribner at "The Birth of Bioethics," conference, University of Washington Medical School, Seattle, September 23, 1992.

23. Alexander followed Scribner at the conference cited above and made this denial immediately after Scribner finished.

24. C. E. Norton, "Chronic Hemodialysis as a Medical and Social Experiment," *Annals of Internal Medicine*, vol. 66, June 1967, pp. 1267–1277.

25. Of course, there were hundreds of moral issues in medicine before this one, and some scholars had tried, though unsuccessfully, to bring them to the public. An example of a pioneering work is Joseph Fletcher, *Morals and Medicine*, Anchor, New York, 1955.

26. *Spare Parts* and *Courage*, cited above.

27. Fox and Swazey, *Courage*, p. 232.

28. Sanders and Dukeminier, op. cit.

29. George Annas, "The Prostitute, the Playboy, and the Poet: Rationing Schemes for Organ Transplantation," *American Journal of Public Health*, vol. 75, no. 2, 1985, pp. 187–189.

30. Nicholas Rescher, "The Allocation of Exotic Medical Lifesaving Therapy," *Ethics*, vol. 79, April 1969.

31. Fox and Swazey, *Courage*, chap. 9.

32. Robert Veatch, "Voluntary Risks to Health: The Ethical Issues," *JAMA*, vol. 243, January 4, 1980, pp. 50–55.

33. Herbert Fingarette, *Heavy Drinking*, University of California Press, Berkeley, 1988.

34. Alvin Moss and Mark Seigler, "Should Alcoholics Compete Equally for Liver Transplantation?" *JAMA*, vol. 265, no. 10, March 13, 1992, p. 1295.

35. C. Cohen and M. Benjamin, "Alcoholics and Liver Transplantation," *JAMA*, vol. 265, no. 10, March 13, 1992, pp. 1295–1301.

36. Michael Bayles, "Allocation of Medical Resources," *Public Affairs Quarterly*, vol. 4, no. 1, January 1990, pp. 1–16.

37. Tracy E. Miller, "Multiple Listing for Organ Transplantation: Autonomy Unbounded," *Kennedy Institute of Ethics Journal*, vol. 2, no. 1, March 1992, pp. 43–57.

38. Ibid., p. 49.

39. M. Michaels et al., "Ethical Considerations in Listing Fetuses as Candidates for Neonatal

Heart Transplantation," *JAMA,* vol. 269, no. 3, January 20, 1993, pp. 401–402.

40. P. Ubell, R. Arnold, and A. Caplan, "Rationing Failure: The Ethical Lessons of the Retransplantation of Scarce Vital Organs," *JAMA,* November 24, 1993, vol. 270, no. 20, pp. 2469–2474.

41. Ibid., p. 2471.

42. Albert R. Jonsen, "(Bentham in a Box)," *Law, Medicine and Health Care,* vol. 14, 1986, pp. 172–174.

43. Gina Kolata, "Doctors Are Questioning the Use of Waiting Lists for Receiving Organs," *NYT,* January 20, 1993, p. B7.

44. Fox and Swazey, *Spare Parts,* p. 10.

45. Thomas Starzl, *The Puzzle People: Memoirs of a Transplant Surgeon,* University of Pittsburgh Press, Pa., 1992, chap. 12.

46. Fox and Swazey, *Spare Parts,* p. 12.

47. Ibid. p. 45.

48. AP, "Lung Recipient, 22, in Good Condition," January 31, 1993. This was also the lead story on *CNN Headline News,* January 30, 1993.

49. Interview, *Good Morning America,* July 9, 1993.

50. David Plank, "Nana Gives Gift of Life," *Newsday,* July 29, 1993, p. 6.

51. A. Bass, "New Liver Transplants: Pressure on Parents," *Boston Globe,* December 17, 1989, p. 1, 75; quoted in Fox and Swazey, *Spare Parts,* p. 52.

52. Michael Kinsley, "Take My Kidney, Please," *Time,* March 13, 1989, p. 88.

53. Fox and Swazey, *Spare Parts,* p. 72.

54. Richard Titmuss, *The Gift Relationship: From Altruism to Commerce,* Pantheon, New York, 1971.

55. Chris Hedge, "Egypt's Desperate Trade: Body Parts for Sale," *NYT,* September 23, 1991, p. A1. India's organ trade was discussed on *Prime Time Live with Diane Sawyer,* "Dignity for Sale," August 1, 1991.

56. Andrew Schneider and Mary Pat Flaherty, "Foreigners Get Kidneys with Flaws," *Pittsburgh Press,* July 8, 1985, pp. A1–A2.

57. Quoted in Michael Kroman, "Dialyzing for Dollars," *Reason,* August 1984, pp. 21–30.

58. N. G. Levinsky and R. A. Rettig, eds., *Kidney Failure and the Federal Government,* National Academy Press, Washington, D.C., 1991.

59. Fox and Swazey, *Spare Parts,* p. 89.

Chapter 13

1. Renée Fox and Judith Swazey, *The Courage to Fail: A Social View of Organ Transplants and Dialysis,* 2d ed., rev., University of Chicago Press, Ill., 1974, 1978; Harmon Smith, "Heart Transplantation," *Encyclopedia of Bioethics,* vol. 2, Free Press, New York, 1978, pp. 654–660; Richard Howard and J. Najarian, "Organ Transplantation—Medical Perspective," *Encyclopedia of Bioethics,* vol. 3, Free Press, New York, 1978, pp. 1160–1165.

2. Smith, op. cit.; Howard and Najarian, op. cit.

3. Denise Breo, "Interview with 'Baby Fae's' Surgeon," *AMN,* November 16, 1984, p. 13.

4. "Baby Fae Stuns the World," *Time,* November 12, 1984, p. 72.

5. Ibid., p. 70.

6. Tom Regan, "The Other Victim," *HCR,* vol. 15, no. 1, February 1985, pp. 9–10.

7. "Pro and Con: Use Animal Organs for Human Transplants?—Interview with Tom Regan," *U.S. News and World Report,* November 12, 1984, p. 58.

8. Thomasine Kushner and Raymond Belotti, "Baby Fae: A Beastly Business," *Journal of Medical Ethics,* vol. 11, 1985, pp. 178–183.

9. Breo, op. cit. p. 18.

10. "Interview with Dr. Jack Provonsha," *U.S. News and World Report,* November 12, 1984, p. 59.

11. Dan Chu and Eleanor Hoover, "Helped by a Baboon Heart, An Imperiled Infant, 'Baby Fae,' Beat the Medical Odds," *People Weekly,* November 18, 1984.

12. Charles Krauthammer, "The Using of Baby Fae," *Time,* December 3, 1984, pp. 87–88.

13. Breo, op. cit. p. 18.

14. Ibid., p. 13.

15. Ibid., p. 14.

16. Thomas Starzl, *The Puzzle People: Memoirs of a Transplant Surgeon,* University of Pittsburgh Press, Pa., 1992, p. 123.

17. "Baby Fae Stuns the World," p. 70.

18. *Animals Voice,* vol. 2, no. 3, December 1984.

19. Jacques Loman, *Journal of Heart Transplantation,* vol. 4, no. 1, November 1984, pp. 10–11.

20. George Annas, "The Anything Goes School of Human Experimentation," *HCR,* vol. 15, no. 1, February 1985, pp. 15–17.

21. *Nature,* vol. 88, no. 312, November 8, 1984, p. 5990.

22. Krauthammer, op. cit.

23. "Judicial Council Offers New Guidelines," *AMN,* vol. 27, December 14, 1984, p. 46.

24. Breo, op. cit., p. 18.

25. Chu and Hoover, op. cit., p. 74.

26. Quoted ibid.

27. Starzl, op. cit.

28. Breo, op. cit., p. 18.

29. Annas, op. cit.

30. Paul Ramsey, "The Enforcement of Morals: Nontherapeutic Research on Children," *HCR,* vol. 6, no. 4, August 1976, pp. 21–30.

31. Richard McCormick, "Proxy Consent in the Experimentation Situation," *Perspectives in Biology and Medicine,* vol. 18, no. 1, Autumn 1974, pp. 2–20.

32. Alexander Capron, "When Well-Meaning Science Goes Too Far," *HCR,* vol. 15, no. 1, February 1985, pp. 8–9.

33. Annas, op. cit.

34. "Celebrity surgery" was a term coined in *New Republic*, editorial, December 17, 1984.
35. Keith Reemtsma, *HCR*, February 1985, p. 10.
36. Alex Capron, *HCR*, February 1985, p. 8.
37. S. Twedl, "Second Recipient of Baboon Liver Dies," *Pittsburgh Post-Gazette*, February 6, 1993.
38. Philip Hilts, "Gene Transfers Offer New Hope for Interspecies Organ Transplants," *NYT*, October 19, 1993, p. B6.
39. Debra Berger, "The Infant with Anencephaly: Moral and Legal Dilemmas," *Issues in Law and Medicine*, vol. 5, no. 1989, p. 68.
40. Medical Task Force on Anencephaly, "The Infant with Anencephaly," *NEJM*, vol. 332, no. 10, March 8, 1990, p. 669.
41. Robert D. Trough and John D. Fletcher, "Can Organs Be Transplanted before Brain Death? *NEJM*, vol. 321, no. 6, 1989, p. 388.
42. A. Kantrowitz et al., "Transplantation of the Heart in an Infant and an Adult," *American Journal of Cardiology*, vol. 22, no. 782, 1968.
43. AP, "Hospital Sets Policy on Organ Donor Use," February 23, 1988.
44. Joan Heilman, "Tiny Gabriel's Gift of Life," *Redbook*, December 1988, p. 162. (I am indebted to Lynn Bondurant for bringing this article to my attention.)
45. J. Peabody et al., "Experience with Anencephalic Infants as Prospective Organ Donors," *NEJM*, vol. 321, no. 6, August 10, 1989, pp. 344–350.
46. AP, "Ethicists Debate Death and Baby's Lacking Brain," March 31, 1992; in *Birmingham News*, p. A1.
47. Brian Udell, quoted in *USA Today*, March 30, 1992, p. 3A.
48. "In Re T.A.C.P.," *Southern (Law) Reporter*, 2d Series, Supreme Court of Florida, November 12, 1992, p. 588–595.
49. D. Shewmon, "Anencephaly: Selected Medical Aspects," *HCR*, vol. 18, no. 5, 1988, pp. 1–9.
50. Laurie Abrahman, "The Use of Anencephalic Infants as Organ Sources," *AMN*, vol. 261, no. 12, March 24–31, 1989, pp. 1773–1781.
51. Debra H. Berger, *Issues in Law and Medicine*, vol. 67, 1989, pp. 84–85; quoted by Estella Moriarty in "In Re T.A.C.P.," p. 595.
52. D. Medearis and L. Holmes, "On the Use of Anencephalic Infants as Organ Donors," *NEJM*, vol. 321, no. 6, August 10, 1989, p. 392.
53. Beth Brandon, "Anencephalic Infants as Organ Donors: A Question of Life and Death," *Case Western Law Review*, vol. 40, 1989–1990, p. 781; quoted by Estella Moriarty in "In Re T.A.C.P."
54. "In Re T.A.C.P.," p. 590.
55. A. Capron, "Anencephalic Donors: Separate the Dead from the Dying," *HCR*, vol. 17, no. 1, February 1987, pp. 5–8; John Arras, "Anencephalic Newborns as Organ Donors: A Critique," *JAMA*, vol. 259, no. 15, April 15, 1986, pp. 2284–2285.
56. Shewmon, op. cit.
57. Gina Kolata, "Baby's Sad Life Highlights Cost of Futile Care," *NYT*, October 6, 1993, p. A1.

Chapter 14

1. Julian Jaynes, *The Origin of Consciousness and the Breakdown of the Bicameral Mind*, Houghton Mifflin, Boston, Mass., 1976.
2. Plato, *The Republic*, in E. Hamilton and H. Cairns, eds., *Collected Works of Plato*, Princeton University Press, Princeton, N.J., 1961.
3. Thomas Szasz, "Involuntary Mental Hospitalization: A Crime against Humanity," in *Ideology and Insanity*, Doubleday, New York, 1970.
4. Ibid.
5. D. Rosenhan, "On Being Sane in Insane Places," *Science*, vol. 179, 1973, pp. 250–258.
6. *O'Conner v. Donaldson*, 422 U.S. 563. 95 S. Ct. 2486, June 26, 1975.
7. John Petrilia, "Mental Health Therapies," *Biolaw*, University Publications of America, Frederick, Md., 1986, pp. 177–215.
8. Quoted in Charles Krauthammer, "How to Save the Homeless Mentally Ill, *New Republic*, February 8, 1988, p. 24.
9. Saul Feldman, "Out of the Hospitals, into the Streets: The Overselling of Benevolence," *HCR*, vol. 13, no. 3, June 1983, pp. 5–7.
10. Paul Chodoff, "The Case for Involuntary Hospitalization of the Mentally Ill, " *American Journal of Psychiatry*, vol. 133, no. 5, May 1976.
11. *NYT*, November 7, 1987, p. B1.
12. *NYT*, November 6, 1987, p. B1.
13. Ibid.
14. *NYT*, November 13, 1987, p. B21.
15. *NYT*, November 14, 1987, p. B1
16. *NYT*, November 13, 1987, p. A1.
17. Ibid.
18. "Brown versus Koch," *60 Minutes*, 1988.
19. "Court Backs Treatment of Woman Held under Koch Plan," *NYT*, December 19, 1987, p. A1. (Why the Appellate Court referred to Joyce Brown as "Ms. Boggs" was unclear.)
20. The previous hospitalizations mentioned in the dissent had been undisclosed; presumably the justices had seen Joyce Brown's medical records.
21. *60 Minutes*, interview with Ed Bradley, 1988.
22. Harold Evans, "Joyce Brown's Freedom," editorial, *U.S. News and World Report*, May 23, 1988, p. 78.
23. *NYT*, January 20, 1988, p. A16.
24. Charles Krauthammer, "Billie Boggs Revisited," *New York Daily News*, December 27, 1988, p. 21.
25. Krauthammer, "How to Save the Homeless Mentally Ill," pp. 22–25.

26. J. Livermore, C. Malmquist, and P. Meehl, "On the Justification of Civil Commitment," *University of Pennsylvania Law Review,* vol. 117, November 1968, pp. 75–96.

27. A. M. Rosenthal, "Questions to a Judge," *NYT,* November 27, 1987.

28. Virginia Abernethy, "Compassion, Control, and Decisions about Competence," *American Journal of Psychiatry,* vol. 141, no. 1, 1984, pp. 53–58.

29. *NYT,* November 13, 1987, p. A1.

30. *The Donahue Show,* Transcript #0128788.

31. *NYT,* November 14, 1987, p. 30.

32. Robert Levy and Robert Gould, "Psychiatrists as Puppets of Koch's Round-Up," *NYT,* November 27, 1987.

33. Chodoff, op. cit.

34. John Doe, personal communication to author, 1987.

35. Harold Evans, "Joyce Brown's Freedom," *U.S. News and World Report,* May 23, 1988, p. 78.

36. Ellen Goodman, "Before They Die with Their Rights On," *WP,* November 21, 1987.

37. Livermore, Malmquist, and Meehl, op. cit., p. 95.

38. Alice Baum and Donald Burnes, *A Nation in Denial: The Truth about Homelessness,* Westview, Boulder, Colo., 1993.

39. C. Dugger, "Judge Orders Homeless Man Hospitalized," *NYT,* December 23, 1992, p. B1.

40. E. Rosenthal, "Who Will Turn Violent? Hospitals Have to Guess," *NYT,* April 7, 1993, p. A1.

41. C. Dugger, "Ruling Draws Debate to Mentally Ill Homeless," *NYT,* February 2, 1993, p. A13.

Chapter 15

1. Alan Guttmacher Institute, "Teenage Sexual and Reproductive Behavior: Facts in Brief," New York, March 15, 1993 (111 Fifth Avenue, New York, NY 10003).

2. Nan Marie Astone, "Thinking about Teenage Childbearing," *Report from the Institute for Philosophy and Public Policy,* vol. 13, no. 3, Summer 1993, p. 9.

3. Ibid.

4. *Bertha,* Joseph P. Kennedy, Jr., Film Service (99 Asylum Avenue, Hartford, Conn., 06105). Quotations from the film are not footnoted.

5. Astone, op. cit.

6. Mimi Abramovitz and Frances Fox Piven, "Scapegoating Women on Welfare," *NYT,* September 2, 1993, p. A13; and Teresa McCrary, "Getting Off the Welfare Carousel," "My Turn" column, *Newsweek,* December 6, 1993, p. 11.

7. Barbara Dafoe Whitehead, "Dan Quayle Was Right," *Atlantic,* April 1993.

8. Lyndon Johnson, quoted in David Popenoe, "The Controversial Truth: Two-Parent Families Are Better," *NYT,* December 26, 1992, p. 21.

9. Quoted in George Will, "Changed Family Structure Ruining Many Young Lives," syndicated column, September 26, 1991.

10. Suzanne Fields, "A Vacuum That Technology Can't Fix," *Washington Times,* December 31, 1992, pp. G1, G4.

11. "Single-Parent Homes Grow by 14.8 Percent," Scripps-Howard News Service, May 13, 1992.

12. Jason De Parle, "Census Reports a Sharp Increase among Never-Married Mothers," *NYT,* July 14, 1993, p. A1.

13. Will, op. cit.

14. Quoted in John Leo, "America Remains in the 'Denial' Stage of a Social Crisis," syndicated column, February 2, 1993.

15. Will, op. cit.

16. *Birmingham News,* June 21, 1992, editorial.

17. Gregory Pappas, *NEJM,* July 8, 1993. See also Robert Pear, "Wide Health Gap Linked to Income Is Reported in U.S.," *NYT,* July 8, 1993, p. A1.

18. Lewis Grizzard, syndicated column, May 28, 1992.

19. Lawrence Mead (New York University), quoted by Will, op. cit.

20. Tamar Lewin, "Rise in Single Parenthood Is Reshaping U.S.," *NYT,* October 5, 1992.

21. Bureau of Census, *Statistical Abstract of the United States,* Superintendant of Documents, Washington, D.C., 1987, table 619, pp. 621–622; and *Statistical Abstract of the United States,* 112th ed., U.S. Government Printing Office, Washington, D.C., 1992, p. 371.

22. Charles Murray, *Losing Ground: American Social Policy 1950–1980,* Basic Books, New York, 1986.

23. Martha N. Ozawa, "Welfare Policies and Illegitimate Birth Rates among Adolescents: Analysis of State-by-State Data," *Social Work Research and Abstracts,* vol. 25, 1989, pp. 5–11.

24. Ellen Goodman, *Boston Globe,* May 25, 1992.

25. *Birmingham News,* June 21, 1992, editorial.

26. Ozawa, op. cit.

27. Hugh LaFollette, "Licensing Parents," *Philosophy and Public Affairs,* vol. 9, no. 2, 1979, pp. 182–197.

28. Stephen Mosher, *Broken Earth,* Free Press, New York, 1983, p. 533.

29. Clennan Ford and Frank Beach, *Patterns of Social Behavior,* Harper and Row, New York 1951; Ford and Beach's study of sexual behavior in 190 societies is quoted in Janet Shibley Hyde, *Human Sexuality,* McGraw-Hill, New York, 1979, p. 15.

30. Tamar Levin, "Baltimore School Clinics to Offer Birth Control by Surgical Implant," *NYT,* December 4, 1992.

31. Astone, op. cit.

32. R. Yaquib, "Norplant Users Say Birth Control Isn't Right for Everyone," *Chicago Tribune*, February 7, 1993.

33. *NYT*, April 30, 1994, p. A8.

34. *NYT*, July 8, 1994.

35. Seth Faison, "Inquiry Finds Bistate Welfare Cheating," *NYT*, March 3, 1994, p. A13.

36. Charles Murray, "Cold Turkey on Welfare," *Wall Street Journal*, October 29, 1993, p. A1.

37. Caroll Bogert, "White Ghetto?" *Newsweek*, May 30, 1994, pp. 46–48.

Chapter 16

1. J. Watson and F. Crick, "Molecular Structure of Nucleic Acids: A Structure for Deoxyribose Nucleic Acid," *Nature*, vol. 171, 1953, pp. 737–738.

2. "Interview with Nancy Wexler," *U.S. News and World Report*, 1985, p. 75.

3. V. A. McKusick, *Mendelian Inheritance in Man: Catalogs of Autosomal Dominant, Autosomal Recessive and X-Linked Disorders*, 11th ed., Johns Hopkins University Press, Baltimore, Md., 1993. (The main reason the 2,500 are only suspected rather than established is not lack of scientific knowledge but lack of families to confirm tests on rare conditions.)

4. Dennis Breo, "Altered Fates: An Interview with Francis Collins," *JAMA*, vol. 209, no. 15, August 21, 1993, p. 2021.

5. Daniel Kevles, *In the Name of Eugenics: Genetics and the Uses of Human Heredity*, Knopf, New York, 1985, pp. 3–19.

6. Ibid., pp. 93–94.

7. Quoted in Kenneth Ludmerer, "History of Eugenics," *Encyclopedia of Bioethics*, vol. 1, Free Press, New York, 1978, p. 460.

8. Robert Lacey, *Ford: The Man and the Machine*, Little, Brown, New York, 1987.

9. Kevles, op. cit., p. 117.

10. Ibid., p. 116.

11. Ibid., p. 97.

12. Ibid., p. 110.

13. *Buck v. Bell*, Superintendent, *United States Supreme Court Reporter*, 1927.

14. Ibid.

15. Kevles, op. cit., p. 53.

16. Richard Herrnstein, "I.Q.," *Atlantic*, September 1971, pp. 63–64; *Crime and Human Nature*, Simon and Shuster, New York, 1985.

17. Hermann J. Muller, *Out of the Night: A Biologist's View of the Future*, Vanguard, New York, 1935; quoted in Kevles, op. cit., p. 164.

18. Ronald W. Clark, *The Life and Work of J. B. S. Haldane*, Coward-McCann, New York, 1968, p. 70; quoted in Kevles, op. cit., p. 127.

19. J. B. S. Haldane, "Toward a Perfected Posterity," *World Today*, vol. 45, December 1924; quoted in Kevles, op. cit.

20. J. Huxley and A. C. Haddon, *We Europeans: A Survey of "Racial" Problems*, Cape, London, 1935, p. 184; quoted in Kevles, op. cit., p. 133.

21. Tabitha Powledge, "Genetic Screening," *Encyclopedia of Bioethics*, Free Press, New York, 1978, pp. 567–572.

22. Gina Kolata, "Nightmare or the Dream: Of a New Era in Genetics," *NYT*, December 6, 1993, p. A1.

23. John Rennie, "Grading the Gene Tests," *Scientific American*, June 1994, p. 91.

24. Quoted ibid.

25. Ellen Clayton, personal communication to author, Ethics Committee Conference, Huntsville, Ala., July 18, 1994.

26. Maya Pines, "In the Shadow of Huntington's," *Science 84*, May 1984, p. 33.

27. Quoted in *Boston Globe*, March 24, 1993; and in *Current Biography*, Wilson, New York, August 1994, p. 53.

28. M. R. Hayden, *Huntington's Chorea*, Springer-Verlag, New York, 1981.

29. Pines, op. cit., p. 33.

30. Ibid., p. 34.

31. Genetic linkage is a major exception to Mendel's law of independent assortment.

32. *Current Biography*, Wilson, New York, August 1994, p. 53.

33. Pines, op. cit., p. 39.

34. J. F. Gusella, N. S. Wexler, P. M. Connealy, et al., "A Polymorphic DNA Marker Genetically Linked to Huntington Disease," *Nature*, vol. 306, 1983, pp. 234–238.

35. Denise Grady, "The Ticking of a Time Bomb in the Genes," *Discover*, June 1987, p. 30.

36. *60 Minutes*, May 1987.

37. "Confronting the Killer Gene," *NOVA*, March 28, 1989.

38. Ibid.

39. S. Wiggins et al., "The Psychological Consequences of Predictive Testing for Huntington's Disease," *NEJM*, vol. 327, no. 20, pp. 1401–1405.

40. M. Hayden, AP, November 12, 1993.

41. Catherine Hayes, "Genetic Testing for HD—A Family Issue," *NEJM*, vol. 327, no. 20, November 11, 1992, pp. 1449–1451.

42. I am indebted to Michael Connealy for this case study.

43. "Jeremy Rifkin," *Contemporary Biography Yearbook 1986*, Wilson, New York, p. 469.

44. *American Journal of Law and Medicine*, special issue on Human Genome Project, 1991.

45. Ibid.

46. *Current Biography*, p. 54.

47. Grady, op. cit., p. 30.

48. G. Meissen et al., "Predictive Testing for Huntington's Disease with Use of a Linked DNA Marker," *NEJM*, vol. 318, no. 9, March 3, 1988, pp. 538ff.

49. Ibid., p. 538.

50. "Preclinical Testing in Huntington's Disease," letter, *American Journal of Medical Genetics*, vol. 27, 1987, pp. 733–734.

51. *Ethics and Mapping of the Human Genome*, Danish Council of Ethics, 1993.

52. Quoted in M. Waldoz, "Probing the Cell: The Diagnostic Power of Genetics Is Posing Hard Medical Choices, " *WSJ*, April 1986, p. A1.

53. D. Craufurd and R. Harris, "Ethics of Predictive Testing for Huntington's Disease: The Need for More Information," *British Medical Journal*, vol. 293, July 26, 1986, pp. 249–251.

54. Grady, op. cit., p. 34.

55. Ibid., p. 30.

56. Waldoz, op. cit.

57. Hayes, op. cit., pp. 1449–1451.

58. President's Commission for the Study of Ethical Problems in Medicine and Biomedical and Behavioral Research, *Screening and Counseling for Genetic Conditions: The Ethical, Social, and Legal Implications for Genetic Screening, Counseling, and Educational Problems*, U.S. Government Printing Office, Washington, D.C., 1983.

59. Arthur Beaudet of Baylor College of Medicine, quoted in Waldoz, op. cit.

60. C. Norton, "Absolutely Not Confidential," *Hippocrates*, March-April 1989, pp. 53–59; see also *Medical Records: Getting Yours*, Public Citizen, Washington, D.C., 1986.

61. Marc Lappe, "The Limits of Genetic Inquiry," *HCR*, vol. 17, no. 4, August 1987, pp. 5–10.

62. Rennie, op. cit., p. 96.

63. Ibid., p. 90.

64. Ibid.

65. Quoted ibid., p. 91.

66. Hayes, op. cit.

67. Waldoz, op. cit., p. A1.

68. Rennie, op. cit., p. 91.

69. Waldoz, op. cit., p. A1.

70. Quoted in Rennie, op. cit., p. 97.

71. Ibid., p. 79.

72. Both quoted in Rennie, op. cit., p. 97.

73. Natalie Angier, "Team Reports Genetic Cause of Huntington's," *NYT*, March 24, 1993, p. A1.

74. Ibid.

75. Natalie Angier, "Gene for Mental Illness Proves Elusive," *NYT*, January 13, 1993, p. B3.

76. Miron Baron, quoted ibid.

77. Sharon Begley, "When DNA Isn't Destiny," *Newsweek*, December 6, 1993, p. 53–54.

78. Sandra Blakeslee, "Genes Tell the Story of Why Some Get Cancer While Others Don't," *NYT*, May 17, 1994, p. B6.

79. Leroy Hood, "Gene Therapy Offers Promise but Holds Pitfalls," Scripps-Howard Papers and *Congressional Quarterly*, November 18, 1991.

80. B. Biesecker, "Genetic Counseling for Families with Inherited Susceptibility to Breast and Ovarian Cancer," *JAMA*, vol. 269, no. 15, April 21, 1993, pp. 1970–1974.

81. Mary-Claire King, "Inherited Breast and Ovarian Cancer," *JAMA*, vol. 269, no. 15, April 21, 1993, p. 1976.

82. Ibid.

83. Natalie Angier, "Vexing Pursuit of Breast Cancer Gene, *NYT*, July 12, 1994.

84. Ibid.

85. Ibid.

86. *NYT*, September 15, 1994, p. A1.

87. Ibid.

Chapter 17

1. Berton Roueché, *The Medical Detectives*, vol. 2, Dutton, New York, 1984, chap. 19; see also, "Thousands Flee Indian City in Deadly Plague Outbreak," *NYT*, September 24, 1994, pp. 1, 5. Some additional information in this section is also from these sources.

2. "Thousands Flee," op. cit.

3. Daniel Defoe, *Journal of the Plague Year* (1723), New American Library, New York, 1960, p. 86.

4. Barbara Tuchman, *A Distant Mirror*, Knopf, New York, 1978, p. 119.

5. Abigail Zuger and Stephen Miles, "Physicians, AIDS, and Occupational Risk," *JAMA*, vol. 258, no. 14, October 9, 1987, pp. 1924–1928.

6. Charles Shepard, "Leprosy," in Maxwell Wintrobe et al., eds., *Harrison's Principles of Internal Medicine*, McGraw-Hill, New York, 1973, pp. 870–873.

7. Roueché, op. cit., chap. 5.

8. Charles Rosenberg, *The Cholera Years*, University of Chicago Press, Ill., 1962, p. 47ff.

9. A. Brandt, *No Magic Bullet: A Social History of Venereal Disease in the United States since 1880*, Oxford University Press, New York, 1985, pp. 43–44.

10. Centers for Disease Control, *Morbidity and Mortality Report*, June 5, 1981.

11. Greg Dixon, "Stop Homosexuals before They Infect Us All," *USA Today*, January 16, 1983.

12. Charles Stanley, Scripps-Howard News Service, *Birmingham Post-Herald*, January 21, 1986.

13. Interviewed on *Cross Fire*, Cable News Network (CNN), November 16, 1987.

14. Quoted in Randy Shilts, *And the Band Played On*, St. Martin's, New York, 1987, p. 311.

15. Seth Berkley, "AIDS in the Global Village," *JAMA*, vol. 268, no. 23, December 16, 1992, pp. 3368–3369.

16. Larry Kramer, "Who Says AIDS Is Hard to Get?" *Newsweek*, 1992.

17. G. Freidland and Robert Klein, "Transmission of the Human Immunodeficiency Virus," *NEJM*, vol. 17, no. 18, October 29, 1987, p. 1127.

18. Institute of Medicine, *Confronting AIDS: Directions for Public Health, Health Care, and Research*, National Academy Press, Washington, D.C., 1986.

19. G. W. Rutherford et al., "Course of HIV-1 Infection in a Cohort of Homosexual Men:

An 11-Year Follow-Up Study, *British Medical Journal*, vol. 301, 1990, pp. 1183–1188.

20. These estimates assumed 750,000 American IV-drug users and relied on Kinsey's estimate that 4 percent of American males (2.5 million) were exclusively gay, but Kinsey overestimated the number of gay males—the accepted figure now is that 1 percent of American men are gay. (See F. Barringer, "Sex Survey of American Men Finds 1% Are Gay," *NYT*, April 19, 1993, p. A1.) A similar study in Britain and France found similar results, i.e., about 1 percent of men had engaged in intercourse with a another man during the previous year. (See Peter Aldous, "French Venture Where U.S. Fears to Tread," *Science*, vol. 257, no. III, July 3, 1992, p. 25.)

21. Quoted in Shilts, op. cit., p. 345.

22. Quoted ibid.

23. Quoted ibid. from *WSJ*.

24. Many patients who received blood transfusions during surgery died before they could develop symptoms of AIDS.

25. Joshua Hammer, "AIDS, Blood and Money," *Newsweek*, January 23, 1989.

26. Bonnie Johnson, "A Life Stolen Early," *People Weekly*, October 22, 1990, pp. 72–78.

27. Dennis L. Breo, "Meet Kimberly Bergalis," *JAMA*, October 17, 1990, p. 2018.

28. Colleen Moore, "I Felt I Was Always Going to Be Here," *Florida Today*, March 15, 1991, p. 1D–2D.

29. *Morbidity and Mortality Report*, July 28, 1990.

30. Ronald Smothers, "Where a Dentist Died of AIDS, Wariness Remains," *NYT*, December 2, 1991.

31. Anthony DePalma, "No Conclusion on Ways Dentist Passed On AIDS," *NYT*, June 26, 1991, p. A9.

32. Tim Golden, "Dental Patient Torn by AIDS Calls for Laws," *NYT*, June 21, 1991.

33. Moore, op. cit.

34. Johnson, op. cit.

35. Robert T. Ferris, quoted ibid. from a letter he wrote to *Palm Beach Post*.

36. AP, June 21, 1991; and "Dental Patient Torn," op. cit.

37. AP, "AIDS Victim's Plight Leads to Revised Rules," January 24, 1991.

38. Centers for Disease Control (CDC), "Estimates of HIV Prevalence and Projected Cases: Summary of a Workshop," *Morbidity and Mortality Report*, vol. 39, 1990, pp. 110–119.

39. See Richard Mohr, *Gays/Justice: A Study of Ethics, Society, and Law*, Columbia University Press, New York, 1988, pp. 251–262.

40. On Socrates, see A. H. Chroust, *Socrates: Man and Myth*, Routledge, London, 1957; and Kenneth Dover, *Greek Homosexuality*, Cambridge University Press, England, 1978. On others, see John Boswell, *Christianity, Social Tolerance and Homosexuality*, University of Chicago Press, Ill., 1980.

41. Boswell, op. cit.

42. See, for example, AP, "Gay Men in Twin Study," *NYT*, January 17, 1991, p. B10; David Gelman et al., "Is This Child Gay? Born or Bred: The Origins of Homosexuality," *Newsweek*, February 24, 1992, p. 46; Laura Allen and Roger Gorski, *Proceedings of the National Academy of Sciences*, August 1, 1992; AP, August 1, 1992. See also an article by Dean Hamer in *Science*, July 16, 1993.

43. Richard Mohr, "Gay Basics," in James Rachels, *Moral Problems*, 5th ed., Harper, New York, 1992.

44. *McCann v. H and H Music Co.*, October 1992. Actually, by declining to review this case, the Supreme Court let stand a decision by the Federal Appeals Court.

45. In Illinois, couples were simply crossing the border to Wisconsin to get married.

46. Bernard Turnock, "Mandatory Testing for Human Immunodeficiency Virus," *JAMA*, vol. 261, no. 23, June 16, 1989, pp. 3415–3418.

47. Ronald Bayer, "Public Health Policy and the AIDS Epidemic: An End to HIV Exceptionalism?" *NEJM*, vol. 324, no. 21, May 23, 1991, pp. 1500–1504.

48. Larry Katzenstein, "When He Has AIDS—And She Does Not Know," *American Health*, January-February 1990, pp. 58–59.

49. Frederick Daniel and Regina Skelly, "Partner Notification in Cases of HIV Infection," letter, *NEJM*, vol. 327, no. 6, August 6, 1992, pp. 435–436.

50. Adam Nossiter, "Man Is the First Convicted for Putting Partner at Risk of HIV," *NYT*, November 28, 1991.

51. M. A. Fischl et al., "The Efficacy of Azidothymidine (AZT) in the Treatment of Patients with AIDS and AIDS-Related Complex," *NEJM*, vol. 317, 1987, pp. 185–191.

52. S. Vella et al., "Survival of Zidovudine-Treated Patients with AIDS Compared with That of Contemporary Untreated Patients," *JAMA*, vol. 267, no. 9, March 4, 1992, pp. 1232–1236.

53. Lawrence K. Altman, "AIDS Study Casts Doubt on Value of Hastened Drug Approval in U.S.," *NYT*, April 6, 1993, p. B6.

54. W. Lenderking, "HIV-Infection and Long-Term Morbidity," *NEJM*, March 18, 1994.

55. L. Altman, "Experts Change Guides to Using Drugs for HIV," *NYT*, June 27, 1993, p. A1; AP, "Benefits of Often-Used AIDS Drug Are Questioned," *NYT*, March 18, 1994, p. A10.

56. Margaret Heagarty and Elaine Abrams, "Caring for HIV-Infected Women and Children," editorial, *NEJM*, vol. 326, no. 13, March 26, 1992, pp. 887–888.

57. Ronald Bayer et al., "Controlling AIDS in Cuba," *NEJM,* vol. 320, no. 15, April 13, 1989.
58. Moore, op. cit.
59. Mary Chamberland et al., "Health Care Workers with AIDS," *JAMA,* vol. 266, no. 24, December 25, 1991.
60. Gene Ann Shelley, "A National Survey of Surgeons' Attitudes about Patients with Human Immunodeficiency Virus Infections and Acquired Immunodeficiency Syndrome," *Archives of Surgery,* vol. 127, February 1992, pp. 206–212.
61. "HIV-Infected Surgeons and Dentists: Looking Forward and Backward," editorial, *JAMA,* vol. 269, no. 14, April 14, 1993.
62. Christine Gorman, "When the Doctor Has AIDS," *Time,* October 21, 1991, p. 83.
63. AP, "32 HIV Cases Linked to Health-Care Jobs," October 30, 1992; and CDC, AIDS Hotline, personal communication to author, October 1994.
64. Roberta Ness et al., "House Staff Recruitment to Municipal and Voluntary New York City Residency Programs during the AIDS Epidemic," *JAMA,* vol. 266, no. 20, November 27, 1991, pp. 2843–2846.
65. Abigail Zuger, "AIDS on the Wards," *HCR,* vol. 17, no. 3, June 1987, p. 16.
66. AP, "Orthopedic Surgeons Not Catching AIDS at Work, Survey Says," May 17, 1991.
67. Martin Shapiro et al., "Residents' Experiences in, and Attitudes toward, the Care of Persons with AIDS in Canada, France, and the United States," *JAMA,* vol. 268, no. 4, July 22–29, 1992, pp. 510–515.
68. Tracie O'Neill et al., "Risk of Needlesticks and Occupational Exposures among Residents and Medical Students," *Archives of Internal Medicine,* vol. 152, July 1992, pp. 1451–1456.
69. Michael Hagen et al., "Routine Screening for HIV," *JAMA,* vol. 259, March 4, 1988, p. 1359.
70. P. Cleary et al., "Compulsory Premarital Screening for HIV," *JAMA,* vol. 258, no. 13, October 2, 1987, pp. 1757–1762.
71. Bruce D. McCarthy et al., "Who Should Be Screened for HIV Infection?" *Archives of Internal Medicine,* vol. 153, May 10, 1993, p. 1107.
72. Ibid. Cost per discovered case is, of course, calculated by dividing total cost of a testing program by number of cases discovered; thus the higher the incidence in a population, the lower the cost per discovered case.
73. "Mandatory Testing: The Illinois Experience," *JAMA,* vol. 261, no. 23, June 16, 1981, p. 3456.
74. Ibid.
75. Tom Ehrenfeld, "AIDS Heroes and Villains," *Newsweek,* October 14, 1991, p. 66.
76. K. Phillips et al., "The Cost-Effectiveness of HIV Testing of Physicians and Dentists in the United States," *JAMA,* vol. 271, no. 11, March 16, 1994, p. 851.
77. *NYT,* September 10, 1991, p. A31.
78. Ronald Smothers, "Teen-Ager with HIV Feels Angry and Alone," *NYT,* May 8, 1993, p. A6.
79. L. Altman, "AIDS Mystery That Won't Go Away: Did a Dentist Infect 6 Patients?" *NYT,* July 5, 1994, p. B6.
80. Ibid.
81. *Lear's,* April 1994, pp. 68–82.
82. Ronald DeBry, "Dental HIV Transmission," *Nature,* vol. 361, February 23, 1993, p. 691.
83. Huntly Collins, Knight-Ridder Newspapers, "Volunteers Enter AIDS Vaccine Test," February 15, 1993.
84. William Haseltine, "For AIDS Treatment, Vaccines, Now Think Genes," *JAMA,* vol. 269, no. 17, May 5, 1993, p. 2189.
85. March Gordon, "Red Cross Privately Felt AIDS Risk to Blood in '83, Documents Say," *Birmingham News* (Alabama), May 15, 1994, p. 7a.
86. Mireya Navarro, "Hemophiliacs Demand Answers as AIDS Toll Rises," *NYT,* May 19, 1993, p. A1, A12.
87. Abigail Zuger, "AIDS Becomes Ordinary," *Medical Humanities Review,* vol. 7, no. 1, Spring 1993.

Chapter 18

1. Betsy Butgereit, "Health amid Poverty," *Birmingham News,* May 3, 1993.
2. "Lisa Belkin, "Victim of Both Cancer and Care System," *NYT,* March 26, 1992, p. B12.
3. Consumers Union, "Does Canada Have the Answer?" *Consumer Reports,* September 1992, p. 580.
4. Richard D. Lamm, "Health Care as Economic Cancer," *Dialysis and Transplantation,* vol. 16, 1987, pp. 432–433.
5. Albert Jonsen, *The New Medicine and the Old Ethics,* Harvard University Press, Cambridge, Mass., 1992.
6. Martha Angle, "Social Security Is Much More Than a Personal Bank," *Congressional Quarterly,* May 18, 1993; reprinted in Scripps-Howard Newspapers, May 19, 1993.
7. Mireya Navarro, "Hemophiliacs Demand Answers as AIDS Toll Rises," *NYT,* May 10, 1993, pp. A1, A12.
8. *60 Minutes,* September 28, 1992.
9. Lawrence K. Altman, "A Surprise in War between Heart Drugs," *NYT,* May 1, 1993, p. A13.
10. Gina Kolata, "Parents of Tiny Infants Find Care Choices Are Not Theirs," *NYT,* September 30, 1991, p. A1.
11. Robert Pear, "U.S. Backs Oregon's Health Plan for Covering All Poor People," *NYT,* March 20, 1993, p. A1.
12. Courtney S. Campbell, "Gridlock on the Oregon Trail," *Hastings Center Report,* vol. 23, no. 4, July-August 1993, p. 6.

13. Interview with James Todd on *Good Morning America,* May 10, 1993.
14. Consumers Union, op. cit., p. 580.
15. Alan Guttmacher Institute, quoted in AP, December 15, 1987.
16. Consumers Union, op. cit., p. 586.
17. Ibid.
18. Robert Pear, "Health Aides Plan to Place Medicare under New System," *NYT,* May 11, 1993, p. A1.
19. "Health Care Costs," *USA Today,* May 12, 1993, p. A2.
20. This has been repeatedly claimed by members of Physicians for a National Health Program; see, e.g., John V. Walsh, *Providence Journal* (Scripps-Howard), column, July 14, 1993.
21. Charles B. Inlander and Charles K. MacKay, *Medicare Made Easy,* Addison-Wesley, Reading, Mass., 1992, p. 7.
22. Consumers Union, "Medicare for All Americans," *Consumer Reports,* September 1992, p. 592.
23. Ibid.
24. Garrett Hardin, "The Tragedy of the Commons," *Science,* vol. 162, 1968, pp. 1243–1248.
25. Pear, op. cit.
26. A. C. Enthoven, "Consumer Choice Health Plan," parts I and II, *NEJM,* vol. 298, March 23 and 30, 1978, pp. 650, 709–720; A. C. Enthoven and R. Kronick, "A Consumer-Choice Health Plan for the 1990s: Universal Health Insurance in a System Designed to Promote Quality and Economy," parts I and II, *NEJM,* vol. 320, January 5 and 12, 1989, pp. 29–37, 94–101.
27. John Inglehart, "National Health Reform and the American Medical Association," *NEJM,* March, 1994.
28. David Orentlicher, "Rationing and the Americans with Disabilities Act," *JAMA,* no. 271, no. 4, January 26, 1994, pp. 308–314.
29. Inlander and MacKay, op. cit., p. 14.
30. Some accountants, such as Peter Peterson, predict that the Medicare Hospital and Insurance fund will be broke when present "baby boomers" retire; instead of the present ratio of 2 workers supporting 1 retiree, Peterson says, the ratio will then be 1 worker supporting 2 retirees. (Peter Peterson, *Facing Up,* Simon and Shuster, New York, 1994.)
31. Paul Starr, *The Social Transformation of American Medicine,* Basic Books, New York, 1982.
32. Paul Menzel, "Equality, Autonomy, and Efficiency: What Health Care System Should We Have?" *Journal of Medicine and Philosophy,* vol. 17, no. 1, February 1992, p. 34.
33. David Blumenthal et al., "The Future of Medical Care," *NEJM,* vol. 314, no. 11, March 13, 1986, p. 723.
34. Michele Davis, "Make Health Insurance More Like Auto Insurance," *Birmingham News,* July 6, 1992.
35. Henry J. Aaron, "The Oregon Experiment," in Martin Strasberg, ed., *Rationing America's Medical Care: The Oregon Plan and Beyond,* Brookings Institute, Washington, D.C., 1991.
36. Lisa Hoffman and Andrew Schneider, "When the House Doubles as a Hospital," *Birmingham Post-Herald* and Scripps-Howard Newspapers, May 18, 1993, p. A1.
37. Consumers Union, "Wasted Health Care Dollars," *Consumer Reports,* July 1992, p. 436.
38. Consumers Union, "The Crisis in Health Insurance," *Consumer Reports,* August 1990, p. 543.
39. Employee Benefit Research Institute, quoted in Marcy Mullins, *USA Today,* May 13, 1993, p. 2A.
40. Robert Wood Johnson Foundation, quoted in AP, May 16, 1993.
41. Consumers Union, "Wasted Health Care Dollars."
42. George Strait, reporting on *ABC World News,* May 11, 1993.
43. Jack K. Shelton and Julia Mann Janosi, "Unhealthy Health Care Costs," *Journal of Medicine and Philosophy,* vol. 17, no. 1, February 1992, p. 8.
44. David Ozar, "Justice and a Universal Right to Basic Care," *Social Science and Medicine,* vol. 15F, 1981, pp. 135–141; Alan E. Buchanan, "The Right to a Decent Minimum of Health Care," in President's Commission for the Study of Ethical Problems in Medicine and Behavioral Research, *Securing Access to Health Care: The Ethical Implications of Differences in the Availability of Health Services* 2, apps., *Social and Philosophical Studies,* Superintendent of Documents, Washington, D.C., 1983, pp. 208–238.
45. Pat Milmoe McCarrick, "Scope Note 20: A Right to Health Care," biblio., *Kennedy Institute of Ethics Journal,* December 1992, pp. 388–405.
46. John Rawls, *A Theory of Justice,* Harvard University Press, Cambridge, Mass., 1971.
47. Sylvia Nasar, "However You Slice the Data, the Richest Did Get Richer," *NYT,* May 11, 1992.
48. Alasdair MacIntyre, *Whose Justice? Whose Rationality?* University of Notre Dame Press, South Bend, Ind., 1988.
49. Ezekiel Emanuel, *The Ends of Human Life: Medical Ethics in a Liberal Polity,* Harvard University Press, Cambridge, Mass., 1992.

Indexes

NAME INDEX

For additional names, see "Further Reading" in each chapter, and "Notes" (pages 469ff).

SUBJECT INDEX